Pharmacotherapeutics in Dentistry

Pharmacotherapeutics in Dentistry

Louis P. Gangarosa, Sr., PH.D., D.D.S.
Professor and Coordinator of Pharmacology
Department of Oral Biology
School of Dentistry
Professor of Pharmacology
School of Medicine
Medical College of Georgia
Augusta, Georgia

Alfred E. Ciarlone, PH.D., D.D.S.
Professor of Oral Biology
Department of Oral Biology (Pharmacology)
School of Dentistry
Associate Professor of Pharmacology
School of Medicine
Medical College of Georgia
Augusta, Georgia

Arthur H. Jeske, PH.D., D.M.D.
Associate Professor
Departments of Pharmacology and Restorative Dentistry
Dental Branch
The University of Texas Health Science Center at Houston
Houston, Texas

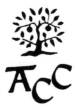

APPLETON-CENTURY-CROFTS / Norwalk, Connecticut

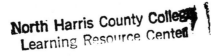

Notice: Our knowledge in the clinical sciences is constantly changing. As new information becomes available, changes in treatment and in the use of drugs become necessary. The author(s) and the publisher of this volume have taken care to make certain that the doses of drugs and schedules of treatment are correct and compatible with the standards generally accepted at the time of publication. The reader is advised to consult carefully the instruction and information material included in the package insert of each drug or therapeutic agent before administration. This advice is especially important when using new or infrequently used drugs.

Copyright © 1983 by Appleton-Century-Crofts
A Publishing Division of Prentice-Hall, Inc.

83 84 85 86 87 88 / 10 9 8 7 6 5 4 3 2 1

Prentice-Hall International, Inc., London
Prentice-Hall of Australia, Pty. Ltd., Sydney
Prentice-Hall Canada, Inc.
Prentice-Hall of India Private Limited, New Delhi
Prentice-Hall of Japan, Inc., Tokyo
Prentice-Hall of Southeast Asia (Pte.) Ltd., Singapore
Whitehall Books Ltd., Wellington, New Zealand
Editora Prentice-Hall do Brasil Ltda., Rio de Janeiro

Library of Congress Cataloging in Publication Data

Gangarosa, Louis P.
  Pharmacotherapeutics in dentistry.

  Bibliography: p.
  Includes index.
  1. Dental pharmacology. I. Ciarlone, Alfred E.
II. Jeske, Arthur H. III. Title. [DNLM: 1. Dentistry.
2. Pharmacology, Clinical. 3. Tooth diseases—
Drug therapy. 4. Mouth diseases—Drug therapy.
QV 50 G197p]
RK701.G36 1983   617.6'061   83-2627
0-8385-7842-X

Design: Jean M. Sabato

PRINTED IN THE UNITED STATES OF AMERICA

Contents

SECTION III: MEDICAL DRUGS IMPORTANT TO DENTISTRY
(SELF-STUDY)

SECTION IV: APPENDICES: SPECIAL PROBLEMS OF DRUG USE
IN DENTAL PRACTICE

Preface

In *Pharmacotherapeutics in Dentistry*, the authors have attempted to develop a balance between a broad survey of basic pharmacology and emphasis on dental therapeutics. The format makes the book valuable to dental students, dental residents, and practicing dentists. The book provides a study guide and reference. The material on pharmacology and therapeutics is ordered in sequence according to priorities related to importance of the information in dental practice. Objectives are presented for all of the self-study material; after self-study, the reader can easily test comprehension by using the testing items at the end of the chapters. The test questions are cross-keyed to the objectives for easy reference. Also, the questions can be used as a pretest, allowing the reader to skip areas already mastered. The therapeutic summaries in Section I allow quick reference to basic facts and prescriptions, which the dentist may wish to review rapidly.

The subdivision of chapters into objectives allows the instructor to eliminate those objectives that are inappropriate for the course. Furthermore, the instructor can choose not to cover chapters (that may have been covered in other courses or otherwise deemed inappropriate for the course) or reorder chapters according to the appropriate course outline.

All of the self-study material was tested in the Pharmacology and Therapeutics course at the Medical College of Georgia School of Dentistry.

Acknowledgments

The authors wish to thank a great number of people who have helped in the preparation of this book. First, we should thank some people who helped train us in pharmacology: Drs. V. DiStefano, H. C. Hodge, James W. Smudski, and R. P. Ahlquist. Secondly, we are grateful to Dean Judson C. Hickey, Medical College of Georgia, who encouraged innovation in dental education and gave us the time and personnel to develop our teaching program based upon self study. Dr. Kenneth Morse, Professor, Ed. Psych., and Dr. Thomas Zwemer, Associate Dean, both from the Medical College of Georgia, were helpful in introducing us to the objective format and encouraged us in preparing our course notes in this format since 1968. Dr. Norton C. Ross, Warner-Lambert Company, although not mentioned as an author, contributed in developing some of the objectives and earlier material for the course notes. Dr. Donald Kroeger, Chairman, Pharmacology, University of Texas Dental Branch at Houston also encouraged and supported Dr. Jeske. Dr. Marshall Shlafer, Department of Pharmacology, University of Michigan Medical School, and Dr. Barbara M. Chang, Assistant Professor of Hematology/Oncology, Medical College of Georgia aided in the review of some of the medical material.

We should like to cite the able work of Dorothy M. Lyons, our Departmental Secretary, who ungrudgingly struggled through many revisions and reminded us of the many deadlines. Others who helped in the typing were Dorothy B. Smith, Dwyane McGahee, Shirl Melton, and Marianna Jones. Milton Burroughs, Lewis Hinely, and Barbara Peebles were helpful in preparation of the artwork. Jan O'Meara, Rhonda Jones, Rhesa Dykes, Jeff Blankenship, and Keith McRae were helpful in proofing manuscripts and organizing references, artwork, and so on.

Finally, the entire staff of Appleton-Century-Crofts was most helpful in encouraging and aiding to make our job pleasant.

We are grateful to all of our dental students who studied our course notes and encouraged us to produce this book. We dedicate this book to all those mentioned above, our families and others who aided but went unmentioned.

How to Use this Book

This book is divided into four sections. Each section contains a segment of pharmacology and therapeutics that is vital to dentistry. The sections are organized by priority of importance to dental practice. A description of these sections follows.

SECTION I. Dental Drug Reference

The purpose of this section is to provide a summary of the salient features of drug therapy in dental practice. Dental drugs are defined as drugs that dentists either prescribe or use in office. Where appropriate, typical prescriptions are presented. The prescriptions do not cover all situations or drug choices. Rather, we chose prescriptions that we feel are useful for most typical situations in dentistry. Dentists must modify these prescriptions to meet various situations, and we expect that the dentist's knowledge and background will allow intelligent choices of other drugs that come on the market later.

SECTION II. Dental Drug Self-Study

This section contains the essential background material for the understanding of dental drugs. Each category of drugs from Section I is studied in an organized manner, and the facts from Section I are cross-referenced for ease of location and review. Since each chapter is designed to stand independently, there may be some repetition of material from Section I.

The material in Section II is classically considered the core material for a minimum basic science course in pharmacology for dentists. If the instructor has only been alloted approximately 45 hours to cover the subject of pharmacology, we would recommend that Section II be the main core for the course. Then, a therapeutics course of at least 11 to 22 hours would be required to cover Section I. However, if the beginning course is alloted approximately 80 to 90 hours, the full range of pharmacology and therapeutics can be covered by studying Section II, interlaced with Section I, and then Section III. All or parts of the Appendices can be woven into closely related chapters of Sections II and III.

SECTION III. Medical Drugs Important to Dentistry (Self-Study)

In this section, the drugs patients take for medical reasons are presented in a self-study format. Such drugs are not used directly in dental therapy, but they give important clues to the patient's health status. In taking a health history, the dentist may discover that the patient is taking one or more drugs for medical purposes. By investigating the drug actions, the dentist gains information about the patient's health that can help his treatment planning and progress. Often this necessitates contacting the patient's physician, but the discussion is much more satisfactory if the dentist knows which medications the patient takes. Finally, it is most important that the dentist understand how drugs prescribed for dental purposes may interact with the drugs used medically.

It was difficult to decide on the content for Section III because of the broad range of chemicals that can be given to a patient for therapeutic purposes. We chose to avoid some topics often covered in medical pharmacology texts (e.g., vitamins and minerals, which we consider a part of biochemistry). The coverage of endocrines is not complete; rather, we selected areas of most interest to dentists. Basically, we tried to provide the minimum core material and then added subjects that were peripherally related.

This gives the instructor maximum flexibility in choosing topics for the appropriate course.

SECTION IV. Appendices

The related appendices are included because of their obvious importance in dentistry. The appendices give information on subjects related to drugs, but which are not always part of a pharmacology or therapeutics course. The appendices may serve as a reference source, but they also may be studied for their value in correlating and summarizing drug information related to special problems of drug use in dental practice. Appendix VIII supplies the answers to questions posed in Chapters 12 through 41.

Pharmacotherapeutics
in Dentistry

SECTION ONE:
DENTAL DRUG REFERENCE

1
Local Anesthetics in Dentistry

11/15

A. INTRODUCTION

Local anesthetics are used in dentistry to reversibly abolish the sensation of pain in a localized area of the oral cavity. There are currently available many local anesthetic preparations, although they can be placed generally into one of two chemical groups: the esters and the amides. Within each of these two categories, individual local anesthetic agents may differ with respect to potency, toxicity, duration of action, vasoconstrictor requirements, or the type of vasoconstrictor used in the solution.

Local anesthetics suppress nerve impulse generation and conduction in peripheral pain fibers and other nerves by blocking the movements of sodium ions across the nerve cell membrane. This action, which prevents depolarization of the nerve, occurs in all excitable tissues, including the heart, vascular smooth muscle, and the central nervous system. Actions on the central nervous system are responsible for the major toxic effects of local anesthetics, including excitement, muscle twitching, convulsions, and coma. With some agents, direct central depression consisting of drowsiness and ataxia has

been described before convulsions occur. The depressant effect of the local anesthetics on the cardiovascular system can result in cardiac depression, cardiac arrhythmias, and hypotension.

Local anesthetics, as used in dentistry, have an excellent safety record. This is probably due to their careful use by most practitioners, who include in treatment a good health history, rational selection of a local anesthetic agent based on the health history and current medications, the use of aspiration in the injection technique, and attention to maximum allowable doses of local anesthetic. In addition, familiarity with the techniques of diagnosing and treating local anesthetic-related emergencies has contributed to the safe use of local anesthetics.

The modern dental practice should be stocked with an appropriate variety of injectable and topical anesthetic agents, as well as emergency drugs. This armamentarium should include both ester- and amide-type agents, agents that can be used without vasoconstrictor, agents that contain reduced amounts of vasoconstrictor, long-acting agents, and agents that do not contain paraben preservatives. When doubt exists about the proper choice in a given

1

patient, the references at the end of the chapter should be consulted. When medical complications are expected, the patient's physician should be consulted.

B. SPECIFICS OF LOCAL ANESTHETIC USE IN DENTISTRY

Indications for Use
1. Topical anesthesia of mucous membranes should be administered to increase patient comfort during the local anesthetic injection.
2. Local anesthesia by nerve block or infiltration should be given prior to all operative procedures where pain is expected.
3. Nerve block may aid in diagnosis of some pain syndromes.
4. Topical anesthesia of mucous membranes may be used for temporary relief of surface oral lesions.

Selection of Local Anesthetic Agent: Patient Factors Include the Following
1. Good health history to identify **allergy, cardiovascular disease, endocrine disease, current medications,** or prior **psychogenic reactions** to local anesthetic injection.
2. Use caution in the following:
   a. Allergy
      (1) avoid anesthetic to which patient is allergic
      (2) consider possibility of allergy to preservatives (paraben)
      (3) always follow-up on patient report of allergy
      (4) always be prepared for unexpected allergic reaction
   b. Cardiovascular disease
      (1) consult physician
      (2) reduce or eliminate vasoconstrictor
      (3) be prepared to handle emergency
   c. Endocrine disease (e.g., hyperthyroidism)
      (1) consult physician
      (2) reduce or eliminate vasoconstrictor
   d. Current medications: possible interactions of local anesthetics with:
      (1) sulfonamides (ester-type agents)
      (2) anticholinesterase agents (esters and amides), such as diisopropyl fluorophosphate (DFP), echothiophate, or stigmine drugs used for glaucoma or myasthenia gravis
   e. Current medications: possible interactions of vasoconstrictors with:
      (1) monoamine oxidase (MAO) inhibitors
      (2) tricyclic antidepressants
      (3) guanethidine
   f. Liver impairment (decreased metabolism of amides)
   g. Genetic cholinesterase deficiency: impaired ester metabolism

Administration and Handling Techniques
1. Use sterile syringe and cartridge (do not touch end that contacts needle).
2. Do not use out-of-date or unmarked cartridges.
3. Use aspiration when injecting.
4. Do not exceed maximum recommended number of cartridges. This varies for local anesthetic chosen, vasoconstrictor chosen, concentration of drugs, age, and presence of disease.
5. Methods of calculating anesthetic dosage. For safety purposes the rule of 5-10-3 is recommended. This means that the adult patient may be given at each appointment: 5 mg/kg of either lidocaine or mepivacaine or 10 mg/kg of procaine, and 3 µg/kg of epinephrine. (NOTE: epinephrine is over 1,000 times more potent than local anesthetics and, thus, is administered in µg rather than mgs.) Children's dosage can be calculated using this rule since weight determines dose. Adults should not be given more than 200 µg epinephrine, according to a New York Heart Association recommendation (1955). The rule of 5-10-3 assumes that some vasoconstrictor is used; when no epinephrine is present, about one-half the dose of local anesthetic should be used.

   Typically, a calculation for an adult is performed as follows:
   a. weight conversion

$$\frac{154 \text{ lb}}{2.2 \text{ lb/kg}} = 70 \text{ kg}$$

lido 2% ~ 1ml → 20mg
1.8ml → 36mg = one cartridge.

b. lidocaine allowance

$$70 \text{ kg} \times 5 \text{ mg/kg} = 350 \text{ mg}$$

c. cartridge calculation

$$\frac{350 \text{ mg}}{36 \text{ mg/cartridge}} = \sim 10 \text{ cartridges}$$

d. epinephrine allowance

$$3 \ \mu\text{g/kg} \times 70 \text{ kg} = 210 \ \mu\text{g}$$
(or 200 μg maximum, see above)

e. cartridge calculation for 1:100,000 epinephrine

$$\frac{200 \ \mu\text{g}}{18 \ \mu\text{g cartridge}} = 11.1 \text{ cartridges}$$ *= 1.8 ml solution.*

f. cartridge calculation for 1:50,000 epinephrine

$$\frac{200 \ \mu\text{g}}{36 \ \mu\text{g cartridge}} = \begin{array}{l} 5.56, \text{ or } 5 \text{ cartridges} \\ (\text{rounded to lower} \\ \text{whole number}) \end{array}$$

These calculations show that epinephrine at 1:50,000 is the limiting factor, and, therefore, the authors favor using 1:100,000 epinephrine. In addition, procaine requires more epinephrine and is marketed with 1:50,000 epinephrine. Thus, although more cartridges can be used based upon procaine, epinephrine still limits the maximum number of cartridges to 5.

Table 1–1 summarizes these calculations for various drugs, giving cartridge limitation. Table 1–2 specifies the number of cartridges that can be used safely in adults and children for various commonly used dental solutions, based on these calculations.

Toxicity

1. Allergy:
   a. rash
   b. itching
   c. urticaria
   d. bronchospasm (difficulty in breathing)
   e. hypotension
2. Psychogenic reaction:
   a. loss of color (pale)
   b. dizziness
   c. rapid, thready pulse
   d. cold sweat
3. Vasoconstrictor:
   a. nervousness, palpitations
   b. talkativeness, elevated blood pressure
   c. anxiety
4. Local anesthetic:
   a. nervousness
   b. excitement
   c. muscle twitching
   d. tremors
   e. convulsions

C. LOCAL ANESTHETICS AVAILABLE FOR DENTAL USE

LIDOCAINE

Description. Lidocaine is an amide-type local anesthetic. The chemical name is diethyl-amino-2, 6-acetoxylidide, and its structure is illustrated in Figure 1–1. Lidocaine is marketed as a hydrochloride salt under the following commercial names: *Alphacaine, Lidocaine, Octocaine, Xylocaine, Dentacaine,* and *Codescaine.*
Indications. Lidocaine can be used for infiltration and nerve block local anesthesia. It is also

TABLE 1–1. MAXIMUM SAFE CARTRIDGE ALLOWANCE FOR AN ADULT USING LOCAL ANESTHETICS CONTAINING EPINEPHRINE

	Epinephrine Concentration		
	1:50,000	*1:100,000*	*1:200,000*
2% lidocaine	5	10	Not available
2% procaine	5	Not available	Not available
4% prilocaine (400 mg limit)	Not available	Not available	5

TABLE 1-2. GUIDELINES FOR CARTRIDGE ALLOWANCE OF VARIOUS DENTAL LOCAL ANESTHETICS

| | Number of Cartridges | | | |
| | Maximum Adult Dose | Child Dose[a] | | Limiting Drug |
		Small (10 kg)	Large (30 kg)	
2% lidocaine, 0 epi[b]	5	0.5	1.5	lidocaine
2% lidocaine, 1:50,000 epi	5	0.5	1.5	epinephrine
2% lidocaine, 1:100,000 epi	10	1.0	3.0	lidocaine
2% procaine, 1:50,000 epi	5	0.5	1.5	epinephrine
3% mepivacaine, 0 epi	3	0.3	1.0	mepivacaine
2% mepivacaine, 1:20,000 levo[c]	7	0.5	1.5	levonordefrin[d]
4% prilocaine, 0 epi	5	0.5	1.5	prilocaine
4% prilocaine, 1:200,000 epi	5	0.5	1.5	prilocaine

[a] These are conservative estimates. For different size children, calculate proportionate dosage on an mg/kg basis.
[b] epi = epinephrine.
[c] levo = levonordefrin.
[d] Assuming levonordefrin to be 1/3 as toxic as epinephrine.

used topically and is supplied in a viscous gel, ointment, and liquid form for topical use (see Topical Anesthetic Agents, p. 7). Lidocaine produces anesthesia of only short duration when used without a vasoconstrictor, and it is recommended that it is routinely used with 1:100,000 epinephrine for dental procedures.

Precautions. Do not use lidocaine in patients with known hypersensitivity to amide-type local anesthetics or in patients with paraben allergy. Preparations containing vasoconstrictor must be used with caution in patients with cardiovascular disease. Lidocaine may be contraindicated in patients with severe liver disease.

Toxicity. Lidocaine is now generally regarded as being the prototype local anesthetic drug

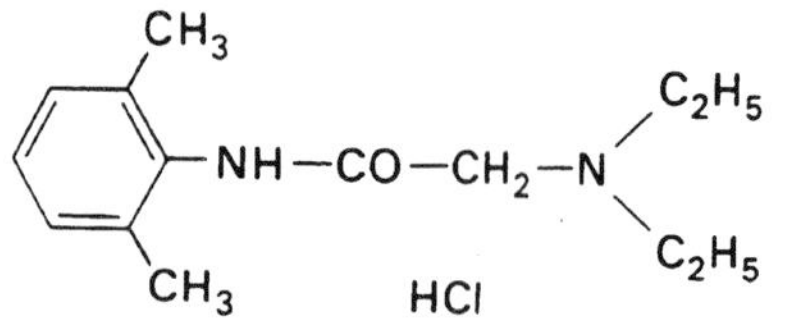

Figure 1-1. Chemical structure of lidocaine. (*From Csáky TZ: Cutting's Handbook of Pharmacology, 6th ed, 1979. Courtesy of Appleton-Century-Crofts.*)

(formerly the prototype was procaine). All other local anesthetics are compared to the prototype. Lidocaine is intermediate in toxicity: twice as toxic as procaine but much less toxic than more potent agents, e.g., tetracaine. The total dose of lidocaine with 1:100,000 epinephrine should not exceed 350 mg (or 5 mg/kg body weight). In adults, therefore, the total number of 1.8 ml cartridges with lidocaine plus 1:100,000 epinephrine should not exceed 10. When significant levels are reached, lidocaine generally produces signs of central depression, including drowsiness, sedation, and ataxia, although tremors and/or convulsions may occur. The total adult dose of plain lidocaine (with no epinephrine) should not exceed 200 mg.

Dosage. One cartridge (1.8 ml) is usually sufficient for block, while one cartridge or less may be sufficient for infiltration, depending on the area of anesthesia desired.

Cartridge Contents. Lidocaine hydrochloride is supplied in 1.8 ml dental cartridges at a 2% concentration with or without epinephrine.

1. Each ml of the plain solution contains:

— 20 mg lidocaine hydrochloride
— 6 mg sodium chloride

1 mg methylparaben
sodium hydroxide to adjust pH

2. Each ml of the solution containing 1:100,000 epinephrine contains:

   20 mg lidocaine hydrochloride
   6 mg sodium chloride
   0.01 mg epinephrine
   sodium bisulfite (0.55 mg) or sodium metabisulfite (0.5 mg)
   1 mg methylparaben
   sodium hydroxide to adjust pH

3. Each ml of the solution containing 1:50,000 epinephrine contains:

   20 mg lidocaine hydrochloride
   6 mg sodium chloride
   0.02 mg epinephrine
   sodium bisulfite (0.55 mg) or sodium metabisulfite (0.5 mg)
   1 mg methylparaben
   sodium hydroxide to adjust pH

MEPIVACAINE

Description. Mepivacaine is an amide-type local anesthetic (1-methyl-2, 6-pipecoloxylidide hydrochloride). The chemical structure is illustrated in Figure 1–2. Mepivacaine is marketed as a hydrochloride salt under the following commercial names: *Carbocaine, Arestocaine, Isocaine,* and *Mepivacaine.*

Indications. Mepivacaine can be used for infiltration and nerve block local anesthesia. It is not used topically. Since mepivacaine can produce acceptable depth and duration without a vasoconstrictor, it may be useful in patients in whom vasoconstrictors are contraindicated. Two mepivacaine preparations are available without

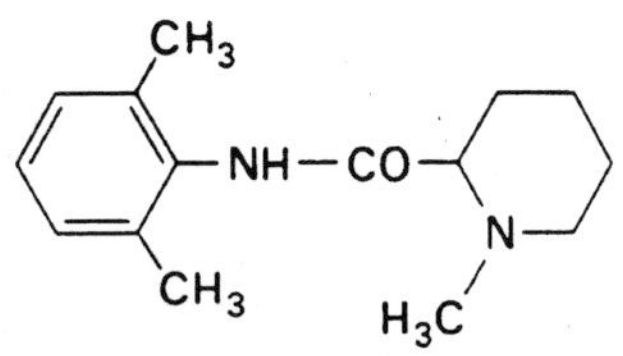

Figure 1–2. Chemical structure of mepivacaine. (*From Csáky TZ: Cutting's Handbook of Pharmacology, 6th ed, 1979. Courtesy of Appleton-Century-Crofts.*)

methylparaben preservative (*Carbocaine* HCl with or without vasoconstrictor and *Arestocaine* HCl with 1:20,000 levonordefrin) and may be used in patients with paraben allergy. However, multidose vials of *Carbocaine* do contain methylparaben.

Precautions. Do not use mepivacaine in patients with known hypersensitivity to amide-type local anesthetics. Preparations containing vasoconstrictor must be used with caution in patients with cardiovascular disease. Mepivacaine may be contraindicated in patients with severe liver disease.

Toxicity. The toxicity of mepivacaine is equal to that of lidocaine. When significant plasma levels are reached, central nervous system excitation can occur, which may terminate in convulsions and postseizure respiratory depression.

Dosage. One cartridge (1.8 ml) is usually sufficient for block, while one cartridge or less may be sufficient for infiltration, depending on the area of anesthesia required. Maximum total dosage should not exceed 5 mg per kilogram of body weight when levonordefrin is present or about one-half that amount with no vasoconstrictor.

Cartridge Contents. Mepivacaine is supplied in 1.8 ml dental cartridges as a hydrochloride salt, at a 3% concentration without vasoconstrictor and at a 2% concentration with 1:20,000 levonordefrin.

1. Each ml of the plain solution contains:

   30 mg mepivacaine hydrochloride
   3 mg sodium chloride
   1 mg methylparaben (except *Arestocaine* and *Carbocaine*)

2. The 2% solution with vasoconstrictor contains (per ml):

   20 mg mepivacaine hydrochloride
   0.05 mg levonordefrin
   4 mg sodium chloride
   1 mg methylparaben (except *Arestocaine* and *Carbocaine*)

   In addition to the above ingredients, the 2% mepivacaine preparations contain sodium metabisulfite or acetone sodium bisulfite as antioxidants, and both the 2% and 3% preparations

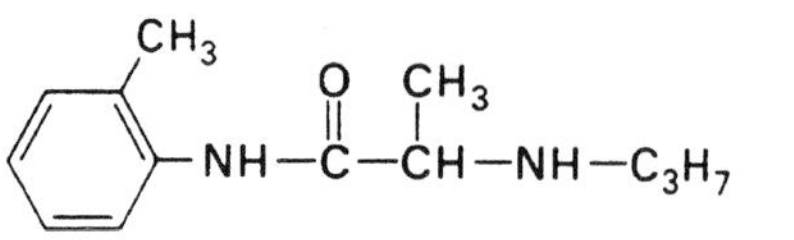

Figure 1–3. Chemical structure of prilocaine. (*From Csáky TZ: Cutting's Handbook of Pharmacology, 6th ed, 1979. Courtesy of Appleton-Century-Crofts.*)

contain various amounts of NaOH or HCl to adjust pH.

PRILOCAINE

Description. Prilocaine is an amide-type local anesthetic (2-propylamino-o-propionotoluidide hydrochloride). The chemical structure is illustrated in Figure 1–3. Prilocaine is marketed as a hydrochloride salt under the commercial name of *Citanest.*

Indications. Prilocaine can be used for infiltration and nerve block local anesthesia. It is not available for topical use. The onset of action of prilocaine is more rapid than that of lidocaine. The manufacturer states that when used in infiltrations, prilocaine has an onset of action of less than 2 minutes, with plain prilocaine producing a duration of soft tissue anesthesia of 26 minutes and prilocaine with 1:200,000 epinephrine lasting approximately 138 minutes. In inferior alveolar nerve block, onset averages less than 3 minutes, with soft tissue anesthesia lasting 162 minutes with plain prilocaine and 180 minutes with prilocaine containing 1:200,000 epinephrine.

Precautions and Toxicity. One of the metabolites of prilocaine is ortho-toluidine, which can produce methemoglobin. The manufacturer states that, in adults, significant levels of methemoglobin are produced only by doses exceeding 400 mg (five and a half cartridges). Therefore, there is little risk of methemoglobinemia when prilocaine is used for routine procedures. However, alternative agents should be used in the debilitated, the elderly, children, or pregnant patients and in patients with heart disease, an existing condition of methemoglobinemia, or respiratory difficulty. Prilocaine is slightly less toxic and less potent than lidocaine, but the

total adult dose should not exceed 400 mg (p. 3). Prilocaine solutions should not be used in patients with known hypersensitivity to amide-type local anesthetics or in patients with paraben allergy. Prilocaine must be used with caution also in patients with liver disease.

Dosage. One cartridge (1.8 ml) is usually sufficient for nerve block, while one cartridge or less may be sufficient for infiltration, depending on the area of anesthesia desired.

Cartridge Contents. Prilocaine hydrochloride is supplied in 1.8 ml dental cartridges at a 4% concentration with or without epinephrine.

1. Each ml of the plain solution (*Citanest Plain*) contains:

   40 mg prilocaine hydrochloride
   6 mg sodium chloride
   1 mg methylparaben
   sodium hydroxide to adjust pH

2. Each ml of the solution with vasoconstrictor (*Citanest Forte*) contains:

   40 mg prilocaine hydrochloride
   0.005 mg epinephrine
   5 mg sodium metabisulfite
   1 mg methylparaben

PROCAINE

Description. Procaine is an ester-type local anesthetic (2-diethylaminoethyl-4-aminobenzoate hydrochloride). The chemical structure is illustrated in Figure 1–4. Procaine is marketed as a hydrochloride salt under the commercial names *Novocain* and *Procaine* hydrochloride.

Indications. Procaine can be used for infiltration and nerve block local anesthesia. Procaine is rapidly metabolized by esterase enzymes and, since it is not metabolized by the liver, may be

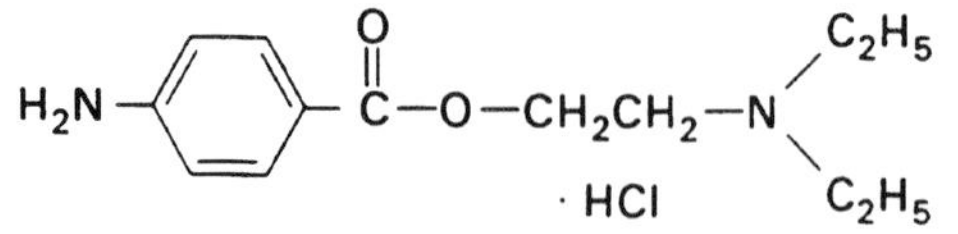

Figure 1–4. Chemical structure of procaine. (*From Csáky TZ: Cutting's Handbook of Pharmacology, 6th ed, 1979. Courtesy of Appleton-Century-Crofts.*)

used in patients with liver dysfunction. Procaine is not effective without a vasoconstrictor for dental applications, and even with a vasoconstrictor, it produces anesthesia of sufficient duration only for routine operative procedures (medium duration).

Precautions. Because procaine is rapidly inactivated in the blood by esterase enzymes, it is one of the least toxic of currently available local anesthetics. However, the incidence of allergy with para-aminobenzoic acid derivatives is substantially greater than that seen with amide-type agents. Furthermore, patients with procaine allergy may also be allergic to other esters, especially tetracaine, and to paraben preservatives. Procaine should be used with caution in patients taking sulfonamides, since one of the metabolites of procaine (para-aminobenzoic acid) can inhibit the action of these antimicrobials.

Dosage. The total dose of procaine hydrochloride with a vasoconstrictor in adults should not exceed 700 mg (or 10 mg/kg) and this limit should be adjusted downward in children according to their body weight. Furthermore, a total of 0.003 mg of epinephrine per kilogram of body weight should not be exceeded when using preparations containing this vasoconstrictor. Epinephrine limits the total dosage to about five cartridges per appointment (p. 3). One cartridge (1.8 ml) is usually sufficient for nerve block, while one cartridge or less may be sufficient for infiltration, depending on the area anesthetized.

Cartridge Contents.

1. Each ml of the 2% procaine HCl preparation with epinephrine 1:50,000 contains:

   20 mg procaine hydrochloride
   0.02 mg epinephrine
   4.5 mg sodium chloride
   2 mg sodium bisulfite
   1 mg methylparaben

2. Each ml procaine HCl 4%, phenylephrine HCl 1:2,500 preparation contains:

   40 mg procaine hydrochloride
   0.4 mg phenylephrine hydrochloride
   4.5 mg sodium chloride
   2 mg sodium bisulfite
   1 mg methylparaben

Cook-Waite Laboratories also markets procaine in combination with tetracaine (*Novocain* 2%, *Pontocaine* 0.15%, *Neo-Cobefrin* 1:20,000) and with propoxycaine (*Ravocaine* HCl 0.4%, *Novocain* 2%, *Levophed* 1:30,000).

Note: tetracaine (*Pontocaine*) and propoxycaine (*Ravocaine*) are not available as single injectable agents in dental cartridges which are approved for use by the ADA Council on Dental Therapeutics. These agents are added to procaine-based preparations to increase the depth and duration of anesthesia in patients in whom it is desirable to use ester-type agents. However, these combinations are more toxic than procaine alone, and the following maximum dosages should not be exceeded in adult patients:

a. tetracaine, 30 mg
b. propoxycaine, 30 mg

These doses should be adjusted according to body weight for younger patients and also reduced because of the procaine concentration.

TETRACAINE
See Procaine, page 6.

PROPOXYCAINE
See Procaine, page 6.

D. TOPICAL ANESTHETIC AGENTS

LIDOCAINE
This is available as a 5% liquid (flavored) preparation), a 5% ointment as the free base, and a 2% viscous preparation (with carboxymethylcellulose) of the hydrochloride salt. When used topically, the total dose of lidocaine should not exceed 200 mg. *Note:* it must be remembered that, when used topically and by injection, a single maximal dose of lidocaine cannot be exceeded and the amount administered by the topical route proportionally reduces the amount that may be injected. The precautions and toxicity of topical lidocaine are the same as those described for the injectable form.

BENZOCAINE

This is available in nonaqueous solutions, gels, and ointments at 5 to 22% concentrations. Benzocaine is poorly absorbed and rapidly metabolized, producing only rare systemic reactions. However, allergy can occur in patients sensitized to benzocaine or other para-aminobenzoic acid derivatives, including procaine and paraben preservatives. Since one of the hydrolysis products of benzocaine is para-aminobenzoic acid, it can antagonize the actions of sulfonamides.

PHENOLS AND PHENOLIC DERIVATIVES

These provide an antibacterial action as well as good topical anesthesia. The concentrations of phenols that can be tolerated are limited by the fact that high concentrations are irritating and corrosive. Preparations containing 0.25% concentrations can be used with minimal side effects. Phenol is well absorbed, and ingestion of sufficient quantities can cause gastrointestinal irritation, central nervous system aberrations, and respiratory failure with death. Care should be taken to keep phenol preparations out of reach of children (see Appendix VI).

DYCLONINE HYDROCHLORIDE

This agent differs sufficiently from other local anesthetic structures so that it may be useful in cases of allergy to other agents. This drug is marketed under the commercial name *Dyclone* as a 0.5% aqueous solution. The total dose should not exceed 200 mg, since it is absorbed.

BUTACAINE

This effective topical anesthetic of the ester-type is marketed under the commercial name *Butyn* as a nonaqueous ointment containing 4% butacaine base. The total dose should not exceed 200 mg (5 gm of ointment) in adults, since it is absorbed (see Appendix VI).

COCAINE

This is an effective topical anesthetic which is still in use in otorhinolaryngology and ophthalmology. In dentistry, the practicality of cocaine is severely limited by its regulation under the Controlled Substances Act and by the fact that it can cause tissue necrosis after repeated applications because of an intense vasoconstriction. The toxicity of cocaine consists of central nervous system stimulation followed by depression. When applied topically, the concentration of cocaine should not exceed 4%.

E. NEWER LONG-ACTING AMIDES

Current Status

These are discussed in Chapter 15. They are generally more potent, more toxic, and of longer duration than lidocaine. Since long duration may be a desirable property in dentistry, the authors believe that there is a role for these amides. The main disadvantage at present is their lack of availability in dental cartridges. (By the time this book is published, that problem may be corrected.) In the meantime, if a long-acting amide is desired for use by a dentist, it will have to be used from a multidose injection vial for medical purposes with a standard needle and syringe.

BUPIVACAINE (*Marcaine*)

This long-acting amide has been approved for dental use and will be supplied in dental cartridges (Ken Dean: Personal communication, 1982). It will be supplied at 0.5% with an epinephrine concentration of 1:200,000.

ETIDOCAINE (*Duranest*)

No information is found as to its future availability in dental dosage form.

F. STATUS OF PARABENS

Parabens (methyl, prophyl, butyl) have a great number of disadvantages and little benefit.

1. They are known sensitizers causing allergy that is cross-reactive with procaine and other ester-type local anesthetics.
2. If parabens are added to amide-type local anesthetics, their usefulness in ester allergy is lost (see above).
3. The bacteriostatic effect of parabens is not

really needed in a unit-dosing system, as used in dentistry. Recently, we have shown (Parker, 1977) that local anesthetic cartridges with epinephrine can be autoclaved, which further controverts the necessity for parabens.

For the above reasons, the authors have recommended for many years that parabens be eliminated from local anesthetic dental cartridges. Recently, the FDA asked manufacturers to remove parabens from pharmaceuticals, wherever possible, for some of the same reasons cited above (DMD, 1981).

REFERENCES

DMD: A Dentists Medical Digest 3(7):6, 1981

Muscholl E: Adrenergic false transmitters. In Blaschko H, Muscholl E (eds): Handbook of Experimental Pharmacology. Berlin, Springer-Verlag, 1972, p 647

New York Heart Association: Report of the Special Committee of the New York Heart Association, Inc., on the use of epinephrine in connection with procaine in dental procedures. J Am Dent Assoc 50:108, 1955

Parker RL: The Effect of Autoclaving on the Stability of Epinephrine Contained in Lidocaine Solutions. MS Thesis, Medical College of Georgia, 1977, p 31

BIBLIOGRAPHY

Accepted Dental Therapeutics, 38th ed. Chicago, American Dental Association, 1979, Sec. II, Local Anesthetics, Vasoconstrictors

Bennett CR: Monheim's Local Anesthesia and Pain Control in Dental Practice, 5th ed. St. Louis, Mosby, 1974, Ch 5, 6, 7

Csáky TZ: Cutting's Handbook of Pharmacology, 6th ed. New York, Appleton-Century-Crofts, 1979, Ch 48

Ritchie JM, Greene NM: Local anesthetics. In Gilman AG, Goodman LS, Gilman A (eds): Goodman and Gilman's The Pharmacological Basis of Therapeutics, 6th ed. New York, Macmillan, 1980, Ch 15

Sollmann T: A Manual of Pharmacology, 8th ed. Philadelphia, Saunders, 1964, pp 322–343

Truant AP, Takman B: Local anesthetics. In DiPalma JR (ed): Drill's Pharmacology in Medicine, 3rd ed. New York, McGraw-Hill, 1965, Ch 11

2

Autonomic Drugs in Dentistry

Autonomic drugs are used to alter sympathetic or parasympathetic function. The autonomic drugs most commonly used in dental practice are: (1) sympathomimetics (epinephrine, norepinephrine, phenylephrine, levonordefrin, and so on), (2) antimuscarinics (methantheline, propantheline, atropine, scopolamine), and (3) the muscarinic agonist, pilocarpine.

Sympathomimetics are used in dentistry for their vasoconstrictor effect in local anesthetic solution and for bronchodilation or cardiovascular stimulation in emergency drug therapy.

Propantheline (or methantheline) is the dental drug of choice for blocking salivary secretions. Other antimuscarinic drugs, such as atropine and scopolamine, are also used for this purpose but usually only during general anesthesia.

The muscarinic drug, pilocarpine, may be used for stimulation of salivary secretion, but side effects limit its usefulness.

(If the words in this introduction seem like a foreign language, it would be best to study Chapters 16 through 18 before proceeding with the therapeutics portion.)

A. SYMPATHOMIMETIC DRUGS

EPINEPHRINE HYDROCHLORIDE (*Epinephrine, USP, Adrenalin hydrochloride*)

Indications. Epinephrine is indicated for the following:

1. Vasoconstriction in local anesthetic solutions in the following concentrations:

   1:50,000 = 20 μg/ml = 0.020 mg/ml
   1:100,000 = 10 μg/ml = 0.010 mg/ml
   1:200,000 = 5 μg/ml = 0.005 mg/ml

The authors prefer the lower concentration because maximum vasoconstriction can be produced by a 1:200,000 concentration (Gangarosa, Halik, 1967; Gangarosa, Larson, 1975). Manufacturers, however, supply only the two higher concentrations with 2% lidocaine. Thus, 1:100,000 appears to be the best available choice. We consider 1:50,000 as an unnecessarily high concentration, which limits the number of cartridges that can be used at a single appointment. Based upon the

New York Heart Association recommendation (1955) of 200 μg as a safe dose of epinephrine per appointment, five cartridges (20 ml) of epinephrine at 1:50,000 (5 × 2 × 20 μg) would be allowed, whereas 10 cartridges of the 1:100,000 (10 × 2 × 10) would be allowed. (NOTE: further details on cartridge limitations in local anesthetic combinations are described in Chapter 1.)

2. Vasoconstriction of gingival tissues
   a. Racemic epinephrine 8% incorporated into gingival retraction cord
      Comment: epinephrine at this concentration is uncalled for and dangerous. According to the New York Heart Association recommendations (1975), the dentist should limit epinephrine to 200 μg per appointment. This is true whether it is given as a vasoconstrictor or by topical application. It has been found that systemic absorption after topical application can be rapid, causing dangerous cardiovascular reactions, and tissue damage due to ischemia is possible (ADT, 1979).
   b. *Ranephrine* 1:500 solution (Pascal Co., Inc.)
      Comment: Epinephrine at this concentration is uncalled for and dangerous (see 2a *Comment*).
   c. Alternate drugs for hemorrhage control and gingival retraction: aluminum chloride, 250 mg/gm, available in 10, 20, and 40 ml bottles or in gingival retraction cord. Higher concentrations of aluminum chloride and the use of zinc chloride or ferric salts, which may cause irritation and coagulation, are not recommended.

3. Acute anaphylactic reactions
   a. For the most severe reactions of anaphylactic shock: 3 to 5 ml of **1:10,000** epinephrine should be injected IV slowly. Observe the patient and repeat the dose if necessary.
   b. For moderate reactions with hypotension: 0.3 to 0.5 ml of **1:1000** epinephrine may be injected IM or subcutaneously (with massage). Observe the patient and repeat the dose if necessary.
   c. For mild reactions (e.g., urticaria, pruritis): 0.3 to 0.5 ml of **1:1000** epinephrine may be injected subcutaneously. Observe the patient and repeat the dose if necessary.
   d. Adjuvant drugs for anaphylaxis (see Appendix I). After breathing and cardiovascular system function are assured by cardiopulmonary resuscitation and after appropriate use of epinephrine, the following may be used:
      (1) If breathing is not well controlled following epinephrine, aminophylline, 250 to 500 mg by slow IV infusion, may be used to help obtain bronchiolar relaxation.
      (2) An antihistamine, such as diphenhydramine 10 to 50 mg IV or IM.
      (3) A steroid, such as methylprednisolone sodium succinate, 125 mg IV or IM, or dexamethasone, 4 to 8 mg IV or IM.

NOREPINEPHRINE (*Levophed*)

Although norepinephrine is a vasoconstrictor like epinephrine, the latter probably performs better in therapeutic situations in dentistry. Epinephrine seems to be a better vasoconstrictor in the oral submucosa than norepinephrine. The use of a higher concentration of norepinephrine (1:30,000 or higher) as a vasoconstrictor by some manufacturers appears unjustified, since norepinephrine is equal in toxicity to epinephrine. The authors see no rationale for replacing epinephrine with norepinephrine as the vasoconstrictor in local anesthetic solutions. If norepinephrine should be chosen, it must be administered at the same maximum dosage as epinephrine (200 μg per appointment, or a maximum of three cartridges containing 1:30,000 norepinephrine).

Norepinephrine may have use in hypotensive shock but should be reserved for later therapy, after the patient is under medical care. It is probably not needed in the dental office, since mephentermine (see the following) is probably a better drug for cardiovascular stimulation. Naturally, norepinephrine would not be valid for bronchodilation because it lacks this β-adrenergic effect. Thus, the use of norepinephrine in anaphylaxis is not indicated.

LEVONORDEFRIN, α-METHYLNOREPINEPHRINE (*Neo-Cobefrin*)

This drug is formed at adrenergic terminals when α-methyldopa is given as a hypotensive drug. Since α-methylnorepinephrine is handled like norepinephrine and may replace it, α-methylnorepinephrine has been called a false transmitter. Levonordefrin is less potent and less toxic than epinephrine but has all of the same actions as epinephrine. Furthermore, at equipotent doses, levonordefrin stimulates the heart to a greater degree than does epinephrine, indicating a lower therapeutic index for the former. Thus, the data do not support superiority of levonordefrin over epinephrine. Levonordefrin (1:20,000) is preferred by some manufacturers as the vasoconstrictor in mepivacaine.

PHENYLEPHRINE (*Neo-Synephrine*)

This is a pure α agonist (no β effect). It is commonly used in over-the-counter nose drops as a nasal decongestant. There has been limited acceptance of phenylephrine as a vasoconstrictor in certain local anesthetic solutions (Chapter 1). It is used at a 1:2,500 concentration as a vasoconstrictor. The relative toxicity on the heart of phenylephrine compared to other sympathomimetic amines needs to be further evaluated.

MEPHENTERMINE (*Wyamine*)

This is a longer acting sympathomimetic which may be useful as a pressor agent in hypotensive states. It may be used at a dose of 10 to 30 mg by IM or subcutaneous injection.

EPHEDRINE (Various Trade Names)

This sympathomimetic acts directly and indirectly (releasing norepinephrine) to give both α and β effects. Its slower metabolism results in a longer lasting effect than that of epinephrine. It is used as an emergency drug in hypotensive states, and the IV dose is 25 to 50 mg. Since the use of ephedrine in hypotension is more complex than the use of mephentermine, ephedrine should be reserved for later use, if needed, and after the patient is under medical care.

B. PARASYMPATHOLYTIC DRUGS

PROPANTHELINE BROMIDE (*Pro-Banthine*)

Propantheline is an atropinelike drug that may be useful to inhibit salivation before a dental procedure. The adult dose is 15 mg as a tablet given 30 to 40 minutes before an appointment. A second tablet is given if the desired effect is not obtained. Children should receive approximately one-half the adult dose.

Prescription 2-1 is a sample prescription for propantheline for the following situation.

Situation: During a prior appointment, this adult male patient produced copious saliva, making prophylaxis somewhat difficult. The patient required about five additional appointments for quadrant amalgams and some composites. *Prescribe* propantheline to control salivary secretion (see page 14).

Contraindications include glaucoma, cardiovascular disease (Chapter 31), and prostatic hypertrophy. Side effects include blurred vision and possible drowsiness, and the patient should be warned not to drive or operate machinery if drowsiness or blurred vision occur. Other possible side effects are tachycardia and decreased intestinal or bladder smooth muscle action. Such side effects may occasionally be noted after a single dose use in dental practice.

METHANTHELINE (*Banthine*)

This is an alternate drug having the same effects as propantheline but generally thought to have slightly more intense side effects. Its dosage in the normal adult is 50 mg po, or 100 mg if needed.

ATROPINE AND SCOPOLAMINE

These are also parasympatholytics, which may be useful in general anesthesia (Chapters 17 and

```
                         JOHN SMITH, D.M.D.
                             BOX 000
                           Maintown, EX
                             11111

Dentist and
Patient            Patient Name_____John Doe_____Date___July 4, 1981___
Identification     Address___1234 5th St., Augusta, GA_____
                                                                 Age____38____

Superscription      R_x

Inscription           Propantheline              15 mg tabs

Subscription          Disp:  10 tabs

Signa                 Sig:   Take one tab on arrival at dental office
                       yes no
                    Label ☒ ☐   Generic Substitution Permitted___John Smith___D.M.D.

Prescriber's
validation and                    Dispense as Written_____D.M.D.
additional
directions
                   Refill 0-1-2-3 (PRN)  State License No._____DEA No. Not required____
                                (Where applicable)              (Where applicable)
```

Prescription 2–1. Prescription for saliva control. (Note: Since this is the first prescription in the book, it is presented as an ideal prescription. All other prescriptions will be presented in an abbreviated format.)

38), but neither is generally recommended for dental office use.

PARASYMPATHOMIMETIC DRUGS

Theoretically, these should be useful for inducing salivation. However, two problems can occur: (1) the salivary glands may be nonfunctional because of disease or destruction (especially after radiation therapy), in which case a stimulant of salivation would not be helpful, and (2) even when the glands are functional, the parasympathomimetics have adverse side effects which may result in the treatment being worse than the condition. Pilocarpine and neostigmine have been tried for stimulation of salivation, with generally unsatisfactory results. Two other approaches are (1) a natural stimulant, such as sugar-free lemon drops or chewing gums, and (2) a lubricant. The latter can be accomplished by increasing fluid intake, by using a glycerol-containing mouthwash, or by using an artificial saliva (see Appendix V).

REFERENCES

Accepted Dental Therapeutics, 38th ed. Chicago, American Dental Association, 1979, p 127

Gangarosa LP, Halik FJ: A clinical evaluation of local anesthetic solutions containing graded epinephrine concentrations. Arch Oral Biol 12:611, 1967

Gangarosa LP, Larson SG: Comparison of blood flow effects of four sympathomimetic amines. J Dent Res 54:L8, L30, 1975

New York Heart Association: Report of the Special Committee of the New York Heart Association, Inc., on the use of epinephrine in connection with procaine in dental procedures. J Am Dent Assoc 50:108, 1955

Luduena FP, Hoppe JO, Oyen IH, Wessinger GD: Some pharmacologic properties of levo- and dextro-nordefrin. J Dent Res 17:206, 1957

BIBLIOGRAPHY

Accepted Dental Therapeutics, 38th ed. Chicago, American Dental Association, 1979, Sect. II, Vasoconstrictors

Accepted Dental Therapeutics, 38th ed. Chicago, American Dental Association, 1979, Sect. II, Hemostatics and Astringents

Accepted Dental Therapeutics, 38th ed. Chicago, American Dental Association, 1979, Sect. II, Other Therapeutic Agents: Anticholinergics, Enzymes and Corticosteroids

Gilman AG, Goodman LS, Gilman A (eds): Goodman and Gilman's The Pharmacological Basis of Therapeutics, 6th ed. New York, Macmillan, 1980, Ch 4, 5, 6, 7, 8.

3
CNS Drugs for Anxiety Control

A. NONPHARMACOLOGIC METHODS OF ANXIETY CONTROL

Nonpharmacologic methods of anxiety control should be practiced by every dentist, and a good chairside manner can sometimes preclude the use of drugs. Moreover, other methods, such as biofeedback and hypnosis, should be used when appropriate, since such methods lack the obvious problems inherent to drug therapy. However, when it is indicated, drug therapy for anxiety control should be used.

B. PHARMACOLOGIC METHODS

CNS drugs for anxiety control during a dental appointment might best be administered IV (or in some cases IM), especially to normal, healthy adults. However, under some circumstances and especially at certain times, e.g., at bedtime, peroral administration of an antianxiety drug is indicated.

C. GENERAL PREADMINISTRATION CONSIDERATIONS

There are a number of factors to be considered prior to CNS drug administration. Each patient must be evaluated before treatment, and drug dosages should be modified accordingly. Modification of dose may be necessary when the patient is:

1. Very young or very old (decreased dose due to reduced drug metabolism and excretion)
2. Obese (increased dose due to greater volume of drug distribution)
3. Chronically ingesting alcohol (increased dose due to increased drug metabolism in early alcoholism, or decreased dose due to liver impairment and liver enzyme induction as in late stages of alcoholism)
4. Agitated (increased dose due to physiologic antagonism in the CNS)
5. Serene (decreased dose due to physiologic addition)

17

6. Dependent on sedative-hypnotic or antianxiety drugs (increased dose due to increased metabolism and tolerance)
7. Taking other CNS depressant drugs, without dependence (decreased dose due to pharmacologic addition or supra-addition)

D. INDICATIONS FOR BARBITURATE SEDATIVE-HYPNOTICS OR BENZODIAZEPINES

Indications include:

1. Preoperative sedation
2. Heavy sedation prior to hospital surgery
3. Induction of general anesthesia in a hospital operating room (ultrashort-acting barbiturates only)
4. Dental or operating room IV sedation
5. Hypnosis (if needed the night before a dental appointment and if needed the first night after dental surgery, as a supplement to an analgesic)
6. Daytime sedation before and during a dental appointment
7. Muscle relaxant for spasms about the TMJ (benzodiazepines only)
8. Anticonvulsant emergency use

E. CONTRAINDICATIONS

Barbiturates
1. Allergy
2. Acute intermittent porphyria
3. Liver or kidney dysfunction
4. Pregnancy
5. Ambulatory patients

Benzodiazepines
1. Allergy
2. Liver or kidney dysfunction
3. Pregnancy
4. Acute narrow-angle glaucoma
5. Open-angle glaucoma (unless the patient is receiving appropriate therapy)
6. Chronic obstructive pulmonary disease
7. Ambulatory patients

F. ADVERSE EFFECTS

Barbiturates
1. Hangover, lassitude, and ataxia
2. Vertigo, nausea, vomiting, and diarrhea
3. Distortions of mood and impairment of judgment
4. Paradoxical excitement
5. Inhibition of REM sleep
6. Hyperalgesia
7. Tolerance, psychologic and physical dependence
8. Laryngospasms (when given IV)

Benzodiazepines
1. Hangover and ataxia
2. Increased hostility and anxiety may occur
3. Psychoses and suicidal tendencies with high doses
4. Weight gain
5. Agranulocytosis
6. Menstrual irregularities
7. Tolerance, psychologic and physical dependence
8. Depression of stage-4 sleep

Chlordiazepoxide
Adverse effects in addition to those under Benzodiazepines, include:

1. Skin rash
2. Nausea
3. Headache
4. Lightheadedness
5. Impaired sexual function

G. COMPARISON AND BASIS FOR SELECTION

Flurazepam is a benzodiazepine that was tested and marketed solely for hypnosis. One source (Med Lett Drugs Ther, 1977) suggests that any one of the many benzodiazepines may be used, not only for hypnosis and antianxiety activity but also for aid in sedation. However, the authors consider that oxazepam, and possibly lorazepam, may be especially suitable for dental sedation because of their relatively short half-lives, which decrease the incidence of hangover or drowsiness beyond the desired duration (Med Lett Drugs Ther, 1978). Exceptions include situations in which diazepam is the drug of first choice: spasms of the TMJ muscles, IV sedation, and to control local anesthetic-induced convulsions.

The benzodiazepines are currently the drugs most frequently used to allay fear and anxiety. However, both barbiturate and nonbarbiturate sedative-hypnotic drugs can also be used. Advantages of the benzodiazepines compared to other sedative-hypnotics are:

1. Wide margin of safety
2. Easier separation of antianxiety effect from sedative effect
3. Higher incidence of amnesia when given IV
4. Lower dependence liability
5. Relatively difficult to produce lethality
6. When used alone, a lesser tendency to depress respiration in healthy adults
7. Lesser tendency to suppress REM sleep

H. PREPARATIONS

Barbiturates, ultrashort-acting

THIOPENTAL (Pentothal)
For IV injection

METHOHEXITAL (Brevital)
For IV injection

Barbiturates, short- to intermediate-acting

AMOBARBITAL (Amytal)
Powder and vehicle for parenteral use
20 or 40 mg/5 ml elixir
50, 65, or 200 mg capsules
15, 30, 50, or 100 mg tablets

PENTOBARBITAL (Nembutal)
Solution for parenteral use
20 mg/5 ml elixir
30, 60, 120, or 200 mg suppositories

30, 50, or 100 mg capsules
50 or 100 mg tablets

SECOBARBITAL (Seconal)
Solution for parenteral use
20 mg/5 ml elixir
30, 60, 120, or 200 mg suppositories
30, 50, or 100 mg capsules
50 or 100 mg tablets

Barbiturates, long-acting

PHENOBARBITAL
Powder and vehicle for parenteral use
20 mg/5 ml elixir
15, 30, or 65 mg suppositories
8, 15, 30, 65, or 100 mg tablets

Benzodiazepines

CHLORDIAZEPOXIDE (Librium and Others)
Solution (nonaqueous) for parenteral use
5, 10, or 25 mg capsules or tablets

CLORAZEPATE (Azene, Tranxene)
3.75, 7.5 or 15 mg capsules

DIAZEPAM (Valium)
Solution (nonaqueous) for IV use
2, 5, or 10 mg tablets

FLURAZEPAM (Dalmane)
15 or 30 mg capsules

LORAZEPAM (Ativan)
Solution (nonaqueous) for parenteral use
1 or 2 mg tablets

OXAZEPAM (Serax)
10, 15, or 30 mg capsules
15 mg tablets

PRAZEPAM (Verstran)
10 mg tablets

Nonbarbiturate sedative-hypnotics
No advantage over barbiturates
Benzodiazepines are better

Patient Name   John Doe   (Address)

Age   28

Rx Oxazepam   30 mg caps

   Dispense 4 caps

   Sig: Take 1 caps at bedtime

Refill <u>0</u>-1-2-3-PRN   (Signature)

DEA No.   <u>required-Schedule IV</u>

Prescription 3–1. Prescription for evening sedation-hypnosis.*

I. SAMPLE PRESCRIPTIONS

There are many choices of drugs, as described above. However, the drugs in these sample prescriptions are suggested by the authors.

Prescription 3–1 is a sample prescription for sedation-hypnosis, for the evening before a dental appointment.

Situation: An adult male patient reports he cannot sleep the night before dental appointments. The patient requires restorations in all

---

Patient Name   John Doe   (Address)

Age   28

Rx Oxazepam   10 mg caps

   Dispense 14 caps

   Sig: Take 1 or 2 caps ½ to 1 hour before appointments

Refill <u>0</u>-1-2-3-PRN   (Signature)

DEA No.   <u>required-Schedule IV</u>

Prescription 3–2. Prescription for antianxiety effect during dental appointment.*

Patient Name   John Doe   (Address)

Age   28

Rx Diazepam   5 mg tabs

   Dispense 12 tabs

   Sig: On the day of dental appointment, take 1 tab on arising and 1 tab at 1 hour before appointment

Refill <u>0</u>-1-2-3-PRN   (Signature)

DEA No.   <u>required-Schedule IV</u>

Prescription 3–3. Prescription for antianxiety effect on day of dental appointment.*

quadrants, and all work will be completed in four appointments.

Prescription 3–2 is a sample prescription for an antianxiety effect before and during the dental appointment.

Situation: This patient is very apprehensive prior to all dental appointments. In addition, he is very fearful of any type of injection. Seven appointments will be required to complete his dental care.

Prescription 3–3 is a sample prescription for an antianxiety effect on the day of the dental appointments.

Situation: This adult patient requires late afternoon appointments and is apprehensive all day prior to each appointment. The patient requires one, two, and three surface restorations in all quadrants plus endodontics. This will take six appointments.

REFERENCES

Med Lett Drugs Ther 19:49, 1977
Med Lett Drugs Ther 20:31, 1978

---

* Go to page 14 where full prescription format is given.

BIBLIOGRAPHY

Bennett CR: Conscious-Sedation in Dental Practice, 2nd ed. St. Louis, Mosby, 1978, Ch 2

Bevan JA (ed): Essentials of Pharmacology, 2nd ed. Hagerstown, MD, Harper & Row, 1976, Ch 26

Gilman AG, Goodman LS, Gilman A (eds): Goodman and Gilman's The Pharmacological Basis of Therapeutics, 6th ed. New York, Macmillan, 1980, Ch 17

Meyers FH, Jawetz E, Goldfien A: Review of Medical Pharmacology, 7th ed. Los Altos, CA, Lange, 1980, Ch 23

4

Treatment of Pain

A. INTRODUCTION

Dental pain can be treated in a variety of ways. According to Bennett (1978), pain can be controlled by (1) removing the cause (this is the treatment of choice if it can be accomplished in the dental office), (2) blocking painful impulses, as with a local anesthetic, (3) raising the pain threshold with analgesics, (4) rendering the patient unconscious, as with a general anesthetic, and (5) using psychosomatic methods, such as biofeedback or hypnosis. Despite the fact that one major thrust of this textbook is the control of pain with drugs, the authors urge practitioners to consider all modalities for the treatment or prevention of dental pain.

Dental treatment often results in postoperative pain. It is up to the dentist to estimate the degree of postoperative pain and prescribe an appropriate analgesic. Preoperative estimation of pain is not an easy task since there are many biologic variables that may contribute to or influence the perception of and reaction to pain.

Postoperative dental pain may be classified as *mild* (expected after scaling and prophylaxis), *moderate* (expected after simple extractions), and *severe* (expected after more extensive surgery, e.g., removal of four impacted third molars). Based on this classification of estimated postoperative pain, the dentist can more intelligently prescribe analgesics. For instance, mild pain is probably best treated with an antipyretic analgesic, such as aspirin (ASA) or acetaminophen (APAP). Moderate pain is more often treated with an antipyretic analgesic plus a narcotic-analgesic, such as codeine. Severe pain may require a strong narcotic-analgesic. Obviously, there is overlap, not only in pain perception but also in the activities of the analgesics chosen. The newer nonsteroidal anti-inflammatory agents (NSAIA), such as ibuprofen (*Motrin*), naproxen (*Anaprox*), or zomepirac (*Zomax*) may radically alter the choice. Not only do they appear to be good substitutes for ASA when indicated, but also they may be useful in all three degrees of pain perception (mild, moderate, severe).

B. PRINCIPLES IN THE USE OF ANALGESICS

1. If an analgesic is needed for a dental patient prior to treatment, the practitioner should diagnose the cause of the patient's dental pain. If the sequence is reversed, i.e., an anal-

gesic is given prior to a diagnosis, the drug may mask certain symptoms, such as pain and fever, thereby making a diagnosis more difficult.

2. It may be best to advise patients to begin taking ASA or other NSAIA after clot formation, subsequent to surgery, since these agents have an anticoagulant effect.

3. It is usually advisable to have patients begin taking pain medication before the effects of the local anesthetic wear off because it may be more difficult to break a pain cycle once it is established.

4. Dental analgesic coverage is best obtained postoperatively with a prescription drug during the first 24 to 48 hours. After that period of time, most patients can switch to a medication they ordinarily use for mild pain, such as for simple headache.

5. When pain medication is required, usually start with an antipyretic analgesic. Add narcotic-analgesics to the regimen only when more severe postoperative pain is predictable or if needed later. One of the newer NSAIA may be used.

6. When severe postoperative pain is expected, prescribe a hypnotic drug in addition to an analgesic, especially for the first postoperative night. Patients apparently have fewer postoperative complaints with this regimen.

7. If vomiting is expected or probable, an antiemetic may be required (see C.6 below). Since antiemetics have prominent sedative effects, they can be used in place of a hypnotic drug.

C. MANIPULATION OF VARIOUS ANALGESICS AND DOSAGES

These are adult recommendations; pedodontic patients are, in general, adequately treated with aspirin or acetaminophen only.

1. The use of ASA or APAP for postoperative pain control has often been underrated. For example, Beaver (1981) has suggested that 650 to 1,000 mg of either drug is approximately equal to the analgesic effect of 50 mg of pentazocine, 32 to 65 mg of codeine, 65 mg of propoxyphene, or 5 mg of oxycodone. However, increased analgesia can be obtained by adding narcotic-analgesics to the ASA or APAP dosage (see 4 and 5).

2. If ASA or APAP are to be used to control postoperative pain, the practitioner can prescribe 975 to 1,000 mg every 4 hours in those adult patients who can tolerate the drugs. More pain relief can be achieved at higher doses compared to the usual recommended dose of 650 mg. However, 4 gm of acetaminophen is the maximum recommended daily dose in healthy adults (Beaver, 1981). Lower dosages are recommended in the presence of hepatic dysfunction.

3. If for some reason a patient can take only ASA or APAP and the patient is estimated to have pain of greater intensity than the mild type, the dentist can prescribe both drugs, to be alternately used every 2 hours. For example, 1,000 mg of ASA at 8:00 AM., 1,000 mg of APAP at 10:00 AM., 1,000 mg of ASA at 12:00 noon, 1,000 mg of APAP at 2:00 PM., and so on.

4. One method of treating a range of intensity of pain is to prescribe 15 mg of codeine and have the patient take, in addition, whatever he usually takes for mild pain. In fact, this method is the most versatile. For example, if needed, the patient may double the codeine dose (30 mg), triple the dose (45 mg), or quadruple the dose (60 mg). (*Note:* dosages of codeine higher than 60 mg produce a high frequency of nausea and vomiting, resulting in noncompliance.) In addition, the patient may take two (650 mg) or three (975 mg) ASA or APAP tablets at the same time as the codeine. However, a word of caution: codeine is a Schedule II drug, while codeine combinations are in Schedule III.

5. The dentist may prescribe one of many antipyretic analgesic-codeine combinations. However, we believe that in order to obtain maximum benefit from each analgesic in the combination, the full dosage of ASA or APAP must be used. This is often overlooked because most combinations contain only 325

mg of the antipyretic analgesic. The dentist can gain more versatility by prescribing the combination with 15 mg of codeine so that he may manipulate dosages, as was discussed above.

6. If nausea and vomiting occur with the use of narcotic-analgesics, the dentist can usually protect the patient from those effects by prescribing one of the phenothiazines to be taken with the narcotic-analgesic or, in some cases, taken 30 min to 1 hr before the analgesic. Phenothiazines have been shown to block receptors that are stimulated by narcotic-analgesics to cause nausea and vomiting. We advise the use of a 5 to 10 mg dose of chlorpromazine as the syrup (5 mg/teaspoon). This can be repeated tid and can be actually increased to 25 mg/dose according to the manufacturer's recommendations. However, because of the probability of a drug interaction causing exaggerated CNS depression, the dose of narcotic-analgesic may have to be reduced accordingly (one quarter to one half of the narcotic-analgesic should be used at the higher dose of chlorpromazine). We advise the use of chlorpromazine and discourage the use of promethazine because of reports by Moore and Dundee (1961) and Dundee et al. (1965). They suggest that chlorpromazine either possesses analgesic effects or is supra-additive with narcotic-analgesics, whereas promethazine is antianalgesic.

An alternative agent to replace chlorpromazine is hydroxyzine (*Atarax, Vistaril*). Hydroxyzine is a good antiemetic, and Beaver and Feise (1976) found that 100 mg IM of hydroxyzine has analgesic activity approximately equal to 8 mg morphine, while the combination hydroxyzine and morphine, given concurrently, causes an additive analgesic effect. Thus, if hydroxyzine is used in combination with a narcotic-analgesic, the dose of analgesic should be reduced by one half.

7. The practitioner may choose to use one of the newer NSAIA, such as ibuprofen, naproxen, or zomepirac. These drugs have a number of advantages. They (1) are useful for a wider range of pain intensities up to and including moderate-to-severe pain, (2) generally do not have CNS depressant effects, and, therefore, patients can remain fully ambulatory to accomplish their daily tasks, (3) apparently do not induce tolerance and dependence, (4) are anti-inflammatory, and (5) are not subject to DEA control.

An additional manipulation might be useful, especially if the pain relieving effect of ibuprofen, naproxen, or zomepirac is just adequate. The practitioner can prescribe a Schedule II narcotic-analgesic (Chapter 6) for use during the patient's leisure hours and an NSAIA to be taken during working hours (when alertness is required).

REFERENCES

Accepted Dental Therapeutics, 38th ed. Chicago, American Dental Association, 1979, pp 171–186

Beaver WT: Aspirin and acetaminophen as constituents of analgesic combinations. Arch Intern Med 141:293, 1981

Beaver WT, Feise G: Comparison of the analgesic effects of morphine, hydroxyzine, and their combination in patients with postoperative pain. In Bonica JJ, Albe-Fessard D (eds): Advances in Pain Research and Therapy, vol 1. New York, Raven, 1976, pp. 553–557

Bennett CR: Conscious-Sedation in Dental Practice, 2nd ed. St. Louis, Mosby, 1978, p 7

Dundee JW, Moore J, Love WT, Nicholl RM, Clarke RSJ: Studies of drugs given before anaesthesia. VI: The phenothiazine derivatives. Br J Anaesth 37:332, 1965

Moore J, Dundee JW: Alterations in response to somatic pain associated with anaesthesia. VII. The effect of nine phenothiazine derivatives. Br J Anaesth 33:422, 1961

5
Drugs for Treatment of Mild-to-Moderate Pain

The treatment of **mild** pain is a common challenge in the dental office and can be effectively dealt with through correct diagnosis and appropriate therapeutic measures. Mild pain frequently occurs after many different types of dental procedures and may accompany, as a symptom, many varied dental problems. Pain should never be treated prior to making a diagnosis of the patient's problem, and the administration of analgesic drugs should not be substituted for definitive dental therapy. For example, a complaint of "painful gums" might best be handled with a complete oral prophylaxis and hygiene instructions. Analgesic drugs should be used only adjunctively for a short period of time. Similarly, other local measures, including protective dressings, topical anesthetics, and removal of etiologic agents, are the best aproach to the relief of mild pain. When indicated, however, mild analgesic drugs are extremely useful, especially in postoperative situations in which mild pain is anticipated.

At the present time, there are two primary agents available for the treatment of mild pain: aspirin (ASA, acetylsalicylic acid) and acetamin-ophen (APAP, acetyl-para-aminophenol). Aspirin should be considered the drug of first choice and acetaminophen as an alternative agent or for use when aspirin is contraindicated. This recommendation is made in view of the relatively low incidence of serious side effects associated with the widespread use of aspirin and the fact that aspirin displays a significant anti-inflammatory action, unlike acetaminophen. When the severity of the patient's pain surpasses the mild level and becomes **moderate,** the mild analgesics can be combined with codeine for higher levels of pain relief. Consideration should also be given to the use of one of the newer nonsteroidal anti-inflammatory agents (NSAIA).

So-called **APC** combinations (aspirin, phenacetin, and caffeine) are now considered to be irrational, since no therapeutic advantage is gained by the combination and since such combinations have been associated with renal toxicity due to the phenacetin. In such preparations, caffeine is provided in subtherapeutic dosages (Chapter 37) and is only effective in certain types of headaches when given at higher doses.

27

A. DRUGS FOR THE TREATMENT OF MILD PAIN

Indications

Indications are pain of a mild nature or pain of mild-to-moderate nature or in combination with more efficacious agents. When severe pain is present, the antipyretic-analgesic should be supplied in full dosage, thereby decreasing the need for higher narcotic-analgesic dosage.

Selection of Appropriate Agents

1. Complete health history to identify:
   a. allergy
   b. systemic diseases
   c. current medications
   d. patient preference
   e. level of pain
2. Contraindications
   a. Aspirin:
      (1) gastric ulcer
      (2) bleeding disorders or anticoagulant therapy
      (3) asthma
      (4) gout
      (5) allergy
      (6) nasal polyps or history of aspirin intolerance
   b. Acetaminophen:
      (1) anemia or other blood dyscrasias
      (2) liver or kidney disease
      (3) anticoagulant therapy
      (4) allergy
3. Level of Pain
   a. Level of pain experienced by patient may be greater (or less) than that anticipated.
   b. In cases of more intense pain, mild analgesics can be used effectively in combination with more efficacious drugs and may be useful in reducing fever and inflammation.

Dosages of ASA and APAP

1. Adults: 650 to 1000 mg, q4–6h, orally, not to exceed total daily dose of 6 gm of ASA or 4 gm of APAP
2. Children: 10 to 20 mg/kg body weight, q6h, not to exceed total daily dose of 3.6 gm of ASA
3. Infants: calculate dose from a nomogram of body surface area (Shirkey, 1966; Tainter, Ferris, 1969).

Dosage Forms

1. 325 mg tablets (ASA and APAP)
2. Elixir (120 mg per teaspoon, APAP only)
3. Chewable tablets (80 mg ASA or APAP)
4. Timed release tablets (650 mg ASA)

Sample Prescription

ASA can be prescribed to relieve mild pain (**Prescription 5-1**). Although these drugs are readily available over the counter, patient compliance with therapy sometimes must be assured by the use of a prescription. The designations "ASA" and "APAP" are used instead of the common names so that the patient does not recognize the over-the-counter medications that he may consider ineffective.

Situation: A patient with mild pain informs you that nonprescription drugs "don't work" for him. To ensure that this patient is provided with pain relief, a prescription for a mild analgesic (ASA or APAP) can be offered. (Prescription may also be used to ensure compliance of institutionalized patients, in whom no medication may be given without the order of a health practitioner.)

Patient Name   John Doe   (Address)

Age   28

Rx ASA   325 mg tabs

     Disp: 20 tabs

     Sig: Take 2 tabs q4–6h as needed for pain

Refill 0-1-2-3-PRN   (Signature)

DEA No.   not required

Prescription 5–1. Prescription for antipyretic-analgesic for relief of mild pain.*

---

* Go to page 14 where full prescription format is given.

Side Effects

1. Nausea and vomiting: both ASA and APAP, more frequently seen with ASA. Can be dealt with by having patient take medication with a full glass of water or small amount of food. Nausea and vomiting are aggravated by alcoholic beverages.
2. Allergy: more frequent with ASA and always necessitates immediate discontinuation of drug.
3. Overdose: acute overdose of either ASA or APAP is an emergency situation (Chapter 23). ASA overdose occurs more frequently, causing respiratory problems, while APAP overdose causes severe liver damage.

Principles of Mild Analgesia

1. Is level of pain really mild?
2. ASA is drug of first choice.
3. Use APAP as an alternative or when ASA is contraindicated.
4. Select dosage (ASA and APAP)
   a. Adults: 650 to 1000 mg (two or three 5-grain tablets) q4–6h
   b. Children: correct for age/body weight. If tablet swallowing is difficult, consider APAP elixir. If GI irritation occurs, encourage use of water and/or small amount of food with drug.
5. Duration of therapy should not usually exceed three days; concurrent dental treatment, if successful, should eliminate need for analgesic.
6. Reevaluate or discontinue therapy if:
   a. allergy occurs
   b. pain relief is not obtained
   c. side effects cannot be tolerated by patient
7. Is patient attitude a problem?
   a. Because mild analgesics are readily available over the counter, patients frequently believe that similar drugs will not work in cases of dental pain, even if it is expected to be at the mild level.
   b. Ensure compliance by writing a prescription in a format that will not be readily identified by the patient as an "OTC" medication (see Prescription 5–1).

Alternate Drugs (NSAIA): Ibuprofen (*Motrin*), Zomepirac (*Zomax*), and Naproxen (*Anaprox*)

1. Indications: patients with mild pain accompanied by inflammation or patients in which pain level may be mild-to-moderate. (Also see Chapter 6 for treatment of moderate and severe dental pain.)
2. Side effects: similar to those of aspirin but less severe and less frequent (this is a major advantage); primarily gastrointestinal irritation (including occult bleeding); prolonged bleeding time (but less of a problem compared with ASA); CNS (tinnitus, dizziness, headache); occasional allergy. (Consult package insert for other side effects.)
3. Drug interactions: protein-bound drugs such as oral anticoagulants, hypoglycemics. (Aspirin taken concurrently reduces effectiveness.)
4. Contraindications: patients allergic to aspirin or to NSAIA. In patients taking anticoagulants or in patients with ulcers or other gastrointestinal disorders use with caution; not recommended for use in pregnancy or in nursing mothers; not recommended for use in children.
5. Dispensing information: these agents require a prescription; these agents are not under DEA controls.
6. Dosage and administration of zomepirac (Zomax)
   a. available in scored 100 mg tablets
   b. adult dose: 100 mg q4–6h prn
   c. do not exceed 600 mg per day for acute dental pain
7. Dosage and administration of ibuprofen (Motrin)
   a. available in 300, 400, or 600 mg tablets
   b. adult dose: 400 mg q6h prn
   c. do not exceed 2400 mg per day for acute dental pain
8. Dosage and administration of naproxen (Anaprox)
   a. available in 275 mg tablets
   b. adult dose: two tablets, then one tablet q6–8h prn
   c. do not exceed 1275 mg per day for acute dental pain
9. Sample prescription

Patient Name   John Doe   (Address)

Age _____28_____

Rx Zomepirac   100 mg tabs

   Disp: 20 tabs

   Sig: Take 1 tab q4–6h prn for pain

Refill 0-1-2-3-PRN   (Signature)

DEA No. __not required__

Prescription 5–2. Prescription for NSAIA.*

Prescription 5-2 is a prescription for NSAIA. *Situation:* An adult patient has two third molars extracted on the right side. After the previous appointment for extraction of left third molars, he had moderate pain with a great amount of swelling. Prescribe an NSAIA.

10. Alternate NSAIA prescription

   a. **Prescription 5-3** is a prescription for ibuprofen.
   b. **Prescription 5-4** is a prescription for Naproxen.

Patient Name   John Doe   (Address)

Age   28

Rx Ibuprofen   400 mg tabs

   Disp: 20 such tablets

   Sig: Take 1 tablet q4–6h prn for pain

Refill 0-1-2-3-PRN   (Signature)

DEA No. __not required__

Prescription 5–3. Prescription for Ibuprofen.*

Patient Name   John Doe   (Address)

Age _____28_____

Rx Naproxen   275 tabs

   Disp: 20 such tablets

   Sig: Take 2 tablets stat and 1 tablet q6–8h prn for pain

Refill 0-1-2-3-PRN   (Signature)

DEA No. __not required__

Prescription 5–4. Prescription for Naproxen.*

REFERENCES

Shirkey HC: Pediatric Therapy. St. Louis, Mosby, 1966, p 234

Tainter ML, Ferris AJ: Aspirin in Modern Therapy. New York, Sterling Drug, Inc., 1969, pp 85–89

BIBLIOGRAPHY

Accepted Dental Therapeutics, 38th ed. Chicago, American Dental Association, 1979, Sec II, Analgesics

Csáky TZ: Cuttings's Handbook of Pharmacology, 6th ed. New York, Appleton-Century-Crofts, 1979, Ch 49

Flower RJ, Moncada S, Vane JR: Analgesic-antipyretics and anti-inflammatory agents; drugs employed in the treatment of gout. In Gilman AG, Goodman LS, Gilman A (eds): Goodman and Gilman's The Pharmacological Basis of Therapeutics, 6th ed. New York, Macmillan, 1980, Ch 29

Kastrup EK (ed): Facts and Comparisons. Central Nervous System Drugs. St. Louis, Facts and Comparisons, Inc., 1981, pp 229–290

* Go to page 14 where full prescription format is given.

6

Drugs for the Treatment of Moderate and Severe Pain

Treatment of pain greater than mild offers several possibilities. First, for moderate pain, a combination of a mild analgesic with codeine may give more relief than the mild analgesic alone. The combination gives greater pain relief because the narcotic analgesic has an additive effect with the antipyretic analgesic. Second, if severe pain is a suspected outcome, codeine will not suffice, and a more potent narcotic-analgesic may be the choice. Since use of potent narcotic-analgesics should be avoided if possible because of habituation and side effects, the dentist now has a third choice, i.e., use of nonsteroidal inflammatory agents (NSAIA). Recent studies have indicated that NSAIA would be the rational first choice because they offer pain relief at least as great as the codeine combinations and possibly better in some cases.

One principle that should be stressed is that pain control is usually simplified by having the patient take the medication while local anesthesia is present. If one waits until pain becomes severe, it may be difficult to reverse.

A. CODEINE

PHARMACOTHERAPEUTICS OF CODEINE

Indications
Moderate pain of dental origin, usually acute pain, including toothache, muscle pain, neuralgia, and headache.

Contraindications

1. allergy to codeine
2. previous history of adverse reaction to codeine
3. drug abuser

Warnings

1. Codeine may be habit-forming.
2. Do not drive since drowsiness will probably occur.
3. Do not operate dangerous machinery.
4. Do not drink alcohol while taking codeine.

Side Effects Are Rare and Include

nausea
vomiting
constipation

Side effects are more severe, including the above plus headache and malaise, when the dosage exceeds 1 grain every six hours.

How Supplied

Codeine sulfate or codeine phosphate tablets

¼ grain or 15 mg
½ grain or 30 mg
1 grain or 60 mg

Prescription

Prescription 6-1 is a sample prescription for codeine without an antipyretic analgesic.

Situation: A 150 lb male, 30 years old, requires codeine after extractions, since moderate pain is expected. Provide a prescription for codeine separate from the antipyretic-analgesic.

B. COMBINATION THERAPY

The details of use of the mild analgesics were described in Chapter 5, and a similar situation applies here. Dosage schedule and therapeutic considerations are the same when treating moderate pain and include the following:

1. A full dose of ASA or APAP must always be used.
2. It may be useful to prescribe 975 to 1000 mg of ASA or APAP (however, 4 gm of APAP is the maximum daily dose in a healthy adult).
3. Codeine can be given by separate prescription or in combination; the former is preferred by the authors because of greater flexibility in dosing.

Pharmacotherapeutics of Combinations

Codeine phosphate and, occasionally, codeine sulfate are supplied in combination with either ASA or APAP (also with APC, which is not recommended; see Chapter 5). For consideration of the pharmacotherapeutics, each drug must be considered (Chapter 4).

How Supplied and Dosage Schedule

Codeine combinations are usually supplied with 325 mg ASA or 300 mg APAP as follows:

1. ASA or APAP + codeine ⅛ gr (7.5 to 8 mg)
2. ASA or APAP + codeine ¼ gr (15 to 16 mg)
3. ASA or APAP + codeine ½ gr (30 to 32 mg)
4. ASA or APAP + codeine 1 gr (60 to 65 mg)

According to the recommendation that no more than 65 mg be given every 6 hours, combination 4 would appear irrational because a full dose of antipyretic-analgesic is not provided. Combination 3 is better because two tablets provide 650 ASA or APAP and a full dose of codeine. However, it is usually best to start with a lower dose of codeine and then increase the dosage if needed. If the patient needs three tablets of ASA or APAP, combination 3 would provide too much codeine. On this basis, the authors prefer use of combination 1 or 2 so that, with one prescription, the patient is provided with full doses of each drug.

Sample Prescriptions

Prescription 6-2 is a prescription for codeine combined with ASA.

Patient Name   John Doe   (Address)

Age____30____

Rx Codeine phosphate   15 mg tabs

Disp: 20 tabs

Sig: Take 1 or 2 tabs q4–6h prn for pain along with 3 aspirin tabs

Caution: Keep out of reach of children

          Do not drive

Refill 0-1-2-3-PRN   (Signature)

DEA No.   Required-Schedule II

Prescription 6-1. Prescription for codeine.*

---

* Go to page 14 where full prescription format is given.

Patient Name John Doe _____ (Address)

Age ___ 30 ___

Rx Codeine phosphate   ⅛ gr tabs

   ASA   325 mg

   Disp: 24 tabs

   Sig: Take 3 tabs q4–6h prn for pain

   Caution: Keep out of reach of children

       Do not drive if you become drowsy

Refill 0-1-2-3-PRN   (Signature)

DEA No. Required-Schedule III _____

Prescription 6–2. Prescription for codeine and aspirin.*

Situation: A 150 lb male, 30 years old, requires codeine after extractions, since moderate pain is expected. Provide a prescription for codeine in combination with aspirin.

Prescription 6–3 is a prescription for codeine combined with APAP.

Situation: A 150 lb male, 30 years old, requires codeine after extractions, since moderate pain is expected. Provide a prescription for codeine in combination with an antipyretic analgesic. (*Note:* Patient is allergic to aspirin.)

Reasons for Adding Third Drug

Adding a third drug to the combination is usually considered irrational because dosing problems become even more complex than described above. However, the dentist may wish to prescribe a third drug separately for the following conditions:

1. sedation or anxiety control (Chapter 3)
2. antinauseant effect (antihistamines, Chapter 7)
3. antacid effect when drugs irritate the stomach—use milk of magnesia or other antacid
4. laxative effect when codeine constipates—use mineral oil or milk of magnesia

Patient Name John Doe _____ (Address)

Age ___ 30 ___

Rx Codeine phosphate   ⅛ gr tabs

   Acetaminophen   300 mg

   Disp: 24 tabs

   Sig: Take 3 tabs q4–6h as needed for pain, not to exceed 12 tabs per day

   Caution: Keep out of reach of children

       Do not drive if you become drowsy

Refill 0-1-2-3-PRN   (Signature)

DEA No. Required-Schedule III _____

Prescription 6–3. Prescription for codeine and acetaminophen.*

C. PENTAZOCINE (Talwin)

Pentazocine is considered a codeine substitute. It is a partial narcotic-antagonist analgesic. The pharmacology of pentazocine is discussed in Chapter 24. A therapeutic review of pentazocine follows.

Indications

1. as a substitute for codeine; 50 mg pentazocine equals 60 mg codeine
2. for relief of pain of dental origin which is moderate-to-severe

Contraindications and Warnings

1. allergy to pentazocine
2. may cause withdrawal symptoms in narcotic drug abusers
3. may cause psychic or physical dependence
4. withdraw slowly if subject is a drug abuser
5. head injuries—may increase intracranial pressure
6. avoid use in pregnancy, especially when delivery is near
7. may cause visual disturbances, hallucinations, disorientation, confusion

---

* **Go to page 14 where full prescription format is given.**

8. not recommended in children less than 12 years old
9. interacts with alcohol and other CNS depressants
10. do not operate car or dangerous machinery
11. avoid in patient with respiratory embarrassment
12. avoid in liver disease (metabolism) or renal disease (excretion)
13. avoid in patient with seizures

Side Effects

Side effects include gastrointestinal effects (e.g., nausea), CNS disturbances (e.g., irritability) autonomic effects, allergy (e.g., rash), cardiovascular symptoms (increased blood pressure, tachycardia), hematologic symptoms, respiratory depression, and other effects.

Dosage and Administration

1. Dosage:

    usual adult dose 50 mg q4h
    double dose if needed
    not to exceed 600 mg daily
    not recommended for children under 12
    parenteral form also available

2. Pentazocine is supplied as 50 mg tablets (*Talwin*) and 12.5 mg plus 325 mg ASA (*Talwin* compound).
3. Prescription

    Prescription 6-4 is a sample prescription for pentazocine.
    Situation: A 70 kg adult patient had headache, nausea, and vomiting when given codeine previously. Prescribe pentazocine for this patient.

D. DRUGS FOR MORE SEVERE PAIN

When severe pain is expected, either from past history or after extensive oral or periodontal surgery, a narcotic-analgesic stronger than codeine may be indicated. If the patient has taken codeine plus ASA (or APAP) with no relief, a stronger narcotic-analgesic should be used,

---

Patient Name	John Doe (Address)
Age	38

Rx Pentazocine HCl   50 mg

   Disp: 12 tabs

    Sig: Take 1 tab q4–6h prn for pain

          Also take 3 aspirins with each dose

          Do not drive, do not drink alcohol

          Keep out of reach of children

Refill 0-1-2-3-PRN   (Signature)

DEA No. Required-Schedule IV

Prescription 6-4. Prescription for pentazocine.*

either as a change at the next dose or for subsequent procedures.

Choice of Narcotic Analgesic

Some of the choices available are listed in Table 6-1. These include:

1. Morphine

    hospitalized patient
    parenteral injection only
    use 8 mg or 15 mg, give stat and q4–6h as needed for pain

2. Meperidine

    hospitalized patient (usually)
    50 to 100 mg IM
    give stat and q4–6h as needed for pain
    for outpatient use, oral form available; use 50 to 150 mg q6h. Ask patient to remain at rest during use. Combinations: 50 mg with APAP (300 mg) and 30 mg with APC are also available.

3. Oxycodone. Oral tablets with aspirin or acetaminophen are available. This is advertised as a more potent codeine, but actually it is more potent than morphine and equitoxic to morphine at equi-analgesic doses. Its only advantage seems to be the availability of and

---

* Go to page 14 where full prescription format is given.

TABLE 6–1. AVAILABLE CHOICE OF STRONG NARCOTIC ANALGESICS

Official Name	Chemical Class	Trade Names	Preparations	Notes
morphine	opium alkaloid	*Morphine*	parenteral solution	use in hospital only
meperidine	opioid	*Demerol* *Meperidine*	parenteral solution 50 or 100 mg tablets 50 mg *Demerol* + 300 mg APAP tablets 30 mg *Demerol* + APC	use in hospital outpatient use (patient should stay at rest)
oxycodone	opiate	*Percodan*	each tablet contains: oxycodone HCl, 4.5 mg oxycodone terephthalate, 0.38 mg aspirin, 325 mg (demitabs contain same except ½ amount of oxycodone)	outpatient use (patient should stay at rest)
		Percocet *Tylox*	same as *Percodan* except 325 APAP same as *Percodan* except 500 mg APAP	
methadone	opioid	*Dolophine*	5 or 10 mg tablets	outpatient use (patient should stay at rest)

satisfactory effectiveness of the oral form. Dentists have been persuaded to use this compound as a substitute for codeine, but it should be used only in severe pain, with the full knowledge that it is pharmacologically equivalent to morphine or meperidine.

4. Methadone. Oral tablets are supplied in 5 and 10 mg sizes; usual adult dose is 2.5 to 10 mg, q4-6h. The advantage of methadone over the other strong narcotic analgesics is its rather good oral effectiveness and relatively long duration of action compared with meperidine. Methadone must be labeled "for analgesia."

Sample Prescriptions

Prescription 6-5 is a sample prescription for meperidine (page 36).

Situation: The patient who was given a prescription for codeine 15 mg and ASA 325 mg calls about midnight and needs something stronger. You may provide a prescription for meperidine by calling the pharmacist. However, the next day you must write the prescription and mail it to the pharmacist.

Prescription 6-6 is a sample prescription for oxycodone (page 36).

Situation: Patient needs third molars extracted, and you expect severe pain. Prescribe oxycodone with ASA for this patient.

Prescription 6-7 is a sample prescription for methadone. The choice among meperidine, oxycodone, and methadone is a toss-up; the authors prefer methadone (page 36).

Situation: After a previous surgical removal of impacted third molars, the patient was given codeine plus ASA but suffered much discomfort. Prescribe methadone for this patient.

Pharmacotherapeutics

We may conclude that all the strong narcotic analgesics are roughly equivalent when used in equi-analgesic doses. Therefore, the same care must be used irrespective of the drug used. Since the narcotic-analgesics are considered therapeutic equivalents, the pharmacotherapeutics of these drugs will be considered together instead of separately for each agent. Any differences between agents will be mentioned if the differences are clinically significant.

Indications and Use

Strong narcotic-analgesics should be used for severe pain only. They may be used for acute pain

---

Patient Name John Doe _____ (Address)

Age ___30___

Rx Meperidine HCl   50 mg

  Disp: 12 tabs

  Sig: Take 1 tab q4–6h, prn for pain with full dose (2–3 tabs) of aspirin

      Do not drive; stay in bed or resting

      Keep out of reach of children

      Do not drink alcohol

Refill 0-1-2-3-PRN   (Signature)

DEA No. ___Required-Schedule II___

Prescription 6–5. Prescription for meperidine.*

Patient Name John Doe _____ (Address)

Age ___30___

Rx Methadone HCl   5 mg

  Disp: 12 tabs

  Sig: Take 1 tab q4–6h as needed for analgesia, also take 2 or 3 aspirins at the same time

      Do not drive, stay in bed or resting

      Keep out of reach of children

      Do not drink alcohol

Refill 0-1-2-3-PRN   (Signature)

Dea No. ___Required-Schedule II___

Prescription 6–7. Prescription for methadone.*

---

of dental origin. Usually, codeine with a full dose of antipyretic-analgesic is tried first, and the strong narcotic is substituted if the former is not sufficient. Occasionally, the dentist may predict that the patient will have severe postoperative pain after massive oral or periodontal surgery. The dentist may then wish to give a strong narcotic analgesic for 48 hours, starting

the first dose while the local anesthetic is still effective. It is recommended that a full dose of antipyretic-analgesic be used along with a strong narcotic-analgesic, because analgesia is obtained by different mechanisms with these classes of drugs. In another situation, a strong narcotic-analgesic may be chosen when codeine has not been sufficient at a previous appointment. One must be wary when the patient asks for the stronger narcotic, as it is well known that narcotic-dependent persons prefer any of the other choices over codeine.

Contraindications

Allergy. A history of allergy to the specific drug is a contraindication. Relative contraindications would occur when the patient has had allergy to chemically similar substances, e.g., oxycodone may be cross-allergenic with codeine, methadone may be cross-allergenic with propoxyphene (*Darvon*), and meperidine may be cross-allergenic with ethoheptazine, anilerdine, or fentanyl.

Abuse potential. Strong narcotic-analgesics are all in Schedule II and are subject to abuse. Use

---

Patient Name John Doe _____ (Address)

Age ___30___

Rx Oxycodone HCl (demi tabs)   2.25 mg

  Aspirin   325 mg

  Disp: 24 tabs

  Sig: Take 2 tabs q4–6h prn for pain

      Do not drive, stay in bed or resting

      Keep out of reach of children

      Do not drink alcohol

Refill 0-1-2-3-PRN   (Signature)

DEA No. ___Required-Schedule II___

Prescription 6–6. Prescription for oxycodone.*

---

* Go to page 14 where full prescription format is given.

in the narcotic-dependent subject or those with a history of narcotic dependence is not recommended. In normal patients (nonaddicted), dental use and prescription should not be for longer than 48 hours unless reevaluation indicates additional use. The dentist should protect his prescription blanks and DEA number and watch for suspicious patients or actions (see App. III).

Head injuries. The narcotic-analgesic may increase intracranial pressure due to respiratory depression. Moreover, the narcotic-analgesic may complicate the diagnosis.

Monoamine oxidase inhibitors. These should be withdrawn at least 14 days before using meperidine. Otherwise, use ASA, APAP, an NSAIA (Chapter 5), or another narcotic-analgesic (cautiously and starting with lower dosages).

Other CNS depressants. Use reduced dosages (low initial dosages) if patient is taking drugs which are narcotic-analgesics, antipsychotics, antianxiety agents, general anesthetics, sedative-hypnotics, antidepressants (tricyclic), and other CNS depressants (including alcohol).

Asthmatics. For these and other patients with respiratory embarrassment, narcotic-analgesic respiratory depression may be additive.

Ambulatory patients. Such patients should not drive or operate dangerous machinery. They may be prone to vomit and have orthostatic hypotension. The best policy is to keep the patient at rest if a strong narcotic-analgesic is required.

Drugs that interfere with blood pressure regulation. These may interact, causing increased hypotensive effect.

Pregnancy. Avoid use of these drugs in pregnancy, especially in the first trimester. This is usually a relative contraindication. The dentist should not use narcotic-analgesics at term. These drugs may get into the milk of lactating mothers.

Convulsive disorders. Avoid in patients with convulsive disorders or seizures.

Abdominal pain. Avoid use in patients with biliary or urinary spasms or other abdominal pain, including prostatic hypertrophy or urinary stricture.

Avoid in liver or renal disease.

Other contraindications. Reduce dosage in hypothyroidism, debilitated and elderly patients, and in Addison's disease.

Adverse Reactions
These include respiratory depression, habituation, and circulatory depression, shock, or cardiac arrest.

Side Effects
These include lightheadedness, nausea, vomiting, sweating, headache, sedation tremors, hallucinations, excitement, euphoria, dysphoria, and others.

Specific Effects of Meperidine
Meperidine can be vagolytic (more care is required in patients with arrhythmias), produces a dry mouth, and may be constipating.

Treatment of Overdose
Establish an airway and respiration, give 100% oxygen, give naloxone (0.4 mg IV), and repeat dose when needed (Appendix I).

E. USE OF NSAIA FOR MODERATE-TO-SEVERE PAIN

The newer NSAIA, especially the propionic acid derivatives (zomepirac, ibuprofen, or naproxen), may be used after major oral or periodontal surgery. The use of these drugs for postoperative discomfort is the same as their use in treatment of myositis or TMJ arthritis, except a shorter course of treatment (72 to 96 hours) should be instituted. A sample prescription was presented in Chapter 5 along with further details (Prescription 5-2). The pharmacotherapeutics of these agents is covered in Chapter 23. Also, as discussed in Chapter 4, the dentist may wish to prescribe a strong narcotic-analgesic at night or during leisure hours and an NSAIA during the day.

BIBLIOGRAPHY

AMA Drug Evaluations, 3rd ed. Littleton, MA, Publishing Sciences Group, Inc, 1977, Ch 20

Gilman AG, Goodman LS, Gilman A (eds): Goodman and Gilman's The Pharmacological Basis of Therapeutics, 6th ed. New York, Macmillan, 1980, Ch 22

Kastrup EK (ed): Facts and Comparisons. Central Nervous System Drugs. St. Louis, Facts and Comparisons, Inc, 1980, pp 743–745

Melmon KL, Morelli HF (eds): Clinical Pharmacology: Basic Principles in Therapeutics, 2nd ed. New York, Macmillan, 1978, Ch 17, pp 874–884

Physicians' Desk Reference, 36th ed. Oradell, NJ, Medical Economics Co, 1982, Insert on meperidine, p 2025; insert on pentazocine, p 2036; insert on methadone, p 1103; insert on oxycodone, p 912

7
Corticosteroids and Antihistamines

Corticosteroids and antihistamines are two diverse groups of drugs which may have some specific usefulness to the dentist in the treatment of inflammation and for histamine reactions. In addition, antihistamines have other effects that may be useful. This chapter concentrates on specific uses for these drugs.

A. CORTICOSTEROIDS

Emergency Use (see also, Appendix I)
Methylprednisolone sodium succinate is a water-soluble preparation intended for IV use during an anaphylactoid reaction or possibly shock. The action of the corticosteroids appears to be on the cardiovascular system by reducing capillary permeability, improving vasomotor response of small vessels, and increasing cardiac output. Methylprednisolone sodium succinate is not the first drug given, since a sympathomimetic is usually chosen as the primary drug. The sympathomimetic may be lifesaving because of bronchodilation (e.g., the β agonist, epinephrine) or by maintaining blood pressure (e.g., mephentermine, a sympathomimetic heart and vascular stimulant). In the case of drug hypersensitivity or an asthmatic attack, there may be evidence of histamine release, and, therefore, an antihistamine may be chosen as the secondary drug (see below) and the corticosteroid becomes the tertiary drug. There appears to be good pharmacologic rationale for choosing the drugs in the following order:

1. sympathomimetic—primary. (*Note:* if epinephrine fails to control respiratory spasms, then aminophylline should be given before the secondary or tertiary agents.)
2. antihistamine—secondary
3. corticosteroid—tertiary (or secondary if no antihistamine needed)

The rationale includes the facts that epinephrine (1) is rapidly acting and (2) attacks the major problems of bronchoconstriction and blood flow. However, there may be a need to provide aminophylline, 200 to 500 mg, slow IV infusion, for its nonspecific relaxant effect on the bronchioles. The antihistamine is slower in action; there is no lifesaving urgency and it can be administered after the bronchodilators. The corticosteroid action on the cardiovascular system

Wyamine

is considered even slower, and it is, therefore, administered later.

Methylprednisolone sodium succinate is marketed as *Solu-Medrol* 50 mg or 125 mg (*Mix-O-Vial*) or under other trade names. The solution is mixed at the time of need, since the drug is not stable in solution. Dexamethasone phosphate, 4 mg/ml IV, is an alternative agent. The only possible side effect, adrenocortical suppression, is not seen with such short-term corticosteroid use.

Topical Application or Iontophoretic Administration

Various anti-inflammatory steroids have been applied topically to noninfected inflamed tissue, such as aphthous ulcers, lichen planus, noninfected burns, traumatic wounds which do not heal, and so on. The rationale for applying anti-inflammatory drugs is that control of inflammation allows for more normal healing. It is true that in higher doses, collagen formation and wound healing can be suppressed, but such high doses are never achieved by topical therapy. Several problems can result from topical therapy:

1. Overuse can lead to adrenal suppression. Topical use beyond 10 days is not recommended except under medical care with adrenocortical monitoring. The authors believe that PO use for longer than 5 days should not be prescribed by the dentist.
2. The drug may be rapidly washed away in the saliva, so that little or no drug is absorbed into the wound. In an effort to overcome this problem, the steroid is often supplied in a sticky vehicle, but adherence is often far from satisfactory, especially in areas of abrasion. Because of slow absorption, it is difficult to build to a sufficient tissue concentration of the drug for effectiveness.
3. All other sources of irritation must be removed, e.g., there is no chance that the drug would be more than marginally effective if the lesion scrapes against a rough restoration each time the cheek moves.
4. Every effort must be made to eliminate all lesions that have a specific, known cause, so

that masking the inflammatory symptoms does not mask the disease.
5. No infection must be present as the infection can worsen in the presence of the steroid.

In an effort to provide a more rational therapy that achieves high tissue levels without the risk of systemic adrenocortical suppression, one of the authors (Dr. Gangarosa) has developed the technique of applying the steroid by iontophoresis. *Solu-Medrol* is a negatively charged, ionic steroid that can be introduced easily under a negative electrode. The drug is mixed just before use, placed on cotton, which covers the lesion for about 4 minutes, and attached to the negative electrode. A positive electrode is placed on the arm. As the current (0.5 mA) passes into the tissue, the drug is carried into the lesion, providing immediate relief and rapid healing. All other precautions of topical therapy with corticosteroids are observed (see above). Iontophoresis is further discussed in Appendix VII.

Available forms for topical therapy include triamcinolone (*Kenalog*) ointment, betamethasone gel (*Uticort*), and methylprednisolone sodium succinate (for iontophoresis).

Systemic Use

Except when emergency therapy is needed, systemic use should be a last resort. Nevertheless, there are some patients with severe oral ulceration who require systemic therapy. Probably, most patients requiring systemic corticosteroids will be under the care of a dermatologist because the lesion may occur not only in the mouth but also on the skin. Occasionally, a patient with many oral lesions but none in other parts of the body will require short-term systemic therapy.

The major reason for using systemic therapy in dentistry is that the lesions are rather inaccessible. When the lesions are accessible, they can be treated by iontophoresis, thus avoiding systemic therapy.

Under the following restricted conditions, the authors would use systemic therapy in dental practice.

1. There should be **no contraindications,** such as history of tuberculosis, pregnancy, peptic ulcer, hypertension, diabetes, systemic steroids prescribed by another practitioner, and long-term use of corticosteroids with suppressed adrenocortical functions.
2. **Consultation with Physician.** The dentist should ascertain that the patient's primary physician has no objection to the therapy.
3. **No active infection present.**
4. **Diagnosis of nonspecific inflammatory disease** is assured, with all other differential diagnostic factors eliminated. It should be ascertained that there are no systemic causes of the disease and no specific local causes (e.g., cancer, infections).

If these four conditions are met, a short course of therapy starting with a high dose and then rapidly lowering the dosage would be indicated. A similar but more intensive therapy is sometimes used in severe poison ivy rash by dermatologists and allergists.

Prescription 7-1 is a sample prescription for methylprednisolone and illustrates the dosage schedule.

Situation: A 37-year-old female weighing 135 lb has acute exacerbations of oral ulcers with multiple ulceration. Prescribe a short

---

Patient Name   Jane Doe   (Address)

Age   37

Rx Methylprednisolone   4 mg tabs

    Disp: 15 tabs

    Sig: Take 5 tabs day 1; 4 tabs day 2; 3 tabs day 3; 2 tabs day 4; 1 tab day 5

      Take correct dosage each day at 8 AM

Refill 0-1-2-3-PRN   (Signature)

DEA No.   Not required

Prescription 7-1. Prescription for methylprednisolone.*

* Go to page 14 where full prescription format is given.

course of methylprednisolone using the 5, 4, 3, 2, 1 dosage schedule.

It would not be advisable to repeat the treatment immediately. We recommend that this treatment be used no more often than once every six weeks, at the time of acute exacerbations. If more frequent therapy is needed, it should be done in collaboration with a dermatologist. Concerning adrenocortical suppression, two points should be noted: (1) giving the full dose each morning at 8:00 AM incurs the least possibility of adrenocortical suppression (Physicians' Desk Reference, 1982), and (2) therapy for five days will probably not cause suppression (Haynes, Murad, 1980). Therapy for longer than 10 days requires monitoring of the plasma steroid level for evidence of suppression and should be performed under medical supervision.

Another consideration is that dental stress may increase the need for systemic therapy when the patient is taking the adrenocorticosteroids for a medical indication. After consultation with the physician, arrangements can be made to increase the dose before, during, and after any major procedures.

Some oral surgery texts (e.g., Bell et al., 1980) recommend short-term steroids for prevention of swelling after major oral surgery. Although many dosage schedules are possible, the prescription provided (Prescription 7-1) would be useful. This therapy appears rational, but long-term evaluation awaits further research.

Another possible use is for control of unexpected postoperative swelling after other types of surgery. In this case and the above, one should ascertain that no infection is present.

B. ANTIHISTAMINES

Antihistamine therapy with classic H_1-blockers (Chapter 19) should be instituted for several reasons.

As an Emergency Measure
An antihistamine may be helpful in drug hypersensitivity or other anaphylactoid reactions, especially if histamine release is a contributing

factor. As described above and in Appendix I, epinephrine is the primary drug because of its lifesaving properties, and antihistamines would be given as secondary drugs when the life-threatening emergency is over. However, if the first symptoms are hives, urticaria, edema, and swelling, an antihistamine should be given in an attempt to prevent further development of the histamine reaction.

For emergency purposes, diphenhydramine hydrochloride (*Benadryl*) should be available in an emergency kit. The solution contains 50 mg/ml, 1 ml per vial. The dose is 50 mg injected IV. For more slowly developing allergic reactions, diphenhydramine can be taken orally.

Prescription 7–2 is a sample prescription for diphenhydramine for a slowly developing allergic reaction.

Situation: This adult patient arrives in your office with urticarial areas on her arms and legs. At her previous appointment, the day before, you prescribed codeine and aspirin for postoperative pain. Prescribe diphenhydramine for this patient in addition to withdrawing the pain medication.

For Nausea and Vomiting

Some of the H_1 antihistamines (e.g., promethazine) are closely related to phenothiazines and have local anesthetic activity. A syrup of the antihistamine may have a dual effect on nausea and vomiting: (1) local anesthetic action can calm the gastric mucosa, and (2) after absorption, the **phenothiazine-like** antihistamines should block the chemoreceptor trigger zone in the medulla. However, in the case of frank vomiting, an analgesic or other oral drug cannot be retained, so that the antihistamine may have to be administered in suppositories. For oral use, promethazine (*Phenergan*) syrup (6.25 mg/5 ml) is available. The dose is up to 25 mg every 4 hours. Suppositories of promethazine are also available in 12.5, 25, and 50 mg sizes. Other antihistaminic syrups, including *Dramamine*, are available, or, alternatively, one may wish to use a phenothiazine syrup, such as *Thorazine*.

Sedation is usually predictable with these products, so the patients should be warned not to drive or operate dangerous machinery.

As Alternate Local Anesthetic

Diphenhydramine (50 mg/ml) has been recommended as a local anesthetic solution for patients allergic to both ester and amide local anesthetics. The predictability of local anesthesia with an antihistamine is not as high as desirable for dental office use. The injection appears to be more painful than with standard drugs, and the duration is shorter. Thus, one should be very certain that the patient cannot tolerate one of the "caine" anesthetics before resorting to the substitution of antihistamines. Roberts and Loveless (1979) recommended adding 1:100,000 epinephrine to the diphenhydramine solution to prolong the duration.

Antihistamines have often been recommended in an oral rinse, presumably for their topical local anesthetic effect. Benzocaine is much better for topical anesthesia, and antihistamines should not be substituted for this pur-

---

Patient Name ___Jane Doe_____ (Address)

Age___37_____

Rx Diphenhydramine HCl   50 mg caps

   Disp: 20 caps

   Sig: Take 1 cap q6h for allergic reaction

       Do not take previous pain medication, take your normal headache medication (APAP) 3 tabs q4–6h

   Cautions: Keep out of reach of children

       Do not drive or operate machinery if you become drowsy

       Do not drink alcohol

Refill _0_-1-2-3-PRN   (Signature)

DEA No. __Not required___

Prescription 7–2. Prescription for diphenhydramine hydrochloride.*

---

* Go to page 14 where full prescription format is given.

pose. Strangely enough, the antihistamines are considered to be high in their ability to cause contact sensitization, and for this reason topical use is not considered rational.

Precautions and Side Effects
These include:

1. drowsiness and sedation
2. interaction with alcohol, other CNS depressants, narcotics, and MAO inhibitors
3. safe use in pregnancy not established
4. children and elderly patients may show exaggerated responses
5. may be unsafe, due to anticholinergic properties of the drug, in narrow-angle glaucoma, asthma, prostatic hypertrophy, peptic ulcer, urethral or GI obstruction
6. may cause blood cell changes
7. may cause excitement, tremors, seizures, catatonia, and extrapyramidal reaction
8. may cause dizziness, blurred vision, incoordination, nausea, or vomiting
9. may cause allergy
10. IV injection may cause thrombosis at injection site
11. cardiac arrhythmias and blood pressure changes have been reported

REFERENCES

Bell WH, Proffit WR, White RP (eds): Surgical Correction of Dentofacial Deformities. Philadelphia, Saunders, 1980, Vol 1, p 207

Haynes RD, Murad F: Adrenocorticotropic hormone; adrenocortical steroids and their synthetic analogs; inhibitors of adrenocortical steroid biosynthesis. In Gilman AG, Goodman LS, Gilman A (eds): Goodman and Gilman's The Pharmacological Basis of Therapeutics, 6th ed. New York, Macmillan, 1980, p 1483

Physicians' Desk Reference, 36th ed. Oradell, NJ, Medical Economics Co, 1982, p 2076

Roberts EW, Loveless H: The utilization of diphenhydramine for production of local anesthesia: Report of case. Tex Dent J 97:13, 1979

BIBLIOGRAPHY

Physicians' Desk Reference, 36th ed. Oradell, NJ, Medical Economics Co, 1982. Insert on methylprednisolone sodium succinate, pp 1967–1969; insert on methylprednisolone, pp 1956–1961; insert on dexamethasone sodium phosphate, pp 1230–1233

8

Principles of Antimicrobial Therapy

INDICATIONS FOR [AN]TIMICROBIAL THERAPY

[Th]ese include:

[1.] Treatment of infections caused by susceptible organisms
[2.] Prophylactic use in patients susceptible to bacterial endocarditis and patients with prosthetic joint replacements, uncontrolled diabetes, glomerulonephritis, or reduced resistance to infections due to advanced age, leukemia, long-term corticosteroid therapy, or antimetabolite therapy

[D]rug selection is determined according to the [eff]ectiveness of the antimicrobial agent against [the] causative organism. Naturally, if a patient is [all]ergic to a particular antibiotic (or group of [ant]ibiotics), it would be eliminated from the se[lec]tion.

[A]ntimicrobial therapy should be continued [for] 10 full days in the case of streptococcal in[fec]tion. For other infections, therapy should be [con]tinued until the patient has been asympto[ma]tic for at least 3 days. Prophylaxis should [be]gin approximately one hour before a proce-

dure and continue for an additional eight doses (Chapter 26 for background and details, Chapter 9 for prescription information).

B. PATIENT'S HEALTH STATUS

Considerations include:

1. antimicrobial allergy
2. prophylaxis for:
   a. heart valve damage from *any* cause
   b. glomerulonephritis
   c. uncontrolled diabetes mellitus
   d. decreased resistance to infection (any cause)

C. ANTIMICROBIAL SELECTION FACTORS

1. If infection is threatening, begin therapy on the basis of clinical judgment.
2. Single-agent therapy is usually best.
3. Agents with an appropriate spectrum should be selected.

4. Etiologic organism is ideally determined by:
   a. gram stain,
   b. culture, if possible.
5. Effective antimicrobial agent is determined by:
   a. antimicrobial sensitivity test (ideally).
   b. clinical judgment—this may be rejected owing to lack of response or after sensitivity tests that indicate organism is not in spectrum

D. ANTIMICROBIAL USE

1. inform patient of value
2. select route of administration, which includes:
   a. oral
      (1) bacteriostatic antibiotics must be taken every 6 hours around the clock
      (2) bactericidal antibiotics can be taken every 6 hours *or* four times a day (during waking hours)
   b. parenteral (or parenteral-oral regimen) if the infection is life threatening
3. determine dosage:
   a. effective blood level needed
   b. provide adequate amount without being wasteful
4. timing of doses:
   a. prophylaxis:
      (1) approximately one hour before procedure
      (2) additional eight doses
   b. infection:
      (1) stat (immediate) dose
      (2) monitor patient response 2 to 3 days after beginning therapy
      (3) continue regular dosage until patient is asymptomatic for 2 days
5. untoward effects include:
   a. development of allergy
      (1) mild: note on chart, inform patient, and treat if necessary
      (2) severe: hospitalize patient
      (3) acute: institute emergency measures
   b. modify treatment plan if needed (use agent of second choice)

E. CAUSES FOR FAILURE

1. Incorrect diagnosis
2. Improper drug selection
3. Improper administration (inadequate absorption)
4. Inadequate dose (low or poorly spaced)
5. Inadequate duration
6. Inaccessible lesion
7. Resistant strain
8. Supra-infection
9. Drug toxicity
10. Host defenses impaired

F. RECORDS NEEDED

These include:

1. notation on patient's chart
2. results (follow-up visits needed)
   a. success of therapy
   b. allergic manifestations
   c. other untoward reactions
   d. any alteration of treatment plan

G. CHARACTERISTICS OF DENTAL INFECTIONS

These are usually:

1. acute (organisms in log phase of growth)
2. gram-positive (of oral origin)
3. manifested by pain, swelling, fever, and lymphadenopathy or combinations of these signs/symptoms

BIBLIOGRAPHY

Accepted Dental Therapeutics, 38th ed. Chicago, American Dental Association, 1979, Sect II, Antimicrobial Agents

Gilman AG, Goodman LS, Gilman A (eds): Goodman and Gilman's The Pharmacological Basis of Therapeutics, 6th ed. New York, Macmillan, 1980, Ch 48

Melmon KL, Morelli HF (eds): Clinical Pharmacology: Basic Principles in Therapeutics, 2nd ed. New York, Macmillan, 1978, Ch 14

Meyers FH, Jawetz E, Goldfien A: Review of Medical Pharmacology, 7th ed. Los Altos, CA, Lange, 1980, Ch 48

9
Penicillins

A. PENCILLIN USE IN ORAL INFECTIONS

Penicillins are the drugs of choice when the infection is caused by penicillin-susceptible organisms (for further details, see Chapter 26). Such infections may include:

1. postextraction infections
2. postsurgical infections
3. pericoronitis
4. dentoalveolar abscess
5. osteomyelitis
6. cellulitis
7. acute necrotizing ulcerative gingivitis
8. periodontitis

B. PENICILLIN (OR PENICILLIN-STREPTOMYCIN) USE IN PROPHYLAXIS

Preventive coverage is always required in the following situations:

1. patient with heart valve damage from any cause
2. patient with previous episode of bacterial endocarditis, even in the absence of clinically detectable heart disease
3. patient with structural abnormalities of the great vessels of the heart, including vascular grafts
4. patient with a heart valve prosthesis (use penicillin-streptomycin)
5. patient with uncontrolled diabetes
6. patient with glomerulonephritis
7. patient with decreased resistance to infection because of
   a. advanced age
   b. leukemia
   c. immunosuppression (corticosteroid or antimetabolite therapy)
   d. any other cause

Preventive coverage may be indicated in the following situations:

1. patient with an indwelling, transvenous pacemaker
2. patient with implanted arteriovenous shunt appliance for dialysis
3. hydrocephalic patient with a ventriculo-atrial shunt
4. patient with a prosthetic joint replacement

C. BASIS FOR SELECTION

1. Take a good medical history. If the patient is allergic to penicillin, use erythromycin.
2. Incise (or open pulp chamber) and drain all abscesses when possible.
3. When possible, take a sample of exudates for antibiotic sensitivity testing.
4. Begin therapy with oral penicillin V. If the infection is severe, begin parenteral penicillin G therapy.
5. If patient does not improve within 48 hours, change to another agent which is suggested by sensitivity testing.
6. The extended-spectrum penicillins (e.g., ampicillin, amoxicillin) should not be used unless indicated by antibiotic sensitivity tests.
7. The penicillinase-resistant penicillins (e.g., cloxacillin, dicloxacillin) should not be chosen initially on the basis of clinical judgment. These agents should be used **only** for the treatment of infection caused by staphylococci that produce penicillinase.

D. CONTRAINDICATIONS

Penicillin is contraindicated in patients who have shown previous hypersensitivity reactions after using the drug.

E. WARNINGS

1. The use of penicillin may cause acute anaphylaxis, which may prove fatal unless promptly controlled. However, the oral route of administration is much less likely to initiate severe hypersensitivity reactions than is the parenteral route. This type of reaction appears more frequently in patients with previous hypersensitivity reactions to penicillin and in those with bronchial asthma or other atopic allergies.
2. If a penicillin-allergic reaction develops, emergency drugs, such as epinephrine, antihistamines, corticosteroids, and aminophylline, should be readily available for paren-

teral administration (see also Chapter 7 and Appendix I).

F. PRECAUTIONS

1. Penicillin should be used with caution in the patient having a history of significant allergies and/or asthma.
2. Reduced dosages should be used in patients with renal dysfunction.
3. Prolonged penicillin therapy, particularly with high dosage schedules, should be accompanied by frequent evaluation of renal and hematopoietic systems.
4. Prolonged use of antibiotics may result in overgrowth of nonsusceptible organisms. Appropriate measures should be taken if suprainfection occurs during therapy.

G. ADVERSE EFFECTS

The penicillins are substances of low toxicity, especially penicillin G, but they do possess a significant index of sensitization. The following hypersensitivity reactions associated with the use of penicillin have been reported: acute glossitis, severe stomatitis, black, brown, or hairy tongue, cheilosis, skin rashes (ranging from maculopapular eruptions to exfoliative dermatitis), urticaria, and serum sicknesslike reactions (including chills, fever, edema, arthralgia, and prostration). Severe and often fatal anaphylaxis has been reported (see warnings). Hemolytic anemia, leukopenia, thrombocytopenia, and nephropathy are rare side effects usually associated with high dosage.

H. ADMINISTRATION AND DOSAGE

1. Maximum absorption of all oral penicillins is obtained if given on an empty stomach (Root, Hierholzer, 1978; Chapter 26). Administration should be one-half hour before, or at least two hours after meals.
2. The usual adult dosage is 500 mg every six

hours or four times a day, continued until the patient is asymptomatic for 2 days. In streptococcal infections, therapy should be continued for 10 full days to guard against the development of rheumatic fever (Prescription 9–1).

3. The prophylactic regimen is 2 gm of penicillin V, one-half to one hour before the procedure, then 500 mg every six hours for an additional eight doses (Kaplan et al., 1977). The practitioner should read in Chapter 26 all pertinent material concerning the prevention of bacterial endocarditis and be familiar with other reference works.

I. PREPARATIONS

These are listed alphabetically.

AMPICILLIN (various brand names)
This is an extended spectrum penicillin available in the following forms:

125 mg tablets, 250 or 500 mg capsules
Oral suspension
125 mg/5 ml in 5, 10, 60, 80, 100, 150, or 200 ml bottles
250 mg/5 ml in 5, 80, 100, 150, or 200 ml bottles
500 mg/5 ml in 5 or 100 ml bottles

Injectable: 125, 250, 500, 1,000, 2,000, or 4,000 mg vials

CLOXACILLIN SODIUM (Cloxapen, Tegopen)
This is a penicillinase-resistant penicillin available in the following forms:

250 mg capsules
Oral solution: 125 mg/5 ml in 80, 100, 150, or 200 ml bottles

DICLOXACILLIN SODIUM (Dynapen and others)
This is a penicillinase-resistant penicillin available in the following forms:

125 or 250 mg capsules

Oral suspension: 62.5 mg/5 ml in 80 ml bottles

PENICILLIN G POTASSIUM (various brand names)
This is available in the following forms:

100,000, 200,000, 250,000, 400,000, 500,000, or 800,000 units (tablets)
Oral solution
125,000 units/5 ml in 60 ml bottles
200,000 or 250,000 units/5 ml in 60, 80, 100, or 200 ml bottles
400,000 units/5 ml in 75, 80, 100, 150, or 200 ml bottles

Injectable: 0.2, 0.5, 1, 5, 10, or 20 million units/vial

PENICILLIN G PROCAINE (various brand names)
This is available in the following form:

Injectable: 300,000, 500,000, or 600,000 units/ml in 1, 2, or 4 ml cartridges and 10 ml vials

PENICILLIN V POTASSIUM (various brand names)
This is available in the following forms:

125, 250, 300, or 500 mg tablets
250 mg wafers
Oral solution
125 mg/5 ml in 40, 80, 100, 150, or 200 ml bottles
200 mg/5 ml in 80, 100, 150, or 200 mg bottles

ALTERNATE PREPARATIONS
Selection of appropriate agent is discussed in Chapter 26.

Amoxicillin (various brand names)
Carbenicillin (*Geocillin*)
Cyclacillin (*Cyclapen*)
Methicillin (*Staphcillin*)
Nafcillin (*Unipen*)
Oxacillin (*Bactocill, Prostaphlin*)
Ticarcillin (*Ticar*)

Patient Name   John Doe   (Address)

Age____28____

Rx Penicillin V potassium USP 500 mg tabs

  Disp: 40 tabs

  Sig: Take 2 tabs immediately, then 1 tab every
     6 hours, either ½ hour before or 2 hours
     after meals, until all tabs are taken

Refill 0-1-2-3-PRN   (Signature)

DEA No.   Not required

Prescription 9-1. Prescription for penicillin V.*

J. SAMPLE PRESCRIPTIONS

Prescription 9-1 is a sample prescription for penicillin V use in dentoalveolar abscess.

Situation: A patient arrives at a dental office with what appears to be an acute dentoalveolar abscess. Radiographs and pulp testing corroborate the diagnosis. The patient does not have a history of allergy to penicillin or a history of atopic allergies. Prescribe penicillin V for this patient.

Prescription 9-2 is a sample prescription for ampicillin, as suggested by sensitivity testing.

Situation: A patient has an acute dento-

Patient Name   John Doe ‘   (Address)

Age____28____

Rx Ampicillin USP   500 mg caps

  Disp: 40 caps

  Sig: Take 2 caps immediately, then 1 caps
     every 6 hours, either ½ hour before or 2
     hours after meals, until all caps are taken

Refill 0-1-2-3-PRN   (Signature)

DEA No.   Not required

Prescription 9-2. Prescription for ampicillin.*

Patient Name   John Doe   (Address)

Age____28____

Rx Dicloxacillin sodium USP   250 mg caps

  Disp: 40 caps

  Sig: Take 2 caps immediately, then 1 caps
     every 6 hours, either ½ hour before or 2
     hours after meals, and until all caps are
     taken

Refill 0-1-2-3-PRN   (Signature)

DEA No.   Not required

Prescription 9-3. Prescription for dicloxacillin.*

alveolar abscess of the maxillary left second bicuspid, accompanied by cellulitis. The dentist attempts to establish drainage by excavating into the pulp chamber of the offending tooth. A sample is taken for culture and antibiotic sensitivity tests. Two days later, the patient shows no signs of improvement. The antibiotic sensitivity test results suggest that an extended spectrum penicillin would arrest the infection. Ampicillin is prescribed for this patient.

Prescription 9-3 is a sample prescription for dicloxacillin, as suggested by sensitivity testing and after failure of penicillin V.

Situation: This patient had been seen three days earlier. He presented with acute pericoronitis of an impacted mandibular right third molar. Penicillin V was prescribed at the first appointment, but the patient shows no signs of improvement. In fact, the infection appears to be worsening. A sample of the exudate was taken at the first appointment for culture and antibiotic sensitivity testing. The test results indicate that the infection is caused by penicillinase-producing staphylococci. Dicloxacillin is prescribed for this patient.

Prescription 9-4 is a sample prescription for penicillin V for prophylaxis of valvular heart damage.

---

* Go to page 14 where full prescription format is given.

Patient Name   John Doe   (Address)

Age   28

Rx Penicillin V potassium USP 500 mg tabs

   Disp: 12 tabs

   Sig: Take 4 tabs ½ to 1 hour before the appointment, then 1 tab every 6 hours until all tabs are taken

Refill 0-1-<u>2</u>-3-PRN   (Signature)

DEA No.   Not required

Prescription 9–4. Prescription for prophylaxis with penicillin V.*

Situation: This patient has a history of rheumatic fever with valvular heart damage. The patient requires a scaling and prophylaxis, numerous restorations, and one extraction. The dentist estimates that three appointments are needed to complete the treatments. The patient is allergy-free. Penicillin V is prescribed for this patient and coverage for three appointments is included.

REFERENCES

Kaplan EL, Anthony BF, Bisno A, et al.: Prevention of bacterial endocarditis: A committee report of the American Heart Association. J Am Dent Assoc 95:600, 1977

Root RK, Hierholzer WJ Jr: Infectious disease. In Melmon KL, Morelli HF (eds): Clinical Pharmacology: Basic Principles in Therapeutics, 2nd ed. New York, Macmillan, 1978, p 745

BIBLIOGRAPHY

Accepted Dental Therapeutics, 38th ed. Chicago, American Dental Association, 1979, Sec. II, Antimicrobial Agents

Gilman AG, Goodman LS, Gilman A (eds): Goodman and Gilman's The Pharmacological Basis of Therapeutics, 6th ed. New York, Macmillan, 1980, Ch 50

Melmon KL, Morelli HF (eds): Clinical Pharmacology: Basic Principles in Therapeutics, 2nd ed. New York, Macmillan, 1978, Ch 14

Meyers FH, Jawetz E, Goldfien A: Review of Medical Pharmacology, 7th ed. Los Altos, CA, Lange, 1980, Ch 49

---

* Go to page 14 where full prescription format is given.

10
Alternate Antimicrobial Agents

A. USES OF ALTERNATE ANTIMICROBIAL AGENTS

Alternate antimicrobial agents are used in dentistry when patients are allergic to penicillin, when culture and sensitivity tests suggest they are indicated, and for special uses. Further details on these drugs are presented in Chapters 27, 28, 29, and 30.

B. DRUGS

ERYTHROMYCIN

Contraindications

1. history of allergy to erythromycin
2. patients with liver dysfunction

Adverse Effects

1. allergic reactions, including cholestatic jaundice induced by the estolate ester (*Ilosone*)
2. epigastric distress
3. ototoxicity with high IV doses

CEPHALOSPORINS

Contraindications

1. history of allergy to cephalosporins
2. history of an immediate allergic reaction to penicillins
3. renal dysfunction

Adverse Effects

1. nausea, vomiting, and diarrhea
2. granulocytopenia and hemolysis
3. full range of allergic reactions

TETRACYCLINES

Contraindications

1. pregnancy
2. children up to 12 years old (possibility of tooth discoloration)
3. renal dysfunction (except doxycycline)
4. danger of use of outdated drug

Adverse Effects

1. a full range of allergic reactions
2. gastric irritation and diarrhea

3. with long-term use, leukocytosis, atypical lymphocytes, granulation of granulocytes, thrombocytopenic purpura
4. phototoxic reaction (especially demeclocycline)
5. hepatotoxic effect with high doses
6. may worsen kidney disease (except doxycycline)
7. negative nitrogen balance (anti-anabolic effect)
8. use of outdated drug results in Fanconi syndrome
9. reversible, increased intracranial pressure
10. minocycline may produce vestibular toxicity
11. increased incidence of supra-infection
12. delayed blood coagulation
13. stained teeth and bones (irreversible effect)

SULFAMETHOXAZOLE PLUS TRIMETHOPRIM

Contraindication

1. history of allergy

Adverse Effects

1. full range of allergic reactions
2. acute hemolytic anemia, agranulocytosis, aplastic anemia, thrombocytopenia, eosinophilia
3. crystalluria and renal damage
4. anorexia, nausea, and vomiting
5. hepatitis, hypothyroidism, arthritis, neuropsychiatric disturbances, and peripheral neuritis
6. possible folate deficiency

NYSTATIN (ANTIFUNGAL)

Contraindications. There are no contraindications.

Adverse Effects

1. occasional nausea, vomiting, and diarrhea
2. occasional irritant effect to oral mucous membranes

STREPTOMYCIN

Contraindications

1. history of allergy
2. presence of myasthenia gravis
3. renal dysfunction

Adverse Effects

1. full range of allergic reactions
2. sterile abscesslike lesions at IM sites
3. ototoxicity (not a problem with short-term use)
4. peripheral neuritis and paresthesia
5. neuromuscular junction blockade
6. nephrotoxicity

VANCOMYCIN

Contraindications

1. history of allergy
2. renal dysfunction

Adverse Effects

1. full range of allergic reactions
2. phlebitis and pain at injection site
3. shocklike state during IV infusion
4. ototoxicity (not a problem with short-term use)
5. nephrotoxicity

CLINDAMYCIN

Contraindications

1. history of allergy
2. severe hepatic failure

Adverse Effects

1. full range of allergic reactions
2. nausea
3. diarrhea (withdraw if it develops)
4. neuromuscular junction blockade
5. erythema multiforme, granulocytopenia, and thrombopenia
6. potentially fatal pseudomembranous colitis

CHLORAMPHENICOL

Contraindication

1. history of allergy

Adverse Effects

1. full range of allergic reactions, including the *potentially lethal* depression of synthesis of all blood cells
2. nausea, vomiting, diarrhea, unpleasant taste
3. blurred vision
4. digital paresthesias
5. supra-infection

C. USES AND BASIS FOR SELECTION

ERYTHROMYCIN

1. Erythromycin is the drug of choice when patients are allergic to penicillin (pending culture and sensitivity tests).
2. Either erythromycin (base) or erythromycin stearate are recommended for peroral use since they are best absorbed (FDA Drug Bull, 1979). The ethylsuccinate ester is preferred for children (suspension or chewable tablets) because it is the only derivative other than the estolate ester available in pediatric formulations.
3. Reduced dosages of erythromycin should be used in the presence of liver dysfunction.

CEPHALOSPORINS

1. Cephalexin is recommended for use because it is well absorbed by the peroral route and is currently the lowest cost cephalosporin derivative available. A number of other cephalosporins are not well absorbed by the oral route.
2. Cephalexin is a possible alternative, pending culture and sensitivity tests, in patients allergic to both penicillin and erythromycin. However, cephalexin is contraindicated if the allergic reaction to penicillin was due to anaphylaxis or another immediate type of allergy (Moellering, Swartz, 1976).

3. Reduced dosages of cephalexin should be used in the presence of renal dysfunction.

TETRACYCLINES

1. Tetracycline is recommended for use because its cost is very much lower than that of other derivatives. Doxycycline is recommended for patients with renal dysfunction.
2. Tetracycline is a possible alternative, pending culture and sensitivity tests, in patients allergic to both penicillin and erythromycin.
3. Tetracycline is the drug of choice, pending culture and sensitivity tests, when infection is present with:
   opening into the maxillary sinus
   compound fracture of the jaws
   traumatic injuries
4. Tetracycline should be avoided in pregnancy and in children up to 12 years old.
5. Tetracycline should not be taken with milk or dairy products, antacids, sodium bicarbonate, or mineral or vitamin-mineral preparations.

SULFAMETHOXAZOLE PLUS TRIMETHOPRIM

1. If a sulfa drug is ever needed in dentistry, sulfamethoxazole plus trimethoprim (*Bactrim, Septra*) would be preferred.
2. In patients with acute dental infections or who require prophylaxis, and who are also allergic to both penicillin and erythromycin, sulfamethoxazole plus trimethoprim may be the next best choice.
3. Sulfamethoxazole plus trimethoprim should be used when the results of culture and sensitivity tests suggest the combination be used, especially when alternate antibiotics may be more toxic.
4. When prescribing sulfamethoxazole plus trimethoprim, water intake must be increased (to avoid crystalluria), such that the patient voids *at least* 1,200 ml of urine per day.
5. Other than for possible uses just cited, sulfamethoxazole plus trimethoprim should be reserved for use by physicians to treat certain gram-negative infections.

NYSTATIN

1. Nystatin is the drug of choice in dentistry for treatment of candidiasis.
2. This is a "super" drug: there are no reports of allergy, no contraindications, no known drug interactions, and no evidence of development of resistant strains in humans.

STREPTOMYCIN

1. Streptomycin is given IM, along with penicillin G (at a separate site), for prevention of bacterial endocarditis in patients with heart valve prostheses. The two drugs may also be useful for prophylaxis in patients taking continuous oral penicillin to prevent recurrent rheumatic fever. Other than these sole uses in dentistry, the agent should be reserved for use in the treatment of tuberculosis.
2. Streptomycin must be used with caution in the presence of renal dysfunction. Dosages must be decreased according to the degree of renal damage.

VANCOMYCIN

1. Vancomycin is used exclusively IV to prevent bacterial endocarditis in patients allergic to penicillin and with a heart valve prosthesis.
2. Vancomycin must be used with caution in the presence of renal dysfunction. Dosages must be decreased according to the degree of damage.

CLINDAMYCIN OR CHLORAMPHENICOL

1. It is possible that clindamycin or chloramphenicol may be the only efficacious drugs in treating certain anaerobic dental infections. In addition, due to clindamycin's excellent penetration into bone, it may be the drug of choice for certain cases of osteitis or osteomyelitis. However, note the cautions and precautions outlined below.
2. One of these agents should be used *only* when indicated, based on culture and sensitivity tests, and when *no* other less toxic drug would be effective. Moreover, the patient's family physician should probably institute therapy due to the potentially *lethal* effects of these drugs. Clindamycin use may require frequent protoctoscopic examinations, and chloramphenicol use requires frequent blood studies.

D. PREPARATIONS

(More important agents are set in bold type)

ERYTHROMYCIN

1. Erythromycin base (various brand names)
   250 or 500 mg tablets
2. Erythromycin ethylsuccinate (various brand names)
   100 mg/2.5 ml drops
   200 or 400 mg/5 ml suspension
   200 mg chewable tablets
   400 mg tablets
3. Erythromycin stearate (various brand names)
   125, 250, or 500 mg tablets

CEPHALEXIN (*Keflex*)

100 mg/ml drops
125 mg or 250 mg/5 ml suspension
250 or 500 mg capsules
1 gm tablets

TETRACYCLINES

1. tetracycline (various brand names)
   100 mg/ml drops
   125 mg/5 ml syrup
   200 mg/5 ml suspension
   100, 250, or 500 mg capsules
   250 or 500 mg tablets
2. doxycycline (*Vibramycin*)
   500 mg/5 ml syrup
   250 mg/5 ml suspension
   50 or 100 mg capsules

SULFAMETHOXAZOLE PLUS TRIMETHOPRIM (*Bactrim, Septra*)

400 mg sulfamethoxazole plus 80 mg trimethoprim tablets, double-strength tablets or suspension

NYSTATIN (*Mycostatin, Nilstat*)

100,000 U/gm powder
100,000 U/gm cream or ointment
100,000 U/ml oral suspension
500,000 unit tablets

ALTERNATE PREPARATIONS

1. Cephalosporins (Chapter 27)
2. Tetracyclines (Chapter 28)

E. SAMPLE PRESCRIPTIONS

Prescription 10–1 is a sample prescription for erythromycin for dental infection in a penicillin-allergic patient.
Situation: A patient has an acute dentoalveolar abscess of a maxillary second bicuspid. The tooth is opened to allow drainage. The patient is also allergic to penicillin.

Prescription 10–2 is a sample prescription for cephalosporin use for a dental infection in a penicillin-allergic patient.
Situation: The patient has an acute dentoalveolar abscess in the first and second mandibular molars on the left side, and drainage is established. The patient reports a history of delayed allergy to penicillin but not to cephalosporins. The patient could not previously comply with erythromycin therapy, due to GI complications.

Patient Name John Doe (Address)

Age 28

Rx Erythromycin stearate 500 mg tabs

  Disp: 40 tabs

  Sig: Take 2 tabs immediately, then 1 tab every 6 hours until all tabs are taken

Refill 0-1-2-3-PRN (Signature)

DEA No. Not required

Prescription 10–1. Prescription for erythromycin.*

Patient Name John Doe (Address)

Age 28

Rx Cephalexin 250 mg caps

  Disp: 30 caps

  Sig: Take 2 caps immediately, then 1 cap 3 times daily until all caps are taken

Refill 0-1-2-3-PRN (Signature)

DEA No. Not required

Prescription 10–2. Prescription for cephalosporin.*

Prescription 10–3 is a sample prescription for sulfamethoxazole plus trimethoprim for prophylaxis of valvular damage when the patient is allergic to both penicillin and erythromycin.
Situation: An adult male patient requires a single extraction. He has a history of heart valve damage and is allergic to both penicillin and erythromycin. The patient's cardiologist suggests the use of sulfamethoxazole plus trimethoprim.

Prescription 10–4 is a sample prescription for tetracycline for a dental infection complicated by penetration of the maxillary sinus.

Patient Name John Doe (Address)

Age 28

Rx Sulfamethoxazole 400 mg

  Trimethoprim 80 mg

  Disp: 10 tabs

  Sig: Take 2 tabs 2 hours before the procedure, then 1 tab every 6 hours for 8 doses. Drink at least 5 glasses of water/day

Refill 0-1-2-3-PRN (Signature)

DEA No. Not required

Prescription 10–3. Prescription for sulfamethoxazole plus trimethoprim.*

---

* Go to page 14 where full prescription format is given.

Patient Name John Doe _____ (Address)

Age ___28___

Rx Tetracycline HCl   500 mg caps

  Disp: 40 caps

  Sig: Take 1 cap every 6 hours until all caps are taken

Refill 0-1-2-3-PRN   (Signature)

DEA No. Not required ___

Prescription 10-4. Prescription for tetracycline.*

Patient Name John Doe, Jr. ___ (Address)

Age ___9___

Rx Nystatin   100,000 U/ml

  Disp: 120 ml

  Sig: Take 1 teaspoonful 4 times a day, swish, hold in mouth as long as possible and swallow

Refill 0-1-2-3-PRN   (Signature)

DEA No. Not required ___

Prescription 10-5. Prescription for Nystatin.*

Situation: A patient arrives with an acute dentoalveolar abscess of the upper left first molar. The tooth has been removed, and careful examination of the socket reveals that the abscess has penetrated the maxillary sinus.

Prescription 10-5 is a sample prescription for nystatin treatment of oral candidiasis.

Situation: A male patient weighing 50 lbs exhibits a clinical picture of oral candidiasis. A culture corroborates this diagnosis.

REFERENCES

FDA begins proceedings to remove erythromycin estolate from market.
FDA Drug Bull 9:26, 1979
Moellering RC Jr, Swartz MN: Drug therapy: the newer cephalosporins. N Engl J Med 294:24, 1976

BIBLIOGRAPHY

Accepted Dental Therapeutics, 38th ed. Chicago, American Dental Association, 1979, Sec II, Antimicrobial agents
Gilman AG, Goodman LS, Gilman A (eds): Goodman and Gilman's The Pharmacological Basis of Therapeutics, 6th ed. New York, Macmillan, 1980, Ch 49, 50, 51, 52, 54
Melmon KL, Morelli HF (eds): Clinical Pharmacology: Basic Principles in Therapeutics, 2nd ed. New York, Macmillan, 1978, Ch 14
Meyers FH, Jawetz E, Goldfien A: Review of Medical Pharmacology, 7th ed. Los Altos, CA, Lange, 1980, Ch 49, 50, 51, 53, 55

---

* Go to page 14 where full prescription format is given.

11
Fluorides

A complete discussion of fluoride therapy in the prevention of dental caries is beyond the scope of this book. Many monographs and books have been written on the subject, and we assume that the student has an adequate background. This chapter emphasizes facts necessary for prescription writing and other uses in dental therapy. The student is advised to consult references if more detailed information is needed.

A. RATIONALE OF FLUORIDE USE AND METHODS OF ADMINISTRATION

Various sources of fluoride ion have been shown to reduce or prevent dental caries when administered (1) in the water supply (1 ppm), (2) as fluoride tablets or solutions for ingestion (in nonfluoridated areas), and (3) by various topical means. Water fluoridation appears to reduce caries about 50%. Sodium fluoride, either as a tablet or as a solution for ingestion, may be used as a supplement but only in low fluoride or nonfluoridated areas. The effectiveness of fluoride tablets and other ingestible supplements in preventing caries appears to be lower than that resulting when optimal amounts of fluoride are available in the drinking water. Topical application (either with neutral solutions, acidified solutions or gels) can be added to systemic use by water fluoridation or to use of tablets. Topical application is considered less effective than water fluoridation, but topicals are especially indicated in nonfluoridated areas or for added benefit in patients with a high caries rate. The exact percentage reduction of caries after topical application depends upon the methods used and the study conditions. Topical application can be accomplished (1) in the dental office, preferably after a prophylaxis, (2) by use of various dentifrices, and (3) by mouth rinses with various fluoride solutions. Sometimes, combinations of methods are helpful.

Generally, the rationale of fluoride application indicates that multiple methods of administration are needed to obtain maximal effects. Thus, the patient would either receive fluoridated water or ingest oral tablets, as well as topical application after prophylaxis by the dentist. In addition, fluoride should be available in dentifrices and mouth rinses. The dentist can judge,

TABLE 11–1. FLUORIDE EFFECTS AND TOXICITY

Fluoride Ion Concentration	Effect
1 ppm[a]	mildly mottled enamel (white spots) with improved calcification and less dental caries
2–10 ppm [a]	mottled enamel (varying in severity according to dose)
20–80 ppm[a]	osteosclerosis
> 80 ppm[a]	crippling osteoarthritis
500 mg NaF swallowed in one dose by a child	acute toxicity, may be fatal
2–5 gm NaF swallowed in one dose by an adult	acute toxicity, may be fatal

[a] Chronic exposure at these levels.

according to the patient's caries experience and exposure to fluoride, how many of these methods are necessary. The only precaution is to remember that fluoride can be toxic and that excessive fluoride solution should not be swallowed.

B. EFFECTS AND TOXICITY OF FLUORIDE

Table 11-1 summarizes the effects and toxicity of various amounts of fluoride in the diet or ingested by other methods. In addition to the symptoms of chronic toxicity shown in Table 11-1, the signs and symptoms of acute toxicity include salivation, nausea, vomiting, abdominal pain, diarrhea, irritability of CNS (including paresthesias, hyperreflexia, and convulsions), muscle pain, hypotension, respiratory stimulation followed by depression, and death due to respiratory paralysis or cardiac failure.

Acute toxicity requires hospitalization as soon as possible, and only the initial care should be performed in a dental office. The treatment of acute toxicity is as follows: institute emergency cardiopulmonary support as needed, start IV infusion with glucose, wash stomach with limewater [0.15% $Ca(OH)_2$] and continue as needed, give Ca^{++} solution IV for tetany, maintain urine volume with IV infusion, and remove vomitus, feces, and urine on appearance.

Since fluoride can be a toxic substance, one should take the following precautions:

1. instruct patient to remove excess from mouth after using rinses (**do not swallow**)
2. suction all excess topical fluoride solutions or gels applied to teeth
3. children under 6 years of age require supervision in use of dentifrices or mouth rinses
4. do not prescribe more than 120 mg fluoride ion (264 mg NaF) in one package

C. PREPARATIONS OF FLUORIDE AVAILABLE FOR PRESCRIPTION AND OTC USE

Prescription Items. These include the following choices:

1. NaF tablets: each scored tablet contains 2.2 mg NaF or 1 mg fluoride ion.
2. Tablets of 0.55 and 1.1 mg NaF are also available.
3. Aqueous solutions of 0.2% NaF with a pH of approximately 7 applied to the teeth as a rinse once a week or every two weeks. Five to 10 ml of the solution should be swished vigorously in the mouth for approximately 1

TABLE 11–2. SUPPLEMENTAL FLUORIDE DOSAGE SCHEDULE[a] ACCORDING TO FLUORIDE CONCENTRATION OF DRINKING WATER

	Concentration of Fluoride in Water (ppm)		
Age (Years)	Less Than 0.3	0.3 to 0.7	Greater Than 0.7
birth to 2	0.25[b]	0	0
2–3	0.50	0.25	0
3–13	1.00	0.50	0

[a] In mg fluoride/day; 2.2 mg sodium fluoride contain 1 mg fluoride.
[b] best supplied by a 1.0 ppm fluoride solution to be used in drinking water and for preparation of the child's food and formula. (*After Accepted Dental Therapeutics, 38th ed., 1979. Courtesy of American Dental Association.*)

minute and the warning **DO NOT SWALLOW,** prominently displayed (Fed Reg, 1974).

4. Premixed solutions for ingestion are also available from various manufacturers. However, any pharmacist can easily mix a solution. Each drop of this preparation should provide 0.1 mg of fluoride ion, and the appropriate number of drops should be specified in the Signa.

OTC Items (see also, Appendix VI):

The following fluoride rinses are considered safe and effective for daily OTC use when marketed in a package containing not more than 120 mg of fluoride ion (Fed Reg, 1980).

1. Aqueous solutions of acidulated phosphate fluoride with a pH of 3.0 to 4.5, yielding a fluoride concentration of approximately 0.02%.
2. Aqueous solution of 0.05% sodium fluoride having a pH of approximately 7.
3. Stannous fluoride as tablets to be mixed for use as a 0.1% dental rinse.
4. Stannous fluoride 0.4% in anhydrous glycerin gel as a nondentifrice rinse.

All OTC fluoride rinses should contain the following statements on labels or instructions. (1) *Do not swallow.* (2) *The rinse does not replace and is not a dentifrice.* (3) Directions for use: *Adults and children 6 years of age and older, use once daily, rinse 10 ml between teeth for 1 minute and expectorate; do not eat or drink for 30 minutes.* (4) Stannous fluoride preparations: *This product may produce staining of the teeth; adequate toothbrushing may prevent these stains which are not harmful or permanent and may be removed by your dentist.*

D. FLUORIDE DOSAGE

Table 11–2 provides information for supplemental fluoride dosing according to the fluoride concentration of the drinking water. It is important to reduce the dosage of fluoride taken orally (by ingestion) as the concentration in the drinking water increases. The objective is that the child receive protection *equal to* 1 ppm in the drinking water.

E. SAMPLE PRESCRIPTIONS

Prescription 11-1 is a sample prescription for a 12-year-old child who will receive fluoride tablets. Using the child's age (Table 11–2, column 1) and concentration of fluoride in the drinking water (column 3), one can find the correct dose.

Patient Name John Doe   (Address)

Age 12

Rx Sodium fluoride   2.2 mg scored tabs

   Disp: 50 tabs

   Sig: One-half (½) tab daily before breakfast

   Caution: Keep out of reach of children

Refill 0-1-2-3-<u>PRN</u>   (Signature)

DEA No. _Not required_

Prescription 11–1. Prescription for fluoride tablets. *

Situation: A 12-year-old patient lives where the drinking water contains 0.4 ppm fluoride. Prescribe sodium fluoride tablets so that the patient receives an optimal amount of fluoride daily.

Prescription 11-2 is a sample prescription for a child, age 30 months, who will receive fluoride in a solution for drinking.

Situation: Prescribe a sodium fluoride solution for a child, age 30 months, living in an area where the drinking water contains 0.1 ppm fluoride.

The method of calculation for this prescription is as follows:

1. determine the amount required in the drinking water, using Table 11-2—*0.5 mg/day* is needed for this child;
2. determine the amount of water ingested per day—**one glassful** is needed for this small child;
3. determine the number of drops of concentrated fluoride solution needed per day (in a glassful of drinking water): concentrated fluoride solution contains 0.1 mg of fluoride/drop; to obtain number of drops, divide as follows:

$$\frac{0.5 \text{ mg F/day}}{0.1 \text{ mg F/drop}} = 5 \text{ drops/day}$$

Patient Name John Doe   (Address)

Age 2

Rx Sodium fluoride   66 mg

   Distilled water to make 15 ml

   Dispense in plastic bottle with dropper which delivers 20 drops per ml

   Sig: Add 20 drops to a quart of water in a plastic container (4-day supply). Keep refrigerated. Give one 8 oz. glassful a day as drinking water. Swish between teeth and swallow.

   Caution: Keep dropper bottle out of reach of children

Refill 0-1-2-3-<u>PRN</u>   (Signature)

DEA No. _Not required_

Prescription 11–2. Prescription for ingestible fluoride solution. *

5 drops of concentrated fluoride are needed/day (or *per glassful of drinking water*).

4. determine a convenient amount of drinking water for mixing and storage:

1 quart = four 8 oz. glasses (4 day supply)

$$\frac{\text{four 8 oz. glasses}}{\text{quart}} \times \frac{5 \text{ drops}}{\text{one 8 oz. glass}}$$
$$= \frac{20 \text{ drops}}{\text{quart (4-day supply)}}$$

therefore, **20 drops concentrated fluoride are needed for 1 quart of mixed solution.**

5. Directions to pharmacists:
   a. Dispense in dropper calibrated to deliver 20 drops/ml.
   b. Concentrated solution will contain 0.1 mg/drop, or:

$$2.0 \text{ mg F/ml} \left(\frac{20 \text{ drops}}{\text{ml}} \times \frac{0.1 \text{ mg}}{\text{drop}} = \frac{2.0 \text{ mg}}{\text{ml}} \right)$$

---

* Go to page 14 where full prescription format is given.

LOCAL FLUORIDATION DATA

Communities with Less Than 0.7 ppm Fluoride in Drinking Water	ppm Fluoride in Water	Fluoride Prescription		
		Child Under 2 Years	Child 2–3 Years	Child 3–13

Figure 11-1. Suggested format for recording water fluoridation and prescription data.

c. Provide patient with a 60-day supply of concentrated fluoride solution:

$$60 \text{ day} \times \frac{1 \text{ quart}}{4 \text{ days}} = 15 \text{ quarts}$$

$$15 \text{ quarts} \times \frac{1 \text{ ml (20 drops)}}{\text{quart}} = \frac{15 \text{ ml conc.}}{\text{fluoride soln.}}$$

d. To make concentrated 0.1 mg fluoride solution, calculate as follows:

$$15 \text{ quarts} \times \frac{2.0 \text{ mg F}}{\text{quart}} = 30 \text{ mg F}$$

$$30 \text{ mg F} \times \frac{2.2 \text{ mg NaF}}{\text{mg F}} = 66 \text{ mg NaF}$$

Therefore, dissolve 66 mg NaF in needed volume, 15 ml.

6. Write prescription as shown in Prescription 11–2.

Since the dentist may serve various communities having different concentrations of fluoride in the water, Figure 11–1 is suggested as a sample chart that should be used so that the proper amount of fluoride can be calculated. County and state public health departments can supply the fluoride levels for various communities. If the concentration is unknown, a sample of drinking water should be analyzed at a chemical laboratory.

Prescription 11-3 is written for a fluoride rinse for an adult.

Situation: A patient with a high caries rate needs extra supplementation with a fluoride dental rinse. Prescribe a rinse for this purpose.

REFERENCES

Fed Reg 39(216): Topical fluoride rinses as prescription drugs or for professional use, 1974, p 39,188

Fed Reg 45(62): Establishment of a monograph on anticaries drug products for over-the-counter human use; proposed rulemaking, 1980, p 20,685

Patient Name   John Doe   (Address)

Age   16

Rx 0.2% Sodium fluoride solution:

Sodium fluoride	0.2 gm
Menthol	0.8 gm
Saccharin	0.4 gm
Distilled water	qs 100 ml

Adjust pH to 7.0

Sig: 10 ml (2 tsp) once weekly before bedtime. Swish between teeth for 1 full minute. *DO NOT SWALLOW.* Do not rinse for at least ½ hour

Caution: Keep out of reach of children

Refill 0-1-2-3-PRN   (Signature)

DEA No.   Not required

Prescription 11-3. Prescription for a fluoride rinse for an adult.*

---

* Go to page 14 where full prescription format is given.

BIBLIOGRAPHY

Accepted Dental Therapeutics, 38th ed. Chicago, American Dental Association, 1979, Sec III, Fluoride Compounds

Fry BW: Toxicology of fluorides. In Picozzi A, Smudski J (eds): Pharmacology of Fluorides, the First Symposium of the Pharmacology, Therapeutics and Toxicology Group, International Association for Dental Research, Atlanta, 1974

Gilman AG, Goodman LS, Gilman A (eds): Goodman and Gilman's The Pharmacological Basis of Therapeutics, 6th ed. New York, Macmillan, 1980, Ch 65

Horowitz HS: Caries prevention and fluoride preparations. In Picozzi A, Smudski J (eds): Pharmacology of Fluorides, the First Symposium of the Pharmacology, Therapeutics and Toxicology Group, International Association for Dental Research, Atlanta, 1974

12
Principles of Pharmacology

A. TERMINOLOGY

Objective 12.A.1. Define and describe drug, medicine, pharmacology, pharmacodynamics, pharmacotherapeutics, pharmacy, toxicology, posology, and pharmacokinetics.

Objective 12.A.2. Describe how drugs are named, including chemical, generic, nonproprietary, and proprietary.

The term **drug** can be broadly defined as any chemical which has an action or effect on animal cells, tissues, or whole organ systems. A name more specific than drug is "medicine," which describes drugs used for the prevention, treatment, or diagnosis of illness and disease. Although the term "drug" is obviously a broader one than "medicine," the therapeutic agents referred to in this text will be generally called "drugs," the more popular term.

Pharmacology
This is broadly defined as the study of drugs, which implies, in modern usage, research into the mechanisms by which drugs act. This in-

cludes the effects of drugs not only on cells, tissues, and animals but also on subcellular organelles and biochemical reactions within cells. It also includes the study of the effects of drugs in human subjects, or "clinical pharmacology." Within the wide scope of pharmacology, there are several subdivisions, as described below.

Pharmacodynamics. This area of pharmacology concerns itself with the actions and effects of drugs on cells and tissues (including the mechanism of action of drugs) and, conversely, the effects of cells on drugs.

Pharmacokinetics. This is the study of the processes of drug absorption, distribution, metabolism, and excretion, usually in a quantitative manner. This area of pharmacology has become extremely important in recent times, as it provides a basis for the study of bioavailability of drug preparations (or the rate at which drugs attain therapeutic concentrations in the blood relative to their dose).

Pharmacotherapeutics. This is the use of drugs in dentistry and medicine for the prevention, diagnosis, and treatment of disease. It includes the study of the indications, contraindications, side effects, and toxicity of drugs.

Pharmacy. Pharmacy is the art of preparing, compounding, and dispensing drugs. The pharmacist is an excellent resource person for the dentist to call upon when questions about specific preparations arise.

Toxicology. This is the science of the adverse effects of drugs and poisonous chemicals. Toxicology also includes the study of the effects of environmental chemicals on living organisms.

Posology. Posology is the study of the dosages of drugs. Doses for specific drugs are usually found in reference works, which should always be consulted before prescribing a drug. (This ends the subdivisions of Pharmacology.)

Drug Names

Drugs have many names. Table 12–1 illustrates the names that have been applied to the local anesthetic, lidocaine. The **chemical name** describes the actual structure in chemical terms. Chemical names are not only cumbersome but also difficult to remember. The **generic name** is actually the pharmacologic classification, but much confusion surrounds the use of the term

"generic." Some authors equate generic with official, which is not technically correct. Nevertheless, the words "generic substitution" on a prescription imply that any official preparation of the same drug can be substituted for a proprietary product.

The **nonproprietary name** is the official name adopted when the drug is accepted by the US Pharmacopeial Convention. (*Note:* the nonproprietary names can vary from country to country, since USP has official status only in the USA.)

The **proprietary** name is the trade name. Trade names are designated in this text by italics with initial capital letters, usually in parentheses, after the nonproprietary name. As a rule, the authors, as well as other pharmacologists, prefer the use of nonproprietary names, but clinicians prefer more commonly known proprietary names. We, therefore, have attempted to satisfy both groups by generally using the nonproprietary names but including trade names whenever feasible.

B. PHARMACOKINETIC TERMINOLOGY

Objective 12.B.1. Define and describe absorption, distribution, biotransformation, and excretion as they relate to drug therapy.

Absorption. This is the process by which a drug enters the circulation. It is dependent on a number of characteristics of the drug and the tissues to which the drug is exposed. These are discussed in detail below.

Distribution. This is the process by which a drug in the circulation enters target tissues, depot tissues, and metabolic and excretory sites. This process, like absorption, depends on a number of characteristics of the drugs as well as those of the body tissues.

Biotransformation. Biotransformation is the process by which metabolic processes in the body, primarily in the liver, convert absorbed

TABLE 12–1. DRUG NOMENCLATURE

Designation (Name)	Lidocaine hydrochloride
chemical	α–diethylamino–2,6–acetoxylidide hydrochloride
generic	local anesthetic, amide type
nonproprietary (official)	lidocaine hydrochloride
proprietary (trade)	*Xylocaine* *Alphacaine* *Lidocaine* *Octocaine* *Codescaine* *Dentacaine*

drugs into different chemical configurations, usually with the end result of making the drug less active and more readily excretable. This process is also frequently referred to as "drug metabolism" or, simply, "metabolism."

Excretion. As the term implies, this is the process by which an absorbed drug is eliminated from the body, usually after it has undergone some chemical modification by the process of biotransformation.

C. ABSORPTION

Objective 12.C.1. Describe the process of drug absorption and list the characteristics of the drugs and of the absorbing tissues which determine the nature and extent of drug absorption.

Drug absorption is dependent on several factors. The properties of a drug that determine its rate of absorption are: (a) the solubility of the preparation (i.e., the rate at which a tablet breaks down); preparations that are administered parenterally are usually given as water soluble solutions; (b) the lipid solubility of the drug molecule (the greater the lipid solubility, the better the absorption; (c) the degree of ionization of the drug molecule (the greater the ionization, the poorer the absorption); (d) the concentration of the drug at the site of administration; and (e) the size (and molecular weight) of the drug molecule (the smaller the molecule, the better the absorption).

The tissue properties which determine drug absorption are: (a) the route of administration of the drug (topical, peroral, sublingual, or parenteral—see discussion below); (b) the surface area of tissues exposed to the drug; (c) the blood flow in the tissue which must absorb the drug; (d) the pH of the tissue fluids at the site of administration. The pH is important for drugs given orally; the stomach pH tends to be acidic, favoring the absorption of weak acids, while intestinal pH tends to be alkaline, favoring the absorption of weak bases.

D. ROUTES OF ADMINISTRATION

Objective 12.D.1. Describe and distinguish between topical, enteral, and parenteral methods of drug administration.

Objective 12.D.2. Describe the possible routes of administration of a drug, and for each route describe the advantages, disadvantages, and tissue characteristics that alter drug absorption.

Topical administration implies that the drug is placed on the skin or mucosa to produce a local effect. There are two types of topical administration: (a) topical, unassisted; and (b) iontophoretic. In topical, unassisted, the drug is placed on the surface and the drug diffuses into the tissues following the law of diffusion (increased gradient causes increased diffusion). In iontophoretic administration, electrical energy is used to propel ionic drugs into surface tissues. Another type of topical, unassisted administration reminds us that systemic effects can occur from topical administration, since some drugs are placed sublingually for diffusion across the mucosa and production of a systemic effect. Thus, sublingual administration is topical application to produce systemic effects.

Enteral administration implies that the drug is placed into the GI tract so that absorption can occur through the stomach, intestine, or rectum. Parenteral administration implies that the GI tract is bypassed, and it includes all types of drug injections (see outline below).

Pulmonary administration can be either for topical treatment (of lungs and bronchi) or for general systemic effect (as in general anesthesia).

The effects of the various routes of administration on the peak blood levels attainable by a drug and the rate at which these levels are reached are illustrated in Figure 12–1. It is evident from this figure that the blood levels following the administration of the same amount of drug but at different sites are markedly altered by the rate of absorption from the various sites. It should also be noted that the toxicity of a given drug can be changed by its route of administration, since the toxicity is generally pro-

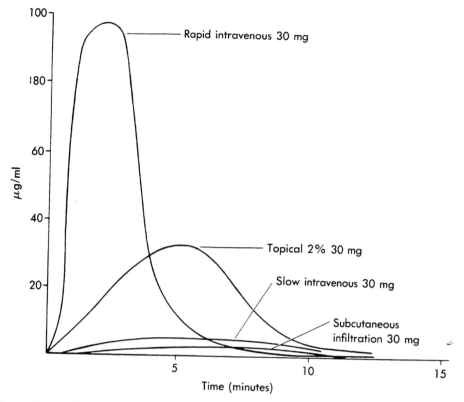

Figure 12–1. Blood levels of the local anesthetic tetracaine following various routes of administration. *Note:* toxic blood level is about 1.5 µg/ml. (*From Adriani J, Campbell B: JAMA 162:1528, 1956. Copyright 1956, American Medical Association.*)

portional to the blood level of the drug. In Figure 12–1, 30 mg of tetracaine exceeds toxic blood levels when given topically because of rapid absorption, but the same amount of drug is not toxic when administered by subcutaneous infiltration.

An outline of methods of drug administration is presented below.

1. Topical
   a. Topical, unassisted (diffusion)
      (1) tissue of absorption: epidermis (skin) or oral mucosa
      (2) advantages:
         (a) simplicity
         (b) patient comfort
         (c) inexpensive
         (d) direct treatment of tissue
      (3) disadvantages·
         (a) poor drug absorption
         (b) unpredictable dosage
         (c) local irritation
         (d) allergy induction is possible
         (e) high blood levels can be achieved with some drugs [e.g., tetracaine (see Fig. 12–1) and epinephrine]
   b. Iontophoretic (electrical assistance)
      Electrical assistance of drug penetration into surface tissues is a preferred method of drug administration when the drug is charged and the condition to be treated is at a body surface. Since most dental treatments are administered upon body surfaces (teeth, gingiva, mucosa, and so on), the use of iontophoresis in dentistry has many applications. Because of the impor-

tance of iontophoresis in dentistry, the subject will be covered in more detail in Appendix VII and, where appropriate, under individual agents.

  c. Sublingual (systemic effect)
    (1) tissue of absorption: oral epithelium
    (2) advantages:
      (a) rapid onset
      (b) avoids gastrointestinal irritation
      (c) avoids first-pass metabolism by liver
    (3) disadvantages:
      (a) poor taste of most drugs limits use
      (b) irritation of sublingual mucosa
      (c) many drugs not well absorbed by this method
    (4) primary use: nitroglycerin for treatment of angina pectoris

2. Enteral
  a. Peroral administration (by mouth)
    (1) tissue of absorption: gastrointestinal epithelium
    (2) enteric pH is either acidic (stomach) or basic (small intestine)
    (3) absorption is proportional to lipid solubility and extent of ionization (weak acids are less ionized and, therefore, absorbed better in the stomach than in the intestine; conversely, weak bases are better absorbed in the intestine)
    (4) mode of absorption: simple diffusion in most cases
    (5) advantages: most convenient, least expensive
    (6) disadvantages: gastrointestinal irritation common, inactivation by gastric acid and by passage through liver (portal circulation) causing first-pass effect of rapid metabolism, inactivation by interaction with food and other agents that can impair or prevent absorption

  b. Rectal
    (1) tissue of absorption: gastrointestinal epithelium
    (2) advantages:
      (a) useful when patient is nauseated, anorexic, or

      (b) unconscious
      (c) avoids gastrointestinal irritation and rapid metabolism
    (3) disadvantages:
      (a) can be irritating to the rectum
      (b) administration inconvenient in dental operatory,
      (c) absorption can be unpredictable

3. Parenteral (by injection)
  a. Intravenous (IV)
    (1) no tissue of absorption (drug placed directly into vein)
    (2) type of drugs: water soluble and sterile
    (3) advantages:
      (a) avoidance of tissue irritation
      (b) rapid effect; the drug can be titrated
      (c) useful for drugs not absorbed by other routes or that undergo rapid metabolic degradation when given by the oral route (e.g., morphine)
    (4) disadvantages:
      (a) drug cannot be recalled once given
      (b) rapidity of effect may give rise to adverse reactions
      (c) possibility of bacterial or pyrogen contamination
      (d) drugs should be soluble in water or at least miscible in blood

  b. Intra-arterial
    (1) no tissue of absorption (drug placed directly into an artery)
    (2) type of drugs: water soluble and sterile
    (3) advantage: drug actions localized to tissues/organs supplied by artery of administration
    (4) disadvantages:
      (a) possible arterial spasm caused by many drugs
      (b) other disadvantages as in IV administration
      (c) arteries to many organs not readily accessible to surface

  c. Intramuscular (IM)
    (1) tissue of absorption: interstitium of skeletal muscle into capillaries

(2) type of drugs:
   (a) water soluble or soluble in other vehicles
   (b) sterile
(3) advantages:
   (a) less hazardous than intravascular routes
   (b) less painful than subcutaneous route
   (c) can be used as a depot if drug is in a highly viscous vehicle or in a slowly dissolving form
(4) Disadvantages:
   (a) erratic rates of absorption depending on cardiovascular status, specific muscle injected, drug precipitation, exercise, volume of injectate
   (b) irritation and/or damage to muscle tissue with pain, possible nerve damage
   (c) possible bacterial contamination
d. Subcutaneous or submucosal
   (1) tissue of absorption: interstitium and connective tissue immediately below the dermis layer of skin (hypodermis) or mucosa
   (2) type of drugs:
      (a) water soluble drugs
      (b) drugs soluble in other vehicles
      (c) sterile pellets, by implantation (e.g., steroids)
   (3) advantages:
      (a) relatively simple injection technique
      (b) rate of absorption can be altered by vehicle, massage of injection site, incorporation of vasoconstrictors or connective tissue enzymes (e.g., hyaluronidase), application of tourniquet, or application of cold or heat
      (c) can serve as depot if slowly dissolving preparation is used
   (4) Disadvantages:
      (a) difficulty in recalling drugs
      (b) requires sterile technique
      (c) many drugs cause pain and tissue irritation

   (d) wide variation in rate of absorption with rate of blood flow, volume drop, and type of vehicle, and other factors
4. Pulmonary (inhalation), topical or systemic
   a. tissue of absorption: respiratory epithelium
   b. type of drugs: gases, volatile liquids, and aerosols
   c. advantages:
      (1) rapid absorption
      (2) can frequently be self-administered by patient
   d. disadvantages:
      (1) many mechanical devices required, as in general anesthesia
      (2) accurate dosages are difficult to attain
      (3) many drugs can irritate the respiratory tract

E. DRUG DISTRIBUTION

Objective 12.E.1. Describe factors which influence the distribution of drugs.

Objective 12.E.2. Describe and list all sites to which drugs may be distributed in the body.

Once a drug is absorbed from its site of administration, the next pharmacokinetic process that alters its activity is that of distribution. This is the process by which the drug, having been absorbed into the blood, reaches its target tissue (at which it exerts its therapeutic action) and other tissues that may serve as metabolic sites, reservoir sites, sites of nontherapeutic actions, and excretory sites. As described in Figure 12–2, the process is a competition for distribution within the blood components and absorption into tissue fluids.

The following factors may influence distribution within the blood:

1. binding to blood cells
2. binding to plasma proteins (primarily albumin)
3. dissolution within the plasma water

For binding to each of these blood compartments, the following factors play an important

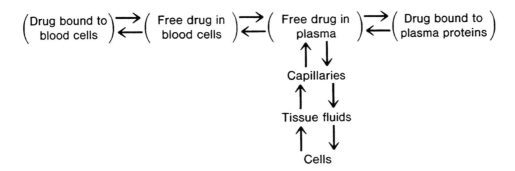

Figure 12-2. Analysis of drug distribution. (*Adapted from Niazi S: Textbook of Biopharmaceutics and Clinical Pharmacokinetics, 1979. Courtesy of Appleton-Century-Crofts.*)

role: (1) the fat solubility of the drug (the greater the degree of fat solubility, the greater will be the entry of the drug into erythrocytes, (2) the water solubility of the drug (generally, nonpolar drugs are bound to a great extent to plasma protein), (3) the acidity or alkalinity of the drug (most drugs are weak acids or weak bases)—basic drugs tend to bind nonspecifically to plasma protein, while acidic drugs usually are bound only to the N-terminal amino acids, and (4) the amount of plasma protein available (hypoalbuminemias occur in a number of disease states, including kidney disease, cancer, hepatitis, and cystic fibrosis).

Objective 12.E.3. Describe the process of protein binding, its effects on drug action, metabolism, and excretion, and its role in drug interactions.

The major distribution sites of drugs within the blood are in the plasma water and the plasma protein. Drugs which bind to plasma protein (most drugs bind to some extent) do so in a manner that depends upon the chemical characteristics of the drug, the concentration of the drug, and the concentration of the plasma protein. The binding of drugs to protein is a two-way (reversible) process, or chemical equilibrium, which can be quantitated using the relationship shown in Figure 12-3.

As drug leaves the plasma, some drug is freed from protein binding to establish a new equilib-

rium. The protein serves as a significant drug reservoir only when a high percentage of a drug is bound. The portion of a dose of a drug that is protein bound is not therapeutically active, nor can it be metabolized in its bound form. Table 12-2 presents examples of drugs used in dentistry which are protein bound to varying degrees. The percent of binding given is only approximate and can vary considerably from one patient to another.

Objective 12.E.4. Recognize the mechanism by which drug interactions occur due to plasma protein binding.

When a significant portion of a drug is protein-bound and another drug with a high affinity

$$[P] + [D] \underset{K_d}{\overset{K_a}{\rightleftharpoons}} [PD]$$

Where: [P] = free protein concentration
[D] = free drug concentration
[PD] = concentration of bound complex
K_a = association constant
K_d = dissociation constant

Figure 12-3. Equilibrium for drug protein binding. (*Adapted from Niazi S: Textbook of Biopharmaceutics and Clinical Pharmacokinetics, 1979. Courtesy of Appleton-Century-Crofts.*)

TABLE 12–2. PROTEIN BINDING OF SELECTED DRUGS USED IN DENTISTRY

Drug	% Binding
acetaminophen	25
cephalexin	22
diazepam	96
erythromycin	19
meperidine	40
oxacillin	94

(From Niazi S: Textbook of Biopharmaceutics and Clinical Pharmacokinetics, 1979. Courtesy of Appleton-Century-Crofts.)

for the same protein-binding sites is given, the first drug may be displaced by the second, resulting in an increased therapeutic action and an increase in toxicity of the first drug. For example, coumarin-type anticoagulants are highly protein bound (e.g., 97 to 99% for dicumarol). Patients on such anticoagulant therapy who receive phenylbutazone, which has a high affinity for plasma protein, may develop severe bleeding tendencies because of displacement of coumarin from protein-binding sites.

Objective 12.E.5. Describe factors involved in drug distribution and the relationship of these factors to tissue levels at various sites.

Once absorbed into the blood, the drug present in the unbound plasma water fraction is available to a number of sites within the body. Figure 12–4 illustrates what can happen to a drug as it passes through a tissue. It may be noted that the distribution of drugs from the blood to other tissues depends upon:

1. the rate of blood flow to a particular tissue
2. capillary penetration
3. permeation of cell membranes
4. the presence of special tissue barriers

Blood Flow
The rate of blood flow to the brain, liver, kidney, and heart is extremely high, while flow to skin and fat is considerably lower. Therefore, drug equilibration with the vital organs occurs very rapidly, while equilibration with poorly perfused tissues requires a relatively long time.

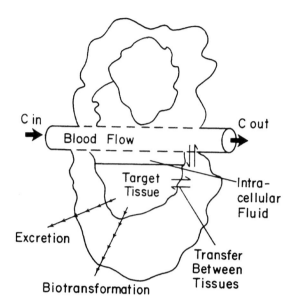

Figure 12–4. Pharmacokinetic model of drug distribution. C, drug concentration. (*From Niazi S: Textbook of Biopharmaceutics and Clinical Pharmacokinetics, 1979. Courtesy of Appleton-Century-Crofts.*)

Capillary Penetration
The movement of drugs from the blood through the capillaries is readily accomplished and is not dependent on the pK_a of the drug or on its relative fat:water solubility. However, drugs with molecular weights greater than 500 to 600 are generally restricted.

Permeation of Cell Membranes
This process is dependent on the relative degree of lipid solubility of a drug, since the cell membranes of target tissues behave as typical lipoidal barriers. Similarly, the degree of ionization of a drug influences cell penetration. Therefore, the pK_a of the drug, as well as the pH of the interstitial fluids and the intracellular fluids, will influence this process. For example, an acidic drug is less likely to be reabsorbed into kidney tubular cells after it has entered the kidney tubules if the pH is elevated, since most of the drug will be in the ionized form. Special transport systems in some cell membranes may limit drug entry, but diffusion accounts for the entry of most drug molecules. Finally, molecular size and weight will influence cellular permeation of a drug.

Special Tissues Barriers

The *blood-brain barrier* is a concept used to describe the relatively high degree of selectivity of the cerebrospinal fluids to accept drug molecules. While some sites within the CNS are readily permeated by polar compounds, most brain tissues behave as highly lipoidal barriers, so that only compounds with a high degree of lipid solubility can enter by diffusion. Special active transport processes account for the entry of some compounds (such as sugars) into the brain, and disease states may alter the permeability of the blood-brain barrier. For example, the penicillin antibiotics can enter the CNS in patients suffering from meningitis but not in normal individuals.

The placenta is also a lipoidal barrier, so that highly lipid-soluble drugs can enter the fetal circulation easily. Other drugs can also enter the fetal circulation, and it is reasonable to assume that the fetus is exposed to all drugs taken by the mother, in varying concentrations, depending on lipid solubility, molecular weight, and the dose taken by the mother (i.e., the drug concentration in the maternal circulation). For this reason, extreme caution should be taken when using drugs while treating pregnant women, especially during the first trimester. Known teratogens must never be used during pregnancy, and most other drugs should be avoided if possible.

F. DRUG METABOLISM

Objective 12.F.1. Describe the sites and mechanisms of biotransformation of drugs.

Objective 12.F.2. Recognize examples of biotransformation reactions which are oxidative, reductive, hydrolytic, or synthetic.

Biotransformation (or more simply metabolism) of drugs is accomplished chiefly in the liver by the liver microsomes, a network of endoplasmic reticulum in hepatocytes. This contains enzymes that accomplish oxidative and reductive reactions with drug molecules. Since this membranous network is of a highly lipid nature, the drug molecules metabolized here are usually lipid soluble. Drug metabolism is also accomplished by nonmicrosomal enzymes present in a variety of tissues. These enzymes include dehydrogenases, oxidases, and peroxidases. They metabolize drugs that are more water soluble. The plasma also contains a number of specific and nonspecific esterases, which hydrolyze a variety of esters, such as procaine.

There are two types of drug-metabolizing reactions: synthetic and nonsynthetic (oxidative, reductive, or hydrolytic). Both processes usually accomplish the same end result: the formation of an altered drug molecule which is less active and/or more readily excretable (more water soluble). In some cases, a drug molecule is activated by metabolism but ultimately is converted to a less active form by subsequent metabolic processes. Drug metabolism may result in one of the following:

1. An active drug is converted into an inactive, more readily excreted one (most of the examples below).
2. An inactive drug (prodrug) is converted into an active one, e.g., prontosil → sulfanilamide.
3. An active drug may be converted into a toxic one (lethal synthesis), e.g., fluoroacetate → fluorocitrate.
4. An active drug may be converted into a different active form e.g., codeine → morphine.

The following reactions* are examples of metabolic drug reactions (*note:* arrows on atoms indicate points of chemical attack).

1. Oxidative reactions (microsomal, requiring O_2 and NADPH)
   a. alkyl side chains:

$$CH_3{-}CH_2{-}OH \xrightarrow{-H_2} CH_3{-}\overset{\overset{O}{\|}}{C}{-}H \xrightarrow{+O} CH_3{-}\overset{\overset{O}{\|}}{C}{-}OH$$

Ethanol   Acetaldehyde   Acetic acid

---

* Reactions 1 through 6 and 8 through 13 are from Csáky TZ: *Introduction to General Pharmacology*, 2nd ed, 1979. Reaction 7 is from Csáky TZ: *Cutting's Handbook of Pharmacology*, 6th ed, 1979. All courtesy of Appleton-Century-Crofts.

b. Aromatic rings:

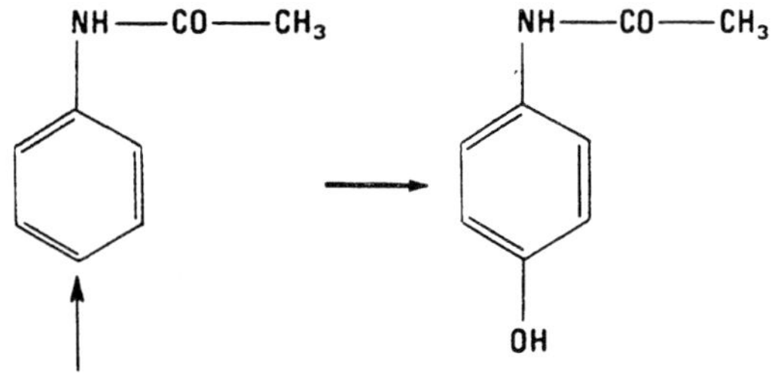

ACETANILID   ACETAMINOPHEN

c. N-dealkylation: This same reaction can occur on sulfur (S) or oxygen (O).

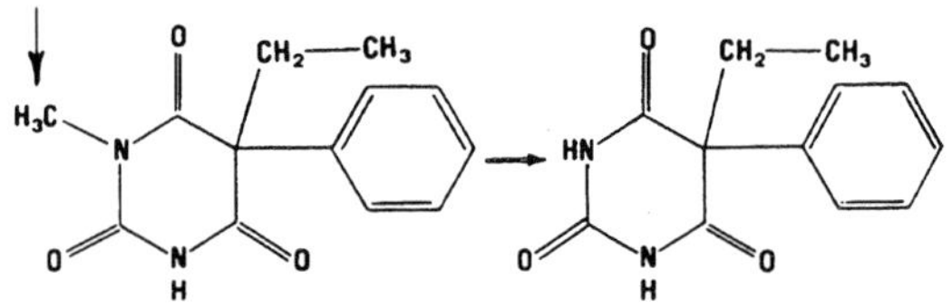

MEPHOBARBITAL   PHENOBARBITAL

d. N-oxidation:

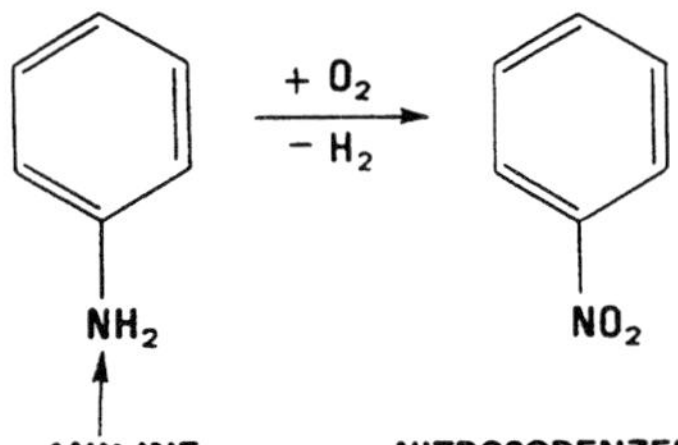

ANILINE   NITROSOBENZENE

e. Amine oxidation (also can be nonmicrosomal):

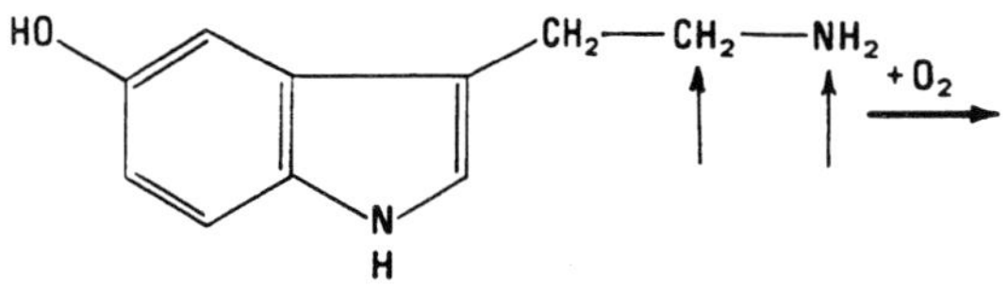

5-HYDROXYTRYPTAMINE

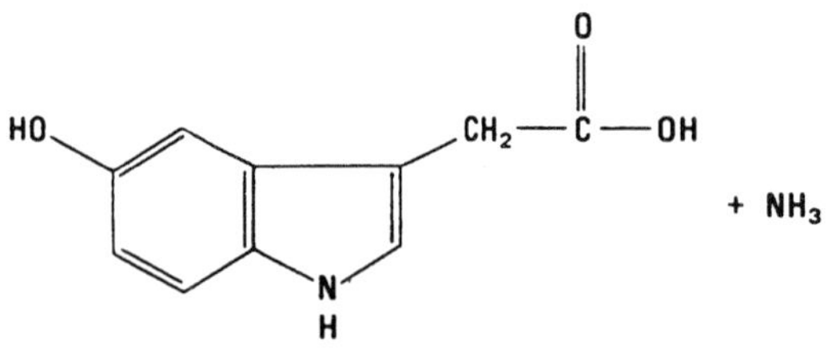

5-HYDROXYINDOLEACETIC ACID

f. Sulfoxidation:

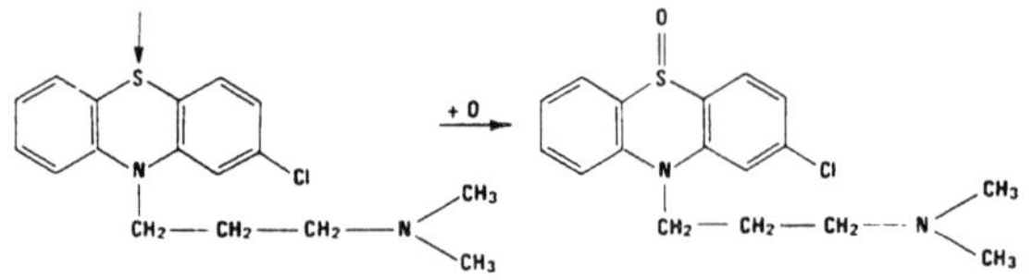

CHLORPROMAZINE   CHLORPROMAZINE SULFOXIDE

g. Desulfuration (replacement of S by O):

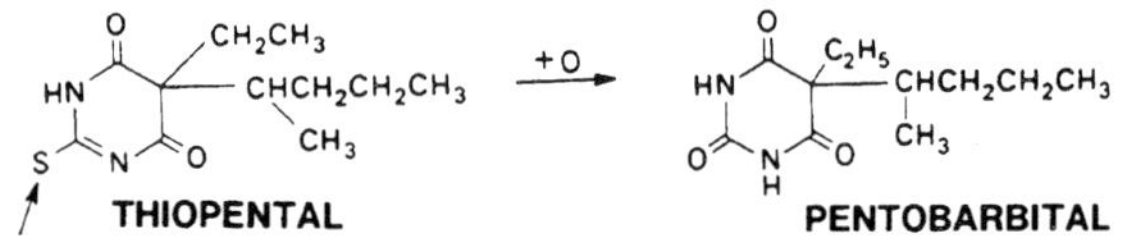

THIOPENTAL   PENTOBARBITAL

2. Reduction (nonmicrosomal):

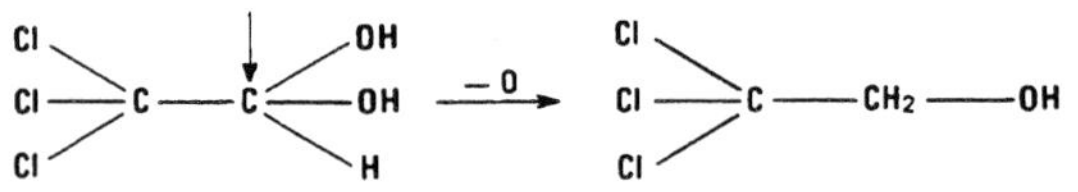

CHLORAL HYDRATE   TRICHLOROETHANOL

3. Hydrolysis (nonmicrosomal):

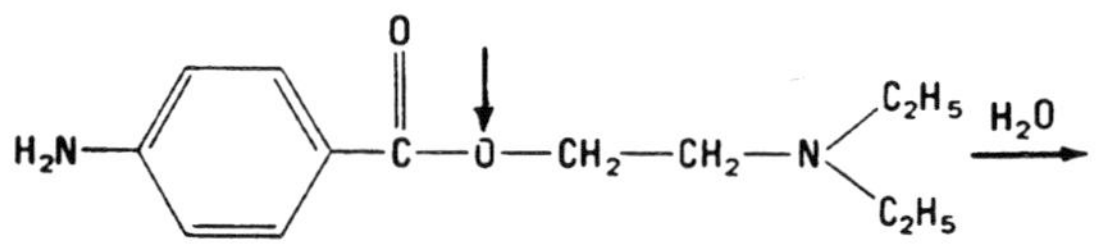

PROCAINE

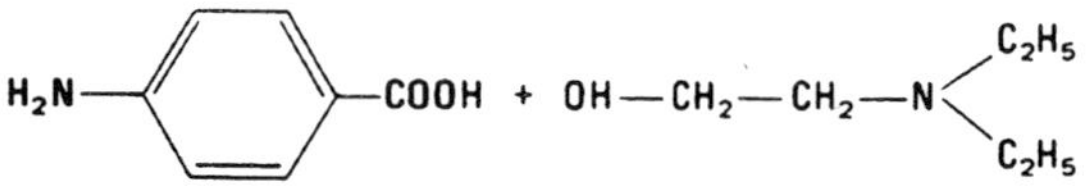

PABA   DIETHYLAMINOETHANOL

4. Synthetic. There are several types of synthetic reactions. In the examples that follow, a chemical moiety is added to a drug molecule to produce a less active and more readily excretable drug metabolite.

a. Acylation or acetylation:

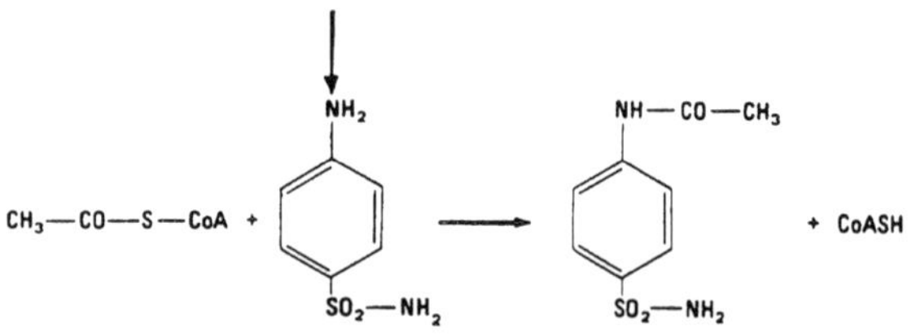

SULFANILAMIDE   ACETYL SULFANILAMIDE

b. O-methylation (an example of O-alkylation):

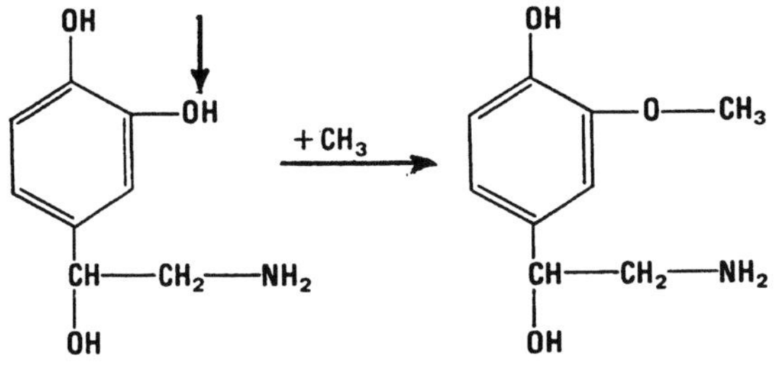

NOREPINEPHRINE   NORMETANEPHRINE

c. N-methylation (an example of N-alkylation):

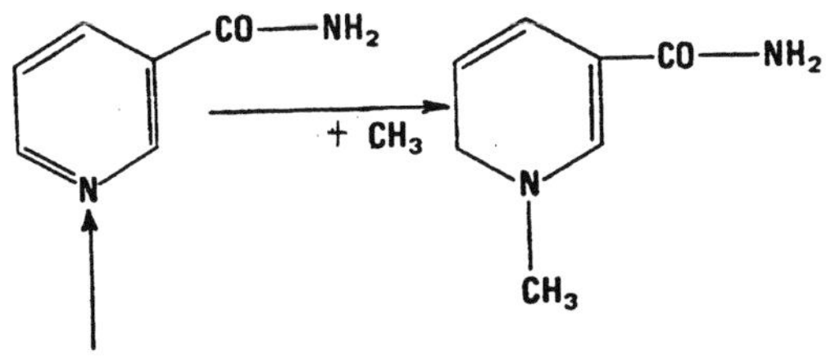

NICOTINAMIDE   N-METHYL NICOTINAMIDE

d. Glucuronide conjugation (microsomal): glucuronic acid is a glucose congener which can combine with a number of drugs. Its structure is shown in Scheme 12-1. Conjugation occurs at the aldehyde linkage of carbon number 1, and some of the drugs with which conjugation occurs are listed on the right.

In addition, similar conjugation reactions occur with sulfate, glutamine, and glycine.

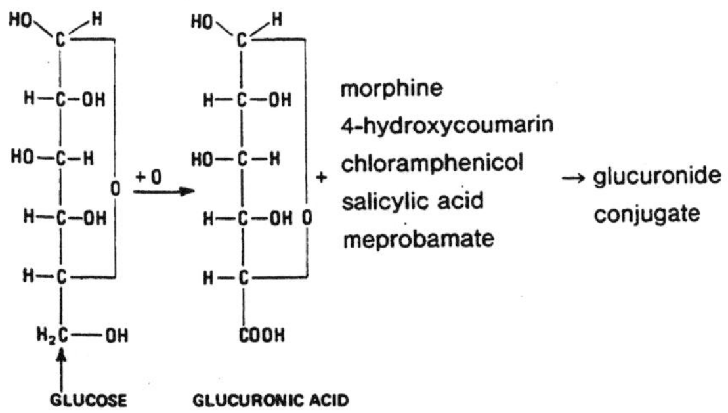

morphine
4-hydroxycoumarin
chloramphenicol
salicylic acid
meprobamate

→ glucuronide conjugate

GLUCOSE   GLUCURONIC ACID

Scheme 12-1. Formation of glucuronide conjugate.

Factors Influencing Metabolism

Objective 12.F.3. Recognize six factors that can influence the metabolism of drugs, including one example of each.

Just as most other processes involving the manner in which a biologic organism handles drugs are influenced by a number of factors, so metabolism can similarly be altered by variations in the tissues that are responsible for drug biotransformation. These factors and examples of each are listed below.

Species Differences. Experimental pharmacology has shown that different species can metabolize drugs at different rates, pesumably because of differences in the rates at which the metabolic reactions occur. An example of this phenomenon is the so-called hexobarbital sleeping time. In the mouse given hexobarbital, the sleeping time is rather brief, since the half-life of the drug in this species is only 19 minutes. In the dog and man, on the other hand, hexobarbital half-lives are 260 and 360 minutes, respectively.

Age. Infants and young children have relatively immature drug-metabolizing capabilities and cannot metabolize drugs as rapidly as can mature individuals. Very old people also tend to have relatively slower rates of drug metabolism, which may be due to hepatic atrophy associated with age.

Pathologic Conditions. Generally, liver pathology tends to reduce the drug-metabolizing capability of an individual. Cirrhosis, partial hepatectomy, and other conditions can greatly reduce the activity of the hepatic, microsomal, drug-metabolizing enzymes.

Genetic Variation. Some individuals are rendered less capable of metabolizing drugs because of genetically associated differences in their enzyme levels. For example, a patient with atypical pseudocholinesterase is less efficient in metabolizing ester-type drugs. Such individuals can experience severe toxic reactions to succinylcholine and tetracaine.

Nutrition. Malnutrition depresses the drug-metabolizing capability. Alcoholic patients may show intolerance to some drugs because of the deficient nutritional state that often accompanies their condition.

Stimulation and Inhibition of Microsomal Enzymes.

1. Stimulation. Phenobarbital is known to stimulate or induce hepatic microsomal enzymes, resulting in more rapid metabolism of a variety of drugs.
2. Inhibition. The enzymatic degradation of a drug may be inhibited by the presence of other drugs in the body. For example, the monoamine oxidase inhibitors (MAOI) diminish the ability of monoamine oxidase to metabolize a number of drugs, including catecholamines. The monoamine oxidase inhibitors also inhibit a number of other enzymes.

G. DRUG EXCRETION

Objective 12.G.1. Describe the mechanisms by which the kidney excretes drugs and metabolites.

Objective 12.G.2. Recognize six nonrenal pathways by which drugs may be excreted.

Objective 12.G.3. Describe examples of drugs used to alter the kidney excretion of (1) penicillin, (2) aspirin, and (3) barbiturates.

Kidney

The major site of drug excretion is the kidney, through which water-soluble compounds are eliminated in the urine. The processes of drug metabolism usually render the inactive metabolite more water soluble (or more polar). When the water-soluble metabolite is filtered out of the blood and into the tubular urine of the kidney, it is less likely to diffuse through the kidney cells back into the blood than the original, active drug. The same principles that govern the processes of drug distribution also apply to excretory processes. The following factors influence drug excretion by the kidney:

1. blood flow to the kidney
2. the relative water/lipid solubility of the drug or its metabolite
3. the pK_a of an acidic or basic drug and urine pH
4. special transport processes within the kidney

In summary, a drug which has been metabolically converted to a more water-soluble form is filtered at the renal glomerulus into the tubular fluid of the kidney (provided that it is not bound to plasma protein). Active, unbound forms of the drug are also filtered. The inactive water-soluble form does not readily diffuse back through the kidney cells into the blood and is, therefore, eliminated in the urine. The more fat-soluble, active form does back-diffuse, however, and reenters the circulation to be carried to other sites, including metabolic ones. A few drugs are actively reabsorbed by carrier-mediated processes, but this is unusual. Several drugs, including penicillin, are actively secreted from the blood into the urine by tubular processes. The latter can be blocked, resulting in increased blood levels of the secreted drug. Probenecid is a drug that blocks the renal secretion of penicillin.

The excretion rates of acids and bases are dependent to a great extent on the pK_a of the drug and the pH of the urine. When urinary pH is elevated, as in sodium bicarbonate infusion, acidic drugs, such as aspirin, are more readily excreted because a greater proportion of the filtered drug is in the ionized state. Conversely, when urinary pH is lowered (as with NH_4Cl), basic drugs, such as amphetamines, tend to be excreted more readily for the same reason—more drug is ionized, and ionized molecules cannot back-diffuse through the lipoidal membranes of the renal tubular cells. Advantage is taken of this ion-trapping effect in drug overdose by deliberately changing urine pH to values which promote drug excretion.

Other Routes of Excretion

These are listed and described below.

Bile. Biliary handling of drugs occurs through the enterohepatic cycle, illustrated in Figure 12–5. Many drugs are secreted by the liver cells into the bile entering the common bile duct. Then the bile enters the duodenum and small intestine, where reabsorption occurs by passive

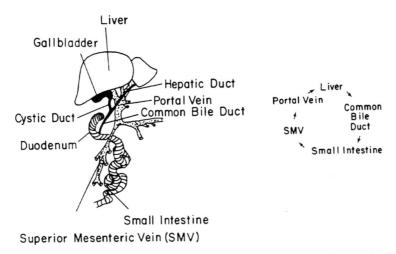

Figure 12–5. Anatomy of the enterohepatic cycle. (*After Niazi S: Textbook of Biopharmaceutics and Clinical Pharmacokinetics, 1979. Courtesy of Appleton-Century-Crofts.*)

diffusion. Such drugs may undergo this cycling several times before being excreted by the kidney (if completely reabsorbed) or into the feces.

Saliva. Some drugs are excreted into the saliva by a process which is pH-dependent, with basic drugs tending to be concentrated in salivary glands to a greater extent than acidic drugs. Drugs that appear in the saliva are also recycled because most of the saliva is swallowed, making the drug available once again to gastrointestinal absorption sites.

Milk. Many drugs are capable of entering the breast milk of lactating mothers, either by pH-dependent processes or by simple diffusion. In most cases, the amounts of a drug transferred from maternal circulation into milk are usually insignificant. However, in some cases, a toxic reaction in the infant may result. Drugs which enter the milk include sulfonamides, ethanol, and tetracyclines.

Lungs. This is primarily a route of excretion for gaseous and highly volatile drugs, including gaseous general anesthetics and alcohol.

Sweat. Some drugs, including alcohol, mercury, and salicylic acid, passively enter the sweat gland secretions.

Feces. Some basic drugs, including nicotine and quinidine, enter the gastric fluids by a pH-dependent ion-trapping effect. While most of these drugs are reabsorbed by the intestine, some of them may be excreted in the feces if they decompose or form a complex with other materials in the GI tract (also see Bile, above).

H. MECHANISMS OF DRUG ACTIONS

Objective 12.H.1. Describe three mechanisms by which a drug may exert a therapeutic action.

Objective 12.H.2. Define the terms **drug receptor, affinity, intrinsic activity, potency, response, effector, agonist, antagonist.**

Drugs may exert their actions in a number of ways. One mechanism is a receptor-mediated mechanism, in which a drug molecule interacts with a receptor located in the target tissue (this **drug receptor** mechanism is discussed below). Another mechanism by which a drug can act is termed a "**physicochemical**" **mechanism,** in which the drug alters the physical properties of a target tissue. This type of action is generally directly dependent on the concentration of drug reached in the tissue. An example of this type of action includes the highly lipid-soluble general anesthetics, which may dissolve within the lipoidal membranes of brain cells to inhibit their electrical activity. A third type involves a simpler **chemical** reaction which accounts for some drug effects, e.g., gastric antacids which neutralize hydrogen ion in the stomach by acid-base neutralization.

The physicochemical and chemical mechanisms of drug action are different from the receptor mechanism in that the latter depends upon a specific chemical moiety in the target tissue combining in a highly specific manner with a drug molecule. A **drug receptor** may be defined as a macromolecular site on or within a cell membrane which, when combined with a drug (agonist), results in a specific change in the activity and/or biochemical behavior of the effector cell (an **effector** cell is simply one that is altered by a drug-receptor interaction to produce a pharmacologic response).

A drug that stimulates an effector through its interaction with a receptor is termed an *agonist.* A drug that occupies a receptor to prevent another drug from exerting its effect, while not causing an effect in itself, is termed an *antagonist,* or blocking drug. Both agonists and antagonists possess chemical structures that are highly specific for a certain type of receptor. Drug molecules and receptors interact in a specific, complementary fashion (lock and key) through a variety of attractive forces—van der Waals, hydrogen bonding, dipole-dipole interactions, and electrostatic (fixed charge) attractions.

Figure 12–6 illustrates the lock and key hypothesis of drug-receptor interaction. Note that the drug receptor model resembles the enzyme substrate interaction in enzyme kinetics. Because of this resemblance, drug-receptor interactions are best studied using enzyme-substrate kinetics.

In this model, the drug fits closely into the receptor, causing a conformational change in the membrane which would trigger further reactions in the cell and eventually cause the response. Antagonists may also be considered in terms of the lock and key model. An antagonist probably has greater attraction to the receptor and, therefore, is less easily removed. Antagonists are of two types: competitive or noncom-

petitive. The competitive types probably bind to the receptor more tightly than does an agonist. For example, in Figure 12–6, competitive antagonists are shown to have additional binding sites either outside the receptor (a) and/or within the receptor (b). A noncompetitive antagonist can bind either at an allosteric site (d), which is removed from the receptor, or by covalent bonding directly to the receptor.

In kinetic terms, the reaction of a drug with its receptor can be represented by the following equation:

$$D + R \rightleftarrows DR \rightarrow \text{Response}$$

This reaction is usually reversible and obeys the law of mass action, i.e., there exists an equilibrium between the reactants and the product at any steady-state concentration of drug and receptor. The reaction between the drug and the receptor can be expressed as an equilibrium constant, which is a reflection of the affinity (or attraction) of the drug for its receptor (affinity = the reciprocal of the dissociation constant). Within a series of drugs acting on the same receptor system, one drug may produce a greater response than another when the two are administered at the same dose. The ratio of this response to the maximal response of which the tissue is capable is termed the "intrinsic activity" (or efficacy) of the drug. Apparently, affinity and intrinsic activity are determined by two different chemical attributes of the drug molecule. To illustrate the concept of affinity and intrinsic activity, consider the dose-response curves in Figure 12–7. Drug A produces the maximal (ceiling) response of the test tissue at a specific dose (10^{-6} molar), while drug B produces the same maximal response at a greater dose (10^{-2} molar). Therefore, drugs A and B have the same **intrinsic activity,** but drug A has a greater **affinity** for the receptors. Drug A also has a greater potency than drug B, since the quantity of drug A required to produce the same effect is less than is required of drug B. **Potency,** then, is an expression of **affinity** and is a term which describes the relative quantity of a drug required to produce a given effect. Drug C has less affinity than drug A; furthermore, since it cannot

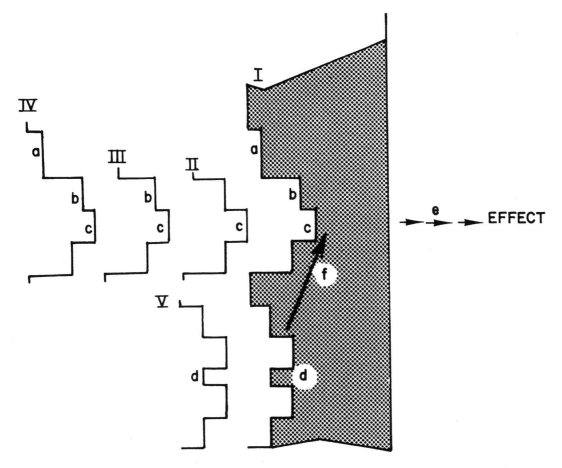

Figure 12–6. Lock and key hypothesis of drug-receptor interaction. I. Receptor surface on membrane (crosshatched area). II. Drug agonist with only c binding site. When the drug interacts with the receptor, a conformational change occurs in the membrane, resulting in one or more actions (e) which eventually result in the drug effect. III. Drug agonist with b and c binding sites. This agonist (III) would have more binding affinity than II. IV. Competitive pharmacologic antagonist (IV) with a, b, and c binding sites. Additional binding sites provide added stability of drug receptor complex. Blockade occurs if the agonist cannot reach the receptor. V. Noncompetitive antagonist (V) usually binds at a nearby (allosteric) site. Binding at d prevents the conformational change (indicated by arrow f). A second type of noncompetitive antagonism results when the receptor is altered, as by covalent binding, although some authors refer to the latter as competitive irreversible.

achieve the same maximal response as either drug A or B, it has less intrinsic activity. Drug C can also be called a partial agonist.

Now consider the concept of an antagonist in similar kinetic terms. A drug that has affinity for the receptor but elicits no response is an antagonist and is said to have no intrinsic activity. Examples of antagonists are shown in the dose-response curves in Figure 12–8. (See legend for explanation.)

The properties of agonists and antagonists follow. An agonist:

1. fits closely to a receptor and has moderate affinity
2. interacts reversibly (so the receptor and the system can regenerate)

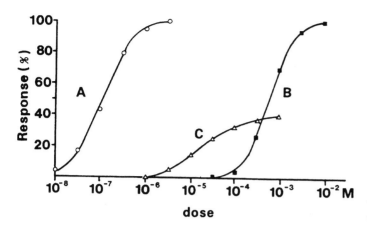

Figure 12-7. Drug dose-response curves. (Adapted from van Rossum J M. J Pharm Pharmacol 15:290, 1963.)

3. follows enzyme-substrate reaction kinetics
4. resembles the primary drug in molecular structure
5. is a partial agonist, if it does not cause the full effect of the primary drug

A pharmacologic antagonist:

1. has a high affinity for receptor site or acts allosterically by preventing the subsequent reactions which result in the observed pharmacologic effect

2. has no intrinsic activity, usually does not cause the agonistic effect (but occasionally an antagonist has some agonistic activity)

3. shows little or no response when used alone (see Fig. 12-8)

4. has a longer duration of effect than the agonist (the system may remain blocked for several hours compared to the agonist effect, which is usually measured in minutes)

Not all drug effects are mediated by a specific receptor for the drug. The following summarizes

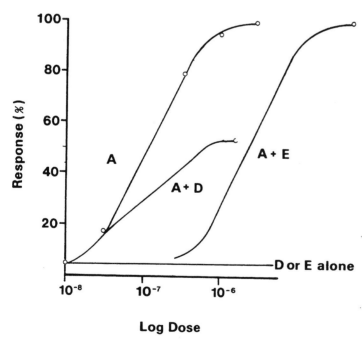

Figure 12-8. Dose-response curves illustrating drug antagonism. Drug D is a noncompetitive antagonist because drug A can no longer exert its maximal effect in the presence of drug D. Drug E is a competitive antagonist because increasing the dose of drug A allows it to exert maximal effect. Drug D and drug E also have no intrinsic activity, as shown in the lowest response curve line. A, typical agonist response without antagonist present; A + D, noncompetitive antagonism; A + E, competitive antagonism.

the types of drug actions and examples of each type.

1. Receptor-mediated action
   a. cellular membrane receptor (e.g., epinephrine acting on a receptor
   b. intracellular receptor (e.g., certain antibiotics acting on ribosomes)
   c. second messenger concept (Fig. 12–6, e). After the drug-receptor interaction, other actions occur in the cellular components, resulting in the ultimate effect. Although these actions are not well known or completely elucidated in all cases, recent evidence indicates that second messengers are important as mediators of the intermediate action. Cyclic AMP (adenosine 3':5'-cyclic phosphate) is the best known example of a second messenger; when epinephrine acts on the heart, a receptor is activated followed by activation of the enzyme adenylcyclase. This enzyme is within the cell membrane and thought to be associated with the receptor. Activation of adenylcyclase results in conversion of ATP (adenosine triphosphate) to cyclic AMP. Cyclic AMP is considered to be the second messenger for the cardiac actions of epinephrine. Many other hormonal and neural activations occur through cyclic AMP, while other substances (such as prostaglandins, Ca^{++}) are known to be mediators of other processes.
2. Nonreceptor-mediated actions (nonspecific)
   a. osmotic effects (e.g., osmotic diuretics)
   b. chemical action (e.g., acid-base)
   c. detergent effects (e.g., benzalkonium chloride)
   d. physicochemical effects (e.g., fat-soluble anesthetics)
   e. chelation (e.g., calcium disodium edetate in treatment of lead poisoning)
   f. antimetabolic effect (e.g., incorporation of 5-fluorouracil and other pyrimidine analogs into DNA metabolites in cancer therapy)

DRUG INTERACTIONS

Objective 12.I.1. List three broad types of drug interactions and give an example of each.

The interaction of an agonist and an antagonist at a drug receptor has already been discussed. In addition to interactions mediated by receptor systems, there are many other ways in which two or more drugs may interact in the body to produce altered therapeutic and/or side effects. Three classes of drug interactions include (1) summation, (2) inhibition, and (3) chemical or physiochemical incompatibilities.

Summation

Simple Addition. The combined effects of two or more drugs that act by the same mechanism equal the sum of the effects that results when each drug is administered alone.

Example. Aspirin and acetaminophen are two mild analgesics which act by the same mechanism to relieve pain; 325 mg aspirin equals about 325 mg acetaminophen. When one aspirin and one acetaminophen are given, the result is the same as giving two tablets of either aspirin or acetaminophen, mathematically, $1 + 1 = 2$.

Simple addition usually requires that each drug be given in a dose on the straight-line portion of the dose-response curve and below the ceiling effect. For example, if the patient has taken six aspirins, he may already be on the upper portion of the dose-response curve, and any further doses of acetaminophen (or aspirin) would probably have no further effect. Another example of simple addition is shown in Figure 12–9A. Notice that the combination gives about twice the response of either drug alone.

Simple addition is not generally recommended in therapy; it is usually better to prescribe a full dose of one medication than half of one and half of the other.

Infra-addition. This implies that the two drug effects do not give the total expected effect, al-

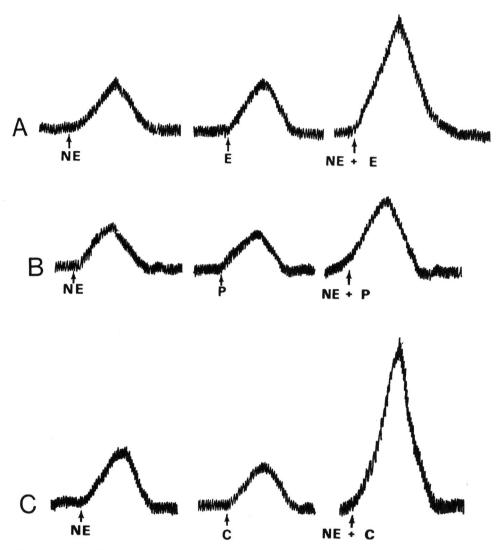

Figure 12–9. Blood pressure response of a cat, illustrating types of summation. The recording shows blood pressure vs time. **A.** Simple addition. **B.** Infra-addition. **C.** Supra-addition. E = epinephrine; NE = norepinephrine; P = phenylephrine; C = cocaine.

though the total effect is greater than the first drug alone. Mathematically:

$$1 + 1 = <2>1$$

Use of infra-addition in therapy would be discouraged because the risks of the second drug are not usually worth taking if the total therapeutic effect of each drug is not obtained. Some authors consider infra-addition as a type of drug antagonism. Figure 12–9B illustrates infra-addition.

Supra-addition. Mathematically:

$$1 + 1 = >2.$$

Other terms for supra-addition are potentiation, positive summation, and synergism. An example of supra-addition is shown in Figure 12–9C.

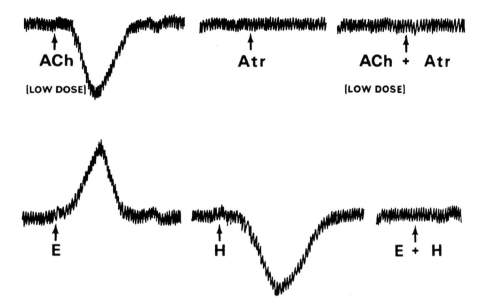

Figure 12-10. Effects of antagonists on blood pressure of a cat. The recording shows blood pressure vs time. **Top.** Pharmacologic antagonism. **Bottom.** Physiologic antagonism. ACh = acetylcholine; Atr = atropine; E = epinephrine; H = histamine.

Inhibition

This includes any type of antagonism.

Competitive Inhibition. The antagonist combines reversibly with the same receptor as the agonist. Increases in the concentration of agonist will reverse the inhibitory or blocking effect of the antagonist. An example of competitive antagonism is illustrated in Figure 12-10A. Acetylcholine lowers blood pressure, atropine generally has no effect on blood pressure, but it prevents the further blood pressure drop caused by the same dose of acetylcholine.

Physiologic Antagonism. Drugs act on different physiologic processes (not the same receptor) to cancel each other's effects. An example of physiologic antagonism is illustrated in Figure 12-10B. Epinephrine acts on adrenergic receptors to increase blood pressure, while histamine acts on histamine receptors to lower blood pressure. If both drugs are given together, the net effect on blood pressure is cancellation of effect. Depending upon dosage, these opposite effects can be titrated so that the net effect is zero.

Noncompetitive Inhibition. The antagonist combines irreversibly with the same receptor as the agonist. Increases in levels of agonist do not reverse the blocking effect of antagonist. An example is shown in Figure 12-8, curve A + D. Norepinephrine increases blood pressure, and phenoxybenzamine blocks this increase irreversibly.

Metabolic Antagonism. An example is *p*-aminobenzoic acid (PABA), which antagonizes the antibacterial effect of sulfonamides (see Chapter 29).

Chemical or Physicochemical Incompatibilities

These include:

1. *Two Solutions Added Together.* Precipitation may result.
2. *Metal Cations.* These prevent absorption of tetracyclines.

Objective 12.I.2. Recognize seven general mechanisms by which drugs may cause unfavorable actions or interactions.

Objective 12.I.3. Describe six ways in which one drug may alter the gastrointestinal absorption of another, and give clinical examples.

Objective 12.I.4. Describe three ways in which one drug may alter the distribution of another, and give clinical examples.

Objective 12.I.5. Describe two ways in which one drug may alter the biotransformation of another, and give clinical examples.

Objective 12.I.6. Describe two ways in which one drug may alter the renal excretion of another, and give clinical examples.

Drugs may cause unfavorable actions or interactions through at least seven mechanisms, which are described below, along with examples of each.

Chemical Interaction. Kanamycin and methicillin inactivate each other chemically if both are added to the same syringe for IV administration.

Modification of GI Absorption

1. Alteration of motility. Cathartics or laxatives speed transit of GI contents (including drugs) and increase mixing action of peristalsis. The results of these two effects on drug absorption are opposite, i.e., faster transit time decreases absorption and increased motility increases absorption. Antispasmodic agents have the opposite effects, slowing transit time and motility.
2. Alteration of bacterial flora: oral antibiotic therapy destroys many microbes of the GI tract. Some GI flora synthesize vitamin K, which is subsequently absorbed. Antibiotic therapy after anticoagulant therapy could result in excessive bleeding.
3. Physicochemical interaction. Tetracycline combined with milk, dairy products, or antacids will form a nonabsorbed product.
4. Alteration of pH. Drugs that are weak acids are more rapidly absorbed in the acidic stomach. Alkalizers usually inhibit absorption of weak acids by ion formation, but sometimes they promote absorption by increasing water

solubility. Weak bases are more rapidly absorbed in more alkaline intestinal tract, and acidification would slow this absorption.

5. Alteration of mucosa by disease. Nontropical sprue causes destruction of intestinal villi and microvilli, resulting in decreased GI absorption.
6. Alteration of transport mechanism. An example is methyldopa, a drug that resembles tyrosine in structure and competes with tyrosine for active transport sites in the GI tract.

Modification of Dermatomucosal Absorption. Many times an agent that is applied topically can achieve significant systemic levels and hence produce a potentially hazardous reaction. This might occur more readily in the presence of inflammation or damaged tissue.

Example. Epinephrine in gingival retraction cord may cause cardiac palpitations and increased blood pressure.

Alteration of Distribution.

1. Fluid flow. Pressor or depressor agents can alter distribution by altering blood flow in certain areas of the body.
2. Transport across membranes (similar to 6 above). Another example is that antidepressant drugs (imipramines) block the uptake of guanethidine into neurons, which is required for guanethidine to have an antihypertensive effect.
3. Displacement of drug from its binding site. Drugs bound to plasma proteins are essentially inactive; free drug is the active portion. Dicumarol (anticoagulant) binds very tightly to plasma proteins. Only 1 to 3% of drug is in free form (unbound) at therapeutic doses. Therefore, a slight shift in the bound: free ratio results in a large change of anticoagulant potency. Phenylbutazone is an example of an analgesic drug that occupies the same sites and will displace dicumarol.

Modification of Action at Receptor Sites. See Competitive and Noncompetitive Inhibition, page 83.

Modification of Biotransformation.

1. Microsomal enzyme stimulation. Phenobarbital stimulates a vast number of liver enzymes. Concurrent use of phenobarbital and an oral contraceptive increases chances of pregnancy.
2. Microsomal enzyme inhibition. Chloramphenicol, an antibiotic, can inhibit a number of liver enzymes, and any other drug metabolized by the same enzymes will be potentiated due to the enzyme inhibition.

Alteration of Excretion. Kidney function is most important in excretion.

1. Alteration of active secretion. Blockade of active secretion by probenecid results in prolonged levels of penicillin.
2. Modification of reabsorption. Alkalinization of urine (NaHCO$_3$) increases the excretion of weak acids, such as barbiturates and aspirin. Acidification (NH$_4$Cl) increases excretion of weak bases, such as amphetamine.

J. ADDITIONAL TERMINOLOGY ASSOCIATED WITH CLINICAL DRUG USE

Objective 12.J.1. Define the following terms: indications, contraindications, onset of action, latent period, duration, site and mode of action, pharmacologic effect, side effect, untoward effect, toxic effect, allergy, idiosyncrasy, hyperreactive, normoreactive, hyporeactive, tolerance, dependence, iatrogenic effect, teratogenic effect, carcinogenic, elimination, first-order kinetics, zero-order kinetics, and biologic half-life.

When discussing drug actions or in pharmacology texts and references, the following terms are frequently used to describe the pharmacologic profile of a drug.

1. **Indications** are the uses of a drug or conditions for which the drug is therapeutically beneficial.
2. **Contraindications** are the conditions under which the drug should not be used, e.g., a disease or the presence of another drug. Contraindications are either relative (use with caution) or absolute (avoid completely).
3. **Onset of action** is the time when the drug begins to show activity, usually calculated from the time of administration until the desired effect is achieved.
4. **Latent period** (latency) is the time from administration until onset of action.
5. **Duration of action** (duration) is the length of time the drug remains active, calculated from administration time until desired effect is lost.
6. **Site of action** is the cell, tissue, organ, or system upon which a drug acts. For example, local anesthetics act on nerve fibers (cellular action), while *Dilantin* acts on connective tissue (tissue action), causing hyperplasia. Morphine acts on the brain (organ action), and epinephrine acts on the cardiovascular system (systemic action).
7. **Mode of action** is the way in which a drug produces its effect. Drugs do not alter physiologic function; they can only stimulate or depress (inhibit) the function.
8. **Pharmacologic effect** is an effect a drug has on cells, tissues, or systems. Usually the **action** is the primary or desired effect, while **effects** are all changes caused by a drug.
9. **Side effects** (sometimes called untoward, undesired, or adverse effects) include any action or effect other than the desired therapeutic effect. These can range from mild to severe.
10. **Untoward effect** is an effect that is difficult to manage and is a type of side effect.
11. **Toxic effects** are adverse effects of a drug that include not only exaggeration of the therapeutic effects (usually excessive dosage) but also induction of other side effects. Overdosage can be either absolute (simply giving more than the usual accepted dose) or relative (giving a normal dose to an individual who is hyperreactive, e.g., children, aged persons, or patients in whom drug metabolism is impaired).
12. **Hyperreactive** refers to a patient who expe-

riences toxic or near-toxic effects from a normal dose of a drug.

13. **Normoreactive** refers to a patient who experiences normal, predictable therapeutic effects from a normal dose of a drug.

14. **Hyporeactive** refers to a patient who experiences little or no therapeutic effect from a normal dose of a drug.

15. **Tolerance** indicates a larger amount of drug is needed to produce its effect (or the usual dose produces less effect).

16. **Dependence** is a need (craving) for the drug.

17. **Psychic dependence** (or psychologic dependence) indicates that no sickness occurs on withdrawal, but a desire and seeking of the drug occur.

18. **Physical dependence** implies that the patient becomes sick (withdrawal syndrome) when the drug is withdrawn.

19. **Addiction** implies a need for the drug, including psychic and physical dependence and drug-seeking behavior which causes harm to the subject or society.

20. **Allergy** is synonymous with hypersensitivity. Allergy implies that a previous exposure to antigen occurred with buildup of antibody. *Cross-sensitivity* implies that related chemicals exhibit the same allergic reactions. Allergy can be immediate (anaphylactoid), accelerated (up to about two days), or delayed (several days or weeks later). The hapten theory indicates that small molecules (such as drugs) can combine with larger molecules, forming antigens that induce antibodies and cause allergy.

21. **Idiosyncrasy** is an unusual, unpredictable reaction.

22. **Iatrogenic** implies a disease or condition caused by the healing agent. This is frequent with drugs, and the more drugs used, the greater the chance of producing such a reaction.

23. **Teratogenic** implies adverse effects on a fetus during pregnancy.

24. **Carcinogenic** means inducing cancer.

25. **Elimination** (elimination rate) is the rate at which a drug is removed from the body and includes both metabolism and excretion.

Elimination, like absorption, often follows first-order kinetics (see below).

26. **First-order kinetics** implies that the rate of absorption or elimination is directly dependent on the concentration of drug in the plasma. When the drug concentration is high, elimination rates are rapid, whereas when drug concentrations are low, elimination rates are slow.

27. **Zero-order kinetics** implies that the rate of absorption or elimination proceeds at a constant rate, regardless of plasma concentration of drug.

28. **Biologic half-life** ($t\frac{1}{2}$) is the time required to eliminate one half of the drug that was initially present.

REFERENCES

Adriani J, Campbell B: Fatalities following topical application of local anesthetics to mucous membranes. JAMA 162:1528, 1956

Csáky TZ: Introduction to General Pharmacology, 2nd ed. New York, Appleton, 1979, pp 18, 46, 47, 48, 49, 50, 51, 52, 53

Csáky TZ: Cutting's Handbook of Pharmacology, 6th ed. New York, Appleton, 1979, pp 521, 581

Niazi S: Textbook of Biopharmaceutics and Clinical Pharmacokinetics. New York, Appleton, 1979, pp 98, 99, 125, 182

van Rossum JM: J Pharm Pharmacol 15:285, 1963

BIBLIOGRAPHY

Csáky TZ: Introduction to General Pharmacology, 2nd ed. New York, Appleton, 1979, Ch 3, 6, 9, 10

Gilman AG, Goodman LS, Gilman A (eds): Goodman and Gilman's The Pharmacological Basis of Therapeutics, 6th ed. New York, Macmillan, 1980, Ch 1, 2

QUESTIONS

1. Posology can be defined as the study of: (Select one.)

   A. Mechanisms of drug action

   B. The preparation of various forms of drugs

C. The pharmacological effects of drugs

D. Drug dosages

2. The process by which a drug in the circulation enters target tissues, depot tissues, and metabolic sites is termed: (Select one.)

A. Absorption

B. Distribution

C. Metabolism

D. Excretion

3. Which of the following tissue properties can determine the rate of drug absorption? (Select one.)

A. Route of administration

B. Surface area of tissues

C. Blood flow

D. All of the above

E. None of the above

4. T F A disadvantage of the oral route of administration is the generally expensive nature of this route.

5. T F The intra-arterial route of drug administration is considered to be a parenteral route.

6. T F Plasma protein binding of a drug does not influence its distribution.

7. The site at which a drug exerts its therapeutic action is termed: (Select one.)

A. Reservoir site

B. Metabolic site

C. Excretory site

D. None of the above

8. The amount of drug bound to plasma protein is: (Select one.)

A. Independent of plasma protein concentration

B. Dependent on plasma protein concentration

C. Dependent on the plasma concentration of the drug

D. All of the above

E. A and C above

F. B and C above

9. Drug interactions at plasma proteins can occur by which one of the following mechanisms?

A. Displacement of one drug by another

B. Precipitation of one drug by another

C. Both of the above

D. Neither of the above

10. T F Most brain tissues are readily permeable to highly polar compounds.

11. T F Generally, the metabolism of a drug results in forms that are less active and/or more readily excretable.

12. Nonmicrosomal hydrolysis of ester-type local anesthetics (e.g., procaine) results in the formation of: (Select one.)

A. Para-aminobenzoic acid and an aminoethanol

B. An aminoethanol and a nitrosamine

C. Benzene and aminoethanol

D. None of the above

13. Phenobarbital can influence the metabolism of other drugs in which one of the following ways?

A. Drug metabolism is impaired because phenobarbital inhibits microsomal enzymes

B. Drug metabolism is unaffected

C. Drug metabolism is enhanced because phenobarbital stimulates microsomal enzymes

D. None of the above

14. **T F** Renal excretion of drugs involves the filtration of water-soluble metabolites into the urine.

15. **T F** In addition to renal excretion, some drugs may be excreted in sweat.

16. **T F** Probenecid increases the rate of penicillin excretion by enhancing its renal secretion.

17. A drug effect which results in an alteration of the physical properties of the target tissue is termed: (Select one.)

   A. Receptor-mediated mechanism
   B. Physicochemical mechanism
   C. Zero-order kinetic effect
   D. None of the above

18. A drug which stimulates an effector through its interaction with a receptor is termed a(an): (Select one.)

   A. Antagonist
   B. Agonist
   C. Partial antagonist
   D. None of the above

19. A drug interaction in which the response to two drugs given simultaneously is much greater than would be expected by adding the effects of the two drugs given alone is termed: (Select one.)

   A. Infra-addition
   B. Supra-addition
   C. Idiosyncrasy
   D. None of the above

20. **T F** Modification of biotransformation of a drug may occur only by stimulation of microsomal enzymes.

21. **T F** A laxative has no influence on the rate of absorption of another, orally administered drug.

22. **T F** If a patient taking dicumarol receives another drug which is highly protein bound, the effect of the dicumarol would be reduced.

23. **T F** Chloramphenicol can enhance the effect of other drugs by inhibiting liver enzymes.

24. **T F** Acidification of the urine would be expected to increase the rate of renal excretion of a basic drug.

25. Toxic effects of a drug can be defined as: (Select one.)

   A. Unusual, unpredictable effects
   B. Adverse effects due to the drug's therapeutic action, but at excessive doses
   C. Any effects other than the desired therapeutic effects
   D. None of the above

13
Principles of Pharmacotherapeutics

A. DEFINITION OF PHARMACOTHERAPEUTICS

Objective 13.A.1. Recognize the definition of pharmacotherapeutics and its relationship to pharmacology.

Pharmacotherapeutics is the use of drugs in human therapy. The principles of pharmacotherapeutics involve application of the principles of pharmacology in actual patient treatment. Chapter 12 covered the principles of pharmacology, including most of the terminology which is useful in pharmacotherapeutics. In this chapter, we describe how these principles are applied when human therapy is the goal of drug application. As an example, dose-response curves are used to define drug safety, effectiveness, and therapeutic index.

B. FACTORS CONSIDERED IN HUMAN DRUG THERAPY

Objective 13.B.1. Describe factors that should be considered before drugs are used in humans and be able to match them to their definitions.

The following factors, related to a drug, should be considered before attempting its use in humans. It is a federal requirement that most or all of this information appear in the drug package insert.

Description. This includes (1) chemical class and type, (2) pharmacologic class and type, (3) chemical form of the drug, and (4) general method of use.

Action. The action describes the beneficial effect which the doctor and patient can expect from using the drug. Sometimes, several actions of the drug contribute to the overall therapeutic benefit. Pharmacodynamic and pharmacokinetic properties that contribute to the beneficial effects are also considered.

Indications. The indications include the conditions for which the drug is useful, either alone or in combination with other drugs.

Contraindications. The contraindications include the conditions under which the drug should *not* be used. A useful subgrouping of contraindications is *relative contraindications* (drug can be used but only with proper precautions or warnings) and *absolute contraindications* (drug must never be used under any circumstances).

Adverse Effects. The patient and doctor must be aware of possible adverse effects of a drug. The package insert will list the adverse effects, classified by organ system, and will usually note whether the adverse effect is rare, occasional, or frequent.

Warnings. Adverse effects of the drug which require caution during therapy include warnings to the patient that must be relayed by the doctor (e.g., do not drive or operate dangerous machinery) and warnings to the doctor (e.g., usage in pregnancy or in small children). The drug may be used in spite of a warning provided that everyone is informed and that the benefit to be obtained by the patient is greater than the risk incurred (low risk:benefit ratio, p. 93).

Precautions. Precautions include tests that should be done or symptoms that may occur. Positive tests or symptoms may warn of impending danger, requiring either avoidance of the drug or its withdrawal if therapy is already instituted.

Dosage and Administration. This is a statement containing the drug dosage schedule under various conditions, how the dosage should be modified, e.g., for patient's age, and how the drug is administered.

Overdosage. This section of the package insert describes symptoms which indicate adverse reactions and which warn that the drug dosage should be modified or the drug should be discontinued.

How Supplied. This describes specific forms in which the drug can be obtained.

The dentist should read the drug package insert to inform himself of the above information. If the package insert is not available, the same information is found in the *Physicians' Desk Reference* (*PDR*), a compendium of drug package inserts.

C. DRUG SAFETY

Objective 13.C.1. Describe methods of screening for drug activity and quantitating safety.

Objective 13.C.2. Describe acute, subacute, and chronic toxicity testing in animals and methods of quantitating toxicity.

Objective 13.C.3. Define lethal dose in animals, including LD_{50}, LD_{95}, LD_5.

Objective 13.C.4. Define IND and NDA.

Objective 13.C.5. Describe three phases of IND investigation.

Objective 13.C.6. Define TD (toxic dose) in humans, including TD_5 and TD_1.

Pharmaceutical manufacturers screen various compounds for desirable pharmacologic activity which may provide a beneficial therapeutic effect. This is performed in animal model screens for such activities as cardiovascular effect and diuretic effect. Antimicrobial activity is defined in microbial cultures.

After desirable compounds are found, they are tested using toxicologic screens. One of the first screens used is the acute lethal effect in the mouse. Mice are injected with various doses of the compound and a graph of log-dose versus lethality (% mortality) is plotted. A typical result for a drug is seen in Figure 13–1. The curve is sigmoidal in shape, showing a threshold (t) below which no animals are killed, a slowly rising phase (I), a rapidly rising, linear phase (II), and a plateau (III) with a ceiling effect (shown by dotted line). Although at first glance this graph resembles the dose-response curves for agonists (see Chapter 12, Fig. 12–7), there is a major difference. The agonist curves are usually graded, that is, the ordinate indicates an increased level of a graded response (for example, percent increase in blood pressure). On the other hand, the lethal dose graph indicates a

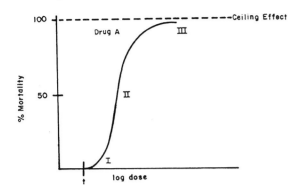

Figure 13–1. Lethal dose-response curve for drug A in mice.

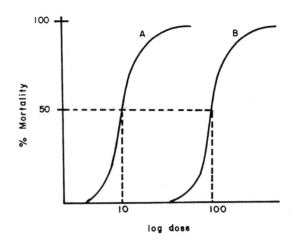

Figure 13–2. Lethal dose curves comparing drugs A and B.

quantal (all-or-none) response. Mortality is an all-or-none response and can be measured only in percentage of animals dead at any particular dose. Whereas an agonist dose-response curve may be obtained in one animal or tissue, the lethal dose-response curve is statistical, requiring many test animals.

The comparison of two lethal dose-response curves is shown in Figure 13–2, which repeats the lethal dose-response curve for drug A and adds a second curve for drug B. The dotted lines indicate the median lethal dose (LD_{50}), the dose that kills 50% of the animals. Similarly, LD_5, LD_{95}, or any other LD can be described. The reason that LD_{50} is usually used, instead of LD_5 or LD_{95}, is that LD_{50} is statistically easier to determine than are the other points (fewer animals are needed to determine the 50% point). These points are determined statistically, by extrapolation from the dose-response curves, since it would be difficult to find a drug dosage that kills an exact percentage (e.g., 50%) of the animals in any one experiment. If the LD_{50} of drug A is 10 and LD_{50} of drug B is 100, which drug has less toxic effect? Since 10 times more of drug B than drug A can be tolerated, drug B should have less toxic effect at any specific dosage. Another way to state this is that drug A is 10 times more potent in causing this effect than is drug B.

Further toxicologic tests might be performed in other species, such as acute LD_{50} in rats, subacute (up to six weeks) and chronic (long-term)

toxicity upon feeding in rats, and, usually, subacute and chronic toxicity in another nonrodent species, such as dog or monkey. Appropriate biochemical and pathologic tests usually are performed in subacute and chronic studies. Tissue irritancy and allergenicity are usually tested on rabbit or guinea pig skin, especially for topical preparations.

After the drug meets the above safety tests, human testing can begin. The human testing program, described below, requires an Investigational New Drug Exemption (IND) from the Food and Drug Administration (FDA). Phase I involves pharmacologic studies of a range of doses, starting at a low dose, in a limited number of human volunteers. At the same time, further animal toxicity testing is required before phase II human testing is started. Phase II is a small-scale trial for therapeutic effectiveness in humans with the disease. During phase II, there is close monitoring of biochemical changes and observation for adverse effects. Phase III is a large-scale trial on the population expected to use the drug. Again, side effects and adverse reactions are closely monitored.

After testing is complete according to submitted protocols, a New Drug Application (NDA) is obtained, and the manufacturer is free to market the drug, providing it continues to monitor it and inform the FDA of any adverse reaction reports received from doctors or patients.

Following a period of drug use in humans (usually more than two years), the drug's true toxicity can be defined in humans by studying observed adverse effects. Since drug toxicity should be minimized, drugs are compared on the basis of the lowest possible acceptable toxic dose (TD) (e.g., a TD for 1 percent or less of the population). Sometimes, when the drug provides an exceedingly beneficial effect, a higher TD level (e.g., TD_5 or higher) might be acceptable. This introduces the concept of risk:benefit ratio, which is discussed under drug effectiveness.

D. DRUG EFFECTIVENESS

Objective 13.D.1. Describe quantitative expressions of effective dose, including ED_{50} (in animals) and EDs in humans.

Objective 13.D.2. Describe the derivation of Therapeutic Index (TI) using LD_{50} and ED_{50}; describe relationship between margin of safety and TI.

Objective 13.D.3. Describe the use of TI in animals and in humans.

Objective 13.D.4. Define MTD (maximum tolerated dose) and risk/benefit ratio (RBR), including an example of a dental drug with a low RBR.

As indicated above (under drug safety), pharmacologists are first interested in the useful effects of drugs, and, therefore, all substances suspected of having therapeutic properties are initially screened for pharmacologic activity. Once the investigators are satisfied that the drug may have some useful benefit, studies of drug safety and effectiveness are performed in parallel in animal models. Drug safety studies were described above and, initially, the LD_{50} will be used to derive therapeutic index (TI).

Drug effectiveness studies are performed to obtain dose-response curves. Usually, an effectiveness dose-response curve is graded because the response is measured in graded intervals. For example, if one wishes to study the hypo-

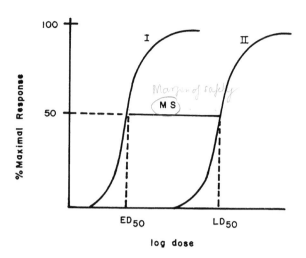

Figure 13–3. Derivation of TI.

tensive effect of a drug, increasing doses of a drug are plotted against increasing fall in blood pressure. The median effective dose (ED_{50}) gives the dose that causes one half of the maximal blood pressure drop. By repeating graded dose-response curves in several animals, the investigator can statistically define the ED curve. The ED_{50} dose is usually the most useful, since it is the easiest point to statistically derive (see above). An ED_{90} or higher dose may be used if one is trying to maximize the benefit of the drug to the patient.

To derive the therapeutic index (TI), two curves are plotted (Fig. 13–3), and calculation of the margin of safety is made as follows:

$$TI = \frac{LD_{50}}{ED_{50}} = MS$$

In Figure 13–3, the MS is shown as the distance between the two curves. Actually, since this is a log scale, the distance MS is equal to the log ratio TI. The greater the separation of the curves (or the greater the TI), the better is the drug. A problem occurs with the MS when the two curves are not parallel. If a greater percentage effectiveness is desired, a greater risk is incurred when the curves are converging. This gives a reduced MS at higher EDs.

The TI is a comparison of safety to effectiveness. However, as there are many measures of safety (see above), there are also many measures of effectiveness, and, therefore, the definition of TI must include the kinds of measures used.

The use of TI is necessary in judging drug usefulness because drug potency alone does not indicate a true value. If a parallel shift occurs in both the toxic and the effective dose curves, no therapeutic advantage may be gained. For example, a manufacturer may find a new drug that is 10 times more potent than the standard drug in its therapeutic effect. If the new drug is also 10 times more toxic, the increased activity is meaningless (both drugs have the same TI).

Other measures of drug effectiveness that can be used to derive TI are the usual adult human dose, ED_{90} (or a higher ED depending on the percentage effectiveness desired). Ideally, one would like to obtain 99% or more effectiveness and only cause adverse effects in 1% or less, (100% and 0 are impossible goals). If the ideal were obtained, the human TI would be defined as:

$$TI \text{ (humans)} = \frac{TD_1}{ED_{99}}$$

In practice, almost no one can agree on which values to use for deriving TI, and sometimes another measure, maximum tolerated dose (MTD), is used. MTD is obtained from studies of human experience and is the dose which will *not* cause adverse effects in almost any member of the population. As a rule, a drug is considered safe when the toxic dose is at least 10 times greater than the therapeutic dose. With drugs that cause a high percentage of adverse effects, another term, risk:benefit ratio (RBR), may be useful. Usually the RBR should be low (low risk to high benefit). As a rule, a greater risk might be acceptable if a great benefit is obtainable. This could be very important in the use of anticancer drugs, which are very toxic but are used to treat a dangerous condition. However, RBR may also be important where the benefit is low, for example a food coloring may be useful, but the benefit is so low, we would not wish to take *any* risk. Thus, only colorings which are ultrasafe are acceptable. Erythrosine (FD&C Red 3) is a food coloring with a long history of use and an extremely safe record as a food additive. Moreover, erythrosine discloses plaque, and although

a patient can live without his teeth ever disclosing plaque, the dye is considered so safe that we are willing to take the almost nonexistent risk.

The relative safety index (RSI) compares merit of a new drug relative to a standard drug.

$$RSI = \frac{TI \text{ new drug}}{TI \text{ standard drug}}$$

RSI usually varies about 0.1 to about 3.0. Any value greater than 1 indicates an improvement over the standard drug. For example, lidocaine has an RSI between 1.5 and 2.0 (the variation is dependent upon how one measures the safety and effectiveness) compared to procaine.

E. PRESCRIBING AND DISPENSING MEDICATIONS

For a general discussion see below, Objectives H–M.

The dentist makes his diagnosis and decides which drugs will be of value in therapeutics. Before making the decision on drugs, the dentist must be familiar with the principles of pharmacology and of pharmacotherapeutics and must have, at hand or in his mind, the detailed facts concerning the use of the chosen drug. The dentist cannot be expected to remember all of the detailed facts that are important in his decision making and should refresh his memory often concerning the use of drugs. Therefore, it is recommended that each time a dentist use a drug, various sources of information should be consulted. These include the package insert, *Physicians' Desk Reference*, various textbooks of pharmacology, and other sources of drug information, as listed in the bibliography for this chapter.

The principles of prescription writing and factors involved in dosing are described on pages 95 through 102.

F. PLACEBO EFFECT

Objective 13.F.1. Define placebo effect.

Objective 13.F.2. List and describe four factors which contribute to the degree of the placebo effect.

Objective 13.F.3. Describe five important considerations for placebos in dentistry.

Placebo literally means "I please" and refers to prescribing a nonactive medication. Although the ethics of deliberately trying to fool a patient with a nonactive compound (e.g., saline injections, sugar pills) may be questioned, the placebo effect plays a role in almost all situations where medications are used. The placebo effect is related to the circumstances surrounding patient medication and may lead to quantitative effects which were not predictable on the basis of the drug's expected performance.

The placebo effect can be explained by at least four factors: (1) patient expectations, (2) practitioner's attitude, (3) drug effects, and (4) nature of the disease.

1. The patient visits the physician or dentist with expectations of obtaining relief. The patient's faith in the situation, as well as his/her confidence in the healer, is very important.
2. The doctor's attitude is also important. As mentioned on page 102, patient suggestibility, the doctor's method of presenting his drug therapy can be the difference between success and failure. The doctor's previous experience with the drug can affect his confidence. If the doctor has had good success (or has acquired confidence through study or other sources), he may display an attitude which positively reinforces the therapeutic situation.
3. The third set of factors involve the drug's actual ability to produce pharmacological effects. Even if the drug has only a limited ability to produce the desired effect, any effect may add positive reinforcement. Sometimes the drug lacks the effect for which it is used, but it has other prominent side effects resulting in the patient's interpretation that the drug is "powerful."
4. The fourth set of factors involve the nature of the disease; e.g., pain and other CNS affective states are extremely susceptible to suggestion and other psychologic factors, while infections, especially of the severe type, are probably less susceptible to suggestion.

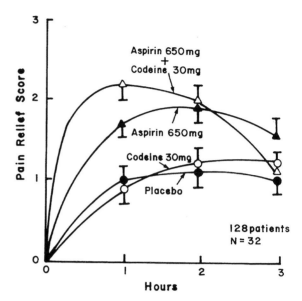

Figure 13-4. Effect of analgesics and placebos on pain relief. (*From Cooper, Beaver: Clin Pharmacol Ther 30:241, 1975.*)

Placebos are often recommended for clinical trials of new drugs for the purpose of eliminating any investigator bias. The extent of the placebo effect can be seen in Figure 13-4. This chart shows that the placebo was 50% as effective as aspirin in relieving this type of pain (*note:* in this study, codeine alone, at a 30 mg dose, was ineffective). In studies of severe postoperative pain after major surgery, placebos provide about 40% relief of severe postoperative pain, while morphine (10 to 15 mg) results in 80% relief. In other words, we can expect placebos to have about 40 to 50% of the desired activity, especially where patient suggestibility is a factor in the therapy (e.g., pain relief).

Controlled clinical trials usually attempt to factor out the placebo effect by determining its extent when tried under the same conditions. Interestingly, in such trials of active drug vs placebo, patients report the same type (and often the same incidence) of side effects from the placebo as from the active drug.

Five important considerations the dentist should remember regarding placebos are described below.

1. Almost any therapy has a certain element of placebo effect. Therefore, the overall effect is equal to the pharmacologic effect plus the placebo effect.
2. The placebo effect is greatest in central nervous system therapy, especially in treating pain, depression, and reaction to stress. Many of these conditions are susceptible to such psychologic therapy as hypnosis because of the importance of suggestibility.
3. The placebo effect may enhance the therapy if one administers the therapy with confidence.
4. You should be aware that any therapy having about a 50% success rate may be dependent upon placebo effect.
5. Prescription of a placebo is seldom necessary or indicated in dentistry. Rather, the placebo effect can be used advantageously by enhancing the effects of moderately active drugs.

G. THE CONTROLLED CLINICAL TRIAL

Objective 13.G.1. Describe five important components of an adequate, controlled clinical trial.

Five important components of an adequate, controlled clinical trial are:

1. Human assurance. The subject must be adequately informed of the nature of the experiment, alternate treatments, and his rights.
2. Double-blind studies. Neither investigator nor subject knows which medication is being given. The code is kept secret until the study is completed.
3. Placebo-controlled study. Usually a placebo is included as one of the blind medications. However, studies comparing two active medications are acceptable.
4. Random assignment. Medications should be randomly numbered and randomly assigned according to a preselected sequence.
5. Statistical analysis of results. Quantitative data should be presented with appropriate statistical analysis.

H. INTRODUCTION TO PRESCRIPTION WRITING

Objective 13.H.1. Recognize the definition of prescription, legend drugs, OTC drugs.

The dental practitioner, in the course of his dental practice, must be capable of correctly prescribing certain drugs. This capability includes (other than the knowledge of the pharmacology of the drug) such items as writing the prescription correctly; suggesting correct methods of administration, including dose, timing, duration, and possible avoidance of food or other drugs; updating the health history to avoid allergic reactions; a listing of potential side effects; and an understanding of federal and state drug laws.

The prescription itself is simply a written or oral order for medication. Prescription drugs (or legend drugs) are agents of sufficient potency and potentially increased toxicity that they are ordered and used only under the direction or supervision of a practitioner (physician, dentist, veterinarian). These agents differ from nonprescription drugs (over-the-counter drugs or OTC drugs), which are judged safe for use by patients without the supervision of a practitioner. Dental OTC drugs are discussed in Appendix VI.

I. LAWS AND REGULATIONS

Objective 13.I.1. Describe federal and state laws and regulations governing the prescribing of drugs.

In 1970, the Controlled Substances Act was enacted. It is a collection of laws designed to regulate the manufacture, distribution, and dispensing of controlled substances for legitimate handlers of these substances. These drugs are categorized into five schedules (see below).

The Drug Enforcement Administration (DEA) is a division of the Department of Justice. This group is charged with the responsibility of controlling abuse of dangerous drugs through enforcement and prevention. Each practitioner must register with the DEA (and pay a fee), thereby permitting the practitioner to prescribe certain drugs. An annual renewal is also necessary. Applications for registration may be requested by writing the DEA at United States Department of Justice, PO Box 28083, Central Station, Washington, DC 20005.

In addition, many states have enacted laws concerning controlled substances. Each practitioner is urged to communicate with his local pharmacist or state board of pharmacy in order to comply with appropriate state laws. If a drug is not listed under federal schedules but is listed under a state schedule, the state law takes precedence, and the drug is to be considered a controlled substance. In other words, the more stringent law, whether federal or state, takes precedence.

Controlled substances have been categorized into five schedules, which were formulated according to three criteria: (1) according to their abuse potential—drugs in Schedule I have the highest abuse potential, and those in Schedule V have the least; (2) according to their ability to produce physical and psychologic dependence—Schedule I drugs exhibit the greatest potential for dependence, while Schedule V drugs have the least; (3) whether or not the drug has a legitimate medical use.(See Table 13–1 for examples of controlled substances in each Schedule.)

Some prescription-writing facts related to federally controlled substances follow:

1. Schedule I drugs have no approved medical use and cannot be prescribed.
2. Practitioner's address must appear on prescriptions for Schedule II drugs.
3. Date is required for Schedule II to IV drugs.
4. Patient's name and address are required for Schedule II drugs.
5. Schedule II drugs cannot be refilled or ordered orally. However, in case of an emergency, the practitioner may telephone an order for a Schedule II drug with a written prescription to follow within 72 hours. The practitioner should prescribe only enough medication to cover the emergency period. If dispensed by the practitioner, Schedule II drugs must be ordered on special DEA forms.

6. Schedule III and IV drugs cannot be refilled more than five times within a six-month period after the prescription is written.
7. Practitioners must enter their DEA number on prescriptions for controlled substances.
8. Concerning Schedule II drugs, the entire prescription must be written in ink, including the practitioner's signature. Typewriter or indelible pencil may be used, but an erasable ballpoint pen is not a valid alternative.
9. Schedule V drugs may be prescribed like other noncontrolled drugs or dispensed without a prescription, depending on state laws.

J. PARTS OF AN IDEAL PRESCRIPTION

Objective 13.J.1. Recognize and describe 11 parts of an ideal prescription.

An ideal prescription is illustrated in Figure 13–5. The parts of an ideal prescription are described below.

Dentist and Patient Identification

1. Federal law requires that the practitioner's address appear on prescription orders for Schedule II drugs. The private practitioner should have his full name, degree, address, and telephone number printed at the top of the prescription blank. This will expedite recognition of the practitioner by the pharmacist and will enable the pharmacist to contact the prescriber quickly and easily if there is some question about the prescription.
2. The date is important on all prescriptions, and it is required by federal law for drugs listed under Schedule II, III, or IV.
3. Accurate identification by name and address of the person to receive the medication is essential. Schedule II drugs require the full name and address of the patient.
4. The age of the patient should be included on the prescription, especially if the patient is a child or an elderly person. This allows the pharmacist to check the dose of the drug, thereby avoiding a possible toxic episode.

TABLE 13–1. SCHEDULE OF CONTROLLED SUBSTANCES

Schedule	Restrictions	Examples
I	All use forbidden except research	heroin dihydromorphine LSD mescaline peyote psilocybin marijuana tetrahydrocannabinols
II	No telephone prescriptions, no refills, written in ink with date	**Narcotic-analgesics** opium, morphine, codeine (alone), hydromorphone (*Dilaudid*), meperidine (*Demerol*), anileridine (*Leritine*), alphaprodine (*Nisentil*), methadone (*Dolophine*), oxymorphone (*Numorphan*), oxycodone (including combinations such as *Percodan*) **Stimulants** cocaine, amphetamines, methylphenidate **Depressants** amobarbital, pentobarbital, secobarbital, methaqualone, phencyclidine (PCP)
III	No more than 5 refills and new prescription after 6 months	**Narcotic-analgesics** (not to exceed 90 mg/tab) ASA, APAP, or APC with codeine ASA, APAP, or APC with dihydrocodeine **Narcotic-analgesic solution** (not to exceed 1800 mg/100 ml) paregoric **Stimulants** chlorphentermine, diethylpropion, benzphetamine **Depressants** Schedule II barbiturates with ASA, APAP, or APC, glutethimide (*Doriden*), methyprylon (*Noludar*), butabarbital (*Butisol*)
IV	Same prescription requirements as Schedule III, but penalties for illegal possession differ	**Narcotic-analgesics** propoxyphene (*Darvon*), pentazocine (*Talwin*) **Stimulants** phentermine, fenfluramine **Depressants** Chloral hydrate, ethinamate (*Valmid*), meprobamate (*Miltown, Equanil*), phenobarbital, ethchlorvynol (*Placidyl*), mephobarbital, chlordiazepoxide (*Librium*), diazepam (*Valium*), oxazepam (*Serax*)
V	Depending on state laws, prescribe like non-controlled drugs or OTC	terpin hydrate/codeine (codeine not exceeding 200 mg/100 ml), loperamide, diphenoxylate

(*After Meyers, Jawetz, Goldfien: Review of Medical Pharmacology, 7th ed, 1980. Courtesy of Lange Medical Publications.*)

Dentist and Patient Identification	JOHN SMITH, D.M.D. BOX 000 Maintown, EX 11111 Phone: QZ5-0012 Patient Name John Doe Date July 4, 1981 Address 1234 Fifth St., Augusta, GA Age 28
Superscription	℞
Inscription	Penicillin V Potassium U.S.P. 500 mg tabs
Subscription	Dispense 40 tablets
Signa	Sig: Take two tabs, immediately, then one tab every 6 hours, either ½ hour before or 2 hours after meals until all tabs are taken.
Prescriber's validation and additional directions	yes no Label [X] [ ] Generic Substitution Permitted John Smith D.M.D. Dispense as Written ________ D.M.D. Refill (0) 1-2-3-PRN State License No. ________ (Where applicable) DEA No. not required* (Where applicable)

*Not a controlled drug.

Figure 13–5. Ideal prescription.

Superscription

This is the symbol ℞, a Latin abbreviation for recipe, which means, "take thou." Some modern prescription blanks no longer contain this preprinted symbol.

Inscription

This is information about the drug(s), i.e., name, dosage, dosage form, and other factors that will aid the pharmacist in filling the order.

Subscription

This contains directions to the pharmacist, e.g., mix, dispense, and the dosage form and amount. The practitioner may want to avoid prescribing odd amounts of medication. For example, penicillin V is available as an oral solution, and it is prepackaged by the manufacturer in 100 ml bottles (as well as other sizes). If the patient needs 80 ml, perhaps the practitioner should prescribe 100 ml, since the patient probably would be charged for the entire 100 ml. Actually, the charge for 80 ml may be greater than for 100 ml, because the pharmacist must take more time to prepare the dose, he may have to supply his own bottle(s), and the other 20 ml will probably be thrown away since shelf life is limited after the preparation is dissolved. Similar concepts apply for other preparations as well. If a patient needs 48 tablets and the preparation is packaged in 50s, it may be better to prescribe 50 tablets. If the patient needs 2 gm of an ointment and it is packaged in 3 gm tubes, the practitioner probably should prescribe 3 gm. However, the practitioner must make the final decision, for there will be times when it is best to prescribe the exact amount of medication, e.g., clindamycin, an expensive antibiotic, is best prescribed as an exact number of capsules. Controlled substances should definitely be prescribed in exact amounts.

Signa (Sig., Label, Let It Be Labeled)

This section of the prescription contains directions to the patient. Directions should be written in readable English, but commonly recognized Latin abbreviations are acceptable (although not necessarily encouraged). The practitioner should **never** label "take as directed," since oral instructions to a patient may result in poor patient compliance if they are not supplemented with written instructions on the label. *Note:* signa is not the same in the Latin as the term signatura (i.e., practitioner's signature).

Prescriber's Validation and Additional Directions

1. Prescriber's signature and degree must appear on every prescription because they represent an authorization for the practitioner to write a prescription and for the pharmacist to fill it. The signature should be written in ink, a requirement for Schedule II drugs.
2. Refill directions (formerly part of the subscription), and label directions (formerly part of the signa) may be convenient for both doctor and pharmacist if placed as indicated on Figure 13–5. The label instructs the pharmacist to affix the name of the medication on the patient's drug container.
   Refills are not allowed for Schedule II drugs. Schedule III and IV drugs cannot be refilled more than five times, and all refills must be within six months of the date on the prescription.
3. Some states require that the practitioner's state license number be written in an appropriate space, and federal law (p. 95, Laws and Regulations) requires the practitioner's DEA number in an appropriate space when prescribing controlled substances. We advise against having the DEA number preprinted.

Instead, the practitioner should insert it only when prescribing controlled substances.

Objective 13.J.2. Recognize the Latin abbreviatons set in bold type in Table 13–2.

A list of more frequently used Latin abbreviations is presented in Table 13–2. Although we do not encourage the use of Latin abbreviations when writing prescriptions, a few commonly recognized abbreviations may be used when convenient. In addition, practitioners who practice in hospitals should be familiar with Latin abbreviations, for many physicians continue to use them on hospital patient charts.

K. MISCELLANEOUS ITEMS ASSOCIATED WITH PRESCRIPTION WRITING

Objective 13.K.1. Recognize six miscellaneous items associated with prescription writing.

1. All prescriptions should be written in ink, for they are medicolegal documents. All prescriptions for Schedule II drugs require ink.
2. An exact carbon copy should be kept on file, or all pertinent information should be transferred to the patient's chart.
3. Many practitioners prefer to dispense some medicines. A complete accounting of controlled substances is required by federal law. At the present time, a listing of controlled substances directly on patient charts is an acceptable method of recording use. An inventory must be made every two years and kept on file. Controlled drugs to be dispensed must be stored in a locked cabinet in an office which also can be locked. In addition, dispensed drugs must be properly labeled, or the patient may be arrested for illegal possession. Such a situation has led to a lawsuit against the dentist.
4. Although we have stressed the need for writing brief, clear, and concise directions to the patient, we believe more information about the drug needs to be related to the patient. For instance, peroral penicillin V may cause

TABLE 13-2. LATIN ABBREVIATIONS FREQUENTLY USED IN PRESCRIPTION WRITING

Abbreviation	Latin	English	Abbreviation	Latin	English
a	ante	before	p	post	after
aa	ana	of each	pc	post cibos	after meals
ac	ante cibos	before meals	prn	pro re nata	as needed
ad lib	ad libitum	at pleasure	q	quaque	every, each
aq	aqua	water	q4h	quaque 4	
b	bis	twice		hora	every 4 hours
bid	bis in die	twice a day	qid	quarter in die	4 times a day
c̄	cum	with	Rx	recipe	take thou
caps	capsula	capsules	rep	repetatur	repeat
d	dies	a day, daily	s̄	sine	without
disp	dispensa	dispense	sig	signa	let it be labeled,
gtt	guttae	drops			label
hs	hora somni	at bedtime	ss	semi	half
m et n	mane et	morning and	stat	statim	immediately
	nocte	night	tab	tabella	tablet
M	misce	mix	tid	ter in die	three times a
no	numero	number, amount			day
nr, non rep	non repetatur	do not repeat			

stomach upset. Therefore, if that side effect should occur, the patient should have been informed of the possibility and told to take the medication either closer to meals or with a light snack, such as tea and crackers. Another potential problem with penicillin V is the possible development of allergy. Although the medical history may reveal that the patient is not allergic to penicillin, it does not mean he cannot become allergic to the drug. Therefore, the patient should be told that if a skin rash, urticarial lesions, wheezing or difficult breathing, or swelling of the oropharyngeal tissues occurs, the medication should be discontinued and the practitioner called immediately. If the reaction is severe, the patient should go to a hospital emergency room for treatment. Such additional directions should be either handwritten or preprinted since verbal communication is difficult to document. The latest publication of the US Pharmacopeial Convention (1982 USP DI) lists such precautions in lay terms. The information is also available in many textbooks and in package inserts.

5. The practitioner should never postdate prescriptions, especially for controlled drugs.

6. Never prescribe a drug, except for use in a dental office or associated with a dental situation. For example, if a neighbor asks you to prescribe an antibiotic for an infected finger and you do, you are in violation of the law. First, you have violated a medical state practice act and are practicing medicine without a license. Second, you have probably violated a dental state practice act, for treating infected fingers is not included in the rights and privileges of said act. Third, if the neighbor has an adverse drug reaction to the medication you prescribed, he may sue you. Your malpractice insurance may not provide coverage under those circumstances.

A worse situation is for dentists to prescribe amphetamines, a Schedule II controlled substance. Amphetamines are occasionally prescribed by dentists, but they should **not** be prescribed because these drugs have no use in dentistry. By so doing, the dentist violates both the Federal Controlled Substances Act and the State Controlled Substances Act (if there is one), even though the dentist may have annually renewed his DEA license to prescribe Schedule II stimulant drugs.

TABLE 13–3. METROLOGY

	Apothecary	Metric
Numerals	Roman	Arabic
Units of weight	grain (gr)	gram (gm or g)
Units of volume	minim (M)	milliliter (ml)

Approximate Equivalents:

Common Liquid Measure	English	Apothecary	Metric
1 drop	—	1–1.5 minim (drop)	0.04–0.06 ml
1 teaspoon	—	1/6 ounce (1 tsp)	4.0–5.0 ml
1 tablespoon	—	½ ounce (1 tbs)	15.0–16.0 ml
		1 ounce	30 ml
1 teacup	—	4 ounces	125 ml
1 cup	—	8 ounces	250 ml
		1 grain	65 mg
1 pint	1 lb	—	454 gm
—	2.2 lb	—	1.0 kg

L. METROLOGY

Objective 13.L.1. Recognize the definition of metrology.

Objective 13.L.2. Understand the conversion of milliliters to drops, teaspoons, tablespoons, ounces, and cups; convert grains to grams, grams to pounds, and pounds to kilograms.

Metrology is the study of weights and measures. All prescriptions should be written with metric values. Table 13–3 lists some important and useful conversions between the metric and apothecary systems.

M. POSOLOGY

Objective 13.M.1. Know the definition of posology.

Objective 13.M.2. Recognize nine factors that may influence drug dosage.

Posology is the study of drug dosages, i.e., the amount of drug to be used under certain circumstances. The drug manufacturers and reference sources, such as USP, list the official, average, or usual adult dosage. These are guides which are not regulations, but they have medicolegal implications.

A drug response, and often the magnitude of response, is related to the concentration of drug at the site of action. This concentration is related to the volume of distribution of the drug. Since the volume of body water is related to body mass, weight has an influence on the amount of drug prescribed, and smaller persons require a lesser amount of drug than larger persons to produce the same effect. The weight of the patient is an important factor concerned with drug dosage and is discussed below.

Factors That Influence Drug Dosage

Age and Weight. The average adult is considered to be 18 to 65 years old and weigh 70 kg (154 lb). Child patients and the elderly deserve special attention, for they generally require reduced dosages. This is because these two groups of patients generally have altered:

1. rates of absorption
2. distribution (fluid volume)
3. metabolism
4. excretion

Methods of Calculating Dosages for Children.
1. Age, use Young's rule:

$$\frac{\text{Age of patient}}{\text{Age of patient} + 12} \times \text{adult dose for child}$$

This method of calculating drug dosage is probably the least reliable compared to Clark's rule or the body surface rule (see below); There often is not a good correlation between body surface areas and age.

2. Weight, use Clark's rule:

$$\frac{\text{Weight of patient}}{150 \text{ lbs}} \times \text{Adult dose} = \frac{\text{Dose for}}{\text{child}}$$

This is a better method of calculating drug dosage than is age. Drug manufacturers' package inserts generally give dosages for children on the basis of mg/kg or mg/lb body weight, which is essentially an application of Clark's rule. Calculation of drug dosage on a mg/kg basis is the best practical method available.

3. Body surface area rule. This is probably the ideal way to calculate drug dosage, but it is also the most difficult method. Several nomograms (e.g., Meyers et al., 1980) have been published, and they can be used for ease of estimation.

Sex. Sex of the patient generally does not alter drug dosages in humans. Since many females are smaller than men, reduced dosages may be advised, but this is based on weight rather than sex. However, adult females generally have a greater percentage of fat than adult males, and this difference may be a factor.

Temperament. This may be a factor, especially when using CNS drugs, for it has been shown that agitated patients more often require increased dosages of CNS depressants than patients who are normal, and vice versa. This concept is discussed in greater depth in Chapter 20.

Route of Administration. Many drugs are partially metabolized by the liver when the agents are taken by the peroral route (the so-called first-pass effect), and they therefore require an increased dose. In addition, lower doses are usually used if the same drug is to be given parenterally, especially IV, rather than perorally. The reason is a decreased rate of absorp-

tion of most drugs by the peroral route compared to parenteral routes.

Concurrent Medications. Some drugs may be supra-additive in the presence of others, and still other drugs may be antagonized (or produce infra-addition). Under these circumstances the drug dose to be used may have to be reduced or increased (see Appendix II, Drug Interactions).

Patient Suggestibility. It is very important to speak in positive terms when discussing a drug with a patient. Certainly, success will be greater and drug dosages may be lower if the practitioner says, when writing a prescription for an analgesic, "Mrs. Jones, I'm *sure* this medication *will* help you with postoperative pain *if* it occurs," rather than, "Mrs. Jones, I think this medication may help you with postoperative pain."

Tolerance. Increasing the dose of a drug is often necessary to achieve the same therapeutic effect. The development of tolerance can occur for a number of agents, especially CNS depressants. When tolerance occurs, increased dosages may be necessary, but this is a danger signal of possible dependence.

Presence of a Disease State. Patients may be more sensitive to a drug in the presence of disease states, such as liver and renal diseases. Since these two organs are responsible for metabolism and excretion of drugs, generally a reduced dose or increased time between doses is required if these organs are compromised.

REFERENCE

Cooper SA, Beaver WT: A model to evaluate mild analgesics in oral surgery outpatients. Clin Pharmacol Ther 30:241, 1975

BIBLIOGRAPHY

Accepted Dental Therapeutics, 38th ed. Chicago, American Dental Association, 1979, Sec I, Prescription Writing

DiPalma JR (ed): Drill's Pharmacology in Medicine, 4th ed. New York, McGraw-Hill, 1971, Ch 2, 6

Gilman AG, Goodman LS, Gilman A (eds): Goodman and Gilman's The Pharmacological Basis of Therapeutics, 6th ed. New York, Macmillan, 1980, App I

Goldstein A, Aronow L, Kalman SM: Principles of Drug Action: The Basis of Pharmacology, 2nd ed. New York, Wiley, 1974

Goth A: Medical Pharmacology, 10th ed. St. Louis, Mosby, 1981, Ch 64

Melmon KL, Morelli HF (eds): Clinical Pharmacology: Basic Principles in Therapeutics, 2nd ed. New York, Macmillan, 1978, Ch 2, 4

Meyers FH, Jawetz E, Goldfien A: Review of Medical Pharmacology, 7th ed. Los Altos, CA, Lange, 1980

1982 USP DI. Rockville, MD, USP Convention Inc., 1982

QUESTIONS

1. **T F** Pharmacology is the application of drugs in human therapy.

2–6. Match

     2. __D__ Actions   **A.** Amount of drug used

     3. __C__ Description   **B.** Cautions

     4. __A__ Dosage   **C.** Chemical class

     5. __E__ Indications   **D.** Pharmacologic response

     6. __B__ Warnings   **E.** Usefulness

7. **T F** A contraindication for a drug describes only conditions where the drug should never be used.

8. **T F** Drugs are usually first screened for pharmacologic properties that may be beneficial in human therapy, and then toxicologic screening is usually started.

9. **T F** Although toxicologic screens in animals are important in drug testing, pharmacologic screens in animals are not helpful because effectiveness can only be determined in human testing.

10. **T F** Chronic toxicity is usually determined in animals, in LD_{50} studies, in which injected drugs cause death within 48 hours.

11. The easiest point to determine on a lethal dose-response curve is the:

     A. LD_5
     B. LD_{50}
     C. LD_{95}
     D. LD_{99}

12. In animal experiments, the easiest dose to determine on a dose-response curve is:

     A. ceiling
     B. threshold
     C. ascending
     D. none of the above

13. Which of the following can be determined in one animal?

     A. lethal dose curve
     B. an agonist dose-response curve
     C. LD_{50}
     D. none of the above

14. In order to effectively use drug A in humans, it has to be used at its TD_5. This means that:

     A. only 5% of the human dose should be given as a starter
     B. if five patients are treated, one will probably show toxicity
     C. after treating a great number of patients, about five out of a hundred will probably show toxicity
     D. if drug A were a "–caine" local anesthetic, it would probably not cause too many problems in dental office use

15. IND refers to:

    A. a Federal agency of the government
    B. laboratory animal phase of testing a new drug
    C. a status where the drug firm can freely market the drug without further testing but with monitoring of adverse reactions.
    D. the human phases of testing a new drug

16. A company must report adverse effects of a drug to:

    A. Food and Drug Administration
    B. Drug Enforcement Administration
    C. a leading journal in the discipline
    D. the American Dental Association

17. A manufacturer may recommend that the dental practitioner may prescribe a drug for humans after:

    A. IND application is approved
    B. NDA application is approved
    C. Phase I clinical studies are completed
    D. animal testing for toxicity is completed

18. T F Phase II testing in humans involves a large-scale clinical trial.

19. Which of the following statements is correct concerning IND investigation?

    A. it occurs in two phases of testing, phase I and phase II.
    B. Phase I involves pharmacologic studies in a limited number of human subjects.
    C. after Phase II is completed the company can receive NDA approval.
    D. the true human toxicity of a drug is usually determined.

20. A drug for human use is best administered at:

    A. the LD_{50} in mice
    B. either the LD_{50} in mice or the LD_{50} in rats, whichever is lower
    C. TD_5 in humans if known and acceptable effectiveness is obtained
    D. TD_1 in humans if known and acceptable effectiveness is obtained

21. A graded dose-response curve can be used to describe all of the following **except:**

    A. hypotensive effect
    B. lethal effect
    C. hypertensive effect
    D. local anesthetic block on nerve

22. T F Plotting data on effectiveness of drugs usually yields a graded dose-response curve.

23. The therapeutic index of a drug is usually first defined as:

    A. $\dfrac{ED_{50}}{LD_{50}}$

    B. $\dfrac{LD_{50}}{ED_{95}}$

    C. $\dfrac{LD_5}{ED_{95}}$

    D. $\dfrac{LD_{50}}{ED_{50}}$

24. The therapeutic advantage of a new drug compared to an older drug is best defined by its:

    A. TI (animal)
    B. TI (human)
    C. Margin of safety
    D. Relative safety index

25. T F The use of erythrosine in disclosing plaque is an example of a drug with a low risk:benefit ratio.

26. T F The placebo effect occurs only when a nonactive drug is used.

27. T F A drug may appear to have a more pronounced desired effect if there are no noticeable side effects.

28. T F A placebo effect is usually more noticeable when treating the central nervous system than when treating infection.

29. In treating pain with morphine, the placebo effect will usually account for:

    A. about 10% of the expected effect
    B. about 40% of the expected effect
    C. almost all of the expected effect
    D. almost none of the expected effect

30. T F The dentist is unethical if he takes advantage of the placebo effect.

31. T F Controlled clinical trials cannot be properly performed unless a placebo medication is used.

32. T F A prescription is simply a written or oral order for medication.

33. T F A legend drug is a drug that can be purchased over-the-counter, i.e., a prescription is not needed.

34. T F The Federal Controlled Substances Act takes precedence over all state acts.

35. According to the Federal Controlled Substances Act, which of the following schedules contains drugs that cannot be prescribed?

    A. Schedule I
    B. Schedule II
    C. Schedule III
    D. Schedule IV
    E. Schedule V

36. According to the Federal Controlled Substances Act, which of the following schedules contains prescription drugs that cannot be refilled?

    A. Schedule I
    B. Schedule II
    C. Schedule III
    D. Schedule IV
    E. Schedule V

37. According to the Federal Controlled Substances Act, certain drugs must be ordered by writing the prescription in ink. Which of the following schedules contains such drugs?

    A. Schedule I
    B. Schedule II
    C. Schedule III
    D. Schedule IV
    E. Schedule V

38. T F Both Schedule III and Schedule IV drugs cannot be refilled more than five times within a six-month period after the prescription is written.

39. Which of the following parts of a prescription includes the R_x symbol?

    A. signa
    B. inscription
    C. subscription
    D. superscription
    E. none of the above is correct

40. Which of the following preprinted parts of a prescription includes the practitioner's name and address?

    A. signa
    B. inscription
    C. subscription
    D. superscription
    E. none of the above is correct

41. Which of the following parts of a prescription includes the age of the patient?

    A. signa
    B. inscription
    C. subscription
    D. superscription
    E. none of the above is correct

42. Which of the following parts of a prescription includes information about drugs, i.e., name of drug, dosage, and dosage form?

    A. signa
    B. inscription
    C. subscription
    D. superscription
    E. none of the above is correct

43. Which of the following parts of a prescription includes directions to the pharmacist?

    A. signa
    B. inscription
    C. subscription
    D. superscription
    E. none of the above is correct

44. Which of the following parts of a prescription includes directions to the patient?

    A. signa
    B. inscription
    C. subscription
    D. superscription
    E. none of the above is correct

45. Which of the following parts of a prescription includes the practitioner's signature and degree?

    A. signa
    B. inscription
    C. subscription
    D. superscription
    E. none of the above is correct

46. Which of the following parts of a prescription includes the date?

    A. signa
    B. inscription
    C. subscription
    D. superscription
    E. none of the above is correct

47. Which of the following parts of a prescription includes the patient's name and address?

    A. signa
    B. inscription
    C. subscription
    D. superscription
    E. none of the above is correct

48. Which of the following parts of a prescription includes the practitioner's DEA number?

    A. signa
    B. inscription
    C. subscription
    D. superscription
    E. none of the above is correct

49. The Latin abbreviation for "at bedtime" is:

    A. a
    B. ac
    C. hs
    D. ss
    E. prn

50. The Latin abbreviation for "immediately" is:

    A. aq
    B. gtt
    C. qid
    D. sig
    E. stat

51. **T F** Ideally, a carbon copy of all prescriptions should be kept on file in every practitioner's office.

52. **T F** A dental practitioner may not legally dispense drugs, even though the drugs are used as part of dental practice.

53. **T F** A dentist may legally order any prescription drug.

54. **T F** Practitioners should never postdate prescriptions.

55. **T F** Metrology is the study of drug dosages.

56. One-half grain from the apothecary system is approximately equal to how many mg of the metric system?

   A. 8
   B. 15
   C. 30
   D. 60

57. One apothecary teaspoon is approximately equal to:

   A. 0.1 ml
   B. 5 ml
   C. 15 ml
   D. 30 ml

58. **T F** Posology is the study of weights and measures.

59. **T F** Infants and elderly patients generally require reduced drug dosages.

60. The usual adult dose of a drug is 90 mg. Therefore, using Clark's rule for a 6-year-old patient weighing 75 lbs, the correct drug dosage would be:

   A. 15 mg
   B. 30 mg
   C. 45 mg
   D. 60 mg

61. **T F** An agitated patient may require an increased dose of a central nervous system depressant drug.

62. **T F** Generally, an IV drug is given at a lower dose than if the same drug is given by mouth.

63. Generally, increased dosages of a drug are required when a patient:

   A. exhibits tolerance
   B. is highly suggestible
   C. takes concurrent medications
   D. has a diseased liver or kidneys

14

Toxicology in Dentistry

A. PRINCIPLES OF TOXICOLOGY

Objective 14.A.1. Recognize the definitions of toxicology, toxicity, acute toxicity, and chronic toxicity.

Toxicology is the science of poisons, their effects, and their antidotes. As it applies to dentistry, toxicology refers to the toxicity of drugs (including chemicals) used in the delivery of dental care and the prevention and treatment of that toxicity. The **toxicity** of a drug or chemical is defined as the adverse effects of the agent which are due to actions at relative or absolute overdosage (relative overdosage refers to induction of adverse effects at a dose considered normal, while absolute overdosage refers to adverse effects when a dose greater than a normal is given). **Acute toxicity** refers to the toxicity of a drug caused by exposure of an individual to a single, excessive dose, e.g., the ingestion of an entire bottle of capsules by a patient who is attempting to commit suicide. **Chronic toxicity,** on the other hand, implies the toxic effects of a drug or other chemical due to exposure to relatively low doses over prolonged periods of time,

e.g., the development of mercury poisoning in dentists working for long periods in operatories contaminated with elemental mercury (see below).

Objective 14.A.2. Recognize the definitions of LD_{50}, ED_{50}, therapeutic index (TI), margin of safety (MS), and threshold limit value (TLV).

Drugs and other chemicals possess varying degrees of toxicity in man and other animals which can be quantitated under experimental conditions. The methodology for such quantitation was described in Chapter 13. In review, you will recall that LD_{50} is the **median lethal dose,** or that dose of a drug which results in the death of 50% of the experimental animals tested, on an acute or chronic basis. The relationship between LD_{50} and the **median effective dose** (ED_{50}, or that dose which produces 50% of the therapeutic response) is the therapeutic index (TI) of the drug. The TI is, therefore, an expression of the relative safety of the drug, and its mathematical development was presented in Figure 13–3. Obviously, the greater the value of the TI, the greater the relative safety of the drug. The use of TI is necessary because no matter how large the lethal dose, if an equally large dose is needed to achieve a therapeutic response, no advantage is gained. The margin of safety of a drug is the absolute difference between the LD_{50} and the ED_{50}, or the same as TI when the two are plotted on a logarithmic scale.

Another term of occupational importance to the dentist is the threshold limit value (TLV). This is the level of an environmental contaminant below which no adverse effects or toxic effects will occur in persons exposed to the contaminant for 40 hours a week.

Relative safety index (RSI) and risk:benefit ratio (RBR) are measures of drug usefulness and were discussed in Chapter 13.

Objective 14.A.3. Describe the factors that determine the toxicity of a drug or other chemical.

There are several factors that determine the toxicity of a given compound, and during a toxic reaction, they all undoubtedly influence the overall toxicologic picture.

Potency of the Agent. Generally, agents of lower potency require greater quantities to produce toxicity than do more potent agents. Toxicity can be produced by most therapeutic agents, however, if sufficient quantities are present.

Time Course of Exposure and Amount of Drug or Chemical Involved. As discussed above, acute toxicity implies exposure to relatively large quantities of a chemical in a single dose. When smaller doses are involved, toxicity usually occurs as a slower developing, chronic event, depending on the cumulation of the effects of the agent and other factors.

Route of Administration. As discussed in Chapter 12, the route of administration of a given agent can determine the rapidity with which its effects are manifested and, indeed, whether the agent exerts any effect at all. For example, the neuromuscular blocking agent, curare, can kill when sufficient quantities are given parenterally, although the drug is not dangerous when ingested by the oral route, since very little is absorbed from the GI tract.

Site of Toxic Action. Toxic agents may exert their actions systemically but also at the site of application or tissue of absorption. Systemic toxicity refers to the toxic effects of an agent that is widely distributed by the circulation, usually involving one or more of the body's organ systems. An example of systemic toxicity is seen when local anesthetics are accidentally injected into a vessel, resulting in central nervous system symptoms and cardiovascular depression. Local toxicity, on the other hand, refers to the toxic effects of an agent in a localized part of the body, usually at the site of application or exposure to the agent. Local toxicity is frequently described as skin irritation, local tissue necrosis, erythema, or abscess formation. An example of local toxicity is seen when vasoconstrictors are infused intravenously. Some vasoconstrictor may escape, producing ischemic tissue necrosis at the injection site.

Pharmacokinetics. Once a toxic agent is absorbed, the processes of distribution, metabolism, and excretion of the compound can determine the blood level of the agent and, hence, the nature and severity of its toxicity. A brief summary of these processes, as they affect toxicity, is presented below:

1. Distribution increases toxicity by:
   a. exposure of target tissues
   b. high blood flow to target tissues
   c. release of toxic agent from protein
2. Distribution processes can decrease toxicity by:
   a. low blood flow rate to target tissues
   b. binding of toxic agent to inert sites (protein)
3. Metabolism can increase toxicity by:
   a. metabolic conversion of nontoxic agent to toxic form
   b. genetic inability to detoxify the agent
   c. pathologic inability to detoxify the agent
4. Metabolism can decrease toxicity by metabolic conversion of toxic form to nontoxic form

5. Excretion processes can increase toxicity by:
   a. impaired renal function
   b. urinary pH which favors reabsorption of the agent
6. Excretion can decrease toxicity by:
   a. enhanced or maintained renal excretion rate
   b. urinary pH which favors excretion of the agent

Administration of Antidotes and Supportive Measures. The nature and severity of a toxic reaction can be greatly influenced by the use of specific antidotes (if they exist), as well as by administration of supportive therapy (IV fluids, correction of blood pH). As an example, an antidote for narcotic-analgesics will reverse the profound respiratory depression. If a narcotic antagonist (e.g., naloxone) is quickly administered, the patient begins to breathe normally. Oxygen and positive-pressure ventilation will also help the patient. However, if respiratory depression is caused by a barbiturate, a good antidote is not known, and a fatal outcome can be avoided only by artificial ventilation and oxygen. Another approach to emergency treatment of drug toxicity is induction of emesis, or vomiting. Caution must be used in this approach, since the vomitus may be aspirated into the lungs. Further discussion of these approaches occurs in various chapters under the appropriate drugs and in Appendix I.

In summary, the blood level of the offending agent plays a great role in determining its toxicity. Pharmacokinetics plays an important role in determining blood levels. Prevention is important, because treatment of toxicity is often difficult.

B. MERCURY

Objective 14.B.1. Describe forms of mercury and the most toxicologically important form in dentistry.

The most widely used heavy metal in dentistry is mercury. Mercury can exist in three forms: elemental mercury, organic mercurial compounds (e.g., mercurial diuretics), and inorganic mercurial salts. Elemental mercury, the form used in dentistry to make silver amalgam, is the most volatile of the three forms and presents the greatest danger to the practicing dentist.

Objective 14.B.2. Describe the routes of absorption and the metabolism of elemental mercury.

Once vaporized, elemental mercury crosses all cell membranes and is usually absorbed as an environmental contaminant through the lung tissues and skin. The dissolved mercury vapor is metabolized to mercuric ion by red blood cells and exerts effects as described below.

Objective 14.B.3. Describe the mechanism of toxicity of mercury.

Divalent mercuric ion is able to form covalent bonds with sulfur. Since many enzymes in the body contain sulfhydryl groups, divalent mercury is capable of reacting with these groups to form mercaptides, resulting in enzyme inactivation with impaired cellular metabolism and synthetic processes. For example, the sulfhydryl group of the amino acid cysteine may combine with mercury (Fig. 14–1).

Since blood flow to the brain is very high, it is likely that large quantities of mercury vapor enter brain tissues before being oxidized, resulting in a greater incidence of central toxic effects than is seen with the other forms of mercury.

Objective 14.B.4. Describe the signs and symptoms of mercury toxicity.

Mercury toxicity in the dental office is usually caused by inhalation of vapor and skin contact over prolonged periods. The severity of the toxic reaction depends, of course, on the blood level of mercury resulting from the exposure and the brain levels of mercury present. The most prominent toxic effects are of a central nature and include the following:

1. psychic disturbances—irritability, paranoia
2. tremors
3. speech difficulties—slurring, stammering

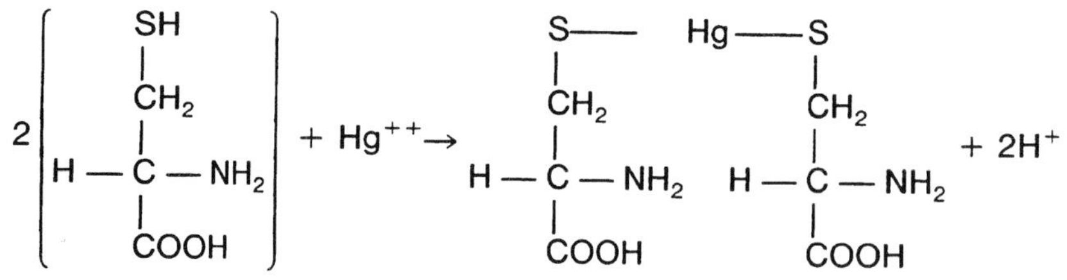

$$2 \begin{bmatrix} SH \\ | \\ CH_2 \\ | \\ H-C-NH_2 \\ | \\ COOH \end{bmatrix} + Hg^{++} \rightarrow \begin{matrix} S-\!\!\!-Hg-\!\!\!-S \\ | \qquad\qquad | \\ CH_2 \qquad CH_2 \\ | \qquad\qquad | \\ H-C-NH_2 \quad H-C-NH_2 \\ | \qquad\qquad | \\ COOH \qquad COOH \end{matrix} + 2H^+$$

Figure 14–1. Chemical Reaction of Hg^{++} with sulfhydryl groups of cysteine.

4. motor disorders and paresthesias—alteration of handwriting, hyperreflexia, numbness
5. visual disturbances
6. renal damage
7. oral manifestations—metallic taste, sialorrhea, gingivitis

Mercury can also cause allergic symptoms in sensitized individuals.

Objective 14.B.5. Describe sources of mercury contamination in the dental office and the means of prevention.

1. Mercury spillage: prevent by safe storage locations, tightly capping mercury containers, using premeasured amalgam capsules, and using nonbreakable mercury containers.
2. Mercury dispersal: prevent by removal of contaminated carpets or rugs, immediate removal of spills using suction with a water trap, using high-volume evacuation and water spray during high-speed removal of old amalgams, covering inaccessible spill sites with powdered sulfur (to prevent vaporization), and avoiding the use of ultrasonic amalgam condensers.
3. Inadequate ventilation: avoid by using open (nonrecirculating) ventilation, change air conditioner filters frequently.
4. Direct skin contact: avoid handling freshly mixed amalgam, use rubber gloves when cleaning mercury spills, wash exposed skin immediately with soap and water.
5. Amalgam scrap: store in tightly closed, nonbreakable containers.

Objective 14.B.6. Describe the treatment of mercury toxicity.

The treatment of chronic mercury intoxication is based on the use of chelating agents and symptomatic measures. Dimercaprol (a dithiol compound, used intramuscularly) and penicillamine or dimethylcysteine (effective orally) are administered to chelate, or bind, mercuric ion, increasing its rate of excretion. Generally, such compounds cannot rapidly or completely reverse cases of chronic intoxication, nor do they effectively reduce brain mercury levels. Reversal of the neurotoxicity of mercury can occur slowly but is often incomplete. Early diagnosis and correction of office conditions offer the best means of dealing with mercury toxicity.

C. NITROUS OXIDE

Although early workers considered nitrous oxide to be innocuous and some clinicians continue to take that view, nitrous oxide has been demonstrated to possess significant chronic toxicity. The acute toxicity of nitrous oxide is rather low and includes potentiation of central respiratory depression (when used with narcotics), simple hypoxia (when used at excessive concentrations), and nausea and vomiting. When chronic exposure occurs, e.g., to dentists and operating room personnel, nitrous oxide is definitely toxic.

Objective 14.C.1. List the chronic toxic effects of nitrous oxide.

The chronic toxic effects of nitrous oxide include:

1. Polyneuropathy, including sensory disturbances (usually numbness), loss of balance, weakness in the legs, and loss of manual dexterity

2. Constipation and spastic bladder—sphincter disturbances
3. Mental depression, impaired memory
4. Depression of spermatogenesis and impotence
5. Spontaneous abortion and fetal malformations
6. Bone marrow changes—megaloblastic anemia, leukopenia

Objective 14.C.2. List sources of nitrous oxide contamination and the means of reducing it in the dental office.

Excessive air concentration, owing to escape of gas, is the major source of nitrous oxide contamination in the dental office. Nitrous oxide is released into the air even when proper technique and equipment are employed. However, other factors may increase this level, such as poor ventilation, lack of a scavenging system, and leaks in tubing and valves. Correction of these problems involves equipment maintenance and use of a scavenging system, in which exhaled nitrous oxide is routed from the nasal mask into the central vacuum system. It is suggested that ambient nitrous oxide concentrations not exceed 50 ppm.

Objective 14.C.3. Describe the possible mechanism of toxicity of nitrous oxide.

While the precise mechanism of action of nitrous oxide toxicity has not been fully elucidated, the neurologic deficits associated with nitrous oxide exposure have been associated with impairment of the neural metabolism of vitamin B_{12}, perhaps by oxidation of the reduced form of the vitamin.

Objective 14.C.4. Recognize the signs and symptoms of the neurologic syndrome which is characteristic of nitrous oxide toxicity.

Layzer (1978) reported a number of neuropathies seen in dentists exposed to prolonged nitrous oxide inhalation, either in the dental operatory or by abuse of the drug. Symptoms included numbness in the extremities, loss of dexterity, poor balance, and weakness. Many of the subjects also showed the Lhermitte sign (an electric-like shock produced by neck flexion), depression, and impairment of thought processes. Laboratory findings included impaired motor and sensory nerve conduction (electromyographically) but no consistent changes in cerebrospinal fluid, blood, or urine. Mercury toxicity was ruled out because of normal urine mercury levels, and chronic mercurial toxicity generally produces more cerebral dysfunction than that noted in these patients.

Objective 14.C.5. Describe the treatment of nitrous oxide toxicity.

The polyneuropathy caused by nitrous oxide is slowly reversible, and this reversal is assisted by the following measures:

1. removal of the victim from further exposure
2. administration of B vitamins (this produces only equivocal results, since there may not be an absolute deficiency of the vitamins)
3. symptomatic support

D. TERATOLOGY

Objective 14.D.1. Define teratology, teratogen, and teratogenicity, and recognize the types of abnormalities drugs may produce in the fetus.

Besides exerting acute and chronic toxicity in patients and practitioners, drugs and other chemicals may have adverse effects on the fetus if given to the mother (Table 14–1). The effects may take different forms, depending on the drug and the phase of pregnancy in which the fetus is exposed. Anatomic malformations may occur if some drugs are given during the third through eleventh weeks of pregnancy. Furthermore, Askrog and Harvald (1970) have shown an increased incidence of spontaneous abortions in nurses and female anesthetists exposed to N_2O and demonstrated a similar risk in the wives of exposed anesthetists.

Generally, all elective dental procedures should be postponed during the first or third tri-

TABLE 14–1. DENTAL DRUGS THAT MAY BE HARMFUL TO THE FETUS AND/OR NEONATE

Period	Drugs	Comment
first trimester	barbiturates	CNS development affected
	narcotic-analgesics	CNS development affected
	tetracyclines	large doses can cause liver damage
second and third trimester	tetracyclines	discoloration of teeth
	aminoglycoside antibiotics	auditory/vestibular nerve damage
neonatal	aspirin	hemorrhage (platelet interference)
(drugs given shortly	phenobarbital	hemorrhage (vitamin K interference)
before birth)	narcotic-analgesics	depressed respiration
	sedatives-hypnotics	depressed respiration
	diazepam	hypotonia and hypothermia
	phenothiazines	extrapyramidal effects
	local anesthetics	neonatal bradycardia
	chloramphenicol	circulatory collapse (gray syndrome)
	sulfonamides	displace bilirubin (kernicterus)
	phenacetin	hemolytic anemia

mester. It is suggested that the dentist consult the mother's physician before administration of drugs during pregnancy, especially if emergency dental procedures are needed late in pregnancy. Nevertheless, small doses of local anesthetics and vasoconstrictors are probably safe for control of pain, as they have not been implicated in teratogenicity. Higher doses of local anesthetics should be avoided if possible, and especially at term (see Table 14–1).

Dental drugs that may be harmful to the fetus are outlined in Table 14–1.

REFERENCES

Askrog V, Harvald B: Teratogenic effect of inhalation anesthetics. Nord Med 83:498, 1970
Layzer RB: Myeloneuropathy after prolonged exposure to nitrous oxide. Lancet 313:1227, 1978

BIBLIOGRAPHY

Berkowitz RL, Coustan DR, Mochizuki TK: Handbook for Prescribing Medications During Pregnancy. Boston, Little, Brown, 1981
Gilman AG, Goodman LS, Gilman A (eds): Goodman and Gilman's The Pharmacological Basis of Therapeutics, 6th ed. New York, Macmillan, 1980, Ch 68

Jastak JT, Greenfield W: Trace contamination of anesthetic gases: a brief review. J Am Dent Assoc 95:758, 1977

QUESTIONS

1. A toxic reaction to a drug produced by a single, above-normal dose of the drug would be considered: (Select one.)

   A. chronic toxicity
   B. relative overdosage
   C. acute toxicity
   D. none of the above

2. Therapeutic index (TI) of a drug is defined as: (Select one.)

   A. ratio of TLV to LD_{50}
   B. ratio of LD_{50} to ED_{50}
   C. ratio of threshold dose to median lethal dose
   D. none of the above

3. T F Generally, agents of lower potency require greater dosages to produce toxicity than do agents with relatively higher potency.

4. **T F** Metabolism of a drug always results in a reduction of its toxicity.

5. The form of mercury which has the greatest potential for causing toxicity in dentists is: (Select one.)

   A. elemental mercury
   B. organic mercurial compounds
   C. inorganic mercurial salts
   D. none of the above

6. **T F** Elemental mercury is usually absorbed via the lungs and skin.

7. Mercuric ion exerts toxic effects by which one of the following mechanisms?

   A. precipitation of anions to form salts
   B. increased cell membrane permeability
   C. combination with sulfhydryl groups of enzyme proteins
   D. none of the above

8. In addition to psychic disturbances and tremors, mercurial toxicity can also be manifested by which of the following symptoms? (Select one answer.)

   A. speech difficulties
   B. metallic taste and sialorrhea
   C. paresthesias
   D. all of the above
   E. none of the above

9. **T F** Amalgam scrap is not considered to be a source of mercury contamination in the dental office.

10. **T F** Reversal of the neurotoxicity of mercury occurs rapidly once the source of mercury contamination is eliminated.

11. **T F** Nitrous oxide toxicity can be associated with mental depression and impaired memory, as well as neurotoxicity.

12. **T F** The major source of nitrous oxide contamination in the dental office is leakiness in valves of storage tanks.

13. **T F** Nitrous oxide toxicity may be associated with alterations in the metabolism of vitamin C.

14. The neurologic syndrome which is characteristic of nitrous oxide toxicity includes which one of the following?

   A. cerebral toxicity identical to that seen with mercury poisoning
   B. marked increases in white cell count in cerebrospinal fluid
   C. loss of dexterity and peripheral numbness
   D. all of the above
   E. none of the above

15. **T F** Besides removal of the victim from the source of nitrous oxide toxicity, specific agents to reverse the syndrome are available as a treatment.

16. **T F** Fetal malformations may occur if teratogens are administered during the third through eleventh weeks of pregnancy.

15
Local Anesthetics

11/15

A. CHEMISTRY AND STRUCTURE-ACTIVITY RELATIONSHIPS

Objective 15.A.1. List three basic components of local anesthetic molecules and describe their importance, including the ester and amide bond.

Local anesthetic drugs consist of three basic components: an aromatic ring which imparts lipid solubility to the molecule, an intermediate aliphatic chain, and a terminal, usually substituted, amino group. This basic structure is illustrated in Figure 15–1. Local anesthetics can be chemically classified into one of two general groups: esters or amides. This distinction is based on the type of chemical bond that links the aromatic residue to the intermediate chain. Ester bonds are formed in the reaction between an aromatic acid and an alcohol, as shown in Figure 15–2. Amide bonds are formed in the reaction between an aromatic amine and an amino acid, as shown in Figure 15–3.

The type of bond present in a given local anesthetic has important clinical implications in that it determines the route of metabolic degradation of the drug, its stability, and, indirectly (by determining the aromatic structure), its allergenicity.

Objective 15.A.2. Describe the general chemical characteristics of the currently available local anesthetics.

Local anesthetics in current use are weak organic bases that are only slightly soluble in water. In the manufacture of injectable solutions of these drugs, the hydrochloride salt is made by treating them with hydrochloric acid, rendering them freely soluble in water. Excess free HCl renders the solution somewhat acidic. Injectable forms of local anesthetics have molecular weights ranging from 270 to 330, although there is greater variation among the topical agents, e.g., the molecular weight of butacaine is 711, while that of benzocaine is 120.

Objective 15.A.3. Describe four structural modifications of local anesthetics that cause increases in potency and toxicity.

The activity of local anesthetics depends on their ability to specifically combine with a critical part of the nerve call membrane, the recep-

117

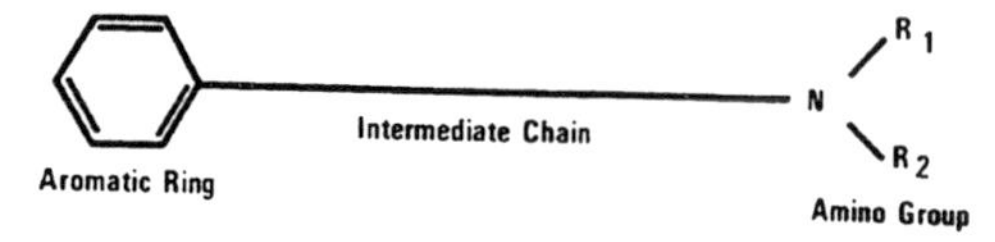

Figure 15–1. The three components of clinically useful local anesthetics.

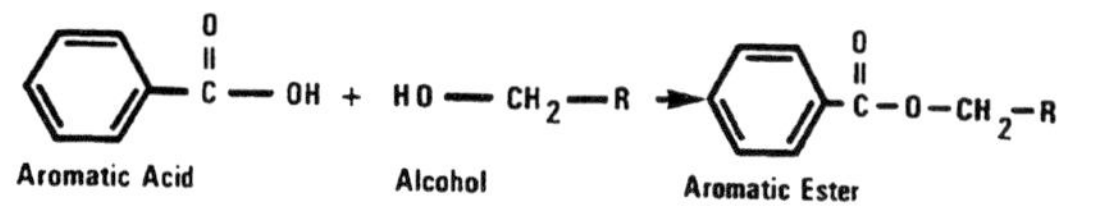

Figure 15–2. Formation of an ester-type local anesthetic molecule.

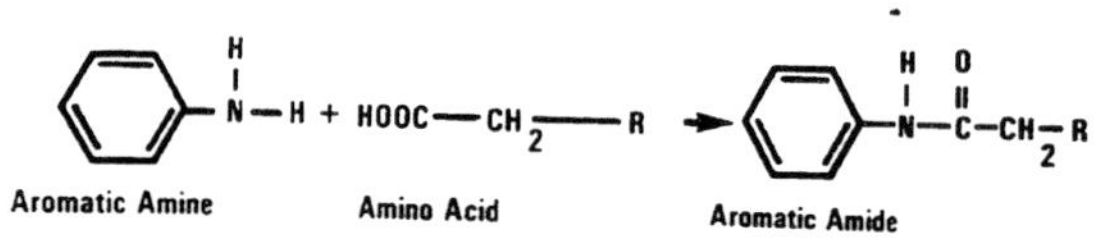

Figure 15–3. Formation of an amide-type local anesthetic molecule.

tor. Because this interaction depends on the spatial and electrical configuration of the drug molecules as well as those of the receptor, alterations of the drug molecule would be expected to change its potency and toxicity. The postulated types of interactions between a local anesthetic and its receptor are diagrammed in Figure 15–4.

Van der Waals interactions are weak, hydrophobic interactions between nonpolar portions of the drug and the receptor. The dipole-dipole interaction between the carbonyl oxygen and the receptor is due to the existence of partial charges, while the electrostatic bond formed at the terminal nitrogen group is due to the presence of fixed charges, with the positive charge on the N atom due to addition of H^+.

The potency and toxicity of local anesthetics may be increased by one of the following measures.

1. Increased length of the intermediate chain (up to five atoms): this presumably increases the hydrophobic (lipophilic) attraction of the drug due to van der Waals forces.
2. Increased length of the terminal nitrogen substituents: this increases potency and toxicity for the same reason as stated above.
3. Addition of electron-donating substituents to the aromatic ring: the effect of this alteration is to push more electrons to the carbonyl oxygen atom, thereby increasing its relative negative charge and, hence, the force of the dipole-dipole interaction.
4. Addition of electron-donating substituents to the intermediate chain: this accomplishes the same effect as in 3.

An example of these structure-activity relationships may be noted by comparing mepivacaine with bupivacaine, as in Figure 15–5. Mepivacaine is approximately equal to lidocaine in potency and toxicity. By increasing the length of the substituent on the terminal nitrogen atom from one carbon to four carbons (e.g., bupivacaine), a large increase in potency and toxicity, as well as duration, occurs. Modifications opposite to those cited above will produce decreases in potency and toxicity. For example, the addition of the electron-withdrawing chlorine atom

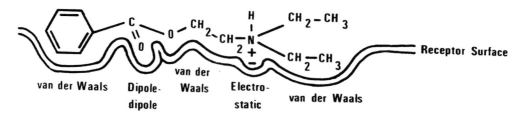

Figure 15–4. Local anesthetic-receptor interaction, showing the potential interactions between various portions of the local anesthetic drug molecule and corresponding sites on the receptor within the nerve cell membrane. (From Buch J, Perlia X: Arzneim Forsch 10:1, 1962.)

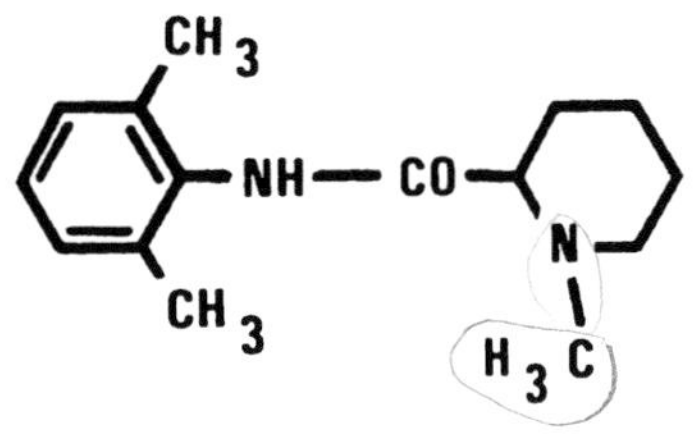

Mepivacaine

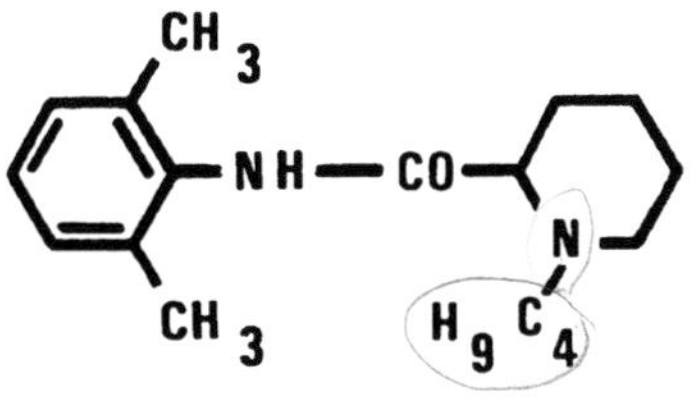

Bupivacaine

Figure 15–5. Chemical structures of mepivacaine and bupivacaine. Note the difference in the length of the N-alkyl group, accounting for the greater potency, toxicity, and duration of action of bupivacaine.

to the structure of procaine (2-chloroprocaine) results in a considerable weakening of the ester bond, with more rapid enzymatic hydrolysis and a radical decrease in toxicity.

B. EFFECTS OF pH

Objective 15.B.1 Be able to describe the qualitative and quantitative effects of pH on the acid-base behavior of local anesthetics.

Since local anesthetics have a tertiary amino nitrogen group, they become positively charged when placed in a relatively acidic environment. The relative quantities of the free base form (uncharged) and the cationic form depend on the pK_a of the local anesthetic and the pH of the solution in which it is placed. The pK_a values of most conventional local anesthetics are between 7.8 and 9.3. The relationship between the free base and the cation is quantitatively described by the Henderson-Hasselbalch equation.

General equation:

$$pH = pK_a + \log \frac{(proton\ acceptor)}{(proton\ donor)}$$

Terms modified for local anesthetics:

$$pH = pK_a + \log \frac{(free\ base)}{(cation)}$$

Since body fluid pH is 7.4, we can use this value in the Henderson-Hasselbalch equation to describe the relative amounts of free base and cation present when a local anesthetic is injected into the body. If we further substitute a mean value of 8.4 for the pK_a of the local anesthetic, we can now predict the relative quantities of the free base and cationic forms of the agent:

$$7.4 = 8.4 + \log \frac{1}{10}$$

The equation is satisfied, because the log of 1/10 is −1. This indicates that at body pH and a local anesthetic pK_a value of 8.4, there is 10 times more of the local anesthetic in the charged form than in the free base form (uncharged). Thus, the more acid the medium, the less free base available.

Objective 15.B.2. Describe the clinical implications of the effect of pH on local anesthetics.

You will recall a general principle of pharmacology that charged molecules do not diffuse through biologic membranes, while uncharged forms (nonpolar) do. This would indicate that in clinical practice the uncharged form of the local anesthetic is the form that actually diffuses into nerves, producing the specific pharmacologic action. The relationship of nerve structure to drug diffusion is shown in Figure 15–6 and explained in the legend.

At normal body pH, there is a sufficient quantity of free base available for diffusion. At reduced pH values, there is correspondingly less free base available, which explains the difficulty in obtaining local anesthesia in an inflamed area, where reduced blood flow and acidic metabolic products reduce tissue pH. Inflammatory changes in nerve membrane structure may also be responsible for this effect (Najjar, 1977).

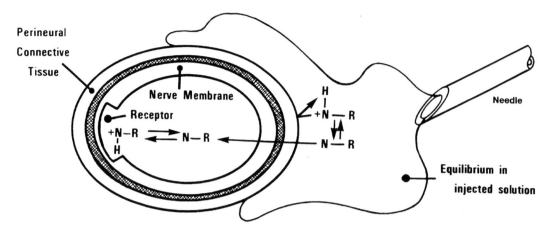

Figure 15–6. Relationship between nerve structure and local anesthetic diffusion. Following injection, the local anesthetic equilibrates in the body fluid (chemical reaction on right), according to the Henderson-Hasselbalch equation, forming free base (N—R) and cation (H—N⁺—R). The latter cannot cross the connective tissue sheaths and nerve cell membrane. Only the free base (uncharged form) can cross. However, once inside the nerve, a new equilibrium between free base and cation is established (chemical reaction on left). The intracellular cationic form is thought to combine with the receptor within the sodium channel (see also Fig. 15–7).

C. THE ACTIVE FORM OF LOCAL ANESTHETICS

Objective 15.C.1. Identify the active (nerve-blocking form of a local anesthetic.

Prior to 1966, the active form of local anesthetics was believed to be the uncharged free base, since isolated nerve preparations were blocked more effectively by local anesthetics when the pH of the bathing medium was basic. Ritchie and Greengard (1966), however, suggested that this observation was explained by the perineural connective tissue barrier which limits the diffusion of the drugs. Increasing the pH in the perineural medium also increases the diffusion of the drug into the neurons. They further demonstrated that when such biologic barriers were circumvented by preloading the nerve with local anesthetic, nerve block was increased by acidic pH and was actually reduced when the bathing medium pH was alkaline. They concluded, therefore, that the cationic form of the local anesthetic was the active form,

since it is the dominant form at lower pH values. Later, this conclusion was supported by experiments demonstrating that quaternary ammonium local anesthetics (which are always charged) were effective in blocking conduction in axons of giant squid only when they were infused intracellularly. (Such drugs must be infused because their charge prevents adequate quantities from diffusing into the nerve from the extracellular space.)

D. ELECTROPHYSIOLOGIC EFFECTS OF LOCAL ANESTHETICS

Objective 15.D.1. Describe the mechanism by which nerve impulse generation and conduction occur.

You will recall from physiology that in the resting state, the nerve cell is polarized. This occurs because a small excess of positive ions (K⁺) diffuses outward from intracellular to extracellular space, leaving a relative excess of

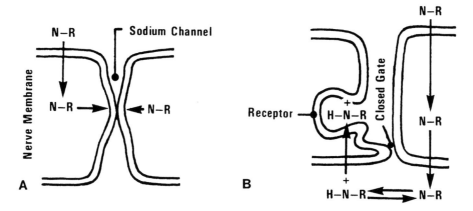

Figure 15–7. Two mechanisms that may explain local anesthesia. **A.** Physicochemical mechanism. In diagram **A**, the free base form (N—R) of the local anesthetic enters the lipid core of the nerve cell membrane. When sufficient quantities of the anesthetic agent have entered the core, lateral pressure deforms the sodium channel, reducing sodium permeability. **B.** Receptor mechanism. In diagram **B**, N—R enters the cell by passing through the entire membrane. On the inside of the cell, N—R equilibrates, forming cations (H—N—R), which can enter the aqueous sodium channel, combining with the receptor, which closes the gate of the sodium channel and results in decreased sodium permeability. *Note:* the gate is illustrated here as being separate from the receptor, but other configurations are possible. (Adapted from Hille B. J Gen Physiol 69:497, 1977.)

negative charges within the nerve cell. The inside of the nerve membrane is, therefore, relatively negatively charged (about −90 mV). In the resting state, the nerve cell membrane is ordinarily impermeable to sodium ions. However, when stimulated, the permeability of the nerve cell membrane to sodium significantly increases, resulting in an inward current of Na⁺, or depolarization. Actually, the influx of Na⁺ is so great that a reversal of membrane potential occurs to about +30 mV. Such changes result in the action potential which is conducted along the nerve because a depolarization in one segment of the membrane excites an adjacent segment, which then becomes sufficiently permeable to sodium for depolarization to continue.

Objective 15.D.2. Describe two mechanisms by which local anesthetics may block nerve impulse generation and conduction.

Local anesthetics block the generation and conduction of the nerve impulses by preventing the transient increase in sodium permeability

that ordinarily accompanies stimulation of the nerve. Sodium permeability is now considered to be a function of a transmembrane sodium channel, which may be opened or closed by a gate mechanism situated on the intracellular aspect of the channel (Fig. 15-7). The evidence for this, recently reviewed by Hille (1977) and Ritchie (1979), indicates that the clinically useful local anesthetics may act to keep the sodium channel closed by two means:

1. Physicochemical mechanism (Fig. 15-7A): the uncharged, free base form of the local anesthetic enters the lipoid, central core of the nerve cell membrane, where accumulation of local anesthetic molecules may increase the lateral pressure against the sodium channel, thereby resisting the forces which tend to open the sodium channel during the action potential.

2. Receptor interaction (Fig. 15-7B): after crossing the cell membrane, the cationic form of the local anesthetic combines with a receptor located near the intracellular aspect

of the sodium channel. Such an interaction presumably results in a change in the conformation of the channel gate, so that the gate remains closed (Fig. 15–7B).

Objective 15.D.3. Describe effects of local anesthetics on electrophysiologic parameters of nerves.

Impairment of sodium movement across the nerve membrane by local anesthetics results in the following effects on single nerves:

1. There is no change in the resting transmembrane potential.
2. There is a decrease in the height of the action potential (the amount of depolarization that occurs).
3. There is a decrease in the rate at which depolarization occurs.
4. There is a decrease in the velocity at which impulse conduction occurs.
5. There is an increase in the amount of depolarization (stimulus strength) that is required to give rise to an action potential (threshold is increased).

When nerve block is complete, the action potential cannot be generated or conducted. However, the effects listed above are a spectrum of events, occurring over a time interval, and if various phases do not proceed to completion, only partial block may occur.

E. PHARMACOLOGIC AND TOXIC EFFECTS

Objective 15.E.1. Describe the actions of local anesthetics on sensory nerves and on neural sensation.

The effect of local anesthetics on nerve impulse generation and conduction is also exerted on other excitable tissues, including cardiac and vascular smooth muscle. When properly used in clinical dentistry, the nerve-blocking effects of local anesthetics are restricted to local areas, and systemic effects are not noted. When locally injected, these drugs block the sensation of pain

first, followed, in order, by the sensations of cold, warmth, touch, and deep pressure. The sensation of deep pressure is seldom completely abolished in clinical practice, and the patient, as well as the dentist, should be aware that a continued sense of pressure should not be mistaken for inadequate anesthesia. The initial abolition of pain is related to the smaller diameter of the pain-conducting fibers. Smaller fibers and those with less myelination tend to be blocked faster and more completely than those of larger diameter and those with relatively greater degrees of myelination. This is probably due to the fact that the smaller fibers and those with less myelin equilibrate with the local anesthetic more rapidly and completely because of a more favorable surface:volume ratio and less membrane barriers to diffusion. However, the sequence of block is reversed when the anesthetic is removed, with pain being the last sensation to reappear.

Objective 15.E.2. Describe pharmacologic actions of toxic blood levels of local anesthetic in the systemic circulation.

Signs of systemic local anesthetic toxicity may be seen when the agent is accidentally injected intravascularly, when excessive doses are used, or when metabolic degradation of the local anesthetic cannot keep pace with its rate of absorption. These signs are initially attributable to effects of the local anesthetic on the central nervous system and may consist of central excitation or central depression. Central excitation begins to manifest itself as restlessness, talkativeness, sweating, and nervousness and may then proceed to muscle twitching, tremors, and, finally, generalized convulsions. The convulsive episode is followed by profound central nervous system depression, and this must be treated by supportive measures, especially respiratory assistance, with an awareness that any central depressant drugs administered during the convulsions may aggravate this postseizure depression, e.g., barbiturates (except for ultrashort-acting forms). Both lidocaine and mepivacaine may produce initial symptoms of CNS depression, but later ataxia and restlessness may occur, followed by the usual, typical local anesthetic convulsion (as seen with procaine) resulting in the same symptoms of excitement, tremors, and convulsions. Initiation of supportive measures, including respiratory assistance and O_2, in any type of local anesthetic overdose is important.

Objective 15.E.3. Describe cardiovascular effects of toxic blood levels of local anesthetics.

During a toxic reaction to an excessive blood level of local anesthetic, a variety of cardiovascular effects may occur. Such cardiovascular effects are due to three concurrent phenomena: (1) central excitation or depression with parallel changes in autonomic drive to the heart and blood vessels, (2) a direct depression of myocardium and vascular smooth muscle by the local anesthetic, and (3) vasoconstriction and cardiac stimulation if a vasoconstrictor is present. Thus, it is difficult to be able to predict the cardiovascular status of the patient during a local anesthetic reaction. However, during the postseizure period of central depression, the cardiovascular system can literally collapse, with hypotension, severe bradycardia, and even possible cardiac standstill.

Objective 15.E.4. List the clinical measures used to treat local anesthetic toxicity.

Local anesthetic toxicity is treated symptomatically. With the onset of any sign of a toxic blood level, the injection should be immediately terminated and intervention begun. Frequently, a psychogenic reaction may be confused with a toxic overdose. Psychogenic reactions are syncopal, with the patient experiencing dizziness, lightheadedness, sweating, loss of color, and fainting, with a rapid pulse rate. Placement of the patient in the Trendelenburg position usually alleviates this type of reaction.

If simple psychogenic reaction is ruled out because of the presence of the signs of central excitation or depression, the patient should be placed in a supine position. If convulsions develop, the dentist should administer O_2 and prevent the patient from possible harm from the movements. If necessary, diazepam (*Valium*) 5 to 10 mg (adult dose) IV may be given and re-

peated in 20 to 30 minutes if needed. This is preferred to most barbiturates, which will produce a greater degree of additional respiratory depression. The airway of the patient must be assured, and cardiopulmonary resuscitation must be instituted if cardiac or pulmonary functions are absent. Resuscitation should be followed by cardiac monitoring with ECG, since the development of cardiac arrhythmias is a likely occurrence. If blood pressure drops, efforts at its restoration should include IV fluid administration and pressor drugs (Appendix I).

F. METABOLISM AND EXCRETION

Objective 15.F.1. Describe the mechanisms by which the ester and amide local anesthetics are inactivated in the body and their major route of excretion.

Local anesthetics are metabolically inactivated by two separate enzymatic mechanisms, depending on their chemical classification. Amide-type agents are broken down exclusively by liver enzymes (e.g., N-dealkylases and amidases). Therefore, the relative toxicity of amide local anesthetics is increased in patients with liver disease. This requires a reduction in the amount of the amide local anesthetic that can safely be used or the alternative use of an ester-type agent. The metabolic breakdown products of the amides are excreted almost entirely by the kidney. Ester-type anesthetics, on the other hand, are metabolized primarily in the blood by plasma pseudocholinesterase, which rapidly hydrolyzes the ester. Since hydrolysis of esters is more rapid than hepatic degradation of the amides, ester-type local anesthetics tend to be somewhat less toxic. Esters are also metabolized by cholinesterase enzymes in other tissues of the body. While esters can be used safely in patients with liver disease, caution must be exercised in patients with genetic deficiencies in plasma pseudocholinesterase. In patients with genetically determined atypical plasma cholinesterase, esters should not be used. Similarly, succinylcholine should be avoided during general anesthesia, since it is also metabolized by the same enzyme. Ester-type local anesthetics which are para-aminobenzoic acid derivatives should not be used in patients taking sulfonamides, as one of the breakdown products, para-aminobenzoic acid, antagonizes the action of this group of antibacterials. The breakdown products of the ester-type local anesthetics are excreted entirely by the kidney.

G. LOCAL ANESTHETIC ALLERGY

Objective 15.G.1. Describe the relative frequency of ester vs amide local anesthetic allergy, the role of local anesthetic preservatives in producing allergic responses, the symptoms of allergic reactions, and an alternative drug to be used in documented cases of local anesthetic allergy.

It is now appreciated that the incidence of true allergy to local anesthetics is extremely low, although the ester-type agents, especially para-aminobenzoic acid derivatives, are known to be allergenic in some individuals. The incidence of documented allergy to amide-type drugs is considerably less. In addition to the local anesthetic drug's acting as an allergen, the paraben preservatives used in many preparations are known allergens. Patients may be exposed to paraben preservatives in injectable drugs, OTC medications, and all forms of cosmetics. A history of contact dermatitis-type reaction to such preparations in a patient should alert the practitioner to the possibility of a reaction to a local anesthetic solution (Luebke, Walker, 1978).

Preventive measures are the best means of dealing with local anesthetic allergic reactions, especially in the form of a good health history with particular attention to reports of allergic reactions. It is your obligation to establish its nature and whether a local anesthetic allergy is really present. If the patient reports that he experienced an "allergic reaction" to a local anesthetic in the form of syncope or simple nausea in the absence of other definitive signs, the reaction was probably not true allergy, and exercising caution by starting with low doses of anesthetic may be all that is necessary. However, if such true signs of allergy as rash, urticaria, hypotension, and bronchospasm were noted, an allergist should confirm the offending allergen before further dental treatment is administered. The dentist should also make certain that specific local anesthetics tested do not also contain parabens.

If allergy is due to an ester, an amide local anesthetic should be used, but the preparation used should not contain paraben preservatives. *Carbocaine* in dental cartridges contains no paraben, but multidose vials of *Carbocaine* do contain paraben. Apparently, the manufacturers (e.g., Astra) are starting to remove the parabens from lidocaine solutions (J. Oakley, personal communication, 1982), which will allow using such solutions when the patient has an ester-type of paraben allergy.

If the patient is allergic to both ester- and amide-types, an alternative agent that can be used is an antihistamine, e.g., 1% diphenhydramine with 1:100,000 epinephrine (Roberts, Loveless, 1979). If an antihistamine is used, you should expect a less reliable onset, less depth, and shorter duration of local anesthesia than are seen with conventional local anesthetics. In addition, pain and tissue necrosis may occur postoperatively.

If an allergic reaction occurs in spite of preventive measures, the type of treatment administered will depend upon the perceived severity of the reaction. A mild allergic reaction, consisting of a rash, itching, or other dermatologic signs, can be treated with an antihistamine injection (e.g., 50 mg diphenhydramine, IM) followed by careful medical follow-up by an allergist. Severe allergic reactions, such as anaphylaxis with severe hypotension, bronchospasm, or laryngeal edema, are life-threatening emergencies and must be managed immediately. This treatment consists of placing the patient in a supine position, administering epinephrine, 0.3 to 0.5 mg (i.e., 3 to 5 ml of 1:10,000 IV or 0.3 to 0.5 ml of 1:1000 IM or subcutaneously), and giving O_2 and CPR as needed. An antihistamine (50 mg diphenhydramine IM) and a steroid may also be needed.

The cardiovascular condition of the patient must be constantly monitored, since profound hypotension usually accompanies anaphylaxis. Similarly, care must be taken when administering epinephrine intravenously, since dangerous increases in blood pressure may occur. It is equally important to determine heart rate and blood pressure before administration of a second dose of epinephrine in order to avoid such adverse elevations of blood pressure. Following stabilization of the patient's condition, an antihistamine may be given, as well as a steroid, and the patient should be hospitalized for follow-up care.

H. VASOCONSTRICTORS

Objective 15.H.1. List three reasons for adding a vasoconstrictor to local anesthetics.

Objective 15.H.2. List four vasoconstrictors that are used in local anesthetic solutions.

Objective 15.H.3. Describe the precautions and dose limitations to be used in conjunction with local anesthetic solutions containing a vasoconstrictor.

Vasoconstrictors accomplish their function by reducing blood flow in the area of local anesthetic injection. In the first place, they reduce the rate of absorption of the local anesthetic into the circulation, thereby allowing the rate of metabolic degradation to keep pace with the rate of drug absorption and preventing accumulation of a toxic blood level of the anesthetic. Second, by reducing the absorption, the local anesthetic remains in the area of injection for a longer period of time, thereby increasing the duration of action of the local anesthetic. Finally, the presence of a vasoconstrictor contributes to a reduction of hemorrhage in the area of surgery, provided the operative site is the same as the injection site. Some clinicians believe that a 1:50,000 concentration of epinephrine may be used for some reduction of hemorrhage in periodontal surgery. This should be restricted in dosage (see Chapter 1), and the use of vasoconstrictors should not be substituted for careful surgical technique and normal hemorrhage control.

Basically, there are four vasoconstrictors in use in dental local anesthetic solutions: epinephrine (*Adrenalin*), norepinephrine (*Levophed*), levonordefrin (*Neo-Cobefrin*), and phenylephrine (*Neo-Synephrine*). The following list identifies the usual concentrations at which these agents are found in dental cartridges:

Epinephrine
   1:50,000 (recommended only for gingival
      infiltration in periodontal surgery)
   1:100,000
   1:200,000
Norepinephrine 1:30,000 (not recommended)
Levonordefrin 1:20,000
Phenylephrine 1:2,500

Epinephrine exerts both alpha and beta adrenergic effects (see Chapters 16, and 18), which produce not only vasoconstriction but also vasodilation and such cardiac effects as increased rate, increased force, and disposition of the myocardium to the development of arrhythmias. Levonordefrin can act on both types of adrenergic receptors (for safety factors, see below). Norepinephrine acts on alpha receptors and beta receptors of the heart. The actions of phenylephrine are due solely to its effect on alpha adrenergic receptors. Vasoconstrictors can cause significant cardiovascular effects during overdose of local anesthetic solutions. Agents that stimulate the beta receptors of the heart will increase heart rate and the force of contraction and, in the presence of other agents, which irritate the myocardium, will produce cardiac arrhythmias. Irritants of the heart include cyclopropane, halogenated hydrocarbon general anesthetics, digitalis glycosides, and the condition of hyperthyroidism. Significant changes in blood pressure and cardiac function are serious in individuals with cardiovascular disease. The New York Heart Association has recommended (1955) that the maximum dose of epinephrine used in adult patients under dental treatment be limited to no more than 0.2 mg per appointment or 0.003 mg/kg per appointment. We recommend the latter dose for healthy adult patients and further recommend that a lower total dose, such as 0.04 mg, be the maximum for patients with cardiovascular disease (Bennett,

1978). The total volume of solution used could be increased by reducing the epinephrine concentration to 1:200,000. Levonordefrin should be limited to 0.009 mg/kg per appointment in the normal patient and to one-fifth that dose in patients with cardiovascular disease. In normal children, the dose of epinephrine can be calculated on a proportional basis (0.003 mg per kg).

Patients taking antihypertensive medication and/or with diagnosed cardiac arrhythmias demand similar attention in the careful use of vasoconstrictors (Chapter 31, Appendix II). It is suggested that the dentist consult the patient's physician if cardiovascular disease is present. While the physician will frequently insist that no vasoconstrictor be used, the dentist should explain that the greater depth and duration of anesthesia produced by a minimal dose of vasoconstrictor can prevent an acute episode of pain and the accompanying adrenal medullary discharge, which can result in even more serious alterations of cardiovascular function. If both practitioners agree that no vasoconstrictor should be used, local anesthetics without vasoconstrictors are available and have proven satisfactory in many situations (Chapter 1). Alternatively, the practitioners may agree that a low dose of epinephrine (0.04 mg) should be used.

Another result of an excess absorption of vasoconstrictors may be so-called vasovagal discharge, with nervousness, sweating, loss of color, syncope, and nausea. This is a mild reaction, and the patient is usually relieved simply by being placed in a supine position. More serious reactions involve elevations of blood pressure, tachycardia, and cardiac arrhythmias and must be quickly diagnosed and treated (Appendix I).

I. PRESERVATIVES

Objective 15.I.1. Describe two preservatives used in conventional local anesthetic solutions and their function.

Many drugs contain one or more preservatives in order to ensure reasonable shelf life. There are two types of preservatives found in local anesthetic preparations used in the dental profession:

1. Parabens (methyl, ethyl, propyl, and butyl forms): these agents are aliphatic esters of *p*-hydroxybenzoic acid and are in widespread use. These are antibacterial and antifungal and are effective in low concentrations (1 mg/ml in most local anesthetic solutions). They are devoid of systemic actions but have been implicated as allergens in cases of contact dermatitis and will induce allergic reactions in sensitive individuals when injected. Patients may already have experienced contact dermatitis due to parabens because of their frequent use in OTC ointments, lotions, and creams. Paraben sensitivity should be suspected in any allergic reaction to a drug containing parabens. Patients sensitive to one paraben show cross-sensitivity to the other forms.

2. While parabens are primarily antibacterial, sodium bisulfite is an anti-oxidant which is added to local anesthetic solutions that contain a vasoconstrictor, thereby protecting the latter from oxidative destruction. This is nonallergenic and is used in 0.5 mg/ml concentrations (e.g., in *Carbocaine*). Bisulfites may irritate skin and mucosa during contact, but apparently have not caused a problem.

J. LONG-ACTING LOCAL ANESTHETICS

Objective 15.J.1. List two currently used long-acting local anesthetics, their clinical advantages and disadvantages, and their duration of action.

Bupivacaine (*Marcaine*) and etidocaine (*Duranest*) are long-acting local anesthetics which have recently been introduced for general medical use. In oral surgery trials, both agents have been shown to produce a significantly longer duration (twice as long) of anesthesia than lidocaine with 1:100,000 epinephrine. Nespeca (1976) and Laskin JL (1978) reported that both agents produce a significantly longer "time to first pain" and reduction in the vasoconstrictor requirement (etidocaine and bupivacaine were shown to be effective with 1:200,000 epinephrine). Two disadvantages of these agents are:

Marcain (Bupivacaine 0.5% + epi 1/200,000)

1. their current availability only in multidose vials. Recently, the Cooke-Waite Company obtained FDA approval for dental use of 0.5% bupivacaine (_Marcaine_) with 1:200,000 epinephrine from the multidose vial, with a maximum recommended adult dose (per appointment) of 90 mg (Dr. Ken Dean, personal communication, 1982). Astra Pharmaceutical Products is evaluating etidocaine (_Duranest_) for use in dentistry (Dr. J. Oakley, personal communication, 1982). Both agents may become available in dental cartridges.

2. the long duration of numbness is uncomfortable for some patients. This problem is easily dealt with by explaining to the patient before treatment begins that there will be a longer duration of numbness.

Long-acting amides are approximately 10 times as potent and toxic as lidocaine, and their total dosage must be reduced accordingly. Toxic reactions to these local anesthetics resemble those described for the other drugs in this class and are attributable primarily to effects on the central nervous system and the cardiovascular system. While of questionable value in routine, short-duration procedures with minimal trauma, these agents may prove to be valuable adjuncts to long procedures, which typically produce a greater degree of postoperative discomfort, such as in endodontics, periodontics, and oral surgery.

REFERENCES

Bennett CR: Moheim's Local Anesthesia and Pain Control in Dental Practice, 6th ed. St. Louis, Mosby, 1978, p 181

Buchi J, Perlia X: Benziehungen zwischen den physikalischchemischen Eigenschaften und der Wirkung von Lokalanasthetica. Arzneim Forsch 10:1, 1962

Hille G: Local anesthetics: hydrophilic and hydrophobic pathways for the drug-receptor interaction. J Gen Physiol 69:497, 1977

Laskin JL: Use of etidocaine hydrochloride in oral surgery: a clinical study. J Oral Surg 36:863, 1978

Luebke NH, Walker JA: Discussion of sensitivity to preservatives in anesthetics. J Am Dent Assoc 97:656, 1978

Najjar TA: Why can't you achieve adequate regional anesthesia in the presence of infection? Oral Surg 44:7, 1977

Nespeca JA: Clinical trials with bupivacaine in oral surgery. Oral Surg Oral Med Oral Pathol 42:301, 1976

New York Heart Association: Use of epinephrine in connection with procaine in dental procedures. J Am Dent Assoc 50:108, 1955

Ritchie JM: A pharmacological approach to the structure of sodium channels in myelinated axons. Ann Rev Neurosci 2:341, 1979

Ritchie JM, Greengard P: On the mode of action of local anesthetics. Annu Rev Pharmacol 6:405, 1966

Roberts EW, Loveless H. The utilization of diphenhydramine for production of local anesthesia: report of a case. Texas Dent J 97:13, 1979

BIBLIOGRAPHY

Bennett CR: Moheim's Local Anesthesia and Pain Control in Dental Practice, 6th ed. St. Louis, Mosby, 1978

Covino BG, Vassallo H: Local Anesthetics: Mechanisms of Action and Clinical Use. New York, Grune & Stratton, 1976

Ritchie JM, Greene NM: Local anesthetics. In Gilman AG, Goodman LS, Gilman A (eds): The Pharmacological Basis of Therapeutics, 6th ed. New York, Macmillan, 1980, Ch 15

Truant AP, Takman B: Local anesthetics. In DiPalma JR (ed): Drill's Pharmacology in Medicine, 3rd ed. New York, McGraw-Hill, 1965, Ch 11

QUESTIONS

1. In addition to an aromatic ring, typical local anesthetic molecules contain which one of the following chemical components?

   A. an ethyl ether linkage

   B. an intermediate carbon chain

   C. a heterocyclic, nitrogen-containing ring

   D. a hydroxyl group

2. Local anesthetics are available for dental injection in which one of the following forms?

   A. water-insoluble free base

   B. alkalinized

C. water-soluble hydrochloride salts
D. dissolved in glycerin

3. Which one of the following chemical modifications will increase the potency and toxicity of a local anesthetic agent?

A. decreased length of the intermediate chain
B. addition of electron-withdrawing substituents
C. increased length of nitrogen substituents
D. addition of chlorine to the aromatic ring

4. According to the Henderson-Hasselbalch equation, raising the pH of a local anesthetic solution should result in which one of the following effects?

A. relative increase in the amount of free base
B. relative increase in the amount of cation
C. no change in the relative amounts of free base and cation
D. the type of change depends on the temperature of the solution

5. Which one of the following forms of local anesthetics is capable of penetrating connective tissues around nerves?

A. free base
B. cation
C. both of the above
D. neither of the above

6. According to the experiments of Ritchie and Greengard, which one of the following is the active (nerve-blocking) form of a local anesthetic?

A. free base
B. cation
C. both of the above
D. neither of the above

7. Under normal conditions, the generation of a nerve impulse results from which one of the following phenomena?

A. An increase in the inward movement of potassium ion
B. a decrease in the inward movement of sodium ion
C. an increase in the inward movement of sodium ion
D. accumulation of calcium ion within organelles

8. In addition to a drug-receptor interaction, local anesthetics may impair nerve function by which one of the following mechanisms?

A. reversible precipitation of nerve membrane proteins
B. increased lateral pressure against the sodium channel
C. occupation of the external opening of the sodium channel
D. chelation of intracellular calcium ion

9. Local anesthetics exert which one of the following effects on the electrophysiologic functions of nerves?

A. increase in resting transmembrane potential
B. increase in the rate of depolarization
C. decrease in the rate of impulse conduction
D. all of the above

10. Which one of the following sensations would be blocked last by local anesthetics?

A. pain
B. cold
C. warmth
D. deep pressure

16

Autonomic Nervous System

11/16

A. IMPORTANCE

Objective 16.A.1. Recognize four reasons why the dentist needs an understanding of autonomic drugs.

Objective 16.A.2. Recognize five situations in dental practice where autonomic drugs are used.

An understanding of the autonomic nervous system (ANS) is useful in dental practice for a number of reasons; four are listed below:

1. Dental patients are in a fearful or stressful situation while anticipating and during dental treatment. Fear and anxiety result in stress, which in turn results in activation of sympathetic nervous activity, resulting in changes in visceral structures, such as glands, smooth muscle, and the heart. As part of the sympathetic discharge, the adrenal medulla secretes a mixture of epinephrine and norepinephrine which can also cause the same visceral changes; this tends to reinforce the overall sympathetic response. A knowledge of the ANS is important, therefore, in understanding the reactions of dental patients during the dental encounter.

2. The parasympathetic division of the autonomic nervous system is the main controlling influence in salivary secretion. An understanding of the mechanism of salivary secretion is most important in oral health, since saliva plays a key role in dental caries, periodontal disease, and other aspects of oral health.

3. The dentist may be administering or prescribing autonomic drugs or drugs with ANS side effects for his patients. Some frequently occurring dental situations requiring a knowledge of ANS drugs are as follows:
   a. Epinephrine or other vasoconstrictors are contained in local anesthetic solutions.
   b. Atropine-like drugs, especially propantheline, are used to reduce excessive salivation.
   c. Epinephrine (in addition to other sympathomimetics) is required as an emergency drug.
   d. Occasionally, drugs are used to treat xerostomia.

e. Drugs having autonomic side effects are used by dentists.

4. The patient may be taking autonomic drugs or drugs with autonomic side effects for medical reasons.

Understanding autonomic homeostatic regulation and drug action depends upon a familiarity with autonomic physiology and pharmacology.

B. GENERAL DESCRIPTION OF ANS

Objective 16.B.1. Distinguish between afferent and efferent, somatic efferent and visceral efferent, voluntary and involuntary, and autonomic and automatic.

Objective 16.B.2. Recognize three synonyms (set in bold type) for the autonomic nervous system.

The physiologic regulation of visceral functions is under control of the ANS through motor (efferent) supply of nerve elements to structures, such as the eye, blood vessels, glands, and internal organs. Therefore, the ANS is referred to as **visceral efferent.** This term is of descriptive value and is useful for studying autonomic nerves. The term **afferent** refers to sensory nerves. The ANS has sensory input, both **somatic** (skin and muscle) and visceral (internal organs), but the ANS is considered a motor (visceral efferent) system.

The term **autonomic** may give the impression that the system acts independently (autonomy). Although there appears to be some independence of action in the ANS, the sensory switching mechanisms and control centers in the brain can influence autonomic function. The hypothalamus is thought to be the center of control of the ANS. The term "autonomic" is still used because it is historically and anatomically important. A better term would be **automatic** instead of autonomic, since the ANS is not under voluntary control and operates without conscious decision (thus, automatically or vegetatively). The ANS has also been called the "involuntary nervous system," another term with descriptive value. (However, note that voluntary nerve fibers are also under reflex or involuntary control.)

We may consider the ANS as a network of nerves having **automatic** activity and exerting a partial, constant, controlling influence upon visceral structures. The terms **visceral efferent system** and **involuntary nervous system** may be considered synonymous with ANS. It should be noted that voluntary (somatic afferent) nerves may participate in involuntary reflex arcs, e.g., the withdrawal reflex. The latter operates involuntarily but still is considered part of the voluntary nervous system because somatic efferent nerves can be controlled, either voluntarily or involuntarily, whereas visceral efferent nerves are only involuntary.

C. CLASSIFICATION OF NEURAL SYSTEMS

Objective 16.C.1. Distinguish between craniosacral and thoracolumbar outflow, parasympathetic and sympathetic nervous systems, and anabolic and catabolic functions of the ANS.

Table 16–1 may help to clarify some relationships between different parts of the nervous system. It may be noted that, anatomically, the nervous system has two major divisions: the central nervous system (CNS) and a peripheral network. The CNS consists of structures enclosed in bony cavities, the cranium and the vertebral canal. The peripheral network extends outside of the bony cavities and consists of nerve pathways which innervate the organs of the body. The peripheral pathways also have ganglia attached or interposed at various points; the ganglia contain neural cell bodies. The ANS has representations in both the CNS and peripheral network. A functional classification of the nervous system is described as voluntary and involuntary. Voluntary fibers supply skeletal muscle and may be controlled by the consciousness. Involuntary nervous system refers to autonomic fibers that control visceral structures and cannot be controlled through operation centers of consciousness. (NOTE: the advent of biofeedback,

TABLE 16–1. CLASSIFICATION OF THE NERVOUS SYSTEM

Classification	Divisions	
anatomic	Central nervous system (CNS) enclosed in bony structure, includes cerebral cortex, cerebellum, brainstem, and spinal cord	Peripheral network* all nerve fibers and ganglia outside of the bony structures, includes nerve fibers, ganglia, and plexuses supplying peripheral organs
functional	Somatic efferent system that controls skeletal muscle and is under voluntary control	Visceral efferent (ANS) system that controls visceral structures and is *not* under voluntary control; synonyms: vegetative (functioning involuntarily or unconsciously), automatic, and autonomic

* It is best not to refer to this network as peripheral nervous system because the initials PNS are used for parasympathetic nervous system.

hypnosis, yoga, and similar systems may alter these generalizations, again emphasizing CNS control of the ANS.)

There are two major subdivisions of the ANS, the parasympathetic (PNS) and the sympathetic (SNS) nervous systems. Table 16–2 compares the two subdivisions. The PNS originates in the cranial or sacral regions of the CNS, following the cranial nerves or sacral plexus, respectively, to reach all of the organs controlled by parasympathetic impulses. The SNS originates in the thoracic or lumbar regions of the CNS and follows the thoracic or lumbar ventral roots, respectively, to form the sympathetic pathways. This major anatomic difference between the subdivisions should be noted: **PNS has a craniosacral outflow** while **SNS has a thoracolumbar outflow.** (See also, Figs. 16–1 and 16–2 with descriptions in text.)

Table 16–2 describes major overall functions for each division of the ANS. The PNS causes discrete, anabolic (synthetic) changes which allow organs to restore themselves, conserving energy and aiding in the preparation for action. The mnemonic, "might and sight," applies to the PNS, since it reminds us of anabolism and control of vision, the major PNS functions. The SNS not only regulates discrete organ adjustments (such as regulation of blood pressure) but also can act by massive activity. This occurs when emotions are stimulated or when one is frightened; thus, the mnemonic, "flight or fight," applies to the SNS. During an emergency situation, the organism attempts to either remove the stimulus or remove itself from the stimulus. Thus, stress results in activation of the SNS, resulting in a pattern of changes in various body organs. The specific SNS changes of different organs and tissues are mostly catabolic (energy yielding) and will be described later.

The differences between SNS and PNS, in structure and function, are emphasized, since this is a basis for understanding the actions of the ANS and related drugs.

TABLE 16–2. COMPARISON OF PNS AND SNS

	PNS (Parasympathetic)	SNS (Sympathetic)
outflow (origin and pathway)	craniosacral	thoracolumbar
function	regulates anabolic functions and vision	regulates protective and catabolic functions
mnemonic	might and sight	flight or fight

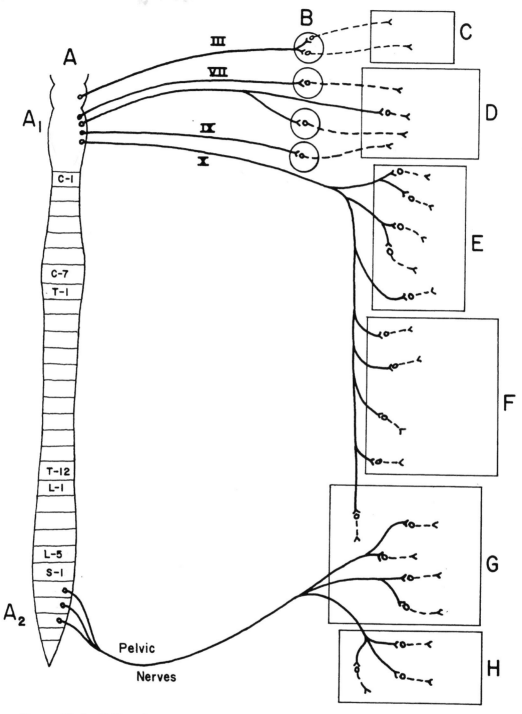

Figure 16–1. PNS pathway to various organs. **A.** CNS and spinal cord. **A₁.** Cranial centers. **A₂** Sacral centers. **B.** Ganglia. **C.** Eye. **D.** Other head and neck organs. **E.** Thoracic organs. **F.** Abdominal organs. **G.** Pelvic organs. **H.** Sex organs. Preganglionic nerves are solid lines; postganglionic nerves are dotted lines.

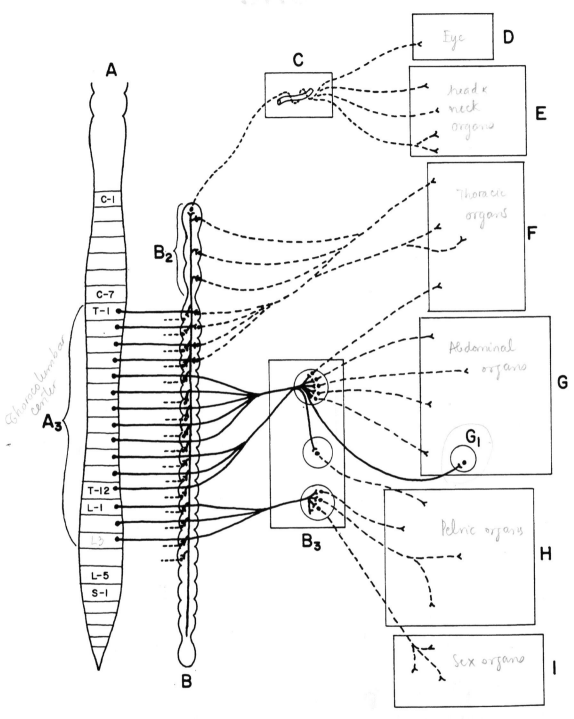

Figure 16–2. SNS pathways to various organs. **A.** CNS. **A₃.** Thorocolumbar centers. **B.** Vertebral chain of ganglia. **B₂.** Cervical ganglia. **B₃.** Abdominal ganglia. **C.** Carotid artery pathway. **D.** Eye. **E.** Other head and neck organs. **F.** Thoracic organs. **G.** Abdominal organs. **G₁.** Adrenal medulla. **H.** Pelvic organs. **I.** Sex organs. Preganglionic nerves are solid lines; postganglionic nerves are dotted lines.

D. PNS PATHWAYS

Objective 16.D.1. Recognize four cranial nerves which have PNS outflow.

Objective 16.D.2. Recognize the distribution of the PNS cranial nerves and their functional relationships.

Objective 16.D.3. Recognize nerve supply containing PNS fibers to the pelvic organs, the abdominal organs, and the thoracic organs.

Objective 16.D.4. Recognize the relative length of PNS pre- and postganglionic fibers.

Figure 16–1 indicates the PNS pathways and the organs innervated by PNS. PNS fibers, which have a craniosacral origin and outflow, follow cranial nerves III (oculomotor), VII (facial), IX (glossopharyngeal), and X (vagus). Other PNS fibers follow the sacral ventral roots from the spinal cord. Nerve III supplies the eye (C) and surrounding structures. Nerves VII and IX supply salivary glands and other facial structures (D), while nerve X supplies the neck (D), thorax (E), and abdominal cavity (F). Nerve X may be considered the great PNS nerve, since it contains the largest number of PNS fibers. The pelvic organs (G and H) are supplied by PNS fibers from sacral nerves. Note in Figure 16–1 how the PNS fibers have a ganglion (B) or intramural ganglion cell interposed. The PNS has long preganglionic fibers (solid lines) and short postganglionic fibers (dotted lines).

E. SNS PATHWAYS

Objective 16.E.1. Recognize the spinal segmental nerves which give rise to the SNS preganglionic fibers.

Objective 16.E.2. Recognize pathways of SNS preganglionic fibers and their relative length compared to PNS preganglionic fibers.

Objective 16.E.3. Recognize pathways of SNS postganglionic fibers and their relative length compared to PNS postganglionic fibers.

Figure 16–2 diagrammatically represents the SNS or thoracolumbar outflow to various organs and structures. Each thoracic and lumbar segment (A_3) of the spinal cord (A) contributes preganglionic fibers (solid lines), which originate in the intermediolateral cell column and follow the corresponding ventral root to the vertebral chain of ganglia (B). These preganglionic fibers can synapse at the ganglion of the same level, rise in the vertebral chain and synapse at a higher level, or pass right through the chain to synapse in a peripheral ganglion. Further details of the SNS pathway are emphasized in the cross section of a thoracic spinal nerve shown in Figure 16–3. Preganglionic cell bodies of the SNS are in the intermediolateral column (A_3) of the spinal cord. Preganglionic fibers exit via the ventral horn (B) and ventral root (C). Attached to the anterior division (E) of the segmental nerve (F) is a ventral root ganglion (D). It is connected by two branches called rami communicantes (G and H). The preganglionic fiber (I) enters the vertebral ganglion by the white ramus (G). It may synapse here on a postganglionic cell (J), which continues as a postganglionic fiber, leaving the ganglion at the same level by the gray ramus (H), enter the spinal nerve (K), and follow the nerve to a visceral structure (effector) in the same segment. The preganglionic fiber may pass through the segmental ganglia without synapsing and then rise in the vertebral chain, synapsing at a higher level or in a peripheral plexus (cervical, thoracic, abdominal, or pelvic).

F. PNS ACTIVITIES

Objective 16.F.1. Recognize at least six organs innervated by the PNS, including the functional changes induced by PNS activity.

As noted above, the PNS participates in physiologic regulation of anabolic functions which restore and conserve body energy, as well as in vision. PNS activities regulate discrete functions necessary for one to adapt to a normal environmental situation or to counteract changes in the environment. Thus, at rest, during digestion, or

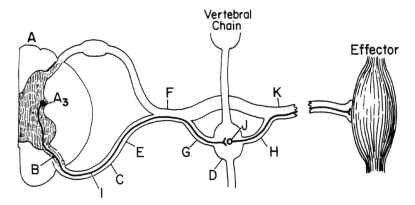

Figure 16–3. Cross-sectional diagram of SNS pathways. **A.** Thoracic or lumbar cross-section. **A₃.** Intermediolateral cell column. **B.** Autonomic nerve axon in ventral horn. **C.** Ventral root. **D.** Ventral root ganglion. **E.** Anterior division of ventral root. **F.** Segmental nerve. **G.** White ramus communicanti. **H.** Gray ramus communicanti. **I.** Preganglionic nerve fiber. **J.** Postganglionic nerve cell body. **K.** Spinal nerve.

when one is participating in purposeful, non-emotional decisions, the PNS predominates and controls our autonomic functions. Examples of organ functions controlled by PNS activity are noted in Table 16–3. (Please learn functional changes by studying Table 16–3.)

G. SNS ACTIVITIES

Objective 16.G.1. Recognize at least six organs or structures innervated by SNS fibers and the functional changes induced during the stress reaction.

Objective 16.G.2. Recognize a reflex for blood pressure regulation involving SNS activity.

When the SNS is massively activated (as by fear, anxiety, or emotion) the body is prepared for the emergency by the changes shown in column 3 of Table 16–3. The pupil of the eye is dilated, glands are generally inhibited (although there may be a secretion of thick, mucous saliva), bronchioles are dilated, GI smooth muscles are inhibited, heart rate is increased (positive chronotropic effect), heart contractile force is increased (positive inotropic effect), and blood pressure is increased. Changes in other organs may be noted in Table 16–3. Blood vessel

changes include either vasoconstriction or vasodilation, which results in decreased or increased blood flow, respectively. This dual mechanism of vascular regulation is quite elegant, since blood vessels in organs that require more flow during an emergency (heart, skeletal muscle, brain) tend to show predominantly dilation, while blood vessels of organs needing less flow (kidney, intestine, skin) show constriction. It should be noted that these mechanisms provide an excellent means of shunting blood during an emergency, which conforms to Dr. Walter Cannon's "wisdom of the body" hypothesis.

Another point to be emphasized is that sympathetic activities do not always have to occur as a massive response; for example, discrete SNS activities occur in control of blood pressure. During all phases of body activity, blood pressure is increased or decreased by sympathetic activity. The carotid sinus baroreceptor reflex corrects lowered blood pressure, since the change is sensed at the carotid sinus by pressorreceptors. They initiate impulses over nerve IX to the vasomotor and cardiac accelerator center in the medulla oblongata. These centers then activate sympathetic pathways to the heart and peripheral blood vessels, causing accelerated heart rate and peripheral vasoconstriction, respectively. This results in a return of the pressure to normal.

TABLE 16–3. FUNCTIONS OF PARASYMPATHETIC AND SYMPATHETIC NERVOUS SYSTEMS

Organ or Tissue	PNS Activity	SNS Activity	SNS[a] Receptor
eye			
pupil	constricts (miosis)	dilates (mydriasis)	α
smooth muscle of lens	thickens lens	flattens lens[b]	β
salivary gland	watery, copious secretion	thick, mucous, and scant secretions	α
other exocrine glands	stimulates	inhibits	—
		stimulates (sweat)	cholinergic
bronchioles	constricts	relaxes (dilates)	β
heart			
rate (chronotropic)	inhibits	stimulates	β
force (inotropic)	inhibits[b]	stimulates	β
GI smooth muscle			
peristaltic	stimulates	relaxes	α,β
sphincters	relaxes	stimulates	α
blood vessels	no innervation	constricts	α
	(ACh causes dilation[c])	dilates	β^{d}
		dilates	cholinergic[c]
metabolism	anabolism	energy utilization	β
	(energy conservation)	(glycogen breakdown, free fatty acid release)	

[a] The concept of α and β receptors is discussed on page 142.
[b] These actions are controversial.
[c] Cholinergic nerves in the SNS cause vasodilation. Further, acetylcholine (ACh) causes massive vasodilation, indicating a noninnervated muscarinic receptor.
[d] Smooth muscle β receptors can cause vasodilation even though innervation is not always present.

H. COMPARISON OF ANS PATHWAYS

Objective 16.H.1. Recognize similarities and differences between sympathetic and parasympathetic pathways.

Figure 16–4 diagrams the pathways of the PNS and SNS. In Figure 16–4, I (recall Fig. 16–1 as you study this section) a typical PNS neuron chain is outlined. The PNS has preganglionic neurons (A_1) which are in the nuclei of cranial nerves III (oculomotor), VII (facial), IX (glossopharyngeal), and X (vagus). Long preganglionic fibers extend from the cranial nerve nuclei and follow nerve III (regulating the eye), nerve VII and IX (regulating salivary glands), and nerve X (regulating visceral organs in the thorax and abdomen). The sacral segments of the spinal cord (A_2) contain preganglionic neurons which supply the pelvic organs via the pelvic plexus. PNS preganglionic neurons usually synapse upon ganglion cells (A_4) within the effector organ (in-

tramural nerve cells) or, less frequently, in discrete ganglia close to the effector organs. A short postganglionic fiber (A_5) then supplies the effector cells (A_6).

In Figure 16–4, II (recall Figs. 16–2 and 16–3 as you study this section), a typical SNS neuron chain is diagrammatically illustrated. The intermediolateral cell column (A_3) from T1 to L5 gives off a short preganglionic fiber proceeding from the CNS to a ganglion and synapses upon a ganglion cell (A_7), which gives off a relatively long postganglionic fiber proceeding to the effector organ and effector cell (A_6). Note the differences in anatomy between PNS and SNS neurons (Fig. 16–4, I and II, respectively). The PNS has relatively *long* preganglionic and *short* postganglionic fibers. The SNS has relatively *short* preganglionic and *long* postganglionic fibers.

The SNS has another important segment (Fig. 16–4, III) which portrays the innervation of the adrenal medulla. The preganglionic neuron (A_3)

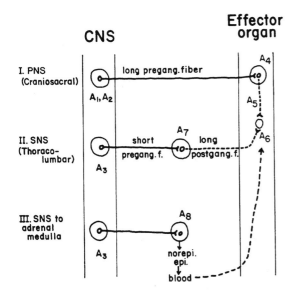

Figure 16–4. Schematic drawing of autonomic nervous system pathways. **A₁.** Cranial PNS centers. **A₂.** Sacral PNS centers. **A₃.** Intermediolateral cell column. **A₄.** Intramural ganglion. **A₅.** PNS postganglionic fiber. **A₆.** Effector cell. **A₇.** SNS ganglion. **A₈.** Adrenal medulla. Preganglionic nerves are solid lines; postganglionic nerves are dotted lines.

is similar to any other SNS preganglionic neuron, but the synapse is upon an adrenal medullary cell (A_8). Activation of the SNS stimulates the adrenal medullary cell, which secretes epinephrine (epi) and norepinephrine (norepi).

I. CHEMICAL MEDIATION OF NEUROTRANSMISSION

Objective 16.I.1. Recognize the five requirements of a chemical neurotransmitter.

Objective 16.I.2. Recognize at least five functional neural connections at which acetylcholine is the neurotransmitter.

Objective 16.I.3. Distinguish between synapse, neuroeffector junction, and neuromuscular junction.

In order to understand the physiology and pharmacology of the autonomic nervous system,

mechanisms of conduction must be described. This involves two mechanisms: electrical and chemical. Electrical conduction occurs within single nerve fibers. The process of electrical conduction is discussed in Chapter 15 (Local Anesthetics). Briefly, when a nerve cell is stimulated, an electrical impulse is generated which can spread electrically over the entire cell in both directions from the point of stimulation; however, the impulse is not intense enough to cross the gap (synapse) between cells. Therefore, another mechanism for transfer of the message must be operative. Impulses have been shown to pass between cells by means of chemical mediators (messengers), which transverse the synapse between cells by the rapid process of diffusion. The chemical messengers then act to stimulate an electrical impulse in the next cell of the chain. Chemical mediators that cause synaptic transmission are called "neurotransmitters." The requirements for a neurotransmitter are that it must:

1. mimic the action caused by normal nerve stimulation
2. be synthesized and stored in the nerve ending
3. be released when the nerve is stimulated
4. diffuse readily across the gap
5. have its action terminated by destruction or diffusion from the effector site

Acetylcholine (ACh) is a chemical substance that has met all these requirements and, therefore, has been identified as a neurotransmitter at many types of nerve synapses. These include lower motor neurons, autonomic ganglion cells, and adrenal medullary cells. ACh is also the neurotransmitter at the parasympathetic neuroeffector junction* and at the neuromuscular junction† (NMJ). ACh is a probable neurotransmitter for many CNS neurons. It has been demonstrated chemically to be a component of synaptic vesicles from presynaptic cells. When PNS postganglionic neurons to the heart are stimulated, an ACh-like substance can be shown

---

* Neuroeffector junction describes the gap between autonomic nerve endings and effector cells.

† Neuromuscular junction (NMJ) describes the gap between a somatic nerve ending and the motor end-plate of a skeletal muscle cell.

in the fluid perfusing the heart. Once released, ACh diffuses readily across the synaptic gap. The administration of ACh mimics the stimulation of PNS nerves, and ACh is readily destroyed by a specific cholinesterase enzyme localized at the postsynaptic membrane. There is a prolongation of effects by drugs which block the breakdown of ACh (cholinesterase inhibitors, Chapter 17). Thus, there is ample evidence to support ACh as a neurotransmitter.

J. AUTONOMIC MEDIATORS AND DRUG ACTION

Objective 16.J.1. Recognize the neurotransmitters of autonomic activity and the location at which they are secreted.

Objective 16.J.2. Recognize definitions of cholinergic, cholinomimetic, adrenergic, sympathomimetic, sympatholytic, anticholinergic, agonist (stimulant), and antagonist (blocker).

Objective 16.J.3. Recognize the chemical differences in structure of norepinephrine, epinephrine, levonordefrin, phenylephrine, isoproterenol, and dichloroisoproterenol.

Objective 16.J.4. Recognize the term "catecholamine" and name four catecholamines.

The action of autonomic drugs can be best understood if one learns the neurotransmitters secreted at the synapses and neuroeffector junctions. All preganglionic neurons secrete ACh, which is the neurotransmitter at all ganglia whether they are PNS or SNS. PNS postganglionic fibers also secrete ACh, which is the neurotransmitter, and ACh is the neurotransmitter at the neuromuscular junction. All nerve fibers that use ACh as the neurotransmitter are referred to as *cholinergic.*

Most SNS postganglionic fibers secrete norepinephrine (NE). These nerves are called *adrenergic,* and NE is the neurotransmitter. Adrenal medullary cells secrete both NE and epinephrine (E). It should be noted that preganglionic cells to the adrenal medulla secrete ACh (cholinergic), which is the neurotransmitter causing secretion of E and NE. Actually, an

TABLE 16–4. TYPES OF AUTONOMIC DRUGS AND THEIR ACTIONS

Drug Type	Action
sympathomimetics	mimic norepinephrine or SNS stimulation
sympatholytics	block norepinephrine action or SNS function
parasympathomimetics	mimic acetylcholine at PNS postganglionic endings
parasympatholytics	block acetylcholine at PNS postganglionic endings
ganglionic stimulants	mimic acetylcholine at ganglia
ganglionic blockers	block acetylcholine at ganglia

adrenal medullary cell is analogous to a ganglionic cell, and the adrenal medulla is analogous to an autonomic ganglion. In summary, all ANS fibers are cholinergic, except for postganglionic SNS fibers, most of which are adrenergic (see 16.N.1.).

If a drug mimics the action of ACh, it may also be referred to as *cholinomimetic* (or an agonist of ACh). Such drugs may be parasympathomimetic, ganglionic stimulants (see 16.O.2.) or neuromuscular stimulants (16.O.3.). Other drugs may antagonize ACh actions; these are either parasympatholytics, ganglionic blockers, or neuromuscular blockers, depending upon their site of action. Any drug that acts on cholinergic mechanisms is referred to as a "cholinergic" drug. Later in this chapter, other cholinergic mechanisms will be discussed in more detail, including ganglionic, NMJ, and cholinergic sympathetic transmission.

A drug that mimics the action of sympathetic nerve stimulation is called a "sympathomimetic" drug. A drug that blocks (antagonizes) sympathetic function or sympathomimetic drugs is called a "sympatholytic" drug (SNS blocking agent). Drugs that act upon sympathetic postganglionic function are called "adrenergic" drugs. Table 16–4 summarizes autonomic drug types and their actions.

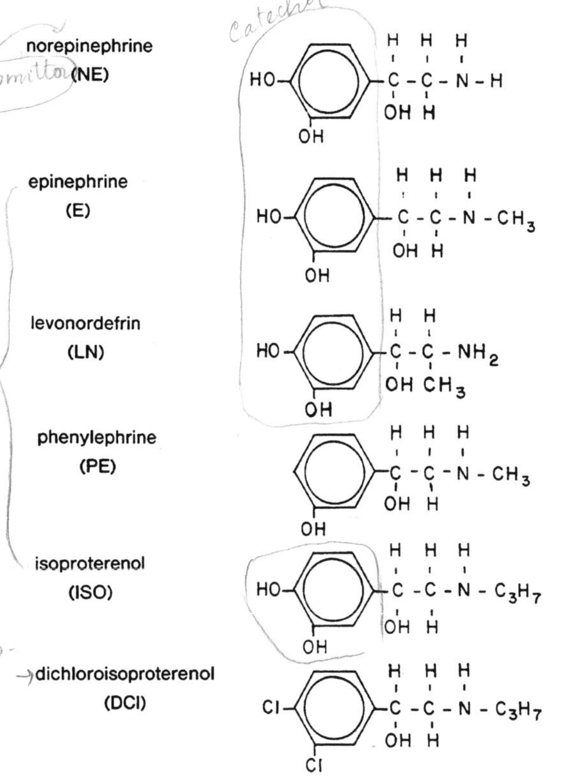

norepinephrine (NE)

epinephrine (E)

levonordefrin (LN)

phenylephrine (PE)

isoproterenol (ISO)

dichloroisoproterenol (DCI)

Figure 16–5. Structures of some adrenergic drugs.

Mimetic (agonist) and lytic (antagonist) drugs not only act by simulating, or blocking the neurotransmitter but also usually resemble it chemically. The similarities and differences in chemical structure of adrenergic drugs is illustrated in Figure 16–5. The first four drugs (NE, E, LN, and PE) are vasoconstrictors that may be added to local anesthetic solutions. NE is recognized as the neurotransmitter of adrenergic activity, while E, LN, and PE are mimetics. Isoproterenol is a sympathomimetic and shares some of the properties of epinephrine (differences will be discussed below). DCI is a sympatholytic, and it may be noted that it also fits a similar chemical pattern.

Another term applied to some sympathomimetics is "catecholamine." Catechol is the dihydroxybenzene portion noted on the left in the structure of NE, E, LN, and ISO (Fig. 16–5). Note that PE is not a catecholamine because it has only one hydroxy group.

K. MECHANISMS OF MIMETIC AND LYTIC ACTION

Objective 16.K.1. Recognize features of the drug-receptor complex which explain both mimetic and blocking actions.

Objective 16.K.2. Recognize seven mechanisms by which a drug can affect neural function.

We have seen above that chemicals with similar structures may be either mimetics or lytics (blockers). The reason for this is explained by the receptor theory. (For a detailed discussion of drug-receptors and the concept of agonist-antagonist, as related to drug-receptor kinetics, refer to Chapter 12, Principles of Pharmacology, Section 12.H.2.) Consider a neuroeffector junction, as in Figure 16–6. The neurotransmitter (M) is stored in vesicles at the nerve ending (B) of the neural cell (A). When an electrical impulse arrives at the ending, some vesicles release the neurotransmitter, which reaches the effector cell (E) by traversing the gap (G). When the neurotransmitter arrives at the effector cell, the message is transferred to the next cell. Pharmacologists believe this is accomplished because the combination of neurotransmitter with receptor (R) initiates a response in the effector cell. Later, the neurotransmitter must be destroyed or removed so that the system can renew itself.

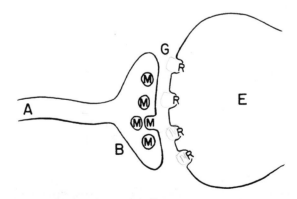

Figure 16–6. Diagram of neuroeffector junction. **A.** Neural cell. **B.** Nerve ending. **E.** Effector. **G.** Gap (neuroeffector junction or synapse). **M.** Neurotransmitter. **R.** Receptor.

Because mimetics resemble the neurotransmitter, they also form a complex with the receptor (drug-receptor complex), which causes the response to occur. The drug-receptor complex of an agonist is rapidly broken, causing restoration of the effector cell to normal activity. A blocker that resembles the neurotransmitter may also form a drug-receptor complex. However, this complex may be so firm that it prevents the neurotransmitter or another agonist from reacting with the receptor.

The seven mechanisms by which autonomic drugs may act on the system of neural transmission are:

receptor action

1. reacting with receptor (drug-receptor complex)
2. blocking receptor (stronger drug-receptor complex)
3. preventing breakdown or reuptake of neurotransmitter
4. decreasing formation of neurotransmitter
5. preventing storage of neurotransmitter
6. depleting stored neurotransmitter
7. preventing release of neurotransmitter

nonreceptor action

Mechanisms 1 and 2 act through receptors and were discussed above as mimetic or lytic actions, respectively. The other mechanisms are nonreceptor actions and are discussed in Chapters 17 and 18.

L. TYPES OF ADRENERGIC RECEPTORS

Objective 16.L.1. Recognize the classification of an adrenergic receptor either α or β.

Objective 16.L.2. Recognize the order of mimetic activity for receptors classified as α or β.

Objective 16.L.3. Recognize classification of β adrenergic receptors into β_1 and β_2, the basis for this classification, and its importance in therapeutics.

Objective 16.L.4. Recognize the classification of α receptors into α_1 and α_2, the basis for this classification, and its importance in therapeutics.

The drug-receptor complex helps pharmacologists to explain why sympathetic stimulation may have either stimulatory or inhibitory effects on various effector cells. For example, SNS stimulation causes constriction of many blood vessels but dilation of some other blood vessels. If one examines the neurotransmitter of sympathetic activity, only norepinephrine is found at the nerve endings. How then can the same transmitter cause opposite effects on blood vessels? R.P. Ahlquist (1948) theorized that, although the neurotransmitter is the same, the receptor may be different in different effector cells. Ahlquist believed that smooth muscle contraction (or vasoconstriction) is due to activation of an α receptor, while smooth muscle relaxation (or vasodilation) is due to activation of a β receptor. It was found that norepinephrine (given as a drug) causes predominantly α responses, while isoproterenol caused β responses. Epinephrine possessed both activities. Thus, the order of activity, NE $\geq$ E $>$ I, was considered α, while the order, I $\geq$ E $>$ NE, was considered β. Ahlquist's theory received strong support when it was found that some sympathetic antagonists blocked only α receptors (e.g., phentolamine), while others blocked only β receptors (e.g., propranolol).

During more recent studies of adrenergic blocking drugs, it became apparent that certain newer beta blocking drugs were selectively antagonizing the heart, while others were selectively blocking bronchiolar smooth muscle. The heart receptors were called β_1, and the bronchiolar receptors were called β_2. Since there is a need to selectively block the heart receptors without blocking bronchorelaxation (propranolol blocks both β_1 and β_2), the discovery of selective β_1 and β_2 receptor blockers led to the development of several new drugs which are β_1 blockers for treatment of cardiovascular disease (see Chapters 18 and 31). Furthermore, it was found that certain newer sympathomimetics were either β_1 or β_2 agonists. The need for a bronchiolar relaxant (β_2) for asthmatic patients that does not affect the heart is obvious. Epinephrine and isoproterenol, although useful bronchiolar relaxants, are nonspecific and react with both β_1 and β_2 receptors. The selectivity is only relative, because increasing concentration of drug tends to cause effects on the other receptor. (The selective β_2 agonists will be de-

Propranolol = Blocks β receptors

Phentolamine = Blocks α Receptors

adrenergic

TABLE 16–5. ALPHA AND BETA RECEPTORS IN VISCERAL STRUCTURES

α Receptors	β Receptors	Both α and β Receptors
vascular smooth muscle (constriction)	vascular smooth muscle (dilation)	GI smooth muscle (relaxation)
pupillary smooth muscle (dilation)	cardiac muscle (β_1) (+ chronotropic) (+ inotropic)	
salivary secretion	bronchiolar smooth muscle (β_2) (dilation)	

scribed in Chapters 18 and 33.) There is no therapeutic usefulness of a β_2 blocker, since bronchoconstriction is never a desirable therapeutic action.

There also seem to be two subtypes of alpha receptors. Alpha$_1$ receptors are located primarily, but not exclusively, at postjunctional sites and are probably responsible for postjunctional events, which are mainly excitatory in nature. Alpha$_2$ receptors are located primarily, but not exclusively, on prejunctional nerve endings, and this receptor regulates release and probably synthesis of transmitter, e.g., stimulation of α_2 prejunctional receptors by NE (an agonist) results in decreased release and synthesis of NE. Conversely, blockade of α_2 receptors results in increased release of NE. This discovery led to eventual introduction of α_1 blockers as antihypertensive drugs (Chapters 18 and 31).

M. CORRELATION OF ADRENERGIC FUNCTIONS TO VISCERAL RECEPTORS

Objective 16.M.1. Recognize three visceral structures which have α adrenergic receptors and three which have β receptors and describe the result of stimulation of these structures.

Objective 16.M.2. Recognize a visceral structure in which α and β adrenergic stimulation cause the same effect.

It would be helpful now to refer back to Table 16–3, reviewing adrenergic activities and learning which of the SNS receptors is responsible for these activities. From the study of Table 16–3, Table 16–5 can be constructed which will aid in the memory of responses to the objectives in 16.M.1. and 16.M.2. (NOTE: more detail on adrenergic pharmacology is found in Chapter 18).

N. OTHER CHOLINERGIC MECHANISMS

Objective 16.N.1. Recognize the cholinergic sympathetic pathway to sweat glands and blood vessels.

Objective 16.N.2. Recognize four differences and one similarity between the somatic efferent and the visceral efferent fibers.

In order to complete the discussion of cholinergic mechanisms and drugs, two other cholinergic pathways should be considered. From Figure 16–4, you should recall the autonomic pathways labelled I, II, and III. Figure 16–7 diagrams these and expands upon the diagram of Figure 16–4 with two additional cholinergic pathways. One of the additional cholinergic pathways is in the sympathetic division; thus, a sympathetic postganglionic ending secretes ACh instead of NE. This pathway (IV) is called **sympathetic cholinergic** and supplies sweat glands and certain blood vessels in skeletal muscles. Figure 16–7, V illustrates the somatic efferent fibers to skeletal muscles. Although somatic efferents are **not** part of the ANS, the neuromuscular junction (NMJ) is cholinergic and responds to mimetics, lytics, and other cholinergic drugs.

(NOTE: there is no ganglionic cell in the somatic efferent nerve.)

Table 16–6 gives a comparison between the somatic efferent system and the visceral efferent (autonomic) system.

O. CHOLINERGIC RECEPTORS

Objective 16.0.1. Recognize the muscarinic and nicotinic effects of ACh.

Objective 16.0.2. Recognize which effects of ACh predominate when either the drug atropine or the drug hexamethonium is given.

Objective 16.0.3. Recognize methods by which pharmacologists can distinguish between the three types of cholinergic receptors.

Although ACh is the mediator for all the cholinergic fibers, there appear to be some differences in the receptors for ACh at the different sites (ganglionic, postganglionic, and NMJ). This was discovered many years ago by pharmacologists who found that the alkaloids muscarine (from a mushroom) and nicotine could mimic ACh. However, each alkaloid acted in a somewhat different manner. Muscarine is a parasympathomimetic; it mimics the action of parasympathetic stimulation. When given to an animal, muscarine causes salivation, gastrointestinal upset, and fall in blood pressure (slowing of the heart and blood vessel dilation). ACh can cause all of these effects. Atropine, another alkaloid which blocks the parasympathetic postganglionic endings, can block both the hypotensive effect and salivation caused by either ACh or muscarine. This action of ACh on smooth muscle, heart, and glands is called the *muscarinic effect.* This usually is considered a postganglionic action, but occasionally it occurs directly on cells which have noninnervated receptors (as in vasodilation). The muscarinic response and its block by atropine are a good example of pharmacologic antagonism. (It would be recommended to review Chapter 12, Objectives 12.H.2. and 12.I.2. at this time.) ACh can directly stimulate ganglionic cells, resulting in both sympathetic and parasympathetic responses. Nicotine causes a similar effect, so

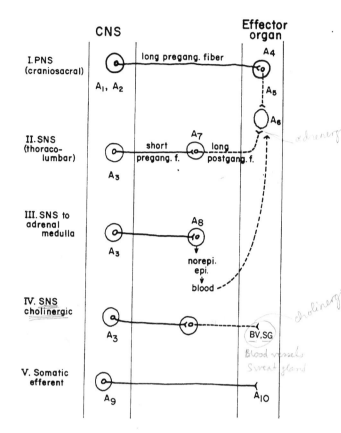

Figure 16–7. Diagrammatic representation of efferent neurons. A_1. Cranial PNS centers. A_2. Sacral PNS centers. A_3. Intermediolateral cell column. A_4. Intramural ganglion. A_5. PNS postganglionic fiber. A_6. Effector cell. A_7. SNS ganglion. A_8. Adrenal medulla. A_9. Ventral horn. A_{10}. Skeletal muscle. SG, Sweat glands. BV, Blood vessels. Preganglionic nerves are solid lines; postganglionic nerves are dotted lines.

ganglionic stimulation is referred to as the "nicotinic actions" of acetylcholine. This response is not blocked by atropine, but a specific blocker, hexamethonium, has been used to block the ganglionic cholinergic receptors (see also Chapter 17).

Pharmacologists have found that curare blocks acetylcholine at the NMJ, indicating a third receptor for cholinergic transmission. On the basis of the specific agonists and antagonists, three types of cholinergic receptors have been recognized (Table 16–7). It can be seen that the receptors are named after the mimetic stimulant, except for the NMJ. The transmitter (ACh)

TABLE 16–6. COMPARISON OF SOMATIC AND VISCERAL EFFERENT SYSTEMS

autonomic nervous system

Property	Somatic Efferent	Visceral Efferent
origin	ventral horn	intermediolateral cell column
numbers of neurons	one	two
supply	skeletal muscle	visceral muscle or gland
neurotransmitter	acetylcholine	acetylcholine or norepinephrine
function	motor	motor

TABLE 16–7. TYPES OF CHOLINERGIC RECEPTORS

Type	Site	Transmitter	Mimetic	Blocker
chol-M	PNS endings	acetylcholine	muscarine	atropine
chol-N	ganglia	acetylcholine	nicotine	hexamethonium
chol-NMJ	NMJ	acetylcholine	PTMA[a]	curare or succinylcholine

[a] PTMA is a phenyltrimethylammonium; it is not necessary to memorize this drug because it is only of interest as a pharmacologic tool.

is the same at all three sites, but the blocking agents are very specific, showing little or no action at the other sites. (NOTE: a detailed discussion of cholinergic drugs occurs in Chapter 17).

P. SUMMARY

This introduction of ANS pharmacology will serve as a basis for more detailed descriptions of cholinergic drugs (Chapter 17) and adrenergic drugs (Chapter 18). Some, but not all, of the concepts discussed here will be reviewed later, but it is assumed that the reader has a sound knowledge of this chapter as a foundation for understanding the material presented later.

An understanding of cardiovascular drugs (Chapter 31) and autonomic agents used in therapy (Chapters 1 and 2) also depends upon the material in Chapter 16.

BIBLIOGRAPHY

Bowman WC, Rand MJ, West GB: Textbook of Pharmacology (2nd ed.), Oxford and Edinburgh, Blackwell Scientific Publications, 1980, Ch. 9, pp. 9.1–9.36

Csáky, TZ (ed): Cutting's Handbook of Pharmacology, 6th ed. New York, Appleton-Century-Crofts, 1979, pp 530–531

DiPalma JR (ed): Drill's Pharmacology in Medicine, 4th ed. New York, McGraw-Hill, 1971, Ch 30, 31, 32, 33, 34, 35, 36

Gilman AG, Goodman LS, Gilman A (eds): Goodman and Gilman's The Pharmacological Basis of Therapeutics, 6th ed. New York, Macmillan, 1980, Ch 4, 5, 6, 7, 8, 9, 10, 11

Crossland J (ed): Lewis's Pharmacology, 4th ed. Baltimore, Williams & Wilkins, 1970, Ch 9, 10, 11, 12, 13, 14, 15

Ahlquist RP: A study of adrenotropic receptors. Am J Physiol 53:586, 1948

QUESTIONS

1. T F Sympathetic nervous activity causes changes in skeletal muscle and sensory receptors.

NE &E

2. T F Acetylcholine secreted into the bloodstream by the adrenal medulla during sympathetic discharge reinforces sympathetic responses induced by SNS neural discharge.

3. T F The parasympathetic nervous system (PNS) is the main controlling influence in salivary secretion.

4. T **F** Autonomic drugs are frequently pre-scribed by dentists for postoperative care.

5. T **F** Dentists cannot legally prescribe drugs which have autonomic side ef-fects.

6. **T** F Atropinelike drugs may be prescribed to reduce excessive salivation.

7. T **F** The parasympathetic division of the ANS includes all cholinergic pregan-glionic fibers.

8–13. Acetylcholine is the neurotransmitter of nerve activity at:

   8. **T** F synapses of lower motor neu-rons

   9. T **F** PNS but not SNS autonomic ganglia

   10. **T** F adrenal medullary cells

   11. **T** F PNS neuroeffector junctions

   12. T **F** all CNS neurons

   13. **T** F all neuromuscular junctions of skeletal muscle

14. T **F** A neuroeffector junction is defined as the gap between two nerve cells.

15. T **F** *NE* Epinephrine is the neurotransmitter at adrenergic postganglionic neuroeffec-tor junctions

16. T **F** Mimetic drugs usually resemble each other chemically, but blockers do not resemble the mimetics.

17. **T** F Cholinergic postganglionic fibers can travel in either PNS or SNS pathways. *sympathetic cholinergic*

18, 19. *ANS* The autonomic nervous system is de-scribed as:

   18. **T** F visceral efferent

   19. T **F** somatic efferent

20, 21. The autonomic nervous system is de-scribed as:

   20. T **F** autonomous of central con-trol

   21. **T** F automatic but centrally con-trolled *(yoga hypnose ...)*

22–30. Indicate

   A. if only A is correct
   B. if only B is correct
   C. if only C is correct
   D. if A, B, and C are all correct
   E. if neither A, B, nor C is correct

22. The autonomic nervous system is consid-ered:

   A. involuntary
   B. visceral efferent
   C. automatic but having central nervous input

23. The PNS is: *straight & right   anabolic*

   A. primarily catabolic
   B. not required for visual acuity
   C. represented in cranial nerves III, VII, IX, and X

24. The SNS:

   A. derives from thoracic and lumbar inter-mediolateral cell columns
   B. has shorter preganglionic fibers relative to the PNS

C. has longer postganglionic fibers relative to the PNS

25. PNS stimulation causes:

   A. miosis

   B. negative chronotropic effect on the heart

   C. bronchiolar constriction

26. Sympathetic stimulation causes:

   A. mydriasis of the pupil

   B. positive inotropic effect on the heart

   C. bronchodilation

27. Epinephrine overdosage may cause:

   A. tachycardia

   B. reduced nervousness

   C. reduced blood flow to heart and brain

28. A neurotransmitter must:

   A. be stored in the nerve ending

   B. be released when the nerve is stimulated

   C. have its action terminated by destruction or diffusion

29. A lytic drug may act by:

   A. forming a drug-receptor complex which is difficult to break

   B. decreasing the formation of neurotransmitter

   C. depleting stored neurotransmitter

30. A smooth muscle response is classified as α adrenergic. When epinephrine is added to the smooth muscle:

   A. contraction is more likely to occur than relaxation

   B. the activity will be greater than if isoproterenol were added

   C. the activity is blocked by propranolol

31-35. Indicate A in the blank if the PNS is involved, B if the SNS is involved

31._____ longer preganglionics

32._____ shorter postganglionics

33._____ craniosacral origin

34._____ thoracic intermediolateral origin

35._____ preganglionic synapse on adrenal medullary cell

36-48. Indicate

   A. if only A is correct

   B. if only B is correct

   C. if both A and B are correct

   D. if neither A nor B is correct

36. The autonomic nervous system is described as:

   A. involuntary

   B. afferent

37. The parasympathetic division (PNS) of the ANS:

   A. has relatively short preganglionic fibers

   B. has relatively long postganglionic fibers

38. Preganglionic parasympathetic fibers follow:

   A. nerve III to the eye

   B. nerve VII to salivary glands

39. Preganglionic parasympathetic fibers follow:

   A. nerve X to the heart

   B. nerve IX to salivary glands

40. Preganglionic parasympathetic fibers follow:

    A. lumbar ventral roots to the pelvic organs

    B. sacral ventral roots to the pelvic organs

41. During a stress reaction:

    A. the blood vessels of the brain dilate

    B. the blood vessels of the kidney constrict

42. The SNS operates:

    A. only through massive outflow to all innervated organs

    B. mainly as in A, but also through discrete reflex regulatory activities

43. Norepinephrine is:

    A. a vasoconstrictor

    B. a cardiac stimulator

44. Norepinephrine is the neurotransmitter of nerve activity at:

    A. adrenergic postganglionic endings

    B. β adrenergic nerve endings

45. The order of activity of three sympathomimetic drugs on a muscle is norepinephrine > epinephrine > isoproterenol. The muscle activity noted is due to activation of:

    A. α receptors

    B. β receptors

46. A cholinergic nerve fiber which has no ganglionic synapse between the spinal cord and the nerve-muscle junction is:

    A. parasympathetic

    B. somatic efferent

47. Propranolol blocks:

    A. sympathetic cardiac stimulation

    B. epinephrine-induced bronchodilation

48. Phentolamine blocks:

    A. sympathetic vasoconstriction

    B. metacholine induced salivation

49-50. Choose the single best answer.

49. The term sympathomimetic applied to a drug indicates that it is:

    A. an agonist of the adrenergic transmitter

    B. an antagonist of the adrenergic transmitter

    C. the neurotransmitter itself

    D. a false transmitter

50. The suffix –ergic indicates:

    A. the nerve is stimulated by the drug in the prefix

    B. the nerve releases the drug implied by the prefix

    C. the drug implied by the prefix is a blocker

    D. the action of the nerve is opposite to the mimetic

51-54. Indicate

    A. if only A is correct

    B. if only B is correct

    C. if only C is correct

    D. if only A and B are correct

    E. if A, B, and C are correct

51. A sympatholytic drug:

    A. blocks sympathetic nerve function

    B. blocks sympathomimetic drugs

    C. blocks cholinomimetic drugs

52. Somatic efferent fibers:

    A. originate in the ventral horn

    B. terminate in the neuromuscular junction

    C. are adrenergic *cholinergic*

53. Atropine blocks:

    A. chol-M activity *anticholinesterase*

    B. physostigmine's stimulation of gastrointestinal smooth muscle

    C. physostigmine's neuromuscular stimulation

54. Acetylcholine causes activity at a synapse as measured by action potential, and hexamethonium blocks this activity. The responding cell is thought to have:

nicotine mimics

    A. chol-M receptors

    B. chol-N receptors

    C. β receptor

(*For Question 55, choose the single best answer.*)

55. If curare blocks an action of acetylcholine, the action is considered:

    A. α receptor

    B. chol-M

    C. chol-N

    D. chol-NMJ

56–62. Indicate:

    A if the activity is α

    B if the activity is β

    C if the activity is both α and β

    D if it is neither α nor β

56. __D__ miosis (pupillary constriction) → (*PNS*)

57. __B__ bronchodilation (*β₂*)

58. __C__ GI smooth muscle relaxation

59. __A__ vasoconstriction

60. __b__ vasodilation

61. __b__ cardiac acceleration (*β₁*)

62. __D__ negative inotropic effect (*ni α ni β*)

17
Cholinergic Drugs

11/17

A. PNS MIMETICS

Definitions

Objective 17.A.1. Recognize definitions of PNS-mimetic and compare to cholinomimetic, cholinergic, muscarinic, nicotinic, and anticholinesterase.

Some of these definitions were presented in Chapter 16. They are repeated here for sake of completeness, for elaboration, and because they are used in a slightly different context.

1. Cholinomimetic literally means acting like choline (that is, acetylcholine). Therefore any drug mimicking the actions of acetylcholine may be considered cholinomimetic. We know that the actions of acetylcholine are very broad and nonspecific because of its multiple sites of action. Therefore, cholinomimetic drugs would have many possible sites of action causing diverse effects. Some authors equate cholinomimetic with PNS-mimetic, but in this text we will use the term "cholinomimetic" in its broadest context: any drug which resembles acetylcholine in its pharmacologic action.

2. Cholinergic literally means having the energy of choline (that is, acetylcholine). Cholinergic nerves are those that secrete acetylcholine, and cholinergic drugs are those that affect the cholinergic system. Cholinergic drugs will, therefore, include any drug that affects cholinergic nerves in any manner. This includes a broad range of drugs displaying the agonistic or antagonistic effects of acetylcholine and acting to depress or stimulate cholinergic nerves.

3. PNS-mimetic drugs are more specific in action because they are agonists at PNS postganglionic nerve endings. The drug, atropine, specifically blocks the actions of PNS-mimetics and PNS postganglionic nerve stimulation.

4. Muscarinic drugs have actions similar to those of the alkaloid muscarine. This drug acts similarly to acetylcholine at PNS nerve endings; therefore, PNS-mimetic and muscarinic are synonymous.

5. Nicotinic drugs have the actions of acetylcholine that are caused by stimulation of ganglia. The actions of nicotinic drugs are unpredictable because both PNS and SNS are stimulated when ganglia are stimulated.

151

6. The anticholinesterase drugs mimic all actions of acetylcholine. By inhibiting the enzyme, cholinesterase, acetylcholine accumulates in all tissues, and the result is massive activity because of activation of all ACh receptors.

PNS-Mimetic Choline Esters

Objective 17.A.2. List four PNS-mimetic choline esters and describe their pharmacologic actions and differences.

ACETYLCHOLINE

This is the natural neurotransmitter at cholinergic nerve endings. It is physiologically important, but it is a poor drug for therapy for two reasons: (1) it is too rapidly hydrolyzed, and (2) it has potent, nonspecific actions. ACh mimics the stimulation of all preganglionic nerves and postganglionic PNS nerves, causing powerful PNS and SNS effects.

METHACHOLINE

This methyl analog of acetylcholine has specific PNS-mimetic actions with little or no ganglionic action. Methacholine has powerful PNS cardiovascular effects as well as smooth muscle effects. It is used in peripheral vascular disorders, including Raynaud's disease (spasms of arteries in the periphery resulting in pain and sometimes gangrene), phlebitis, varicose ulcers, and Buerger's disease (progressive arterial obliteration in feet and legs).

Symptoms of toxicity of methacholine are marked hypotension, abnormalities of cardiac rhythm, cardiac arrest, and asthmatic attack. Methacholine is relatively resistant to cholinesterase attack and is not used for GI or bladder stimulation because of CNS effects.

BETHANECHOL (Urecoline)

This drug is similar to methacholine except that bethanechol is a carbamic acid ester and is, therefore, only slowly hydrolyzed by cholinesterase. Bethanechol has minimal nicotinic effects and preferentially acts on smooth muscle with fewer cardiovascular effects than methacholine. Therefore, bethanechol is used to treat atony of the GI tract and urinary bladder.

CARBAMYLCHOLINE (Carbachol)

This drug is the carbamic acid ester of acetylcholine. Carbachol is very stable in the presence of cholinesterase and has significant nicotinic effects on ganglia. It is used principally as a miotic in ophthalmology in the treatment of glaucoma (increased intraocular pressure due to poor drainage through the canal of Schlemm). Mydriasis (the opposite of miosis) aggravates the condition by causing further restriction of the opening of the canal of Schlemm.

PNS-Mimetic Alkaloids

Objective 17.A.3. List two PNS-mimetic (cholinomimetic) alkaloids and describe their importance.

MUSCARINE

An alkaloid present in the mushroom, *Amanita muscaria*, muscarine causes one form of mushroom poisoning. The usual type of mushroom poisoning, unrelated to PNS stimulation, is caused by *Amanita phalloides*. Muscarine is not used clinically but is important in pharmacology and toxicology.

PILOCARPINE

This is a tertiary amine (most PNS-mimetics are quaternary amines). The tertiary amine penetrates eye tissues more readily, making it more useful for producing miosis for therapy of glaucoma. Pilocarpine is used often in a diagnostic test for cystic fibrosis. It is applied to the skin by iontophoresis and causes sweating. After collection, the sweat is analyzed for sodium and chloride. Very high chloride levels indicate the presence of cystic fibrosis. Pilocarpine may also be used as a sialagogue for the treatment of xerostomia. However, the side effects (PNS stimulation) limit its usefulness.

Characteristics of PNS-Mimetics

Objective 17.A.4. Compare the relative hydrolysis rate, the principal uses, the muscarinic potency, and the nicotinic potency of five clinically useful PNS-mimetics.

Table 17–1 lists characteristics of useful PNS-mimetics. Study of the table allows comparison

TABLE 17–1. SUMMARY OF USEFUL PNS-MIMETICS AND THEIR CHARACTERISTICS

Drug	Relative Hydrolysis Rate	Principal Use	Muscarinic Effect	Nicotinic Effect
acetylcholine	rapid	pharmacologic	powerful	powerful
methacholine	medium	cardiovascular	powerful	weak
bethanechol	slow	GI and bladder stimulant	moderate	weak
carbachol	slow	miotic (pupil constriction)	powerful	powerful
pilocarpine	none	miotic	powerful	weak

of the various aspects of PNS-mimetics thus fulfilling the objectives.

B. CHOLINESTERASE INHIBITORS (ANTICHOLINESTERASES)

Activity

Objective 17.B.1. Describe the activity of cholinesterase inhibitors.

These drugs increase the concentration of acetylcholine at cholinergic junctions. The resulting actions are nonspecific because of multiple effects and widespread build-up of acetylcholine. Stimulation of the bladder, GI and respiratory smooth muscle, glandular activity, ganglia (stimulation causes both PNS and SNS effects), and skeletal muscle occur when cholinesterase inhibitors are given.

Reversible Cholinesterase Inhibitors

Objective 17.B.2. Name three reversible cholinesterase inhibitors and describe their importance in medicine.

PHYSOSTIGMINE (*Eserine*)
This is a tertiary amine that is well absorbed from the GI tract and readily penetrates the **blood-brain barrier.** Side effects limit its usefulness. Physostigmine sulfate may be used in glaucoma treatment. Physostigmine may be used for smooth muscle atony and, rarely, in myasthenia gravis. It may be useful in reversing some of diazepam's toxicity.

NEOSTIGMINE (*Prostigmin*)
This is a synthetic quaternary analog of physostigmine. Neostigmine is less readily absorbed from the GI tract but also has fewer CNS effects. It is the drug of choice for myasthenia gravis (abnormal fatigue of skeletal muscle due to impairment of NMJ transmission).

EDROPHONIUM CHLORIDE (*Tensilon*)
This has a rapid action with short duration. It is used to establish the diagnosis of myasthenia gravis: if improvement of muscle strength occurs within five minutes after IV administration, the diagnosis is confirmed. Edrophonium may also be used to counteract curariform blockade of NMJ.

Irreversible Cholinesterase Inhibitors

Objective 17.B.3. Name one irreversible cholinesterase inhibitor, describe the importance of this group of drugs, and name a drug that can reverse the irreversible inhibitors.

Organophosphorus compounds are highly toxic cholinesterase inhibitors. **Diisopropylfluorophosphate** (DFP) is the only useful drug in the group. DFP is sometimes used in glaucoma therapy.

Thousands of organophosphorus compounds have been synthesized as insecticides and chemical warfare agents (i.e., nerve gases). They are important in toxicology because of human exposure to insecticides and the desire of nations, engaged in warfare, to find antidotes. The reason for the irreversible action of these drugs is that they form covalent bonds with the cholinesterase enzyme. During World War II, the drug 2-PAM (**pralidoxime**) was synthesized to break the covalent bond and regenerate the enzyme.

C. ANTICHOLINERGIC DRUGS

Definition

Objective 17.C.1. Define and distinguish between parasympatholytic, ganglionic blocker, and neuromuscular junction blocker.

Parasympatholytic refers to drugs that block the postganglionic cholinergic receptors or the actions of acetylcholine that mimic postganglionic parasympathetic stimulation. The prototype drug of this class is atropine, which acts by combining with acetylcholine receptors, preventing attachment of the PNS-mimetics (e.g., acetylcholine) and thereby blocking the effect of nerve stimulation. The receptors for acetylcholine at the PNS postganglionic endings are called Chol-M, because the drug, muscarine, mimics the actions of PNS postganglionic stimulation (Chapter 16). Therefore, parasympatholytic drugs are also called antimuscarinic or Chol-M blockers.

Ganglionic blocking drugs combine with acetylcholine receptors at the postganglionic cell body. Thus, ganglionic blockers will prevent transmission in all autonomic ganglia whether SNS or PNS. Since nicotine stimulates all autonomic ganglia, the acetylcholine receptors at

ganglia are called Chol-N. It is thought that ganglionic blockers attach to Chol-N receptors just as parasympatholytics attach to Chol-M receptors. The prototype ganglionic blocking drug is hexamethonium.

The neuromuscular junction (NMJ) is also a site of cholinergic transmission, since acetylcholine is secreted by somatic nerves and acts as the neurotransmitter of skeletal muscle activity. The receptors for ACh at the NMJ resemble the nicotinic (Chol-N) receptors in some respects, but since there are pharmacologic differences, they are better named "Chol-NMJ receptors." The major difference is that NMJ blockers are selective, affecting the NMJ transmission but having little or no effect on ganglionic transmission. The prototype drug for NMJ blockade is *d*-tubocurarine (curare), a drug which is often used to paralyze skeletal muscles during anesthesia.

Effects of Atropine

Objective 17.C.2. Describe the pharmacologic and toxicologic effects of atropine.

Atropine blocks all PNS activities. Thus, atropine blocks all secretions (salivary, sweat, GI tract, respiratory tract, and so on), increases the heart rate (by blocking vagal activity), decreases smooth muscle tone (GI and bronchiolar), dilates the pupil, and paralyzes accommodation of the eye. Table 17–2 may help the reader to re-

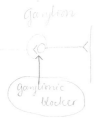

TABLE 17–2. EFFECTS OF ATROPINE

Effector	Therapeutic Use	Toxic Effect
glands	drying secretions in anesthesia	**"dry as a bone"** (secretions dried)
cardiovascular	relief of heart block	**"red as a beet"** (vasodilation)
glands and cardiovascular	see above	**"hot as fire"** (combination of no sweat and vasodilation)
eye	pupillary dilation (eyedrops for ophthalmologic examination)	**"blind as a bat"**
CNS	antiparkinson drug	**"mad as a hatter"**[a]
smooth muscle	peptic ulcer	(atony)

[a] Hatters actually became maniacal because of mercury ingestion that occurred as a result of licking their fingers.

member atropine's effects. In the column on the left, the organ effectors are listed; in the center column the therapeutic usefulness of the effect is listed; and, in column 3, the toxic result of overdose is listed. The mnemonic in column 3 is given as an aid to memory.

In general, toxic doses of atropine cause exaggerated therapeutic responses. Side effects of atropine include dry mouth, blurred vision, gastric atony, palpitations, and urinary retention. Almost all of the therapeutic and side effects of atropine are due to blockade of Chol-M receptors, except cutaneous vasodilation (a direct effect), and reduced sweating (a blockade of cholinergic sympathetic innervation).

There appears to be a dose-related order of sensitivity of the Chol-M receptors to atropine. At small doses, the patient has xerostomia and lack of sweating. Larger doses block the vagus, causing cardiac effects. Still larger doses inhibit GI and urinary tract smooth muscle. Extremely high doses are needed to block gastric secretion in humans, which makes the achievement of this therapeutic goal difficult. Atropine causes ganglionic blocking effects in extremely high doses.

Belladonna

Objective 17.C.3. Describe the term belladonna-alkaloid.

Atropa belladonna (the deadly nightshade) is the plant from which atropine was originally isolated. Tincture of **belladonna** is often used for its atropinic effects because it contains the alkaloid, atropine, and some related alkaloids, including scopolamine. In modern medicine, the pure, synthetic drug is preferred to the impure tincture. Belladonna is the Italian word for beautiful lady, and the plant was given the name, belladonna, because of the practice of using the extract for the purpose of causing pupillary dilation in Venetian ladies, which apparently was a sign of beauty.

Other Parasympatholytics

Objective 17.C.4. Name three parasympatholytic drugs which are closely related to atropine and compare them to atropine.

Scopolamine, methantheline (*Banthine*), and **propantheline** (*Pro-Banthine*) are parasympatholytic drugs related to atropine. Scopolamine is similar to atropine in most respects. It has a shorter duration of action and a more pronounced CNS depressant effect. Scopolamine may have some selectivity on certain Chol-M receptors, having more activity than atropine on the eye and in blocking secretions. Atropine seems to be more potent on heart and smooth muscle. Anesthesiologists often prefer scopolamine over atropine because of scopolamine's CNS depressant and amnesic effects. Scopolamine is also preferred for motion sickness.

While atropine and scopolamine are tertiary amines, methantheline and propantheline are synthetic quaternary amines. Thus, the quaternary drugs have fewer CNS side effects, such as drowsiness, due to lack of penetration of the **blood-brain barrier.** They are used at higher adult dosages (2 to 15 mg) than is atropine (0.6 mg). Propantheline is considered the drug of choice for saliva control in dentistry because of its relative lack of side effects. Propantheline is effective orally. The usual adult dose is 15 mg, but occasionally 30 mg are needed. The drug is given 30 to 45 minutes preoperatively. Contraindications include glaucoma and prostatic hypertrophy. Drowsiness may occur, and the patient should be forewarned (see also, Chapter 2).

Contraindications of Parasympatholytics

Objective 17.C.5. Lilst two absolute contraindications for atropinelike drugs.

Atropine and related drugs, including propantheline, are contraindicated in patients having **glaucoma** or **prostatic hypertrophy.** In glaucoma, pupillary dilation caused by parasympatholytics can have disastrous results, leading to blindness. As the pupils dilate, the drainage canals in the eye are obstructed, which leads to increased intraocular pressure. In prostatic hypertrophy, the decreased ability to micturate can be aggravated by urinary tract atony caused by atropinelike drugs.

Antidotes to Atropine and Anticholinesterase Poisonings

Objective 17.C.6. Name an antidote for atropine poisoning and for anticholinesterase poisoning; list unfavorable results occurring when using these antidotes.

Atropine and anticholinesterase drugs are antagonists, and one drug will reverse the effect of the other. Atropine has been recommended to counteract the symptoms of nerve gas and organophosphorus insecticide poisoning which have a pronounced anticholinesterase effect. (Remember DFP? If not, see 17.B.3.) Although atropine may make the patient comfortable by relieving unpleasant effects of acetylcholine, the real danger is respiratory paralysis due to Chol-NMJ stimulation, which leads to depolarization blockade of respiratory muscle.

On the other hand, physostigmine can be used to increase acetylcholine by an anticholinesterase action, thus competitively overcoming the blockade caused by atropine poisoning. Problems may occur if too much anticholinesterase drug is used, resulting in excess ACh stimulation, and possible paralysis of the respiratory muscles.

Ganglionic Stimulants

Objective 17.C.7. Name and describe the effects of two ganglionic stimulant drugs.

Nicotine and **lobeline** are ganglionic stimulants. Nicotine is the main drug in cigarettes, while lobeline is sold OTC as a drug used for breaking the cigarette habit. Both drugs have similar effects, stimulating ganglionic cells and generally causing vasoconstriction and increased heart rate. The vasoconstriction can be harmful in subjects with peripheral vascular disease where the blood supply is already compromised. The ganglionic stimulant action of nicotine is the basis for naming acetylcholine receptors in ganglia as Chol-N receptors. Nicotine in low doses will stimulate ganglia and reverse the effects of ganglionic blockers, but in high doses nicotine depolarizes the ganglion cell, thus causing a depolarizing blockade.

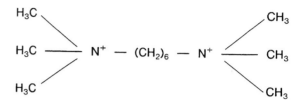

Figure 17-1. Chemical structure of hexamethonium

Ganglionic Blockers

Objective 17.C.8. Describe two ganglionic blocking drugs and their general effects.

Hexamethonium is a quaternary bisonium ion shown in Figure 17-1. (*bis* means two, *onium* means quaternary amine). The six carbon separation of the onium ions seem to be important for fit on the Chol-N receptor. **Mecamylamine** differs in structure because it has tertiary amine groups instead of quaternary groups. Mecamylamine is well absorbed and has clinically important ganglionic blocking action.

It is difficult to predict with certainty the action of ganglionic blockers, since they nonselectively block both PNS and SNS ganglia. In many systems, the mixed effects tend to cancel each other out, and the net effect may be related to the status of the system at the time of injection. However, since the SNS is predominant in controlling vascular tone, ganglionic blockers tend to reduce vascular tone, causing vasodilation and reduction of blood pressure. This was considered important after their discovery for possible use in therapy of hypertension, but frequent side effects and discovery of better hypotensive drugs, e.g., adrenergic neuron blockers (Chapters 18 and 31), has led to a loss of popularity of ganglionic blockers as antihypertensive drugs. They are used only to produce controlled hypotension during surgery.

Side Effects of Ganglionic Blockers

Objective 17.C.9. List the side effects of ganglionic blocking drugs.

Postural hypotension, smooth muscle atony, blurred vision, dry mouth, lack of sweating, and

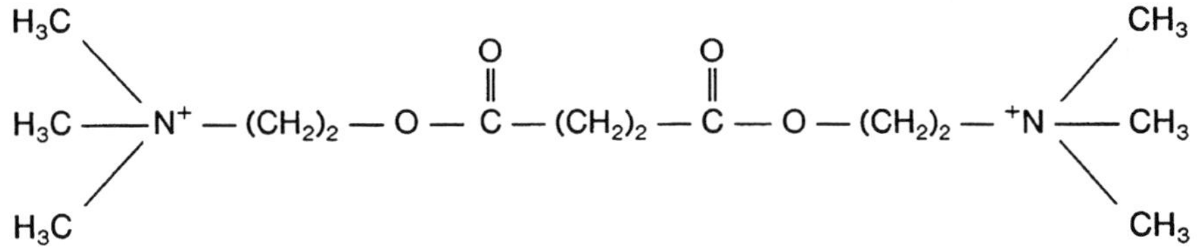

Figure 17-2. Chemical structure of succinylcholine.

interference with sexual function are the major side effects of ganglionic blocking drugs.

Neuromuscular Blockers

Objective 17.C.10. Name five neuromuscular junction (NMJ) blocking drugs and describe their mechanisms and durations of action.

d-TUBOCURARINE (CURARE)

This is a bisonium compound with a 10-atom distance between its two positive ionic centers. Its relaxing effect on skeletal muscle is transient, the drug being rapidly excreted and metabolized. d-Tubocurarine causes **nondepolarizing,** competitive antagonism of acetylcholine's action at the NMJ. Therefore, depolarizing drugs (acetylcholine or cholinesterase inhibitors) tend to reverse the block of curare. Curare is also a potent histamine releaser.

GALLAMINE

This drug is like curare but is shorter acting and lacks the histamine-releasing action. However, gallamine has a vagolytic (atropine-like) action that causes tachycardia.

DECAMETHONIUM

This is a relative of hexamethonium with a 10-atom separation of the two onium groups, as in curare. Decamethonium causes **depolarization** blockade of the NMJ. Thus, other depolarizing drugs (acetylcholine or cholinesterase inhibitors) tend to increase the block of decamethonium.

SUCCINYLCHOLINE

This drug is two acetylcholine molecules connected, with about a 10-atom distance between the two positive (quaternary amine) centers. The chemical structure can be noted in Figure 17-2. Succinylcholine causes considerable muscle fasciculation when injected, then a short-

lived (about 5 min.) paralysis with a rather rapid recovery. The NMJ block is **depolarizing** and noncompetitive, causing respiratory arrest. Artificial respiration must be used when giving succinylcholine for muscular relaxation, and, therefore, this drug is used only during general anesthesia or for electroshock therapy to prevent convulsions.

Unlike the other NMJ blockers, succinylcholine is rapidly metabolized by plasma cholinesterase, which accounts for its short duration of action. Rarely, a patient is encountered who has hereditary absence of a plasma cholinesterase; succinylcholine would be extremely dangerous in such a patient.

PANCURONIUM

Pancuronium is a **nondepolarizing agent.** Ganglionic blockade and histamine-releasing actions of d-tubocurarine are essentially absent with use of this drug. In addition, pancuronium's action is more easily reversed, compared with gallamine, and it is approximately five times as potent as d-tubocurarine.

BIBLIOGRAPHY

Csáky TZ: Cutting's Handbook of Pharmacology, 6th ed. New York, Appleton-Century-Crofts, 1979, Ch 43, 44, 45, 46

Gilman AG, Goodman LS, Gilman A (eds): Goodman and Gilman's The Pharmacological Basis of Therapeutics, 6th ed. New York, Macmillan, 1980, Ch 5, 6, 7, 10

QUESTIONS

1. **T** F Cholinomimetic refers to any drug that resembles acetylcholine in its pharmacologic action.

2. **T** F Cholinergic drugs have an effect on nerves that secrete acetylcholine.

3. **T** *F* A cholinergic nerve secretes the chemical, choline. *Acetylcholine*

inhibits

4. **T** *F* Atropine specifically stimulates the action of PNS-mimetics and PNS post-ganglionic nerve stimulation.

5. A PNS-mimetic drug can also be classified as all of the following *except:*

   A. muscarinic
   B. cholinomimetic
   C. atropinic → *Parasympatholytic*
   D. cholinergic

   ganglionic blocker < *PNS / SNS*

6. **T** *F* A nicotinic drug will cause parasympathetic effects but no sympathetic effects.

7. A cholinesterase inhibitor causes:

   A. massive stimulation of PNS receptors
   B. massive stimulation of ganglia
   C. both A and B are correct
   D. neither A nor B is correct

   anti-cholinesterase   PNS-mimetic (ester)

8. Physostigmine and methacholine are:

   A. direct-acting parasympathomimetics
   B. cholinergic drugs which act by different mechanisms
   C. blocked by hexamethonium
   D. all of the above are correct
   E. none of the above is correct

   bronchiolar constriction

9. Methacholine would be contraindicated in a patient who has:

   A. asthmatic attacks
   B. glaucoma
   C. both A and B are correct
   D. neither A nor B is correct

10. Acetylcholine is a poor therapeutic agent because:

    A. it is extremely stable, resulting in long duration of action
    B. it has highly nonspecific actions
    C. both A and B are correct
    D. neither A nor B is correct

11. A patient under your care has been diagnosed as having atony of the GI tract. What would be the drug of choice for treatment?

    A. methacholine → > *cardiovascular effect*
    B. bethanechol → *GI & urinary bladder stim*
    C. carbachol → *↑ glaucoma (miosis)*
    D. pilocarpine

12. All of the following apply to methacholine *except*:

    A. slow hydrolysis rate
    B. contraindicated in vascular spasms → *↑ vascular spasm*
    C. little or no ganglionic activity
    D. PNS-mimetic

13. **T** *F* Carbachol is a useful miotic which has minimal nicotinic effects. *(significant)*

14. **T** *F* Pilocarpine and atropine are naturally occurring parasympathomimetics.

    toxicity

15. **T** F Muscarine is used clinically more often than pilocarpine.

    alkaloid

16. Pilocarpine causes all of the following *except*:

    A. sweating
    B. xerostomia → *↑ = xerostomia*
    C. prominent side effects
    D. miosis

17. All of the following are clinically useful PNS-mimetics *except*:

    A. methacholine
    B. pilocarpine

C. muscarine
D. bethanechol

18. Cholinesterase terminates the action of all of the following *except:*

A. acetylcholine
B. succinylcholine — *neuromuscular blocker*
C. pilocarpine *(alkaloid)*
D. methacholine

19. Which of the following drugs is the most slowly hydrolyzed by cholinesterase action?

A. acetylcholine
B. methacholine
C. carbachol → *stable*
D. pilocarpine → *is most slowly hydrolyzed*

20. Which of the following drugs has the lowest nicotinic effect?

A. lobeline ~ *nicotine*
B. methacholine *very little or no*
C. carbachol *significant*
D. acetylcholine

21. Cholinesterase inhibitors cause:

A. increased concentration of acetylcholine at cholinergic nerve junctions
B. specific PNS effects but no SNS effects
C. inhibition of most smooth muscle
D. skeletal muscle relaxation

22. Each of the following drugs is a reversible cholinesterase inhibitor *except:*

A. physostigmine
B. neostigmine
C. diisopropylfluorophosphate → *irreversible*
D. edrophonium chloride

23. Which of the following drugs is used for the diagnosis of myasthenia gravis?

A. physostigmine
B. edrophonium chloride → *very short duration (5')*

→ *Δ + myasthenia gravis*
↓
(NMJ impairment)

C. both A and B are correct
D. neither A nor B is correct

24. **T** F *Tensilon* Edrophonium may be used to counteract curariform blockade of NMJ.

25. Irreversible cholinesterase inhibitors are so named because:

A. they form covalent bonds with the cholinesterase enzyme
B. they have no known antidote
C. both A and B are correct
D. neither A nor B is correct

only (DFP → A glaucoma)

26. T **F** Thousands of organophosphorus compounds are useful irreversible cholinesterase inhibitors.

2-PAM → world war II

27. **T** F Pralidoxime is a drug that can reverse the effects of DFP.

28. Which of the following is not considered an anticholinergic prototype drug?

A. atropine
B. decamethonium
C. hexamethonium
D. *d*-tubocurarine *(curare)*

29. **T** F *d*-tubocurarine is used to paralyze skeletal muscle during anesthesia.

gan
30. **T** F Nicotine blocks receptors on the postganglionic cell body.

chol-NMJ
31. T **F** Chol-N blockers are known for their effect in blocking NMJ transmission.

32. Pilocarpine would be antagonized by:

A. atropine
B. muscarine
C. both A and B are correct
D. neither A nor B is correct

33. Atropine is an antidote for:

A. cholinesterase inhibitors
B. vagal hyperactivity

C. both A and B are correct
D. neither A nor B is correct

34. Atropine causes:

    A. pupillary dilation
    B. accommodation of the eye
    C. both A and B are correct
    D. neither A nor B is correct

35. An effect of atropine correlated to PNS blockade is:

    A. cutaneous vasodilation (direct effect)
    B. decreased sweating → cholinergic sympathetic
    C. both A and B are correct
    D. neither A nor B is correct

36. Which of the following effects is most easily blocked by atropine?

    A. ganglionic transmission
    B. gastric secretion
    C. urinary tract muscle
    D. salivation

37. T F Belladonna contains not only atropine but also scopolamine and some other alkaloids.

38. T F Scopolamine, methantheline, and propantheline are parasympatholytic drugs related to atropine.

39. Which of the following drugs is a quaternary amine?

    A. atropine
    B. propantheline (pro Banthine)
    C. both A and B are correct
    D. neither A nor B is correct

40. Scopolamine may be more useful than atropine, because scopolamine:

    A. causes more amnesia
    B. prevents motion sickness better

C. both A and B are correct
D. neither A nor B is correct

41. Which is considered the drug of choice for saliva control in dentistry?

    A. atropine
    B. scopolamine
    C. methacholine
    D. propantheline (Pro Banthine)

42. T F A contraindication for propantheline is glaucoma.

43. T F Atropinelike drugs are contraindicated in prostatic hypertrophy because the decreased ability to micturate can be aggravated by urinary tract atony caused by atropinelike drugs.

44. T F The main danger for a patient with DFP poisoning is the parasympatholytic effects of acetylcholine build-up.

45. T F Anticholinesterase is not perfect as an antidote for atropine, and the converse is also true. (because of side effects)

46. T F Either atropine or scopolamine might serve as antidotes for anticholinesterase drugs.

47. Each of the following drugs has an effect on Chol-N receptors except:

    A. carbachol → significant ganglionic effect
    B. norepinephrine
    C. nicotine
    D. lobeline

48. T F Nicotine can stimulate ganglia and cause depolarizing blockade.

49. T F Lobeline is a nicotinelike substance found in cigarettes.

ganglionic stimulant → vasoconstriction. ↑ heart rate.

50. (T) F Nicotine is contraindicated in a patient with peripheral vascular disease.

51. Mecamylamine's activity most closely resembles that of:

A. methacholine
(B.) hexamethonium → *ganglionic blocker*
C. decamethonium → *neuromuscular blocker*
D. all of the above are correct
E. none of the above is correct

52. T (F) Mecamylamine is a useful drug for most patients with hypertension.

53. Side effects of ganglionic blocking drugs include all of the following *except:*

A. interference with sexual function
B. lack of sweating
C. blurred vision →
(D.) hypertension

54. *d*-Tubocurarine's use involves all of the following *except:*

A. respiratory paralysis
B. neuromuscular junction blockade
C. histamine release → *potent histamine releaser*
(D.) cholinesterase inhibition

55. Competitive nondepolarizing neuromuscular blockade is produced by:

(A.) *d*-tubocurarine
B. succinylcholine
C. both A and B are correct
D. neither A nor B is correct

56. T (F) Physostigmine antagonizes the neuromuscular blocking action of succinylcholine.

57. (T) F Succinylcholine's action is terminated by metabolism due to activity of the enzyme cholinesterase.

58. Each of the following drugs is a neuromuscular blocking drug *except:*

A. *d*-tubocurarine
B. decamethonium
C. succinylcholine
(D.) mecamylamine → *ganglionic blocking drug (& hexamethonium)*

59. Physostigmine will reverse NMJ blockade of:

A. neostigmine
(B.) gallamine
C. succinylcholine
D. decamethonium

18

Adrenergic Drugs

¹¹/₁₈

A. SNS DRUGS AND ADRENERGIC MECHANISMS

Objective 18.A.1. Define and differentiate between sympathomimetic (SNS-mimetic) and sympatholytic, adrenergic and noradrenergic.

Objective 18.A.2. Classify adrenergic drugs into sympathomimetic, sympatholytic, and adrenergic neuron blockers.

Sympathomimetic is an adjective which means "resembling sympathetic." In other words, an SNS-mimetic drug has activity similar to stimulation of sympathetic nerves. On the other hand, **sympatholytic** drugs are those that block sympathomimetic drugs or block SNS activity. When stimulated, the sympathetic nerves cause norepinephrine (NE) release from postganglionic endings and a mixture of epinephrine (E) and NE from adrenal medulla. Thus, massive SNS stimulation causes a syndrome of SNS effects related to both neural release and adrenal outpouring of E-NE into the bloodstream. Effects of sympathomimetic drugs can resemble SNS stimulation in one or more respects.

The term **adrenergic** comes from adrenaline, the official British name for epinephrine. Historically, the neurotransmitter of SNS activity was thought to be an adrenaline-like substance, and the nerves causing effects similar to epinephrine administration were called adrenergic. Many early pharmacologists noted that nerve stimulation did not always cause the same effects as epinephrine. Therefore, the substance was called "sympathin." Later, pharmacologists discovered that the neurotransmitter of sympathetic nerve activity was NE, which helped account for some of the differences between nerve stimulation and epinephrine administration. Actually, because SNS nerves secrete NE, they should have been called *noradrenergic* instead of adrenergic. Nevertheless, the term "adrenergic" has been used synonymously with sympathetic. Thus, we classify adrenergic drugs as all those having an action upon sympathetic (adrenergic) nerves or related adrenergic function. We could also call them sympathetic drugs. The classification of adrenergic drugs includes (1) **sympathomimetic drugs,** (2) **adrenergic receptor blockers,** and (3) **adrenergic neuron blocking agents.**

163

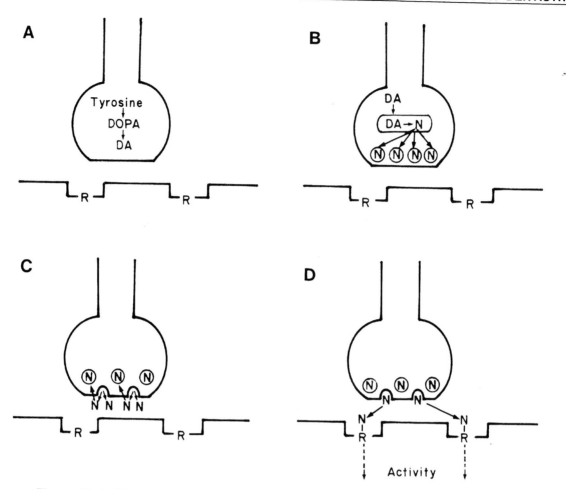

Figure 18–1. Mechanisms of adrenergic transmission. **A.** DA synthesis. **B.** NE synthesis and granular storage. **C.** Release and reuptake. **D.** Receptor activation. Dopa, L-dihydroxyphenylalanine; DA, L-dopamine; N, norepinephrine; R, receptor (can be either α or β); N→R, receptor complex.

Objective 18.A.3. Describe the adrenergic neuron in terms of neurotransmitter synthesis, storage, release, reuptake, and reaction with receptor.

Figure 18–1 diagrams an adrenergic neuron, showing its function of synthesis (A and B), storage (B), release and reuptake (C), and receptor activation (D). Figure 18–1, A, and Figure 18–2 show that tyrosine is converted by an enzyme (tyrosine hydroxylase) to dihydroxyphenylalanine (dopa) or L-dopa. Dopa is then decarboxylated by an enzyme to dopamine (DA). The decarboxylation enzyme is L-aromatic amino acid

(L-AAA) decarboxylase. It is nonspecific, acting on almost any L-AAA (see Chapter 19). The next step is in the granule (Fig. 18–1, B), where DA is converted to NE by the granule-bound enzyme DA β-hydroxylase. After NE is synthesized, it is stored in the granules (Fig. 18–1, B), which are located near the presynaptic membrane (Fig. 18–1, C). During activity, the vesicles coalesce with the membrane, releasing their contents of neurotransmitter into the synaptic cleft. In Figure 18–1, D, the neurotransmitter traverses the cleft and reacts with the postsynaptic receptor (either α or β). The receptor activation results in further reactions in the postsynaptic cell,

$$\text{tyrosine} \xrightarrow[\text{tyrosine hydroxylase}]{\text{add OH to ring}} \text{DOPA} \xrightarrow[\text{L-AAA}]{-CO_2} \text{DA} \xrightarrow[\text{DA } \beta\text{-hydroxylase}]{\text{add OH alkyl chain}} \text{NE}$$

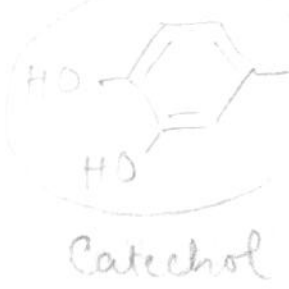

Figure 18–2. Formation of NE.

causing contraction, relaxation, or secretion. (NOTE: in the adrenal medulla up to 80% of the NE may be methylated to form epinephrine. It is known that granular NE must be released into the cytosol before being converted to epinephrine and subsequent restorage.) In addition to reacting with the receptors, some of the NE is returned to the neurons and is reincorporated into the storage granules (a process called reuptake, Fig. 18–1, C).

Objective 18.A.4. Describe how SNS-mimetics act.

The agonists which resemble NE or E act by combining with the receptor, causing a loose drug-receptor complex and resulting in similar events which follow SNS activity when NE is released. It should be noted that epinephrine is the best overall drug for mimicking SNS stimulation, even though NE is the neural transmitter. For example, epinephrine inhibits vascular smooth muscle, causing vasodilation (a β response), while NE is devoid of this activity.

Objective 18.A.5. Describe mechanisms for termination of action of NE and its reuptake.

Reuptake
When NE is released, not all of the mediator reacts with the receptor. Some (about one half) is returned to the neuron by an active reuptake mechanism. After reuptake, the mediator may be returned to granules or follow other pathways (e.g., metabolism). Reuptake is blocked by cocaine (the only local anesthetic which is active in blocking reuptake) or by nerve section. Increased availability of NE for the receptor is thought to be the reason for cocaine's potentiating action on adrenergic activity. Denervation sensitivity, due to nerve section, is thought to potentiate NE by the same mechanism, blocking the pump and making more NE available for re-

ceptor action. However, other explanations are possible, including change in the state of, or number of, receptors on the effector cell.

Catechol-O-Methyl Transferase (COMT)
This enzyme inactivates NE or E by methylation. This mechanism seems to act as a scavenger for catecholamines which are absorbed into the bloodstream because the COMT activity is found mainly in vascular walls and liver. Thus, enzymatic termination of synaptic activity by COMT is not important; reuptake and diffusion seem to be the important processes for termination of neurotransmitter activity. There are no important drugs that act by inhibiting COMT.

Monoamine Oxidase (MAO)
This enzyme is found intracellularly in mitochondria and may act on NE which has been taken up from extracellular space, on other amines taken up from extracellular space, and on excess stored NE. There is an important category of drugs called MAO inhibitors (MAOI).

Monoamine Oxidase Inhibitors (MAOI). Pargyline is the prototype MAOI drug. Strangely, pargyline produces hypotension (opposite of the expected result, assuming that catecholamines accumulate). The MAO inhibitors appear to have other actions, some of which may be central, and MAO may be necessary to maintain the adrenergic neuron. Therefore, MAOI could act as adrenergic neuron blocking agents, possibly allowing false transmitters to accumulate.

Since MAOI do not potentiate adrenergic nerve activity, MAO must not be important for deactivation of NE at the neuroeffector junction. Again, the importance of reuptake and of diffusion seem to be emphasized for termination of SNS activity.

MAOI are rather toxic drugs causing many side effects and drug interactions and generally

TABLE 18–1. COMPARISON OF SYMPATHOMIMETICS

Drug	Trade Name	α	β	CNS	Main Therapeutic Use
norepinephrine	*Levophed*	√	heart only	±	vasopressor
epinephrine	*Adrenalin*	√	√	+	anaphylactic shock, vasoconstrictor
levenordefrin	*Neo-Cobefrin*	√	√	±	vasoconstrictor in local anesthetic
phenylephrine	*Neo-Synephrine*	√	0	±	vasoconstrictor (mainly nasal)
ephedrine	—	√	√	+	long-acting bronchodilator
amphetamine	*Dexedrine*	√	√	++	obesity, CNS stimulant
mephentermine	*Wyamine*	√	heart only	0	shock
isoproterenol	*Isuprel*	0	√	±	bronchodilator by inhalation

0, none or minimal; ±, not expected but may occur; +, reported; ++, pronounced.

are difficult to use. One adverse effect of MAOI is increased SNS activity due to accumulation of amines absorbed from food. Tyramine is a naturally occurring amine in such foods as cheese and wine which is normally metabolized and inactivated by MAO, but in the presence of MAOI, tyramine accumulates and exerts hypertensive and other SNS effects.

Norepinephrine and epinephrine and other SNS-mimetics (including levenordefrin) are contraindicated for use with local anesthetics when the patient is taking MAOI. (We believe this is a relative contraindication; by using about one-third the normal dose and injecting carefully, the dentist can use the anesthetic with vasoconstrictor.) An absolute contraindication is the use of indirect-acting sympathomimetics (such as ephedrine) because of a possible hypertensive crisis.

B. SNS-MIMETICS

Objective 18.B.1. List eight adrenergic receptor agonists, describing their similarities and differences, therapeutic usefulness, and side effects.

Eight important adrenergic receptor agonists are described below. Their activities on α and β receptors and on the CNS and their usfulness in therapeutics are summarized in Table 18–1.

NOREPINEPHRINE (*Levophed*)
This catecholamine is the neurotransmitter in adrenergic neurons. NE is a potent stimulator of all α receptors and of cardiac β receptors. It is almost devoid of activity on β receptors for vasodilation and bronchiolar dilation. When it is given to man by IV infusion, there are pronounced effects on blood pressure because NE constricts blood vessels without causing vasodilation in any vascular beds. As a result, pronounced reflex bradycardia may occur after administration of NE. The main therapeutic use of NE is as a vasopressor, but some other SNS-mimetic may be preferred.

EPINEPHRINE (*Adrenalin*)
This is a naturally secreted catecholamine from the adrenal medulla. Epinephrine is not a known adrenergic neurotransmitter. Epinephrine has pronounced α and β actions, thus having a broader range of activity than NE. Because epinephrine causes vasodilation, it does not cause the pronounced reflex bradycardia usually caused by NE. Epinephrine and NE are about equipotent on most adrenergic structures where both are active (i.e., α receptors and cardiac β receptors). Epinephrine is the most useful vasoconstrictor for local anesthesia, since vasodilation probably does not occur in the submucosa. Epinephrine is a useful emergency drug for treating bronchiolar constriction, as in asthma and allergy.

LEVONORDEFRIN (*Neo-Cobefrin* α-methylnorepinephrine)
This SNS-mimetic is considered a false neurotransmitter in adrenergic nerves because it is readily stored in place of NE, when α-methyldopa is given to an animal. The synthesis would be as follows:

α-methyldopa $\rightarrow$ α-methyl DA $\rightarrow$ α-methyl NE

These reactions use the same enzymes that form NE (Fig. 18–2). This observation led pharmacologists to attribute the hypotensive action of α-methyldopa to formation of a false transmitter, which is weaker than NE and replaces it. Actually, α-methyl NE is a rather strong agonist (about one fifth to one tenth the potency of NE). There are many other arguments against the concept of the false transmitter mechanism. Some pharmacologists favor a central (CNS) action as an explanation of the hypotensive action of α-methyldopa.

Levonordefrin is used as a vasoconstrictor in mepivacaine solutions.

PHENYLEPHRINE

Phenylephrine (PE) is an agonist with no β activity, which makes it helpful in pharmacologic investigations. PE is used clinically in nosedrops to constrict the nasal mucosa and relieve congestion. The problem with this therapy is a possible rebound effect, i.e., after action of the drug is terminated, the vessels overreact and are more dilated than before the drug was administered. PE is much less potent and much less toxic than NE.

EPHEDRINE

The actions of ephedrine resemble those of epinephrine more closely than those of NE. Its main action is to release stored NE (indirect effect), but a direct effect on the receptors has also been described. Ephedrine is known for its tachyphylactic effect and produces more CNS stimulation than does epinephrine. *CNS Broncho dilator*

AMPHETAMINE

This drug is similar to ephedrine, but amphetamine's CNS stimulatory effects are more pronounced. Amphetamine stimulates wakefulness and elevates mood. Side effects are frequent, including nervousness, insomia, and, in high doses, hallucinations and exhaustion. Amphetamine has been used therapeutically in obesity (anorexic effect) and as a stimulant for treatment of depression. Both of these therapeutic uses are questionable, and the use of amphetamine is fraught with danger because of the ease with which it causes psychic dependence. Phenylpropanolamine is an OTC diet suppressant drug related to amphetamine and having all of the possible side effects, although it requires a higher dosage in milligrams.

MEPHENTERMINE (*Wyamine*)

This may be a preferred drug for hypotension because it is longer acting and has little CNS activity. Mephentermine increases blood pressure by both vascular and cardiac action.

ISOPROTERENOL

This is the prototype β agonist. It stimulates all β receptor activities, including cardiac acceleration, increased cardiac contractility, vasodilation, and bronchodilation. The drug is used therapeutically mainly for bronchodilation. Isoproterenol is short acting and potent, with side effects due to cardiac stimulation and hypotension (vasodilation). Terbutaline, a more specific β_2 agonist is discussed in 18.C.6.

Objective 18.B.2. Distinguish between direct- and indirect-acting sympathomimetics and list four direct- and three indirect-acting drugs.

Direct-acting sympathomimetics act by combining with the receptor. NE, E, PE, and isoproterenol are direct acting. Indirect-acting sympathomimetics act by displacing NE from storage granules, thus releasing NE from the adrenergic terminals. **Tyramine** is an amine found in food and is only indirect acting. **Ephedrine** and **amphetamine** are classified as indirect acting because they release NE. However, they also combine directly with receptors in some situations.

C. ADRENERGIC RECEPTOR BLOCKING AGENTS

Objective 18.C.1. Distinguish between α-adrenergic receptor blocking agents and β-adrenergic receptor blocking agents.

Alpha adrenergic receptor blocking agents (α blockers) are drugs that react with α receptors not only blocking adrenergic transmission but also blocking action of α adrenergic receptor agonists. Some α activities include vasoconstriction, pupillary dilation, and GI relaxation. Beta adrenergic receptor blocking agents are drugs that have an analogous activity on β receptors as α blockers on α receptors. Some β activities are cardiac acceleration, increased cardiac force, vasodilation, bronchodilation, and smooth muscle relaxation (see Chapter 16, Table 16–3).

Objective 18.C.2. Describe two types of α blockade and name three α receptor blockers, identifying their type.

Alpha blockers can be divided into **reversible, competitive** antagonists and **irreversible, noncompetitive** antagonists. Reversible implies that increasing the concentration of agonist will overcome the block and, therefore, a full response can be obtained. With irreversible blockers, no response or only a partial response can be obtained. The dose response curves for these drugs would appear as is shown in Figure 18–3.

Three α blockers and their types are:

1. ergot alkaloids—reversible
2. phentolamine—reversible
3. phenoxybenzamine—irreversible

Ergot alkaloids were the first α blockers known and are important historically and pharmacologically. **Phentolamine** (*Regitine*) is marketed for human use mainly to diagnose pheochromocytoma (an adrenal medullary tumor that secretes catecholamines). Phentolamine may also be used in peripheral vascular disease and sometimes in shock to increase organ perfusion by blocking SNS tone. **Phenoxybenzamine** is used mainly as a pharmacologic tool.

Objective 18.C.3. Describe epinephrine reversal and three differences in the actions of antagonists compared to agonists.

Epinephrine reversal is illustrated in Figure 18–4. It is mentioned because some of your patients may be taking drugs which have α blockade as a side effect (e.g., chlorpromazine, an antipsychotic drug, which has substantial α

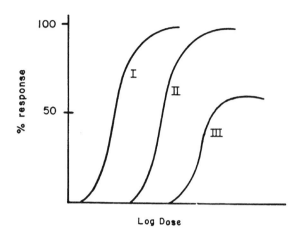

Figure 18–3. Dose-response curves for competitive and noncompetitive antagonism. **I.** Dose-response curve of agonist with no antagonist present. **II.** Dose-response curve of agonist with reversible, competitive antagonist present. **III.** Dose-response curve of agonist with a noncompetitive antagonist present.

blocking activity). In addition, β blockers are becoming more popular (see Chapter 31), and a patient taking a β blocker would have more prominent α responses. Referring to Figure 18–4, when no α blocker is present, epinephrine causes vasoconstriction, and the blood pressure increases. However, after α blockade, epinephrine causes only β vasodilation (since α vasoconstriction is blocked), and the blood pressure drops. When this epinephrine reversal was first discovered, it was somewhat of a mystery. More recently, the α,β receptor theory has explained the reversal quite clearly. Actually, it should probably be called "unmasking," because epinephrine causes both vasoconstriction and vasodilation with no blocker present, but only one activity predominates (depending on the magnitude of the two vectors which are opposite and tend to cancel each other). After blockade of the predominant vector (vasoconstriction), the less dominant vector becomes noticeable. However, alternate explanations are possible (see Chapter 36, p. 391).

Figure 18–4 is instructive about the differences between agonists and antagonists (see explanation in legend). Study of the explanation

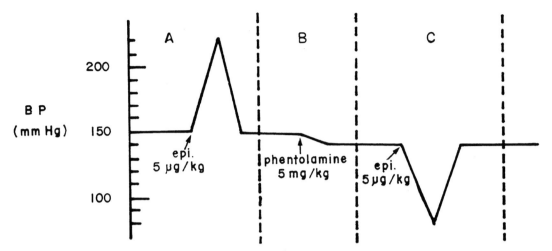

Figure 18–4. Epinephrine reversal. **A.** Epinephrine (epi.) raises the cat's blood pressure. **B.** The α blocker, phentolamine, is given. Three differences in action of antagonists and agonists are shown: (1) the blocking drug is usually used at higher concentration than the agonist, (2) the blocker causes very little effect on its own (in this case only a slight fall in BP), and (3) the blocker's action is of relatively long duration, while the agonist's duration is short. **C.** Epinephrine reversal. Instead of raising the BP, epinephrine lowers it after α blockade. Alpha blockade unmasks β vasodilation, which was present but not apparent in the absence of the blocker.

should satisfy the second part of Objective 18.C.3. This will serve also to reinforce Chapter 12 (Objective 12.H.2).

Objective 18.C.4. Recognize the classification of α receptors into α_1 and α_2, the basis for this classification, and an important useful drug (set in bold type) developed from studying this classification.

As described in Chapter 16 (Objective 16.L.4), there appear to be two subtypes of alpha receptors. Alpha$_1$ receptors are located primarily but not exclusively at postjunctional sites and are probably responsible for postjunctional events, which are primarily excitatory in nature. Alpha$_2$ receptors are located primarily but not exclusively on prejunctional nerve endings, and these receptors regulate release and probably synthesis of transmitter (e.g., stimulation of α_2 prejunctional receptors by NE, an agonist, results in decreased release and synthesis of NE). Conversely, blockade of α_2 receptors results in increased release of NE. How this information relates to therapy is unknown at this time, except that the drug, **prazosin,** a pure α_1 blocker, is an antihypertensive drug that produces little or no reflex tachycardia. Of lesser importance, but still interesting, is the finding that yohimbine, a pure α_2 blocker, has been shown to antagonize the blood pressure-lowering effect of some antihypertensive agents.

Objective 18.C.5. List two β blockers (set in bold type) and describe their effects, therapeutic usefulness, and side effects.

Dichloroisoproterenol was the first drug discovered which blocked β receptors. The drug was not clinically useful because it has considerable β **agonistic** activity as well as **antagonistic** activity. **Propranolol** (*Inderal*), an important β blocking drug, is useful in cardiac arrhythmias, for angina pectoris and hypertension, and is recommended for migraine headaches. Propranolol is contraindicated in asthmatic patients because it increases bronchiolar tone. Side effects include symptoms related to the CNS, GI tract, skin (rash), and the heart (hypotension, and cardiac failure).

Objective 18.C.6. Recognize classification of β adrenergic receptors into β_1 and β_2, the basis for this classification, and the two drugs set in bold type related to this classification which are therapeutically useful.

During the study of adrenergic blocking drugs, it became apparent that certain newer drugs were selectively blocking the heart and others were selectively blocking bronchiolar smooth muscle. The heart receptors were called β_1 and the bronchiolar β_2. This finding resulted in discovery of a selective β_2 agonist and a selective β_1 antagonist. (NOTE: the selectivity is only relative because increasing concentration of drug tends to cause effects on the other receptor.)

The need for a bronchiolar relaxant in asthmatic patients which does not affect the heart is obvious. Epinephrine and isoproterenol, although useful bronchiolar relaxants, are nonspecific and react with both β_1 and β_2 receptors. Therefore, pharmacologists became very interested in the selective β_2 agonists, **terbutaline,** metaproterenol, and albuterol (these drugs are further described in Chapter 33). There appears to be no therapeutic use for a β_2 blocker, since bronchoconstriction is never therapeutically desirable.

There is a need for cardiac blockade without bronchoconstriction. Thus, the selective β_1 blockers, **atenolol** and metoprolol, were developed for use in treatment of cardiovascular diseases, such as hypertension, arrhythmia, and angina (see also Chapter 31).

D. ADRENERGIC NEURON BLOCKING AGENTS

Objective 18.D.1. Describe the usefulness of adrenergic neuron blocking agents.

Drugs of this class are useful in lowering blood pressure in patients with excessive sympathetic tone. Adrenergic neuron blockade has been found to be more effective therapeutically than ganglionic blockade in lowering blood pressure because the latter action is accompanied by many side effects and disappointing quantitative effects. Therefore, adrenergic neuron blockers (e.g., guanethidine and reserpine) have assumed more important roles in controlling hypertension.

Objective 18.D.2. List three adrenergic neuron blocking mechanisms.

Objective 18.D.3. Describe four drugs (set in bold type) that act by these mechanisms.

Adrenergic neurons are blocked when there is interference with synthesis, release, or storage of NE and when there is release (or depletion) of NE.

RESERPINE
This drug has been used as an antipsychotic drug but was found to deplete all adrenergic neurons of stored transmitter. The release is slow, and after 24 hours (usually two doses), depletion is relatively complete. **Reserpine** also depletes DA and serotonin. Reserpine acts centrally and peripherally to cause depletion and also blocks reaccumulation. Enzymes destroy the released catecholamine. Side effects are rather severe, including sedation, severe depression, hypotension, other CNS disturbances, and drug-induced parkinsonism. Peptic ulcers may be aggravated. Because of its side effects, reserpine is used only as an adjunct to other hypotensive agents in order to keep the doses of each drug lower.

GUANETHIDINE
This drug has effects on adrenergic nerves very similar to those of reserpine but without the CNS effects. The adrenergic neurotransmitter is depleted only in the periphery. **Guanethidine** is thought to interfere with synthesis and storage as well as possibly causing release. The net effect is depletion of norepinephrine and adrenergic neuron blockade.

Guanethidine was formerly the most popular hypotensive agent, but several newer agents (see Chapter 31) are now the drugs of choice. Side effects include orthostatic hypotension, bradycardia, diarrhea, and others. Guanethidine causes supersensitivity, and vasoconstrictors should be avoided if guanethidine is being used.

METHYLDOPA
This drug is handled like L-dopa (see synthesis of NE p. 165). It causes a false transmitter, α-methyl NE, to appear in the adrenergic storage granules, but its hypotensive action is thought to be central (see also levonordefrin p. 166).

PARGYLINE
This drug is an MAO inhibitor. MAOIs block many other enzymes, leading to side effects and drug interactions. The mechanism of the hypotensive effect is not known, but it may be central and/or related to false transmitter storage. Patients taking MAOIs would have a relative contraindication for epinephrine because its action may be potentiated. It is recommended that a small dose be used, for example, a child's dose for an adult.

BIBLIOGRAPHY

Csáky TZ: Cutting's Handbook of Pharmacology, 6th ed. New York, Appleton-Century-Crofts, 1979, Ch 41, 42

Gilman AG, Goodman LS, Gilman A (eds): Goodman and Gilman's The Pharmacological Basis of Therapeutics, 6th ed. New York, Macmillan, 1980, Ch 8, 9

Goth A: Medical Pharmacology, 10th ed. St. Louis, Mosby, 1981, Ch 15, 16

QUESTIONS

1. T F When direct-acting sympathomimetic drugs are administered, the sympathetic nerves release NE.

2. Adrenergic drugs include all of the following *except:*
   A. sympathomimetics
   B. sympatholytics
   C. adrenergic neuron blockers
   D. ganglionic blockers

3. Sympatholytic drugs may be all of the following *except:*
   A. adrenergic neuron blockers
   B. blockers of sympathomimetic drugs
   C. blockers of adrenergic receptors
   D. cholinesterase inhibitors

4. The adrenergic neuron can be blocked by all of the following *except:*
   A. blockade of dopa decarboxylase
   B. release of granular storage
   C. prevention of transmitter storage
   D. ganglionic blockade

5. T F Of all the SNS-mimetics, injected norepinephrine best simulates the results of massive sympathetic discharge.

6. Norepinephrine's action after release from adrenergic endings may be increased by:
   A. blocking reuptake into the neuron
   B. blocking the enzyme monoamine oxidase (MAO)
   C. blocking the enzyme catechol-O-methyltransferase (COMT)
   D. blocking the enzyme acetylcholinesterase

7. MAO is an enzyme responsible for:
   A. breakdown of catecholamines in the extracellular space
   B. breakdown of intracellular amines
   C. reuptake of norepinephrine
   D. termination of the adrenergic mediator released during SNS nerve activity

8. Ephedrine and amphetamine are sympathomimetics with:
   A. indirect and direct activity
   B. CNS activity

C. both A and B are correct
D. neither A nor B is correct

9. For a patient with hypotension the choice of sympathomimetic vasopressor may be:

    A. mephentermine (Wyamine)
    B. isoproterenol
    C. both A and B are correct
    D. neither A nor B is correct

10. T F Levenordefrin is α-methylnorepineph-
    rine.

11. T F Isoproterenol is a sympathomimetic which is useful as a vasopressor.

12. Amphetamine's pharmacologic actions most closely resemble that of:

    A. norepinephrine
    B. ephedrine
    C. α-methyldopamine
    D. phentolamine

13. When given IV, the pharmacologic activities of phenylephrine are most closely related to the activities of which one of the following drugs (given by the same route of administration)?

    A. isoproterenol
    B. norepinephrine
    C. diphenhydramine
    D. phentolamine

14. Levenordefrin (α-methylnorepinephrine):

    A. is used in local anesthetic solutions as a vasoconstrictor
    B. is considered a false transmitter
    C. has both α and β activity, but has less affinity than epinephrine
    D. all of the above
    E. none of the above

15. Amphetamine acts:

    A. on the CNS to a greater extent than ephedrine
    B. partially by direct action on the receptor
    C. paritally by releasing norepinephrine (indirect)
    D. A, B, and C are all correct
    E. neither A, B, nor C is correct

16. Which of the following is a valid test for α receptors?

    A. activated by phenylephrine
    B. norepinephrine more active than epinephrine more active than isoproterenol
    C. blocked by phentolamine
    D. A, B, and C are all correct
    E. neither A, B, nor C is correct

17. Two cats were tested for blood pressure effects of tyramine.

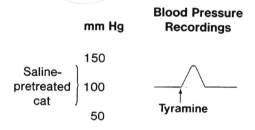

Result: The BP started at 100 mm Hg; when tyramine was given (at arrow) the BP rapidly rose to 150 and then returned to normal.

	mm Hg	Blood Pressure Recordings
	150	
Reserpine-pretreated cat	100	
	80	
	50	

Result: The BP started at 80 mm Hg; when tyramine was given there was no effect on BP.

The above experiments and your knowledge of adrenergic drugs indicate that:

A. reserpine is a releaser of stored norepi-nephrine

B. tyramine may act by releasing stored norepinephrine

C. both A and B are correct

D. neither A nor B is correct

α-blocker

18. After a cat is pretreated with a blocking dose of phentolamine, the injection of a pressor dose of epinephrine should cause:

A. a fall in blood pressure

B. bronchodilation

C. both A and B are correct

D. neither A nor B is correct

19. Phentolamine and phenoxybenzamine are:

A. both α adrenergic receptor blockers

B. both β adrenergic receptor blockers

C. both A and B are correct

D. neither A nor B is correct

20. Alpha receptor blockade is a form of:

A. competitive, pharmacologic antagonism

B. noncompetitive, depolarizing blockade

C. physiologic antagonism

D. local anesthesia

21, 22. The following results are obtained in a cat blood pressure experiment:

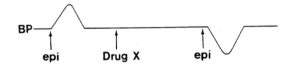

21. The interaction is known as:

A. physiologic antagonism

B. epinephrine reversal

C. both A and B are correct

D. neither A nor B is correct

22. Drug X may be:

A. either ephedrine or phenylephrine

B. either phentolamine or phenoxybenza-mine

C. phentolamine or phenylephrine

D. dichlorisoproterenol or propranolol

β-blocker *SNS ginmetic (prototype β agonist)*

23. A patient taking which one of the following drugs may show epinephrine reversal?

A. cocaine

B. chlorpromazine *(antipsychotic drug → α blocking activity)*

C. curare

D. carbachol

24. Which of the following drugs would serve as a replacement for propranolol?

A. DCI (dichloroisoproterenol)

B. DFP (diisopropylfluorophosphate)

C. phenoxybenzamine

D. phentolamine

25. T **F** Propranolol blocks epinephrine-in-duced bronchodilation.

26. T **F** Alpha receptors can be classified into two types called H_1 or H_2.

27. Hypertension can be controlled by:

A. propranolol

B. guanethidine

C. both A and B are correct

D. neither A nor B is correct

28. Which of the following drugs is useful to lower blood pressure of an ambulatory pa-tient?

A. a ganglionic blocker

B. an adrenergic neuron blocker

C. both A and B are correct

D. neither A nor B is correct

29. Adrenergic neuron blockade occurs when there is:

   A. interference with transmitter release
   B. transmitter release (depletion)
   C. both A and B are correct
   D. neither A nor B is correct

30. Guanethidine is an:

   A. adrenergic neuron blocking agent
   B. MAO inhibitor
   C. both A and B are correct
   D. neither A nor B is correct

31. T F Guanethidine and reserpine both deplete norepinephrine from adrenergic nerve terminals.

32. The blood pressure-lowering activity of guanethidine is probably related to:

   A. adrenergic neuron blockade
   B. blocking of synthesis and storage of norepinephrine
   C. depletion of stored norepinephrine
   D. A, B, and C are all correct
   E. neither A, B, nor C is correct

19
Autoregulatory Substances (Autacoids) and Antagonists

HISTAMINE, SEROTONIN, BRADYKININ, ANGIOTENSIN, PROSTAGLANDINS

The human body contains a number of active substances which have profound pharmacologic effects and which are suspected of playing a role in normal physiologic regulation as well as in pathologic processes. Such substances are formed and, in some cases, stored in the body. For some of these substances, the amount available would be fatal if released into the bloodstream all at one time. Naturally, such active substances aroused great interest among physiologists and pharmacologists, resulting in many studies attempting to discover possible functions. While such studies have not always been productive of complete answers, they have led to interesting knowledge concerning the role of autacoids in physiology and pathophysiology. Studies of autacoids resulted in some completely unexpected discoveries of other classes of useful therapeutic agents, e.g., many antipsychotic agents were discovered after investigations of the properties of structural analogs of promethazine, an antihistamine.

In this text, we consider autopharmacologic agents (autacoids) as active substances which are naturally formed in the body and are *not* hormones. Autacoids include histamine, serotonin, angiotensin, bradykinin, and other substances that are discussed elsewhere (e.g., enkephalins) or are not discussed at all (e.g., substance P).

A. DEFINITIONS

Objective 19.A.1. Define and contrast autopharmacologic agent, hormone, autacoid, and neurotransmitter.

Objective 19.A.2. Name two autacoids which are polypeptides and one which is a derivative of fatty acid metabolism.

Objective 19.A.3. Define biogenic amine and name five important substances in this group.

Objective 19.A.4. Recognize the important enzymatic reactions in formation of the biogenic amines.

The term "autacoids" will be used synonymously with autopharmacologic agents. Since

175

autacoids is the simpler term, it will be used more frequently in this text. A hormone has been classically defined as a substance secreted by an organ and having a biologic effect on a distant organ. Autacoids, on the other hand, have less respect for locality; they may be formed at the site of action or at distant sites. They may be formed on the spot and as needed, or they may be stored and then released. They may regulate important physiologic processes, or an excess may result in development of pathologic processes.

As discussed in Chapter 16, neurotransmitters are specific messengers formed in nerve endings and released at the exact time that they are needed for transmission of the nerve impulse. Thus, norepinephrine is the adrenergic neurotransmitter when stored in nerve endings. However, norepinephrine is also an autacoid when released from the adrenal medulla. Norepinephrine is an example of a biogenic amine. Autacoids include not only biogenic amines but also several other types of active substances, e.g., polypeptides and lipid derivatives. Autacoids include **bradykinin,** other kinins (including **angiotensin**), **prostaglandins,** and a host of other substances.

Some of the more recently discovered polypeptide autacoids, although interesting from a theoretical standpoint, are not discussed in this text. An effort was made to select only agents that have been well studied and appear to have a role in physiology or pathophysiology. If study of an autacoid has led to the development of other pharmacotherapeutic agents, the autacoid is emphasized in this chapter.

Prostaglandins are derivatives of fatty acid metabolism and are discussed because of their possible role in pain and inflammation, as well as in other biologic functions.

A biogenic amine is a decarboxylation product of an amino acid which is formed by enzymatic reactions in living cells. Biogenic amines have biologic activity as either neurotransmitters or autacoids.

Important biogenic amines include **norepinephrine, epinephrine, dopamine, histamine, and serotonin.** The three major catecholamines, norepinephrine, epinephrine, and dopamine,

are mentioned in this chapter only to relate them to autacoids. For further details about these biogenic amines, the reader is referred to Chapters 16, 18, and 40. Histamine and serotonin receive more emphasis in this chapter since they are not covered elsewhere in this text, and, for the sake of discussion, they are here classified as autacoids.

The common enzymatic step in formation of histamine, serotonin, and dopamine is the decarboxylation reaction catalyzed by the enzyme L-aromatic amino acid (L-AAA) decarboxylase as follows:

$$\text{L-AAA} \xrightarrow[\text{decarboxylase}]{\text{L-AAA}} \text{L-aromatic amine} + CO_2$$

This enzyme is fairly ubiquitous in the tissues and is rather nonspecific, since it can decarboxylate most of the aromatic amino acids. On the other hand, histidine decarboxylase appears to be more specific, using mainly histidine as its substrate (see the following). Norepinephrine is formed from dopamine by alkyl hydroxylation, and epinephrine is formed from norepinephrine by N-methylation (see also Chapter 18).

B. HISTAMINE

Distribution and Formation

Objective 19.B.1. Recognize the distribution of histamine and enzymes for its biosynthesis and biodegradation.

Histamine is widely distributed in the body. It is contained in most tissues, but especially in the lungs, skin, and GI tract. The GI mucosa is very rich in histamine, with a high concentration around glandular cells. The bloodstream contains much histamine in basophils, and mast cells, found in many tissues, also have high concentrations. Both basophils and mast cells contain histamine, along with heparin and protein, in their basophilic granules. Histamine appears to be bound with heparin, and both are released simultaneously by certain drugs (see the following). Bacteria in the GI tract can also form histamine, which can then be absorbed. Blood platelets can scavenge histamine from the serum.

Histamine is formed by histidine decarboxylase (HDC), which converts histidine to histamine as follows:

$$histidine \xrightarrow[HDC]{-CO_2} histamine$$

Histamine is deactivated by diamine oxidase and histamine methyltransferase. Thus, biodegradation of histamine occurs by oxidation or by methylation as follows.

$$histamine \xrightarrow[oxidase]{diamine} acetic\ acid\ derivative$$

$$histamine \xrightarrow[transferase]{methyl} methylhistamine$$

Histamine Release

Objective 19.B.2. Describe possible physiologic significance of histamine release and some methods which result in release.

Histamine is released by tissue injury, drugs (e.g., narcotic-analgesics), large molecules (e.g., dextrans, polypeptides, surfactants), enzymes (e.g., those in venoms, trypsin), and antigen-antibody reactions. There are some characteristic responses of histamine effects which resemble reactions in allergy, anaphylaxis, and inflammation that have been demonstrated by either injection of histamine or by release. These similarities have led scientists to associate these states with the release of histamine and subsequent actions on the tissues.

Histamine Receptors

Objective 19.B.3. Recognize which actions of histamine are associated with H_1 receptors and which with H_2 receptors.

There are two types of histamine receptors: H_1 receptors and H_2 receptors. The difference between the receptors was not obvious until the recent discovery of H_2 blockers, such as cimetidine. Before this, it was thought that all hista-

mine responses were related to the same receptor but that the classic antihistamines (now called H_1 receptor blockers) were not very effective against some histamine responses (e.g., gastric acid secretion).

Based upon studies of H_1 and H_2 receptor blockers, H_1 receptor activation by histamine mediates increased capillary permeability, bronchiolar constriction, and intestinal smooth muscle contraction, and, conversely, activation of H_2 receptors by histamine mediates the gastric secretory effect, cardiac acceleration, and uterine relaxation. Vascular dilation may be related to activation of both H_1 and H_2 receptors.

H_1 receptors are antagonized by the classic antihistamines (e.g., diphenhydramine). These antihistamines were discovered about 1938, and many analogs have since been synthesized to find better blocking agents. It was found that the classic antihistamines blocked most of the actions of histamine but had no effect on gastric secretion. Recently, H_2 blockers (e.g., cimetidine) were discovered and were found to block the histamine stimulation of gastric secretion. They were named H_2 receptor blockers, and all activities inhibited by them were related to H_2 receptor activation. There was a great interest in blocking gastric acid secretion in peptic ulcer patients, which led to this discovery of the H_2 blockers.

C. ANTIHISTAMINES

Types of Antihistamines

Objective 19.C.1. Recognize four H_1 blockers, one H_2 blocker, and two motion sickness antihistamines.

The two classes of antihistamines are H_1 blockers and H_2 blockers. H_1 blockers include **diphenhydramine** (*Benadryl*), **chlorpheniramine** (*Chlor-Trimeton*), **promethazine** (*Phenergan*), and **hydroxyzine** (*Vistaril*) (these trade names are included because they are well known and widely used). H_2 blockers include **cimetidine** (*Tagamet*) and metiamide. Some H_1 antihistamines appear relatively specific for controlling motion sickness; they include: **meclizine** (*Bonine*) and **dimenhydrinate** (*Dramamine*).

Uses of Antihistamines

Objective 19.C.2. Describe four dental uses and recognize the medical uses of H_1 antihistamines.

Objective 19.C.3. Recognize the medical use of H_2 blockers.

H_1 blockers are used in dentistry for allergic reactions, for their sedative effect, as alternate local anesthetics, and for treatment of drug-induced extrapyramidal reactions.

Allergies, especially drug allergies, are a significant problem in both dentistry and medicine. Whenever a drug is administered, the practitioner must be prepared to treat an allergic reaction. If it is mild (e.g., when the symptoms are pruritis, rash, hives, or urticaria), an H_1 antihistamine may be the only drug needed, and it may be given orally. However, severe, immediate allergic reactions of the anaphylactoid type require, first, epinephrine as a life-saving drug and, then, an H_1 antihistamine (such as diphenhydramine), followed by a corticosteroid. Antihistamines and corticosteroids are considered secondary and tertiary agents because any beneficial response develops more slowly, and they are not considered life-saving during the acute emergency (see also Chapter 7). Delayed-type hypersensitivities are more difficult to treat. The H_1 antihistamines may control skin reactions but are ineffective against fever, arthralgia, and so on and do not seem to shorten the course of the disease.

The use of topical antihistamines for contact dermatitis or local allergic responses is *not* considered rational because of penetration problems and the known fact that patients can become allergic to the antihistamine after topical use. Like other drugs, the antihistamines probably combine with skin protein to form a hapten complex which can induce allergy.

The sedative effect of H_1 antihistamines is usually considered a side effect, but sometimes it may be used as a therapeutic effect. As a matter of fact, numerous OTC remedies for sleep (e.g., *Nytol, Sominex*) contain H_1 antihistamines.

For each patient, the dentist will have to decide whether sedation is useful and make his choice accordingly. In any event, the differences in sedative effect among various preparations may be only relative and are usually not clearcut. Antihistamines which have the greatest sedative effect include promethazine and hydroxyzine. Chlorpheniramine is considered to have a low incidence of sedative action, while diphenhydramine has an intermediate (some sources say "high") incidence. In all cases, antihistamines should be suspect regarding their sedative effects because it is difficult to predict when or how severe the effect will be until the patient has had some experience with the drug in question. The sedative antihistamines are sometimes used as antiemetics and, if the patient is vomiting, may have to be given by suppository.

H_1 antihistamines are sometimes used as alternative local anesthetics. They have reasonable local anesthetic activity and are sufficiently different from procaine or lidocaine in structure that cross-allergy would not be expected. However, injection for block anesthesia is reported as painful, the duration is shorter, and the percentage of success is not as high as for "–caine" anesthetics (see also Chapter 7).

In the treatment of drug-induced extrapyramidal reactions caused by antipsychotic drugs, diphenhydramine is considered one drug of choice. Sometimes, the dentist is called upon for consultation in this emergency, because the patient's TMJ may be totally immobilized with the teeth in malocclusion during the reaction.

H_1 antihistamines are used in medicine for allergic drug reactions, chronic allergic states, atropinelike effects, sedative effect, motion sickness, antiemesis, and treatment of cold or flu symptoms. The uses in allergy, sedation, and antiemesis were described above. The atropinic effects may be useful (1) in treatment of drug-induced extrapyramidal reactions, (2) as an antiparkinson drug (see Chapter 40), (3) for motion sickness (this appears to be related to CNS cholinergic activity), and (4) for treatment of cold or flu symptoms (infectious rhinitis). The cold remedy action of H_1 blockers (*Contac, Coricidin*) is a symptomatic effect that probably helps the patient to feel better without actually helping to cure the common cold or flu in any way. Sometimes, the side effects (e.g., sedation) and possible rebound effect (symptoms worse after drug action is over) are worse than suffering with the symptoms.

Uses in chronic allergic states deserve some further discussion. H_1 antihistamines may be effective in hayfever (seasonal rhinitis) and in perennial (nonseasonal) rhinitis. The use of H_1 antihistamines in infectious rhinitis is extremely questionable. H_1 antihistamines may or may not be effective in the treatment of asthmatic patients, depending upon the role of histamine in that particular allergy. If other mediators are involved, the antihistamine may be ineffective.

H_2 blockers are used mainly for reduction of gastric acid secretion. Cimetidine, the most useful member of this class, has recently become extremely popular as an inhibitor of gastric acid secretion. Its effects are very specific (H_2 blockade), and there are few side effects.

Side Effects of Antihistamines

Objective 19.C.4. Recognize the side effects and toxicity of H_1 and H_2 blockers.

Side effects and toxicity of H_1 blockers are:

1. atropinelike (dry mouth)
2. sedation in lower doses (additive with other sedatives)
3. excitation and convulsions in higher doses
4. skin sensitization (allergenic)
5. blurred vision and incoordination
6. teratogenic effect
7. nausea, vomiting, and diarrhea

The H_2 blocker, cimetidine, is usually well tolerated but may cause dizziness, diarrhea, muscle pain, and rash. In addition, cimetidine is known to inhibit liver microsomal enzymes.

D. ROLE OF HISTAMINE IN PHYSIOLOGY AND PATHOLOGY

Objective 19.D.1. Recognize three pathologic functions of histamine and at least three postulated physiologic functions.

Pathologic Functions

1. Vasodilation and increased capillary permeability can lead to redness (with itching), wheal, and edema. In excessive doses, histamine may cause shock, with death due to hypotension. Blood vessel effects are usually treated with H_1 blockers and not with H_2 blockers.
2. Inflammation can be caused by injection of histamine. However, most inflammatory reactions or phases of inflammation are not influenced by either H_1 or H_2 antihistamines.
3. Hypersensitivity (allergic) reactions include anaphylaxis, allergy, and drug reactions, which often respond well to H_1 antihistamines but not to H_2 antihistamines.
4. Excessive gastric acid secretion (leading to peptic ulcer) responds well to H_2 antihistamines.

Postulated Physiologic Functions

1. gastric secretion
2. regulator of vasodilation
3. regulator of bronchiolar constriction
4. neurotransmitter
5. local hormone

E. HISTAMINE ACTION AND ITS MEDICAL USES

Objective 19.E.1. Recognize three effects of injected histamine and two medical uses.

Actions

Actions of injected histamine include the following:

1. Intracutaneous administration results in the Lewis triple response:
   a. local vasodilation (redness),
   b. swelling resulting in a wheal (edema), and
   c. peripheral vasodilation (flare).
2. Intravenous administration, in animals, results in arteriolar dilation, venular constriction, increased capillary permeability to large molecules, and heart rate increase (H_2). Excessive dose may result in vasomotor collapse (histamine shock).

3. Bronchiolar smooth muscle is constricted; this is especially serious after sensitization (allergy induction), in anaphylaxis, and in asthmatic patients.
4. Gastric secretion is stimulated, especially hydrochloric acid, but other glands are also stimulated.

Medical Uses

The only medical uses of histamine are for diagnosis of pernicious anemia and pheochromocytoma.

1. Histamine, after IV administration, causes no HCl secretion in pernicious anemia.
2. Histamine (IV) causes an increased blood pressure (instead of decreased) due to stimulation of catecholamine secretion from adrenal medullary tumors (pheochromocytoma).

F. SEROTONIN (5-HYDROXYTRYPTAMINE)

Formation, Distribution, Metabolism

Objective 19.F.1. Recognize mechanism of formation and deactivation of serotonin and its biologic distribution.

Serotonin (5-HT) is a biogenic amine formed from 5-hydroxytryptophan by action of L-AAA decarboxylase. Serotonin is deactivated by the monoamine oxidase enzyme, which also inactivates epinephrine, norepinephrine, dopamine, and other biogenic amines. Serotonin is distributed in GI mucosa (90%), platelets, mast cells, lung, and certain areas of the brain.

Pharmacologic Effects

Objective 19.F.2. Describe the pharmacologic effects and possible physiologic functions of serotonin.

Serotonin inhibits gastric secretion, stimulates vascular and other smooth muscle, and has a CNS effect. Administered serotonin or circulating serotonin does not penetrate the **blood-brain barrier.** This is fortunate, since serotonin appears to have some powerful CNS effects. Serotonin probably is a neurotransmitter in the brain and spinal cord and possibly at other sites.

Serotonin has no pharmacologic use, but many drugs that alter CNS serotonin levels have therapeutic uses, as well as providing evidence for CNS functions of serotonin.

Serotonin-Altering Drugs

Objective 19.F.3. Recognize the possible relationships of serotonin-altering drugs to effects of these drugs.

Reserpine releases serotonin as well as norepinephrine. During the release phase, transient mental stimulation occurs. However, after prolonged use, reserpine exhausts serotonin supply, as well as many other neurally active substances, and also causes CNS depession. Tryptophan, a serotonin precursor, causes increased serotonin in the brain, but serotonin itself does not cross the blood-brain barrier. MAO inhibitors also cause a serotonin build-up in brain tissues. There appears to be some evidence for serotonin as a CNS neurotransmitter which is involved in sleep, behavior, release of pituitary hormones, body temperature regulation, and other CNS functions.

Antiserotonin drugs include (1) cyproheptidine, which may be used for treatment of excessive serotonin secretion (also called carcinoid syndrome), and (2) methysergide, which may prevent migraine. Both drugs have side effects that are alarming, and methysergide causes a severe side effect, retroperitoneal fibrosis, which limits its use. LSD (lysergic acid diethylamide) apparently interacts with serotonin receptors. Whether this is responsible for LSD's hallucinogenic effects is still uncertain.

G. BRADYKININ

Chemistry, Formation, and Inactivation

Objective 19.G.1. Recognize the chemistry, formation, and inactivation of bradykinin, including the factors necessary for activation.

Bradykinin is a polypeptide chain containing nine peptide units. Bradykinin can result from two sources that will be discussed. (1) Alpha$_2$ globulin of serum (prekallikrein) can be cleaved to form kallikrein. This cleavage is thought to be caused by enzymatic activity of activated Hageman factor. Trypsin or enzymes in tissues (other than glandular) can also act on α_2 globulin, giving the same result. Thus, clotting, tissue damage, changes in pH, inflammation, and immunologic factors can stimulate formation of plasma kallikrein. Once activated, kallikrein cleaves kininogen, by its enzymatic activity, to bradykinin. (2) In glandular tissue, there is a high concentration of glandular kallikrein, which can act on glandular kininogen to form kallidin, an active decapeptide. Kallidin can then be cleaved to the nonapeptide, bradykinin, by a peptidase.

Bradykinin is inactivated either by kininase to form the inactive octapeptide or by peptidyl dipeptidase (PDP) to form a heptapeptide.

The biochemical reactions for generation and breakdown of bradykinin can be summarized by the reactions below:

Activation.

1. Prekallikrein $\xrightarrow{\text{activators}}$ kallikrein
   (α_2 globulin,
   tissue pre-
   kallikrein)
       1. Hageman
          factor
          (activated)
       2. Trypsin
       3. Tissue factors

   plasma $\xrightarrow{\text{kallikrein}}$ bradykinin
   kininogen   (nonapeptide)

2. Glandular $\xrightarrow[\text{kallikrein}]{\text{glandular}}$ kallidin
   kininogen   (decapeptide)

   kallidin $\xrightarrow{\text{peptidase}}$ bradykinin
   (decapeptide)   (nonapeptide)

Metabolism.

1. bradykinin $\xrightarrow{\text{kininase}}$ octapeptide
   (active)   (carboxypeptidase) (inactive)

2. bradykinin $\xrightarrow{\text{PDP}}$ heptapeptide
   (active)   (inactive)

Pathophysiologic Roles and Status in Therapeutics

Objective 19.G.2. Describe possible pathophysiologic roles of bradykinin and the status of bradykinin and its analogs in therapeutics.

Bradykinin is considered a possible inflammatory mediator. It causes vasodilation and capillary permeability. It is also a pain-producing substance. Bradykinin causes slow (*brady* means "slow") relaxation of all smooth muscle except in bronchioles, which are constricted. The search for blockers of bradykinin from structural analogs has not been fruitful in finding useful therapeutic agents, probably because of the pharmacokinetics of the polypeptide analogs. However, captopril may cause accumulation of bradykinin by blocking PDP, but its effect in hypertension is more related to blocking angiotensin conversion (see the following) than to blocking breakdown of bradykinin.

H. ANGIOTENSIN (RENIN-ANGIOTENSIN-ALDOSTERONE SYSTEM)

Renin Secretion

Objective 19.H.1. List and describe the factors that result in secretion of renin.

Secretion of renin can take place by stimulation of nerves that originate in the CNS and by local factors that either stimulate the juxtaglomerular cells (JG) of the kidney directly to secrete renin or indirectly via the macula densa (MD), which is also located in the kidney.

Factors that stimulate the system include sodium depletion (MD), decreased perfusion pressure or blood pressure to the kidney (JG), and decreased plasma volume (JG). Figure 19–1 diagrams the role of these factors in the renin-angiotensin-aldosterone system.

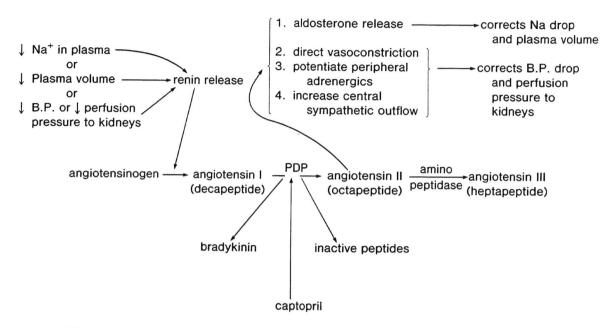

Figure 19–1. Biologic interactions in the renin-angiotensin-aldosterone system. PDP, peptidyl dipeptidase.

Types of Angiotensin

Objective 19.H.2. Recognize the three angiotensins and describe the generation of angiotensin II.

Figure 19–1 illustrates the formation of angiotensins. The renin enzyme is released into the bloodstream, and it attacks the aminoterminus of an α-globulin fraction called angiotensinogen(s), producing the decapeptide angiotensin I. Angiotensin I has only slight pharmacologic activity, but it is coverted to angiotensin II (an octapeptide) by the converting enzyme, which is now more correctly termed peptidyl dipeptidase (PDP). This is the same enzyme that deactivates bradykinin into inactive peptides. PDP is located on the endothelial surface of blood vessel walls throughout the body, but it is found in greater concentration in the pulmonary bed.

Angiotensin II is converted in the plasma to angiotensin III (a heptapeptide) by an aminopeptidase. Angiotensin III also has some pharmacologic activity. Other peptidases present in plasma are available to convert all three angiotensins to inactive peptides.

Pharmacologic Effects of Angiotensin

Objective 19.H.3. List and describe the pharmacologic effects of angiotensin II.

Angiotensin II is the most potent pressor agent known; it is also the most important form of angiotensin. Angiotensin II causes vasoconstriction by a direct effect on blood vessels, mostly arterioles. It potentiates the peripheral sympathetic nervous system by increasing the secretion of NE from adrenergic nerve endings and by increasing central sympathetic outflow (a central action). All of these effects are capable of correcting decreased blood pressure (or perfusion pressure), and the secretion of renin is inhibited.

Angiotensin II is also capable of releasing aldosterone. Aldosterone causes increased reabsorption in the kidney of sodium and chloride, followed by passive water reabsorption. This function tends to correct decreased plasma vol-

ume or hyponatremia, which also results in inhibition of renin secretion.

Captopril

Objective 19.H.4. Recognize captropril and its
primary and secondary mechanisms of action.

Some cases of hypertension are thought to result from an imbalance of the renin-angiotensin-
aldosterone system. A new antihypertensive
drug, captopril (*Capoten*), has recently been
marketed. Captopril has been shown to inhibit
converting enzyme or PDP, thereby blocking
the generation of angiotensin II. A second and
probably less important effect is that the vasodilator bradykinin accumulates, since bradykinin
is affected by the same enzyme. This new group
of agents (PDP inhibitors), represented by the
prototype captopril, may prove to be a valuable
addition to antihypertensive therapy (see also,
Chapter 31).

I. PROSTAGLANDINS

Chemistry and Naming

Objective 19.I.1. Recognize the chemistry of
prostaglandins and the methods of naming PGs.

Prostaglandins (PGs) are a series of naturally
occurring substances found throughout the body
and formed in every tissue. They are compounds
derived from 20-carbon, essential fatty acids,
and in the case of humans, the only precursor is
probably arachidonic acid (Fig. 19–2). Various
chemical or mechanical stimuli are thought to
activate the enzyme phospholipase A_2, resulting
in the release of arachidonic acid from cell
membranes. Microsomal enzymes then trans-
form arachidonic acid into one of a series of active PGs, which are analogs of the **unnatural**
compound, prostanoic acid (Fig. 19–3). The active compounds are lettered A through F, depending on various substitutions in the five-
membered ring (labeled **a** in Fig. 19–3). In addition, each compound, A through F, has an assigned number (e.g., F_2), indicating the number
of double bonds in the fatty acid structure. The

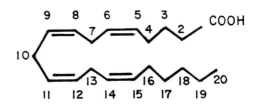

Figure 19–2. Arachidonic acid.

double bonds can be one to three in number, but
only two double bonds (sub-2 series) appear to
be found in human PGs. The subscript number
also may have an α or β associated, which relates to the orientation of the double bonds.
Only the α series is found in humans.

Biologic Formation and Synthesis

Objective 19.I.2. Recognize a general description of PG synthesis in the biologic system.

After phospholiphase A_2 releases arachidonic
acid from membrane phospholipids, PG synthesis can be initiated by action of cyclooxygenase
on arachidonic acid. The generation scheme is
diagramatically illustrated in Figure 19–4.
Many intermediates are possible, but most authorities agree that PGG_2 and PGH_2 are formed
and give rise to other PGs of the E and F series.
The enzyme prostaglandin synthetase, now
more correctly termed "fatty acid cyclooxygenase," is inhibited by a number of therapeutically
useful drugs. For example, aspirin and indomethacin, referred to as nonsteroidal anti-in-

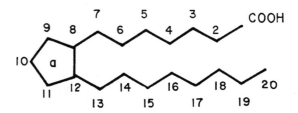

Figure 19–3. Prostanoic acid. This unnatural intermediate is the basis of the naming of prostaglandins. The five-membered ring (**a**) can take on
many configurations, leading to the series A-F
prostaglandins. Since the number of double bonds
is usually two in humans, the E series is designated PGE_2.

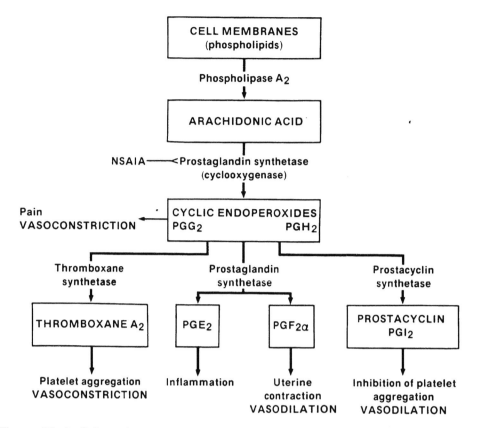

Figure 19–4. Schematic representation of the production of prostaglandins. (*After Di-Palma JR: Basic Pharmacology in Medicine, 2nd ed, 1981. Courtesy of McGraw-Hill Book Company.*)

flammatory agents (NSAIA), are known to block PG synthetase. NSAIA and their effects are further described in Chapter 23.

Cyclic endoperoxides can be enzymatically converted not only into PGE and PGF (by further action of enzymes categorized as prostaglandin synthetase) but also into two other series of compounds, the thromboxanes (TBA_2 and TBB_2) and prostacyclins. The latter can be converted to leukotrienes and related active substances. Leukotrienes are chemotactic substances which attract leukocytes. Thromboxanes are vasoconstrictive and cause platelet aggregation.

Important Compounds and Drugs

Objective 19.I.3. Name the most important PGs and name two PG-derived drugs which are useful in abortions.

PGE and PGF are probably the most important PGs generated in humans, and, in fact, both are marketed drugs that are used for induction of abortion. Their trade names are *Prostin E2* (as a vaginal suppository) and *Prostin F2 Alpha* (for intra-aminiotic administration). The agents are used locally so as to lessen the incidence of systemic side effects, which may be unpredictable, widespread, and annoying (see the following).

Actions and Side Effects

Objective 19.I.4. Describe the actions and side effects of PGs.

The actions of PGs are very broad. They have actions on many organs, and sometimes different PGs have opposite actions. The variability of action is dependent on the type of PG, the animal species tested, the state of activity of the organ or tissue at the time of exposure, and the presence or absence of other hormones or mediators.

In the cardiovascular system, PGs produce vasodilation of blood vessels, but vasoconstriction is also encountered. Cardiac output is often increased, and the increase is usually reflexly mediated. Decreased blood pressure is usually the overall effect.

PGs inhibit platelet aggregation, as do prostacyclins, which results in an anticoagulant effect. However, thromboxanes tend to induce platelet aggregation. PGs have also been shown to produce erythema, increased local blood flow, increased vascular permeability, and edema (all of which are reminiscent of inflammation). PGs induce increased production of red blood cells.

The response of the kidney to PGs is an increased renal blood flow and diuresis. Prostacyclins may mediate the release of renin in the renal cortex. In the central nevous system, PGs produce either sedation or stimulation. Induction of fever is also produced by the PGs, and the site of action is the hypothalamus. Fever is a frequent side effect seen in women who are having an abortion and have been given either PGE or PGF.

Smooth muscle is affected by PGs throughout the body. Contraction or relaxation can occur in bronchi, gastrointestinal smooth muscle, and the uterus, although contraction is the predominant effect in the latter. PGs apparently protect the mucosal surface of the gastrointestinal tract.

Numerous endocrine effects have been noted and include stimulation or release of ACTH, growth hormone, prolactin, gonadotropins, thyrotropin, insulin, and adrenocortical steroids. Subnormal levels of PGs in male seminal fluid correlate with decreased male fertility.

PGs are thought to increase or decrease lipolysis, and to produce hypoglycemia and hypercalcemia. Sensory nerve endings become sensitized by PGs, resulting in the amplification of pain mechanisms. In addition, PGs have been shown to produce hyperalgesia; at high doses, PGs produce intense pain at the injection site. PGs produce only slight effects on the autono-mic nervous system, but inhibition or enhancement of norepinephrine release has been noted at adrenergic nerve endings.

Two somewhat unusual functions in pathologic conditions have been assigned to PGs. PGs may be needed to maintain the patency of the ductus arteriosus. They may be responsible for most of the symptoms of Bartter syndrome, suggesting that increased synthesis of PGs may be the cause of the syndrome.

In conclusion, the exact role of PGs relative to bodily functions is sometimes unknown. However, as has been noted for histamine, PGs obviously have either a physiologic or pathophysiologic function (or both), with their main effects probably related to inflammation.

REFERENCES

DiPalma JR (ed): Basic Pharmacology in Medicine, 2nd ed. New York, McGraw-Hill, 1981, p 156

BIBLIOGRAPHY

DiPalma JR (ed): Drill's Pharmacology in Medicine, 4th ed. New York, McGraw-Hill, 1971, Ch 14

Gilman AG, Goodman LS, Gilman A (eds): Goodman and Gilman's The Pharmacological Basis of Therapeutics, 6th ed. New York, Macmillan, 1980, Ch 26, 27, 28

QUESTIONS

1. **T F** Another name for autopharmacologic agent is autacoid.

2. Corticosteroids are defined as:

   A. autacoid
   B. hormone
   C. neurotransmitter
   D. all of the above are correct

3. Norepinephrine, secreted under different circumstances, may be:

   A. a neurotransmitter
   B. an autacoid
   C. both A and B are correct
   D. neither A nor B is correct

4. Which of the following is both an autacoid and a derivative of fatty acid metabolism?

   A. arachadonic acid
   B. prostaglandin $G_{2\alpha}$
   C. captopril
   D. angiotensin II

5. Which of the following is a polypeptide?

   A. histamine
   B. serotonin
   C. bradykinin
   D. all of the above are correct

6. Biogenic amines include:

   A. histamine
   B. serotonin
   C. epinephrine
   D. all of the above are correct

7. T F Biogenic amines are formed by the action of L-aromatic amino acid decarboxylase.

8. Norepinephrine is formed from:

   A. dopamine
   B. epinephrine
   C. both A and B are correct
   D. neither A nor B is correct

9. Histamine is distributed in:

   A. GI mucosa
   B. blood cell basophils
   C. tissue mast cells
   D. lungs
   E. all of the above are correct

10. H_2 blockers are used mainly to:

    A. inhibit gastric secretion
    B. relieve asthma
    C. both A and B are correct
    D. neither A nor B is correct

11. Which of the following autopharmacologic agents appears to be involved in inflammation?

    A. histamine
    B. bradykinin
    C. prostaglandins
    D. all of the above are correct
    E. none of the above is correct

12. Histamine can be released by:

    A. narcotic-analgesics
    B. antigen-antibody reaction
    C. both A and B are correct
    D. neither A nor B is correct

13. H_1 receptor blocking agents inhibit histamine-induced:

    A. gastric secretion
    B. bronchoconstriction
    C. cardiac acceleration
    D. all of the above are correct

14. The following actions of histamine are blocked by H_2 receptor blocking agents:

    A. bronchoconstriction and edema
    B. gastric secretion and cardiac acceleration
    C. both A and B are correct
    D. neither A nor B is correct

15. T F Histamine and bradykinin are considered bronchoconstrictors.

16. Which of the following is a classic H_1 blocking agent?

    A. amphetamine
    B. mecamylamine
    C. phentolamine
    D. diphenhydramine
    E. phenylpropanolamine

17. Which of the following is an H_2 histamine blocker?

    A. cimetidine
    B. chlorpheniramine
    C. dichlorisoproterenol
    D. meclizine

18. Which of the following drugs would be most useful of inhibiting motion sickness?

    A. meclizine
    B. metiamide
    C. tripelennamine
    D. phenoxybenzamine

19. **T F** The use of sedative drugs at the same time as diphenhydramine may counteract the most common side effect of diphenhydramine.

20. **T F** Drug-induced muscular spasticity (extrapyramidal reaction) is treated by injection of cimetidine.

21. Which of the following drugs are H_1 antihistamines?

    A. chlorpheniramine
    B. diphenhydramine
    C. promethazine
    D. all of the above are correct
    E. none of the above is correct

22. Diphenhydramine (*Benadryl*):

    A. has a sedative effect
    B. is effective in counteracting drug-induced extrapyramidal reaction

C. both A and B are correct
D. neither A nor B is correct

23. Side effects of H_1 antihistamines include possible:

    A. drowsiness
    B. dry mouth
    C. excitation and convulsions
    D. all of the above are correct
    E. none of the above is correct

24. Side effects of H_1 antihistamines include:

    A. arousal at low dose
    B. excessive salivation
    C. both A and B are correct
    D. neither A nor B is correct

25. **T F** Cimetidine is known to inhibit liver microsomal enzymes.

26. Histamine is considered a mediator of:

    A. inflammation
    B. gastric secretion
    C. both A and B are correct
    D. neither A nor B is correct

27. Injection of histamine may cause:

    A. redness
    B. wheal
    C. flare
    D. all of the above are correct

28. Serotonin is formed from:

    A. angiotensin
    B. 5-hydroxytryptophan
    C. dopamine
    D. none of the above is correct

29. Serotonin:

    A. stimulates gastric secretion
    B. penetrates the blood-brain barrier

C. both A and B are correct

D. neither A nor B is correct

30. Build-up of serotonin in the brain can occur by giving:

A. MAO inhibitors

B. tryptophan

C. both A and B are correct

D. neither A nor B is correct

31. Aspirin has been shown to inhibit the enzyme:

A. kallikrein

B. peptidyl dipeptidase

C. histidine decarboxylase

D. prostaglandin synthetase

E. L-aromatic amino acid decarboxylase

32. **T F** Activation of clotting factors results in activation of enzymes which cause increased bradykinin in the blood.

33. **T F** Chemical activation of bradykinin results from activation of a proenzyme in plasma to kallikrein.

34. Bradykinin is considered a:

A. possible inflammatory mediator

B. vasodilator and causative of increased capillary permeability

C. pain-producing substance

D. all of the above are correct

35. Renin secretion occurs by:

A. CNS stimulation

B. low sodium at the kidney macula densa

C. low perfusion pressure at the juxtaglomerular apparatus

D. all of the above are correct

36. **T F** Angiotensins are formed after renin enzymatically attacks an α globulin, angiotensinogen.

37. **T F** Of the three angiotensins, only angiotensin I has any pharmacologic activity.

38. Peptidyl dipeptidase acts to decrease:

A. bradykinin

B. angiotensin II

C. both A and B are correct

D. neither A nor B is correct

39. Angiotensin II is:

A. the most potent pressor agent known

B. releases aldosterone

C. both A and B are correct

D. neither A nor B is correct

40. Captopril:

A. blocks the generation of angiotensin II

B. counteracts hypertension due to pheochromocytoma

C. both A and B are correct

D. neither A nor B is correct

41. Captopril's **primary** antihypertensive effect is due to:

A. inhibition of the conversion of angiotensin II to angiotensin III

B. accumulation of histamine

C. both A and B are correct

D. neither A nor B is correct

42. **T F** Prostaglandins are only formed in lungs, GI tract, and uterus.

43. **T F** Prostaglandin synthetase releases arachidonic acid from cell membranes.

44. Products of arachidonic acid metabolism include:

A. prostaglandins

B. leukotrienes

C. thromboxanes

D. all of the above are correct

45. T F Prostaglandins are still considered theoretical, and no useful drugs have been developed from their study.

46. T F The response of the kidneys to prostaglandins is an increased renal blood flow and diuresis.

47. By action on neural tissue, prostaglandins may produce:

A. fever

B. amplification of pain

C. both A and B are correct

D. neither A nor B is correct

20
Introduction to Use of CNS Drugs

A. INTRODUCTION

CNS drugs have their primary effects on the brain and spinal cord, although peripheral effects are sometimes observed. Peripheral effects can be indirect via the CNS or by direct effect on the organ or tissue.

The CNS drugs produce a wide variety of actions, including such diverse effects as antipyretic (fever-lowering), analgesic, cough suppressant, general anesthetic, anticonvulsant, and antipyschotic. CNS drugs are also the most abused drugs, since they affect behavior, consciousness, and mood.

B. DIVISIONS

Objective 20.B.1. Recognize anatomic and functional divisions of the CNS.

Gross Anatomic Divisions

1. brain
   cerebrum (cortex)
   cerebellum
   brainstem
   medulla
2. spinal cord

The peripheral nervous system (both somatic and visceral) has connections to the CNS. The autonomic nervous system (visceral efferent) and the somatic efferent were covered in detail in Chapter 16, with additional information in Chapters 17 and 18.

Functional Divisions

Functional divisions are difficult to identify anatomically because CNS pathways are extremely branched, with many interconnections between centers. However, a brief list of functions may be in order:

1. sensory
2. motor
3. emotional or behavioral
4. memory
5. vegetative
6. sleep–arousal

C. Blood-Brain Barrier

Objective 20.C.1. Recognize the **blood-brain barrier** and its properties.

Objective 20.C.2. Recognize two mechanisms of drug-induced vomiting.

The blood-brain barrier is an ill-defined structure associated with central vascular structures. This barrier is capable of preventing the passive diffusion of a number of drugs from blood to brain. Simply stated, the barrier prevents transfer of charged drugs while allowing the movement of uncharged or lipid-soluble agents. In fact, the more lipid soluble the drug, the more readily it will diffuse into the brain. However, several brain structures are located outside the **blood-brain barrier.** Two such structures are a portion of the hypothalamus and the area postrema (which is located in the medulla oblongata).

Drug-induced vomiting involves two mechanisms: (1) the chemoreceptor trigger zone (CTZ) located in the area postrema, which when activated, sends impulses to the vomiting center, resulting in the vomiting reflex. Since the CTZ is located outside the **blood-brain barrier,** all drugs are capable of reaching the area, and as a result, certain agents specifically stimulate or block receptors in the CTZ. For example, narcotic analgesics are thought to stimulate CTZ receptors, resulting in vomiting. On the other hand, phenothiazines (antipsychotic drugs) have been shown to specifically block (competitively) the same receptors, resulting in an antiemetic effect. (2) A second mechanism of drug-induced vomiting involves the direct irritation of the upper GI tract by the drug. The irritation causes increased sensory nerve traffic to the vomiting center, and vomiting occurs by reflex activation of efferent nerves to the appropriate tissues and muscles.

D. COMPLEXITY

Objective 20.D.1. Recognize the cellular complexity of the CNS.

Objective 20.D.2. Recognize the significance of the terms EPSP and IPSP.

Objective 20.D.3. Distinguish between the terms neurotransmitter, second messenger (neuromediator), and neuromodulator.

The CNS is extremely complex, and it is thought that the human brain contains 10 to 100 billion neurons plus supporting cells (Hubel, 1979). In addition, each neuron probably receives thousands of synapses. Histologic study suggests that a single neuron may have 1,000 to 10,000 synapses, and, therefore, potentially 10,000 neurons can influence activity of one nerve cell (Stevens, 1979), while one nerve cell may influence 10,000 other synapses. Further, it is believed that each neuron contains at least one neurotransmitter, similar to the mediators studied under the autonomic nervous system (see Chapter 16). Recent evidence suggests there may be more than one neurotransmitter present in some neurons (Iversen, 1979).

Neurotransmitters are thought to be either excitatory transmitters or inhibitory transmitters. When an excitatory transmitter combines with a receptor on a postsynaptic neuron, pores are thought to open on the membrane, probably allowing the influx of sodium ions, which causes depolarization or an excitatory postsynaptic potential (EPSP), resulting in generation of an action potential in the postsynaptic neuron. Conversely, an inhibitory transmitter combines with a receptor on the postsynaptic neuron, pores are thought to open in the membrane, probably allowing the influx of chloride ions, causing hyperpolarization or an inhibitory postsynaptic potential (IPSP) and inhibition of action potential activity in the postsynaptic neuron. (NOTE: IPSPs may also occur through a presynaptic mechanism.) Therefore, each neuron is thought to receive excitatory and inhibitory input. The activity (rate of firing) of the postsynaptic neuron is dependent on the algebraic sum of excitatory (EPSP) and inhibitory (IPSP) input.

More recently, postsynaptic activity other than the classic changes of membrane potential (EPSP or IPSP) have been identified. Slow synaptic potentials (SSP) have been shown to occur in both the CNS and periphery. These slow synaptic potentials are thought to occur as a result of activation of a mediator-receptor complex. However, there is some question whether the mediator of SSP should be referred to as "neurotransmitter."

Recently, two new terms have been introduced to describe chemicals that influence neurotransmission but are not classified as neurotransmitters: (1) neuromodulators (such as

TABLE 20–1. CNS NEUROTRANSMITTERS

Excitatory	Inhibitory	Unknown
acetylcholine	alanine	**endorphin**
aspartic acid	**γ-aminobutyric acid (GABA)**	**enkephalin**
cysteic acid	**dopamine**	histamine
glutamic acid	epinephrine	
homocysteic acid	**glycine**	
substance P	**norepinephrine**	
	serotonin (5-hydroxytryptamine, 5-HT)	
	taurine	

the prostaglandins) do not directly affect the postsynaptic receptor, but they are thought to quantitatively modify the effect of action of a neurotransmitter, and (2) second messengers (neuromediators), such as cyclic AMP, act within the postsynaptic cell. Some evidence exists that either neuromodulators or second messengers may influence neurotransmission by regulation of SSPs (Bloom, 1980).

E. NEUROTRANSMITTERS

Objective 20.E.1. Recognize the neurochemicals (Table 20-1) that may qualify as CNS neurotransmitters.

Many compounds have been shown to be CNS transmitters; some are very strong candidates and others have been proposed. The list presented in Table 20–1 includes CNS neurotransmitters recognized by many neuropharmacologists (Cooper et al., 1978) and includes all of those for which some supportive evidence exists. In addition, the list is divided into transmitters that are believed to be excitatory, inhibitory or unknown in effect.

F. MECHANISMS OF ACTION

Objective 20.F.1. Recognize seven proposed mechanisms by which CNS drugs may act at the level of the synapse.

Mechanisms by which CNS drugs act at the synapse are probably very similar to mecha-

nisms known to take place in the autonomic nervous system (Objective 16.K.2., p. 141), including the following:

1. reacting with receptor (drug-receptor complex)
2. blocking receptor (stronger drug-receptor complex)
3. preventing breakdown or reuptake of neurotransmitter
4. decreasing formation of neurotransmitter
5. preventing storage of neurotransmitter
6. depleting stored neurotransmitter
7. preventing release of neurotransmitter

G. MODEL OF CNS ACTIVITY

Objective 20.G.1. Recognize a theoretical model of CNS activity.

In addition to known excitatory and inhibitory neurons and their respective neurotransmitters, we know that these neurons are part of excitatory and inhibitory pathways, or outflows, from the CNS, and the pathways are often antagonistic to each other, much as in the system of autonomic neurons. In Figure 20–1, a simplified model of CNS activity is presented which attempts to explain neural interactions. Although the model is obviously oversimplified, it is nevertheless useful for explanation of general mechanisms of stimulant and depressant drugs. Surprisingly, when the model is used to test the theoretical outcome of a CNS drug, the results of the model almost always agree with the effects found in biologic systems. (For a more specific discussion of antagonistic CNS pathways

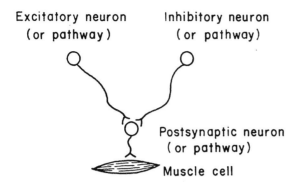

Figure 20-1. Theoretical model of CNS excitation and depression.

and drug treatments, see Chapter 40, Antiparkinson Drugs.)

H. CLASSIFICATION OF CNS DRUGS

Objective 20.H.1. Recognize a classification of CNS drugs and cite examples of each.

CNS drugs may be broadly classified into stimulants or depressants. In addition, each broad classification can be subdivided into general and specific. General implies that all CNS cells are affected, while specific implies that only certain functions are affected. Further subdivision results in breakdown into therapeutic categories. This breakdown readily conforms to the proposed model (Fig. 20-1).

1. General (nonspecific) CNS depressants
   a. general anesthetics
   b. alcohols
   c. barbiturates
   d. nonbarbiturate sedative-hypnotics
2. General (nonspecific) CNS stimulants
   a. **Convulsive** or respiratory stimulants: these agents have no use in dentistry nor in medicine and are now obsolete. In order to achieve their proposed therapeutic effect (respiratory stimulation), a dose close to a toxic (convulsive) dose is required; therefore, they are not discussed further in this book.
      (1) bemegride—respiratory stimulant
      (2) nikethamide—respiratory stimulant

      (3) pentylenetetrazol—experimental (mimics convulsive states)
      (4) picrotoxin—stimulant to treat poisoning by CNS depressants
      (5) strychnine—convulsant and poison
   b. **Strong** stimulants
      (1) amphetamines (dextroamphetamine, methamphetamine)
      (2) methylphenidate
   c. **Mild** stimulants
      (1) xanthines (e.g., caffeine)
3. Specific CNS drugs (usually depressants but may be stimulant)
   a. anticonvulsants
   b. antipyretic analgesics
   c. narcotic analgesics
   d. psychopharmacologic agents

I. GENERAL PRINCIPLES OF STIMULATION AND DEPRESSION

Objective 20.I.1. Recognize principles of stimulation and depression.

The CNS at any given moment exhibits a certain degree of balance between excitability and depression, or a normal state, even without the influence of drugs. Certainly, during non-REM sleep, the CNS is depressed. After lack of sleep, the CNS probably remains somewhat depressed throughout the following day, a state that can manifest itself clinically by yawning, decreased reaction time, grogginess, ataxia, stupor. Similar symptoms may be noted on awakening. Conversely, on being notified of having won the Irish Sweepstakes, one might expect to be hyperexcitable and exhibit symptoms opposite to those just cited. In Figure 20-2, a spectrum of CNS excitability is diagrammed. It can be readily understood how a patient may move under physiologic circumstances or under the influence of a drug from a state of hypoexcitability to hyperexcitability or vice versa. Using this scheme and our previous model of CNS activity (Fig. 20-1), the following principles apply to drug action on the CNS:

1. Drug action is seldom restricted to one functional or anatomic set of neurons, since there

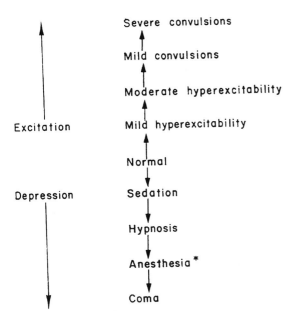

Figure 20–2. Spectrum of excitability of the CNS.

* This scheme was purposely oversimplified. General anesthesia may be caused by either depression or overexcitement. General depressants that cause general anesthesia usually produce an excitement stage, probably due to depression of inhibitors. Excitement may also be seen with alcohol (inebriation) or barbiturates (paradoxical).

are extensive interrelationships among these neurons. Thus, a drug may produce not only multiple effects but also many side effects (e.g., narcotic-analgesics Chapter 24).

2. Individual drugs having qualitatively similar effects may differ greatly in potency and efficacy (e.g., compared to chlordiazepoxide, diazepam is both more potent and a better muscle relaxant, Chapter 22).

3. A drug effect will exhibit addition (summation) with the physiologic state of the CNS and with the effects of another CNS drug that acts in the same direction (e.g., increased CNS depression is known to occur when barbiturates are combined with benzodiazepines, Chapters 21 and 22).

4. Antagonism between stimulant and depressant drugs occurs, but this can be more variable than the expected additive effect when both drugs act in the same direction.
   a. Antagonism is usually physiologic, i.e., by action on opposing systems of the CNS. For example, anticholinergic drugs counteract phenothiazine-induced extrapyramidal effects (the anticholinergic drug is thought to act on excitatory neurons, while phenothiazines act on neurons that are inhibitory, Chapter 36).
   b. There is increasing evidence of true (receptor-mediated) pharmacological antagonism, e.g. (1) phenothiazine antiemetics prevent or reverse narcotic-induced nausea and vomiting (Chapters 24 and 36), and (2) naloxone reverses all the effects of morphine (Chapter 24).

5. Low concentrations of some depressant drugs commonly cause excitation (e.g., alcohol, Chapter 39). This could occur by inhibition of inhibitors. The converse is usually not true, i.e., low concentration of exciters does not cause depression. However, an exception seems to occur in hyperkinetic children where a stimulant, dextroamphetamine, brings about control of the hyperkinetic state. Further, some subjects claim that a cup of coffee puts them to sleep. Thus, perhaps low concentrations of excitatory drugs can cause depression.

6. Potent drug stimulation of the CNS is usually followed by depression after convulsions are controlled. This is thought to be related to a tired state of overworked neurons. This type of depression is additive with the effects of CNS depressant drugs, and, therefore, it may be dangerous to treat local anesthetic convulsions (which are followed by depression) with a barbiturate drug (Chapter 21).

7. Acute, drug-induced depression is not usually followed by stimulation, but chronic, drug-induced depression may be followed by a period of hyperexcitability when the drug is withdrawn (e.g., sudden withdrawal from a barbiturate that was used on a chronic basis often results in a convulsion (Chapter 21, and Appendix II).

8. Two CNS depressant drugs with different mechanisms, given concurrently, may produce a supra-additive effect (e.g., an antipsychotic drug used concurrently with a narcotic analgesic see Chapters 24 and 36).

Summary

This introductory chapter should serve as a background for studying CNS drugs. Excitations and inhibitions based on drug effects on neurotransmitter systems appear to be the basis of neuropharmacologic mechanisms and interactions.

REFERENCES

Bloom F: Neurohumoral transmission and the central nervous system. In Gilman AG, Goodman LS and Gilman A (eds): Goodman and Gilman's The Pharmacological Basis of Therapeutics, 6th ed. New York, Macmillan, 1980, p 241

Hubel DH: The brain. Sci Am 241:45, 1979

Iversen LL: The chemistry of the brain. Sci Am 241:134, 1979

Stevens CF: The neuron. Sci Am 241:55, 1979

BIBLIOGRAPHY

Cooper JR, Bloom FE, Roth RH: The Biochemical Basis of Neuropharmacology, 3rd ed. New York, Oxford, 1978

Gilman AG, Goodman LS, Gilman A (eds): Goodman and Gilman's The Pharmacological Basis of Therapeutics, 6th ed. New York, Macmillan, 1980, Ch 12

QUESTIONS

1. Gross anatomic divisions of the brain include:

    A. brainstem
    B. cerebellum
    C. cerebrum
    D. all of the above are correct
    E. none of the above is correct

2. **T F** Functional divisions of the CNS include sensory pathways.

3. **T F** The blood-brain barrier is more permeable to uncharged than charged drugs.

4. Nausea and vomiting induced by drugs can occur by:

    A. stimulating vagal receptors
    B. direct action on the vomiting center
    C. a direct irritating effect on the upper portions of the gastrointestinal tract
    D. all of the above are correct
    E. none of the above is correct

5. **T F** The human brain is thought to contain 10 to 100 billion neurons plus supporting cells.

6. An excitatory postsynaptic potential (EPSP) is associated with the influx of:

    A. chloride ions, resulting in depolarization
    B. choride ions, resulting in hyperpolarization.
    C. sodium ions, resulting in depolarization
    D. sodium ions, resulting in hyperpolarization

7. **T F** Prostaglandins are examples of neuromediators.

8. **T F** Neuromodulators act as secondary messengers.

9. Which of the following neurotransmitters are thought to be excitatory in nature?

    A. acetylcholine
    B. dopamine
    C. norepinephrine
    D. serotonin

10. CNS drugs may act at the level of the synapse by:

    A. depleting the transmitter from their storage sites
    B. mimicking the transmitter by acting at a postsynaptic receptor
    C. preventing the release of the transmitter

D. all of the above are correct

E. none of the above is correct

11. According to a simplified model of CNS activity, CNS excitation (stimulation) can be accomplished by:

   A. inhibition of the excitatory pathway

   B. inhibition of the inhibitory pathway

   C. inhibition of the postsynaptic pathway

   D. stimulation of the inhibitory pathway

12. General CNS depressants (nonspecific) include:

   A. antipyretic analgesics

   B. barbiturates

   C. methylphenidate

   D. narcotic analgesics

13. T F CNS drug effects exhibit summation (addition) with the physiologic state of the CNS and with the effects of other CNS stimulant and depressant drugs.

14. T F Antagonism between CNS stimulant and CNS depressant drugs is based entirely on receptor-mediated antagonism.

15. T F High concentrations of some CNS depressant drugs commonly cause excitation.

16. T F Potent drug stimulation of the CNS is usually followed by depression, and the depression is additive with the effects of CNS depressant drugs.

21
Sedative-Hypnotics

Sedative-hypnotic drugs are relatively old drugs, having been introduced in the nineteenth century (chloral hydrate). Barbiturates, the most important group, were introduced into the practice of medicine in 1903 (barbital). The major portion of this chapter deals with barbiturates, with a very minor discussion of nonbarbiturate sedative-hypnotics. Ethanol, an agent also considered to be a sedative-hypnotic drug, is discussed at length in Chapter 39.

In some circles, there is a move underway to pressure the FDA into withdrawing most of these agents from the market. Exceptions are the ultrashort-acting barbiturates (used for induction of general anesthesia) and long-acting agents (with specific anticonvulsant activity). The reason for withdrawal is that the short-to-intermediate-acting drugs are the primary agents used for adult suicides. These drugs are now thought to be inferior in sedative properties to the benzodiazepines, which were more recently introduced. Also, it is difficult to commit suicide with benzodiazepines, which have a wide margin of safety.

The authors do not recommend the routine use of barbiturates in the dental office but instead recommend the use of benzodiazepines, which are discussed in Chapter 22. Benzodiazepines seem to be superior drugs in their antianxiety, sedative, and hypnotic effects. For example, the benzodiazepines have low potential for abuse, are less likely to produce dependence, do not induce liver microsomal enzymes, have much less effect on REM sleep, and so on. Under certain circumstances, however, the barbiturates may be indicated, and we recommend their judicious use under such circumstances. Possible indications include reported allergy to benzodiazepines, induction of hospital general anesthesia, and practitioner experience with the use of barbiturates.

A. DEFINITIONS OF SEDATION AND HYPNOSIS

Objective 21.A.1. Recognize the definitions of sedation and hypnosis.

Sedation is defined as the process of calming. Under the proper circumstances, sedation may lead to drowsiness, and the patient may tend to

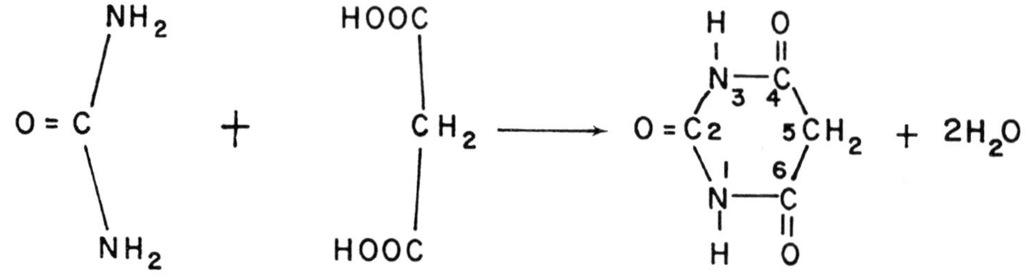

$$
\begin{array}{ccc}
\text{urea} & \text{malonic acid} & \text{barbituric acid}
\end{array}
$$

Figure 21–1. Chemical formation of barbituric acid. (*After Harvey SC: In Goodman LS, Gilman A (eds): The Pharmacological Basis of Therapeutics, 5th ed, 1975. Courtesy of Macmillan Publishing Company.*)

become sleepy. However, induction of drowsiness and sleep is not a part of the definition of sedation. Drug-induced sleep is referred to as "hypnosis." In Chapter 20, CNS excitement and depression were described on a scale through which the subject moves. In this concept, small doses of drug may depress slightly, causing an excited subject to become calm, while larger doses would cause more depression, resulting in sleep. Thus, the drugs in this group are referred to as sedative-hypnotic, and the ultimate effect is dose-dependent.

B. CHEMISTRY

Objective 21.B.1. Recognize the reaction product of urea and malonic acid.

Objective 21.B.2. Recognize the difference between oxybarbiturates and thiobarbiturates.

Barbituric acid can be formed by chemically reacting urea and malonic acid (Fig. 21–1). Barbituric acid itself is not a sedative-hypnotic agent, but when certain groups are added to carbon 5 (C5), the resultant chemicals are usually sedative-hypnotic. All the barbiturates have groups attached to carbon 5. The nitrogen at position 3 may sometimes be substituted, and the oxygen on carbon 2 may be replaced by a sulfur. Barbiturates with an oxygen at carbon 2 are referred to as oxybarbiturates, and when the oxygen is replaced by a sulfur atom, the drugs are known as thiobarbiturates.

C. CLASSIFICATION OF BARBITURATES

Objective 21.C.1. Recognize the classification of barbiturates (Table 21–1), i.e., long-, short-to-intermediate-, and ultrashort-acting.

Barbiturates are most often classified as long-acting, short-to-intermediate-acting, and ultrashort-acting (Table 21–1). This classification has been criticized in the past because it may be quite difficult clinically to distinguish between phenobarbital (a long-acting agent) and pentobarbital (a short-to-intermediate-acting agent) when either drug is given perorally for hypnosis. However, we believe there is some utility in the classification. For instance, if phenobarbital (long-acting) were used as an IV sedative agent by titration (small increases of dosage while observing the patient), it could take as long as a half-hour to achieve sedation. Usually this difficulty is encountered because the drug takes a relatively long time to reach adequate levels in the brain. Conversely, thiopental (ultrashort-acting) can be titrated to a correct level in seconds to minutes, but the duration is so short that the drug is not useful for the average dental appointment. Pentobarbital or secobarbital (short-to-intermediate-acting barbiturates) is consid-

TABLE 21-1. CLASSIFICATION OF BARBITURATES

Agent	Duration	Lipid Solubility
hexobarbital	ultrashort	high
methohexital (*Brevital*)	ultrashort	high
thiamylal	ultrashort	high
thiopental (*Pentothal*)	ultrashort	high
amobarbital (*Amytal*)	short-to-intermediate	intermediate
butabarbital (*Butisol*)	short-to-intermediate	intermediate
pentobarbital (*Nembutal*)	short-to-intermediate	intermediate
secobarbital (*Seconal*)	short-to-intermediate	intermediate
mephobarbital	long	low
metharbital	long	low
phenobarbital (*Luminal*)	long	low

ered a satisfactory compromise because the patient can be titrated in minutes, and the duration is adequate for accomplishment of many dental procedures. The classification of sedative-hypnotic barbiturates is described in Table 21-1.

D. STRUCTURE-ACTIVITY-RELATIONSHIP (SAR)

Objective 21.D.1. Recognize six SARs of barbiturates (refer to Fig. 21-1).

The addition or substitution of various atoms or groups to the barbituric acid molecule yields structures of varying activities. It has been found that the following general rules apply:

1. Increased lipid solubility → increased potency and decreased latency. Increased lipid solubility usually causes decreased duration and increased rate of metabolic breakdown.
2. Increased polarity of alkyl substitutions on C5 → decreased hypnotic potency and decreased lipid solubility. (*Note:* substitution of polar groups occurs during metabolism.)
3. Alkyl substitutions on C5 tend to shorten duration due to increased lipid solubility, but a longer chain (over 7 carbons) substitution may change the activity to a convulsant.
4. N-methylation at N3 → increased lipid solubility, but substitutions on both Ns → convulsant activity

5. Phenyl substitution on C5 → anticonvulsant activity (thus, phenobarbital is used as an antiepileptic, Chapter 38).
6. Sulfur substitution (thiobarbiturates) for oxygen at C2 → increased lipid solubility.

E. MECHANISM OF ACTION OF BARBITURATES

Objective 21.E.1. Describe the mechanism of action of barbiturates.

Barbiturates are general depressants; they are capable of depressing all excitable tissues. Synapses are usually more easily affected than are nerve bundles. Since the CNS is composed of excitable tissues with many synapses, therapeutic doses produce pronounced effects on the CNS without affecting the peripheral nerves. The ascending reticular activating system (ARAS) is thought to be especially sensitive to barbiturates. ARAS is responsible for modulating the level of consciousness, as well as selection of which stimuli should be processed as meaningful. ARAS is, therefore, most important in maintaining wakefulness, and slight to moderate depression of ARAS can result in calming effects and induction of sleep. This selectivity for ARAS is further shown by considering barbiturate effects on vital functions, such as cardiovascular and respiratory. These remain essentially unaffected in doses less than those necessary to produce general anesthesia. At dosages that produce sedation and hypnosis, vital signs are slightly depressed and are approximately equal to vital signs during natural sleep.

The actual mechanism of action of barbiturates is unknown. There is evidence to suggest that barbiturates are capable of depressing (1) central and peripheral synaptic events, including interneurons of the spinal cord, (2) transmission across neuromuscular junctions of both the sympathetic and parasympathetic divisions of the autonomic nervous system, and (3) transmission in nerve fibers (local anesthetic activity).

F. ABSORPTION, DISTRIBUTION, METABOLISM, AND EXCRETION

Objective 21.F.1. Recognize factors involved in absorption of barbiturate drugs.

In general, the barbiturates are well absorbed from all sites of the body. The more lipid-soluble agents (ultrashort-acting) will be absorbed more rapidly than the less lipid-soluble types (Table 21–1). However, when drugs are injected into body fluids, aqueous solubility becomes important. The sodium salts, when administered IM or PO, are more rapidly absorbed because the sodium salts are more soluble in the aqueous body fluids. In fact, it is claimed for barbiturates that the degree of water solubility increases their absorption more than does their lipid solubility. The presence of food in the stomach delays absorption of barbiturates, including their sodium salts.

Objective 21.F.2. Recognize the distribution of barbiturate drugs.

The barbiturates are distributed to all tissues, including across the placenta to the fetus. Due to certain physicochemical characteristics of each drug (see the following), the transfer to all tissues may be slowed but not prevented. The distribution of the agents is primarily dependent on lipid solubility, protein binding, and extent of ionization.

As with absorption, the more lipid soluble the

drug (see Table 21–1), the more rapidly it will be distributed to all tissues, including the brain, the major target organ for these agents. This factor may be the most important factor with regard to transfer of drug from blood to tissue. With increased lipid solubility, there will be an increased probability of the drug's being reabsorbed in the kidney tubule.

Plasma protein binding follows a similar pattern, but this factor does not correlate with the pharmacologic properties of the drugs. The ultrashort-acting agents bind to plasma proteins more completely than do the long-acting agents, with the short-to-intermediate types falling somewhere in between.

The extent of ionization at body pH is extremely important, since the more ionized the drug the less likely that it will traverse membranes. The ultrashort-acting agents are inherently highly lipid soluble, and hence their extent of ionization probably does not affect the distribution of these agents. However, the ionization of the short-to-intermediate and long-acting agents is definitely affected by body pH. At the pH of plasma, the long-acting agents are highly ionized, with only a small fraction unionized (remember, the unionized portion crosses membranes more readily). This is part of the reason for a delayed onset of action of long-acting agents. Another reason is delayed absorption of the agents. They tend to remain in plasma and tissue for a longer period, which accounts for their longer duration. The ionization of the short-to-intermediate types falls between the ultrashort-acting and the long-acting agents.

Knowledge of the ionization of barbiturates in the urine is an additional important factor. Barbiturates are weak acids; patients with acute toxicity may benefit from alkalinization of the urine. Alkalinization, which results in an increased ratio of ionized to unionized drug, favors excretion, aiding in detoxification.

In conclusion, although all the barbiturates produce the same pharmacologic effects, they do differ, principally by speed of onset and duration of action. These two factors are functions of tissue storage, lipid solubility, protein binding, extent of ionization in tissue fluids, redistribution, metabolism, excretion, and blood flow.

(NOTE: the IV route will bypass the gastrointestinal tract, giving immediate distribution in the blood compartment.)

Objective 21.F.3. Recognize the metabolism of barbiturate drugs and their effect on the body's metabolism.

The barbiturates are metabolized almost entirely by the liver. Other tissues are also thought to participate, but to much less a degree. In general, the more lipid soluble the drug or the more unionized the drug is at body pH, the more readily will the drug be metabolized. There is a correlation between the ability of a barbiturate to cross cell membranes and the degree of metabolism of the drug. Therefore, ultrashort-acting agents are metabolized almost completely, long-acting agents only slightly or not at all (and, therefore, a good deal of long-acting drug is excreted unchanged), and the short-to-intermediate types fall somewhere in between.

All the barbiturate drugs induce liver microsomal enzymes, and, therefore, any drug that is administered along with a barbiturate will be metabolized more rapidly than normal. Of course, the second drug must be metabolized primarily by the liver. In addition, barbiturates increase their own metabolism.

Metabolism of barbiturates occurs by four known processes: (1) oxidation on one of the side chains at carbon 5 (all barbiturates can be metabolized by this process, and the oxidized metabolite may then be excreted, or further metabolism may occur by glucuronide conjugation), (2) N-demethylation at nitrogen 3 (only hexobarbital, mephobarbital, metharbital, and methohexital are metabolized by this process), (3) replacement of a sulfur with an oxygen atom (only thiamylal and thiopental are metabolized by this process), and (4) fracture of the barbituric acid ring (all barbiturates can be metabolized by this process).

Objective 21.F.4. Recognize the route of excretion of barbiturate drugs.

Barbiturates are excreted almost entirely by the kidney. Metabolites and free drug appear in the urine, with a relatively high fraction of the long-acting drugs being excreted unchanged (especially barbital). Depending upon urine pH and lipid solubility of the drugs, a certain portion of the filtered agent will be reabsorbed in the kidney tubule.

Fecal excretion via bile secretion is minor, but a significant amount of drug may be secreted (excreted) in milk by nursing mothers.

G. TERMINATION OF ACTIVITY

Objective 21.G.1. Recognize the process responsible for the termination of pharmacologic effects (activity) of the barbiturates.

Termination of activity is responsible for the loss of pharmacologic effects (CNS effects). The processes involved in termination of activity are metabolism, excretion, and redistribution of drugs. The last factor is probably the most important involved in the termination of activity of the IV, ultrashort agents and probably also for the short-to-intermediate types when these agents are used for IV sedation.

H. PHARMACOLOGIC EFFECTS

Objective 21.H.1. Recognize the pharmacologic effects of barbiturate drugs.

Pharmacologic effects are almost entirely on the CNS. However, anesthetic and higher dosages will depress all excitable tissues, both peripheral and central.

Barbiturates will depress the CNS in a dose-dependent fashion, that is, with increasing dose, there is an increased CNS depression. Typically, there is a relief of anxiety, then sedation, then hypnosis. Increasing doses can cause coma and death. Depending upon the subject and the dose, ataxia, excitement (disinhibition), and drunkenness can occur. Anesthesia with barbiturates is difficult to control, but all stages of anesthetic depression can be produced (see also General Anesthesia, Chapter 35). Relief of anxiety and sedation are difficult to separate, especially with the use of short-to-intermediate-acting barbiturates. Fortunately for the practitioner, the depression begins at higher centers of the CNS (cortex) and progresses caudally, with the pons and medulla oblongata being the last sites to be depressed. This brain area contains the centers for vital functions, i.e., cardiovascular and respiratory. The most sensitive CNS site is the ARAS, which is involved with arousal and sleep (p. 201).

The therapeutic index or margin of safety of barbiturates is considered to be satisfactory when they are used as sedative-hypnotics; however, the TI is not favorable for general anesthesia (p. 203).

Certain barbiturates (phenobarbital, mephobarbital, and metharbital), when administered prophylactically, have a specific anticonvulsant effect, and they can be used to treat certain types of epilepsy (Chapter 38). Although all of the barbiturates are anticonvulsant when given IV, the ultrashort-acting barbiturates are the most useful barbiturates for control of an acute convulsive episode, including local anesthetic-induced convulsions. However, the short-to-intermediate or long-acting types are not recommended because their CNS depressant effects are additive, with postconvulsive depression. Diazepam is the recommended drug for an acute convulsive episode that may occur in a dental office (Chapter 22).

I. ADVERSE EFFECTS

Objective 21.I.1. Recognize the adverse effects of barbiturate drugs.

Hangover (recurring drowsiness) is frequently reported, as are lassitude, vertigo, nausea, vomiting, and diarrhea. Distortions of mood and impairment of judgment and fine motor skills can also occur. Paradoxical excitement occurs (idiosyncrasy), with increased frequency with phenobarbital and the N-methylated derivatives, especially when given PO. Inhibition of REM sleep occurs frequently, but rebound occurs after drug withdrawal.

Barbiturates are not analgesics; in the presence of pain, there is good evidence that they are hyperalgesic. The only usefulness of barbiturates in pain control is the sedative-hypnotic effect, but an analgesic drug is usually required simultaneously for optimal effect.

Tolerance, physical dependence, and psychologic dependence can and do occur with continued use. One potentially dangerous aspect of barbiturates is that tolerance develops to the sedative-hypnotic effect but not to the respiratory depressant effect. Thus, the lethal dose remains essentially the same, and the margin of safety becomes less and less.

With high doses, depression of peripheral organs occurs, including the bronchial tree, heart, and blood vessels, GI structures, ureter, urinary bladder, uterus, and kidney. However, death is usually due to respiratory depression, which occurs at moderate to high doses.

When given IV, induction of laryngospasms is a frequent occurrence. Laryngospasms may be prevented by pretreatment with an anticholinergic drug, such as atropine.

J. DRUG INTERACTIONS

Objective 22.J.1. Recognize the drug interactions of barbiturates.

All the barbiturates may cause drug interactions when given with oral anticoagulants, tricyclic antidepressants, β blockers, CNS depressants, oral contraceptives, corticosteroids, digitalis, griseofulvin, MAO inhibitors, phenothiazines, phenytoin, primidone, quinidine, rifampin, doxycycline, and theophylline. A more complete discussion of this topic occurs in Appendix II.

K. CONTRAINDICATIONS

Objective 21.K.1. Recognize the contraindications of barbiturates.

Absolute contraindications are allergy, acute intermittent porphyria, and presence of uncontrolled pain. Relative contraindictions are liver, respiratory, or kidney dysfunction, pregnancy, and use in ambulatory patients, especially those operating motor vehicles or dangerous machinery.

L. THERAPEUTIC USE AND BASIS FOR SELECTION

Objective 21.L.1. Describe the basis for selection of barbiturate drugs, especially as they relate to therapeutic use.

Before considering the use of a barbiturate, the practitioner should be advised to try all other methods of reducing anxiety and to avoid these drugs as much as possible. Certainly, dependence upon sedative-hypnotics as a primary method of patient control would be ill-advised.

There are other factors to be considered prior to selection and drug administration. Each patient needs to be evaluated beforehand. For example, there may be an exaggerated CNS depressant effect in infants and elderly persons. Other situations that may require dosage adjustment are obese patients (increased dose), patients with a history of chronic ethanol ingestion (increased dose), patients who are agitated (increased dose) or serene (decreased dose) at the time of administration, patients who are dependent on sedative-hypnotic or antianxiety drugs (increased dose), and whether another CNS depressant drug will be used concurrently (decreased dose). Hyperthyroid patients usually require increased dosage, while the opposite is true for patients with hypothyroidism.

Actual dental uses are listed below, followed by the recommended agents. The agents are chosen on the basis of the pharmacologic profiles of each category.

1. Preoperative sedation (IM or PO): use a short-to-intermediate-acting agent.
2. Hypnosis the night before a dental appointment (PO): use a short-to-intermediate-acting agent.
3. Heavy sedation prior to hospital surgery (IM): use a short-to-intermediate-acting agent.
4. To induce general anesthesia in a hospital operating room (IV): use an ultrashort-acting agent.
5. Office IV sedation: use a short-to-intermediate-acting agent.
6. Hypnosis, if needed the first night after dental surgery, always along with an analgesic (PO): use a short-to-intermediate-acting agent.
7. Daytime sedation or antianxiety effect (PO): use a long-acting agent.

M. NONBARBITURATE SEDATIVE-HYPNOTICS

Objective 21.M.1. Recognize names (set in bold type in Table 21–2) of nonbarbiturate sedative-hypnotic drugs.

There are a number of nonbarbiturate sedative-hypnotics on the market and available for use by dentists (Table 21–2). The nonbarbiturates are of many chemical classes, including potent antihistamines, which have prominent sedative-hypnotic side effects. Most OTC sleep remedies are antihistamines or contain an antihistamine. One other drug, flurazepam, is a benzodiazepine and is marketed for use as a sedative-hypnotic. This agent is discussed along with other benzodiazepines in Chapter 22.

None of the nonbarbiturate sedative-hypnotic agents offer an advantage over the barbiturates for the purpose of sedation and hypnosis. The OTC antihistamines are convenient from a patient standpoint because no prescription is needed. Nevertheless, pharmacologists, physicians, and dentists should not encourage this OTC use. On the other hand, the benzodiazepines are probably the best sedative-hypnotics discovered to date.

The complete pharmacology of nonbarbiturate sedative-hypnotic agents will not be presented. Briefly, all are allergenic, all (except antihistamines) can produce dependence, many produce blood element changes, some have autonomic effects, a few are antihistamines, a few have antispasmodic and antiemetic activity. A list of agents is presented in Table 21–2, and

TABLE 21–2. NONBARBITURATE SEDATIVE-HYPNOTICS

Agent	Chemical Class	Duration
chloral hydrate (Noctec, Somnos)	chloral derivative	short-to-intermediate
ethchlorvynol (Placidyl)	alcohol	short-to-intermediate
ethinamate (Valmid)	carbamate	short-to-intermediate
glutethimide (Doriden)	piperidinedione	short-to-intermediate
hydroxyzine (Atarax, Vistaril)	piperazine (AH)	short-to-intermediate
meprobamate (Miltown, Equanil)	carbamate	short-to-intermediate
methaqualone (Quaalude, Sopor)	quinazolone	short-to-intermediate
methyprylon (Noludar)	piperidinedione	short-to-intermediate
paraldehyde	cyclic ether	short-to-intermediate
promethazine (Phenergan)	phenothiazine (AH)	short-to-intermediate
propriomazine (Largon)	phenothiazine	short-to-intermediate

AH, antihistamine (Chapter 19).

practitioners are urged to learn the complete pharmacology of any of the agents that may be chosen for dental practice, if a rationale for use is found.

REFERENCES

Harvey SC: Hypnotics and sedatives. In Goodman LS, Gilman A (eds): The Pharmacological Basis of Therapeutics, 5th ed. New York, Macmillan, 1975, p 102

BIBLIOGRAPHY

Accepted Dental Therapeutics, 38th ed. Chicago, American Dental Association, 1979, pp 171–186
Bevan JA (ed): Essentials of Pharmacology, 2nd ed. Hagerstown, MD, Harper & Row, 1976, Ch 26
Gilman AG, Goodman LS, Gilman A (eds): Goodman and Gilman's The Pharmacological Basis of Therapeutics, 6th ed. New York, Macmillan, 1980, Ch 17
Goth A: Medical Pharmacology, 10th ed. St. Louis, Mosby, 1981, Ch 26
Meyers FH, Jawetz E, Goldfien A: Review of Medical Pharmacology, 7th ed. Los Altos, CA, Lange, 1980, Ch 23

QUESTIONS

1. **T F** Sedation is drug-induced sleep, while hypnosis is a state of calmness that often includes drowsiness.

2. **T F** The combination of urea and malonic acid produces phenobarbital.

3. **T F** Oxybarbiturates are a series of agents that contain an oxygen at C2, while thiobarbiturates contain a sulfur atom attached to the same carbon.

4. Which of the following agents are classified as short-to-intermediate-acting barbiturates?

   A. methohexital
   B. pentobarbital
   C. phenobarbital
   D. thiopental

5. **T F** Methylation of a barbiturate at N3 results in a compound with increased lipid solubility.

6. **T F** Addition of a phenyl group at C5 confers anticonvulsant activity.

7. **T F** Barbiturates are general CNS depressants that are most active in the pons-medulla oblongata of the brain.

8. Absorption of barbiturate drugs is increased when:

   A. the free base is administered
   B. the sodium salt is used in the presence of food

C. ultrashort-acting agents are used

D. all of the above are correct

E. none of the above is correct

9. T F The distribution of barbiturate drugs throughout the body is primarily dependent on lipid solubility, protein binding, and extent of ionization.

10. The metabolism of barbiturate drugs is thought to be by:

A. fracture of the barbituric and acid ring

B. N-demethylation at N3

C. oxidation on one of the side chains of C5

D. replacement of an S with an O

E. all of the above are correct

F. none of the above is correct

11. T F Barbiturates are excreted as free drug and metabolites, almost entirely by the kidney.

12. T F Redistribution of barbiturate drugs is the most important factor involved in the termination of activity of the IV ultrashort-acting agents.

13. T F The sedative effect is easily separated from relief of anxiety when administering pentobarbital to dental patients.

14. T F All barbiturate drugs have some degree of anticonvulsant activity.

15. Adverse effects of barbiturate drugs include:

A. hangover

B. inhibition of REM sleep

C. laryngospasms when given IV

D. physical dependence

E. all of the above are correct

F. none of the above is correct

16. T F Barbiturates, when taken concurrently with other CNS depressants, could result in a drug interaction.

17. T F One absolute contraindication to the use of barbiturates is the presence of uncontrolled pain.

18. The selection of a short-to-intermediate-acting barbiturate is best for:

A. induction of daytime sedation

B. induction of general anesthesia

C. preoperative sedation

D. all of the above are correct

E. none of the above is correct

19. All of the following agents are nonbarbiturate sedative-hypnotics *except:*

A. chloral hydrate

B. methaqualone

C. glutethimide

D. meprobamate

E. thiamylal   *ultrashort*

22
Antianxiety Drugs

A. INTRODUCTION

This chapter is devoted almost entirely to the benzodiazepines. The benzodiazepines are currently the best agents available for the treatment of anxiety. Although all of the sedative-hypnotic drugs (e.g., barbiturates) have an antianxiety effect, it is difficult or impossible to separate this action from sedation and drowsiness. Conversely, it has been shown that the benzodiazepines can be more reliably administered at an antianxiety dose while avoiding the problem of sedation and drowsiness.

Often, pharmacologists will include a few other drugs as antianxiety agents in this category (e.g., meprobamate), but such drugs are quite similar pharmacologically to the sedative-hypnotic agents described in Chapter 21. In other words, the benzodiazepines constitute a unique category of drugs.

Clarification of terminology is probably necessary at this time. In recent years, the antianxiety agents were called "minor psychosedatives" or "minor tranquilizers." Neither term seems very helpful in pharmacologic terminology. Psychosedative is a fancy term that is not

needed, since all sedatives naturally work on the psyche. The term tranquilizer is a lay term and is another fancy term that has been exploited by the pharmaceutical industry. Tranquilize means to calm or relax, an effect that can be produced by many classes of CNS depressant drugs. Later, the term "antineurotic" was assigned to the antianxiety drugs, because they were frequently and successfully used to treat neurosis. The term "antineurotic" is also considered passé. Similarly, the antipsychotic drugs were previously referred to as "major psychosedatives" or "major tranquilizers," but the currently accepted term is antipsychotic drug (these drugs will be presented in Chapter 36).

The group of agents discussed in this chapter is best referred to as "antianxiety drugs."

Antianxiety drugs are extremely popular in medicine and dentistry. It has been estimated that diazepam and chlordiazepoxide (two benzodiazepines) accounted for 80% of the prescriptions written worldwide during one year of the mid-1970s. One reason for their popularity is their wide margin of safety, or high TI (comparing the lethal dose to the therapeutic dose). For example, approximately 10 to 15 times the seda-

TABLE 22–1. BENZODIAZEPINE DRUGS

Official Name	Trade Name
chlordiazepoxide	Librium
clonazepam	Clonopin
clorazepate	Tranxene, Azene
diazepam	Valium
flurazepam	Dalmane
lorazepam	Ativan
oxazepam	Serax
prazepam	Verstran

Short Acting (handwritten bracket beside lorazepam and oxazepam)

TI = 70-150 (handwritten in left margin)

tive-hypnotic therapeutic dose of barbiturates can result in high toxicity and, in many cases, death. Conversely, for diazepam, the lethal dose in humans is somewhere between 70 and 150 times the therapeutic dose. Apparently, it is difficult (but not impossible) to commit suicide with the benzodiazepines.

B. CLASSIFICATION AND CHEMISTRY

Objective 22.B.1. Recognize the classification and names (set in bold type in Table 22–1) of benzodiazepines.

Objective 22.B.2. Recognize the chemical structure of diazepam, as a representative of the benzodiazepines.

The benzodiazepines can be classified much like the barbiturate sedative-hypnotics, except that no ultrashort-acting derivatives are available. Only oxazepam and lorazepam are considered short-acting or short-to-intermediate-acting. All the others are considered to be long acting because they have relatively long half-lives, which may be due to the generation of active metabolites (p. 210). Diazepam is the prototype drug of this group. Table 22–1 contains the official and trade names of popular benzodiazepines.

The benzodiazepines contain two six-member rings and one seven-member ring. Various atoms or groups of atoms are attached to the rings (see Fig. 22–1). Metabolism by the liver microsomal enzymes often results in active metabolites.

C. MECHANISM OF ACTION

Objective 22.C.1. Recognize the mechanism of action of diazepam.

There is good evidence that the benzodiazepines interact with CNS receptors that have been classified as GABA-ergic (receptors associated with neurons using gamma-aminobutyric acid as a neurotransmitter). Apparently, the benzodiazepines facilitate GABA-ergic transmission by binding to an area adjacent to the receptor (or part of its functional unit) and allowing for increased GABA receptor binding.

D. ABSORPTION, DISTRIBUTION, METABOLISM, AND EXCRETION

Objective 22.D.1. Recognize the absorption of benzodiazepines.

Objective 22.D.2. Recognize the distribution of benzodiazepines.

Objective 22.D.3. Recognize the metabolism of benzodiazepines.

Objective 22.D.4. Recognize the excretion of benzodiazepines.

All the benzodiazepines are rapidly absorbed when given orally. Diazepam is often used IV, the preferred parenteral route, especially for immediate onset of effect.

The agents are distributed to all tissue, and they readily cross the **blood-brain barrier.**

The metabolism of most benzodiazepines is complex. For example, a portion of diazepam is metabolized to hydroxydiazepam, desmethyldiazepam (or nordiazepam), and oxazepam, all active products. In addition, there is good evidence that diazepam goes through an enterohepatic cycle, i.e., it is secreted in bile into the small intestine, then reabsorbed (see Chapter 12). Thus, the half-life of diazepam and active products is quite long. However, metabolism of diazepam to inactive, water-soluble products also takes place and includes glucuronide conjugation. Apparently, only oxazepam and loraze-

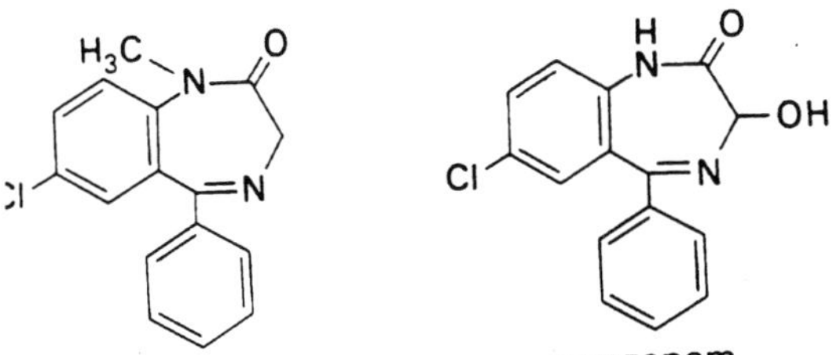

Figure 22-1. Chemical structures of diazepam and oxazepam. (*From Csáky TZ: Cutting's Handbook of Pharmacology, 6th ed, 1979. Courtesy of Appleton-Century-Crofts.*)

pam are *not* transformed to active products and they have relatively short half-lives.

Excretion of unchanged drug and metabolites is accomplished mostly by the kidneys.

E. PHARMACOLOGIC EFFECTS

Objective 22.E.1. Recognize the pharmacologic effects of diazepam.

Diazepam is currently the most popular agent, and its effects will be described. The same effects can be ascribed to the other agents, but the effects may vary in degree or duration or in other ways.

Although pharmacologic effects are listed as (1) CNS, (2) cardiovascular, and (3) respiratory, all the effects originate from the CNS, with two possible exceptions: coronary vasodilation and a neuromuscular junction blockade, the latter with very high IV dosages.

CNS Effects

1. Relief of anxiety, sedation, hypnosis with easy arousal. Increased dosages do *not* result in general anesthesia, as noted with the sedative-hypnotic drugs. (Sedation and hypnosis are thought to occur by depression of the RAS in the central core of the brain.)
2. Central skeletal muscle relaxation. The most important site for this action is subcortical, but there is evidence that spinal cord interneuronal sites are also affected. Sedation also contributes to a skeletal muscle relaxant effect.
3. Amnesia is possible when the drug is administered IV, especially at higher doses.
4. There is clinical evidence of an antineurotic effect, but experimental evidence is lacking (however, there is evidence that diazepam has an action in the limbic system).
5. Anticonvulsant activity.
6. Anticholinergic activity.
7. Hypnosis with slight loss of REM sleep. There is evidence of depression of stage-4 sleep, although there is an increase in total sleeping time.

Cardiovascular Effects

Usual PO therapeutic doses depress cardiovascular function only slightly, i.e., approximately equal to the depression noted with natural sleep. When diazepam is administered IV, a transient but prominent fall in blood pressure may be occasionally noted; the cardiovascular effect is induced by vasodilation and depression of myocardial function, with the heart rate reflexly increased. There is some evidence that the decreased blood pressure is caused, at least partially, by the diluent used for diazepam and chlordiazepoxide. Even though this complication has been reported, it can usually be avoided by proper IV technique and careful titration.

Respiratory Effects

As with cardiovascular function, when diazepam is administered alone PO, respiration is depressed approximately equally to that noted with natural sleep. With good IV technique, respiration is only slightly depressed.

F. ADVERSE EFFECTS

Objective 22.F.1. Recognize adverse effects of benzodiazepines.

1. allergy (rare)
2. drowsiness and ataxia, hangover
3. paradoxical effects: increased hostility, increased anxiety, insomnia, hallucinations, seizures, rage, paranoia, and depression

4. psychoses and suicidal tendencies with high dosages
5. weight gain
6. hepatotoxic or hematologic disorders (rare)
7. menstrual irregularities
8. tolerance and psychologic and physical dependence can occur, and with a more rapid onset when supratherapeutic dosages are used (i.e., greater than 30 mg/day with diazepam)
9. nausea, vomiting, epigastric distress
10. xerostomia
11. with use of chlordiazepoxide, skin rash and impairment of sexual function

G. DRUG INTERACTIONS

Objective 22.G.1. Recognize drug interactions.

1. An increased CNS depressant effect (including respiratory) when the drugs are combined with **all** other CNS depressants, especially with alcoholic beverages.
2. Cigarette smoking may decrease drug effectiveness.
3. Diazepam should not be used when patients are taking levodopa.
4. Benzodiazepines with valproic acid, an antiepileptic drug, have produced psychotic episodes.

H. CONTRAINDICATIONS

Objective 22.H.1. Recognize contraindications to diazepam.

1. allergy
2. caution is required in patients with liver or kidney dysfunction
3. pregnancy (there is evidence of increased incidence of cleft lip and cleft palate)
4. acute narrow-angle glaucoma (also open-angle glaucoma, unless patients are receiving appropriate therapy)
5. chronic obstructive pulmonary diseases

I. THERAPEUTIC USES

Objective 22.I.1. Recognize medical and dental uses of diazepam.

Medical Uses

1. relief of anxiety
2. alcohol withdrawal, especially chlordiazepoxide
3. preoperative sedative
4. drug of first choice for treatment of muscle contractions of tetanus
5. drug of first choice for treatment of status epilepticus
6. spastic musculoskeletal disease, e.g., cerebral palsy
7. muscle strain and/or spasm, especially in conjunction with aspirin
8. hypnosis
9. IV administration for bronchoscopy, esophagoscopy, and cardioversion
10. chronically, to prevent epileptic seizures (clonazepam only)
11. emergency drug for local anesthetic convulsions

Dental Uses

1. preoperative sedation, PO
2. hypnosis, the night before a dental appointment
3. IV sedation
4. hypnosis along with an analgesic, postoperatively
5. daytime sedation (daytime antianxiety effect)
6. anticonvulsant, as an emergency drug for local anesthetic convulsions
7. muscle relaxant for spasms about the TMJ

J. DENTAL IMPLICATIONS, BASIS FOR SELECTION

Objective 22.J.1. Recognize dental implications and basis for selection.

1. For hypnosis the night before a dental appointment, flurazepam is the drug that was tested and is marketed solely for this purpose.

Dalmane

However, one source (Med Lett Drugs Ther 19:49, 1977; Med Lett Drugs Ther 23:41, 1981) suggests that any of the benzodiazepines would be useful for an antianxiety effect, sedation, or induction of hypnosis. We (and others) believe oxazepam or lorazepam should be considered, for they are not metabolized to active products, and their half-lives are relatively short; therefore, the incidence of hangover may also be decreased (Med Lett Drugs Ther 20:31, 1978; Med Lett Drugs Ther 23:41, 1981). Exceptions to the use of oxazepam or lorazepam are listed below.

Apparently, most or all benzodiazepines, in lower dose ranges, do not interfere with REM sleep. However, they do depress the amount of time spent in stage-4 sleep. This may be an advantage in those patients that have nightmares, which occur in stage 4. However, some investigators believe that loss of stage-4 sleep is as much of a disadvantage as the loss of REM sleep.

2. With regard to IV use, only chlordiazepoxide, diazepam, and lorazepam are marketed for parenteral administration. Of the three agents, diazepam appears to be superior for IV sedation. One disadvantage is that the agents are not water soluble and cannot be diluted except with the recommended diluent.

Diazepam IV is an excellent drug for induction of conscious sedation, and this use is frequently and easily taught to dental students and practitioners in many dental schools. However, we believe that if combinations of diazepam with other drugs are to be used IV, further, more intensive training is recommended.

A comparison of pharmacologic profiles of pentobarbital and diazepam is presented in Table 22–2.

TABLE 22–2. COMPARISON OF PHARMACOLOGIC PROFILES OF SEDATIVE AGENTS

Pentobarbital or Secobarbital	Diazepam
Some General Properties	
anticonvulsant (at higher doses)	potent anticonvulsant
some amnesic activity	potent amnesic (especially IV)
some central muscle relaxation	good central muscle relaxation
no analgesic	transient analgesic in man (IV)
With Gradually Increasing Dosage	
relief of anxiety	relief of anxiety
sedation	sedation
hypnosis	hypnosis
general anesthesia—all stages	no general anesthesia
respiratory depression	Rare[a]
cardiovascular depression	Occasional[a]
death	Rare[a]
With Continuous Use	
physical dependence	physical dependence
psychologic dependence	psychologic dependence
Schedule II drug	Schedule IV drug

[a] Poor IV technique using therapeutic dosages can occasionally result in cardiovascular depression, but respiratory depression or death has only rarely been reported. Very high dosages (e.g., 700 mg PO) may result in respiratory depression, cardiovascular depression, or death.

3. There is some evidence that dental postoperative patients have a more restful night if a hypnotic is prescribed along with an analgesic. Oxazepam or lorazepam would probably be best. If the analgesic to be used has significant CNS depressant effects, especially respiratory depression, the dosage of the analgesic should be reduced about one quarter to one half.

4. Dental patients who are anxious prior to an appointment are better treated with benzodiazepines than with barbiturates because the antianxiety and sedative effects are more easily separated. Again, probably oxazepam or lorazepam is best to avoid cumulative effects of hangover.

5. If an anticonvulsant drug is needed (epilepsy or local anesthetic toxicity) due to an acute convulsive episode in the dental chair, diazepam is the drug of choice to stop the seizure. The drug is best given IV, but that may not be possible, and other sites may be considered, e.g., IM.

6. These drugs are of no value for patients with a problem of the temporomandibular joint (that is, within the joint itself). However, if the problem is due to a spasm of the muscles near or around the joint, diazepam will probably be the antispasmodic drug of choice. Aspirin or other analgesics may also be needed for pain relief. Long-term treatment with diazepam should be avoided, as dependence may develop.

7. Patients must be cautioned about driving motor vehicles or operating dangerous machinery, especially patients who continue to be under the influence of the drug. It is the dentist's responsibility, medicolegally, to ensure a safe trip home and provide instructions for drug use after reaching home. Included in such instructions should be warnings against the use of these drugs with other CNS depressant drugs, including alcohol.

8. Clonazepam probably should not be used in dentistry; it should be reserved for treatment of epilepsy and convulsive disorders.

K. CENTRAL MUSCLES RELAXANTS

Objective 22.K.1. Recognize the names of central skeletal muscle relaxant drugs.

Objective 22.K.2. Recognize their mechanism of central skeletal muscle relaxation.

A number of drugs are capable of producing central skeletal muscle relaxation and are reported to be useful for muscle spasms associated with arthritis, fibrositis, myositis, and muscle sprains. The major problem with all agents is that they act nonspecifically, and, therefore, ataxia can occur.

Mechanisms of action include depression of spinal cord interneurons (probably all of the agents have this property), an action in the brain that is thought to be at a subcortical site (benzodiazepines), and in muscle itself (dantrolene). All sedative-hypnotics have some central skeletal muscle relaxant effect, and some authors believe that the relaxation is the result of sedation, rather than a specific action in the CNS.

Table 22–3 contains a list of agents that are currently marketed for use as central skeletal muscle relaxants. The list does not include sedative-hypnotics (Chapter 21), nor does it include the antianxiety agents that were just described in this chapter.

A popular combination that is frequently used by many physicians is diazepam plus 650 to 975 mg of aspirin. The anti-inflammatory action of aspirin undoubtedly aids in controlling muscle

TABLE 22–3. CENTRAL SKELETAL MUSCLE RELAXANTS

Official Name	Trade Name
baclofen	Lioresal
carisoprodol	Soma
chlormezanone	Trancopal
chlorphenesin	Maolate
chlorzoxazone	Paraflex
cyclobenzaprine	Flexeril
dantrolene (direct and CNS)	Dantrium
metaxalone	Skelaxin
methocarbamol	Robaxin

spasm. Other physicians are using aspirin plus either of the two recently marketed drugs, baclofen or cyclobenzaprine.

The FDA (FDA Drug Bull 9:27, 1979) has recently approved dantrolene for the treament of malignant hyperthermia; the drug is apparently very efficacious for this problem. This genetically related syndome occurs when susceptible patients are exposed to inhalation anesthetics and often in conjunction with neuromuscular blocking drugs. Symptoms of the syndrome include tachycardia, tachypnea, hypercarbia, fever, rigidity, profuse sweating, and cardiac arrhythmias. Treatment includes IV dantrolene and supportive measures, such as administering oxygen, correcting metabolic acidosis, cooling the patient when necessary, maintaining urinary output, and monitoring electrolyte balance. Prior to dantrolene treatment, the condition had a mortality rate of 50 to 70%, despite the use of supportive measures.

REFERENCES

FDA Drug Bull 9:27, 1979
Med Lett Drugs Ther 19:49, 1977
Med Lett Drugs Ther 20:31, 1978
Med Lett Drugs Ther 23:41, 1981

BIBLIOGRAPHY

Accepted Dental Therapeutics, 38th ed. Chicago, American Dental Association, 1979, Sec II, Agents for the Control of Anxiety

Bevan JA (ed): Essentials of Pharmacology, 2nd ed. Hagerstown, MD, Harper & Row, 1976, Ch 26

Csáky, TZ: Cutting's Handbook of Pharmacology, 6th ed. New York, Appleton-Century-Crofts, 1979, Ch 54

Gilman, AG, Goodman, LS, Gilman A (eds): Goodman and Gilman's The Pharmacological Basis of Therapeutics, 6th ed. New York, Macmillan, 1980, Ch 17

Goth A: Medical Pharmacology, 10th ed. St. Louis, Mosby, 1981, Ch 24

Meyers FH, Jawetz E, Goldfien A: Review of Medical Pharmacology, 7th ed. Los Altos, CA, Lange, 1980, Ch 23

QUESTIONS

1. T (F) Benzodiazepines may be classified much like the barbiturates, because there are ultrashort-, short-intermediate-, and long-acting agents.

2. T F Diazepam probably produces at least part of its effects by interacting with GABA receptors in the CNS.

3. T F Body handling of diazepam is not unique, for it is readily absorbed, distributed to most tissues, biotransformed by the liver, and excreted by the kidneys.

4. Which of the following drugs is considered to be long acting because it forms active metabolites?

   A. diazepam
   B. oxazepam
   C. both A and B are correct
   D. neither A nor B is correct

5. The pharmacologic effects of diazepam include:

   A. anticholinergic activity
   B. central skeletal muscle relaxation
   C. relief of anxiety
   D. all of the above are correct
   E. none of the above is correct

6. T F There is little or no effect on cardiovascular or respiratory function with therapeutic doses of peroral diazepam.

7. Adverse effects of diazepam include:

   A. drowsiness and ataxia
   B. increased anxiety
   C. increased hostility
   D. all of the above are correct
   E. none of the above is correct

8. **T F** An increased CNS depressant effect can occur if diazepam is taken along with any other CNS depressant.

9. **T F** One contraindication to the use of diazepam is the presence of acute narrow-angle glaucoma.

10. Dental uses of diazepam include:

   A. anticonvulsant
   B. IV sedative
   C. muscle relaxant
   D. all of the above are correct
   E. none of the above is correct

11. A preferred benzodiazepine for hypnosis is:

   A. chlordiazepoxide
   B. clonazepam
   C. diazepam
   D. oxazepam
   E. prazepam

12. **T F** A benzodiazepine may be preferred for hypnosis because, at lower therapeutic doses, they have little effect on REM sleep.

13. **T F** Sedation is the sole mechanism by which diazepam produces its central muscle relaxant effect.

14. All of the following drugs produce a central muscle relaxant effect *except:*

   A. baclofen
   B. chlorpromazine
   C. cyclobenzaprine
   D. metaxalone
   E. methocarbamol

23

Antipyretic-Analgesics, Combinations, and Other Nonnarcotic Analgesics

The drugs used in treating mild pain are commonly referred to as **antipyretic-analgesics** and comprise one of the most frequently used groups of agents in existence today. We are all familiar with the use of aspirin and acetaminophen in headache, hangover, neuralgia, and so on. Mild pain of dental origin is readily relieved with the same drugs. When combined with other analgesics, such as codeine, antipyretic-analgesics can be used to treat moderate pain. Even in severe pain, these drugs should be used as a supplement to strong narcotic-analgesics (Chapter 24). Another group of drugs, **nonsteroidal anti-inflammatory** agents (NSAIA), can be used in treating mild or even higher levels of pain intensity.

A. ANALGESIA AND MECHANISMS

Objective 23.A.1. Describe analgesia and mechanisms by which analgesia is obtained pharmacologically.

Analgesia means "without pain." Drugs that cause analgesia reduce or eliminate the sensation of pain without necessarily altering consciousness. Mechanisms of analgesia are (1) alteration of pain threshold (more stimulus needed to cause the same amount of pain), (2) alteration of pain interpretation (e.g., focusing attention away from painful situation), and (3) anti-inflammatory effect. In addition, some drugs may cause drowsiness, which may be a useful therapeutic property in some situations. Aspirin (acetylsalicylic acid) is the prototype not only of antipyretic-analgesics but also of NSAIA, while morphine is the prototype of narcotic-analgesics. Table 23–1 compares the two prototype analgesics, aspirin and morphine, for properties that make them useful in the clinical situation of pain.

B. ANTIPYRETIC-ANALGESICS AND RELATED DRUGS FOR THE TREATMENT OF MILD PAIN

Objective 23.B.1. List antipyretic-analgesic drugs and compare their activities.

Aspirin (a salicylate) and acetaminophen (a para-aminophenol) are the most commonly used drugs for pain of mild intensity. They are called

TABLE 23-1. COMPARISON OF ASPIRIN AND MORPHINE

	Aspirin	Morphine
prototype for	antipyretic-analgesics or NSAIA	narcotic-analgesics
pain threshold	no change	increased
interpretation	altered	altered
anti-inflammatory	yes	no
drowsiness	no	yes

antipyretic-analgesics because of their ability to reduce fever as well as pain. They are sold OTC and used for integumental pain (as opposed to visceral, which is probably best treated with narcotic-analgesics), such as mild dental pain, headache, hangover, neuralgia, joint pain, muscle aches, and so on. Other drugs effective against mild pain are NSAIA (e.g., ibuprofen, zomepirac) and fenamic acid derivatives (mefenamic acid). Phenylbutazone (a pyrazolone) and indomethacin (an indene derivative) are pharmacologically related drugs that are anti-inflammatory and antipyretic but are seldom used in dentistry because of their high toxicity. Table 23-2 compares representatives of the mild analgesic drug groups.

C. ASPIRIN (ACETYLSALICYLIC ACID)

Objective 23.C.1. Describe the chemistry of aspirin.

Aspirin is the acetic acid ester of benzoic acid (Fig. 23-1). Its acidic nature accounts for the corrosive effect of aspirin when it is applied topically (aspirin burn). Salicylates have been in use for centuries, primarily in the form of a plant extract, for the treatment of fever. Salicylic acid was isolated and purified in the middle of the nineteenth century, and the synthetic derivative acetylsalicylic acid has been in use for pain, inflammation, and fever since that time. Aspirin is the prototype of salicylate drugs, as well as the classes **antipyretic-analgesics** and NSAIA.

Therapeutic Actions

Objective 23.C.2. List three therapeutic actions of aspirin and describe the usefulness of these actions.

Analgesia. This is the chief use for aspirin in dentistry. While the mechanisms of this action remain uncertain, experimental data indicate that it involves central, peripheral, and placebo alterations of the perception of pain. Aspirin is effective in the treatment of pain of a mild intensity, resulting from superficial wounds and irritations, arthralgia, myalgia, and other conditions of an integumentary origin.

Antipyresis. Aspirin lowers the body temperature in febrile individuals by an action on the hypothalamus. This action is thought to occur by aspirin inhibition of prostaglandin (PG) synthesis in the hypothalamus. The result is increased sweating and dilation of cutaneous blood vessels, which in turn increases heat loss.

Anti-inflammatory. This effect is important in the treatment of arthritis and probably involves inhibition of PG formation, reduction of local edema, and/or stimulation of adrenocorticosteroid secretion. Relatively large doses (6 gm per day) are used in treating inflammatory diseases.

Side Effects

Objective 23.C.3. List six side effects of aspirin and describe their clinical implications and the types of patients in whom aspirin is contraindicated.

The side effects of aspirin are described below, along with their clinical implications.

Gastrointestinal irritation. Since aspirin is an acidic tissue irritant, it frequently produces epigastric distress, nausea, and vomiting. Vomiting may also be due to an effect of aspirin on the chemoreceptor trigger zone in the medulla. GI irritation contraindicates use of aspirin in patients with ulcers and may necessitate normal patients taking the drug with a small amount of

TABLE 23-2. REPRESENTATIVES OF MILD ANALGESIC DRUG GROUPS

Group	Prototype	Other Drugs	Anal-gesic	Anti-pyretic	Anti-inflammatory (NSAIA)	Uricosuric[a]
salicylates	aspirin	sodium salicylate	yes	yes	yes	weak
anilines	acetaminophen	phenacetin	yes	yes	no	no
NSAIA	ibuprofen	zomepirac, naproxen	yes	yes	yes	no
fenamic acid derivatives	mefenamic acid	meclofenamate	yes	yes	yes	no
pyrazolone derivatives	phenylbutazone	(antipyrine)[b] (aminopyrine)	yes	yes	yes	weak
indene derivatives	indomethacin	sulindac	±	yes	yes	no
—	probenecid	—	no	no	no	potent

[a] Causing uric acid excretion.
[b] Parentheses indicates drug is no longer used.

food or a full glass of water or other beverage. This gastrointestinal irritation also results in a small amount of bleeding from the gastrointestinal mucosa, which is manifested as an increase in fecal blood content from a normal value of 0.6 ml to 3 to 8 ml per day (occult bleeding). This situation is especially detrimental to patients with bleeding ulcers or with defects in their blood clotting processes.

Prolongation of bleeding time. It is now commonly known that a single dose (two 5-grain aspirin tablets) can double the bleeding time for a period of from four to seven days. By inhibiting the release of ADP from platelets, aspirin inhibits platelet aggregation and delays clot formation. Aspirin should, therefore, be avoided in patients with liver damage, hypoprothrombinemia, vitamin K deficiency, hemophilia, and in patients taking anticoagulants. Aspirin therapy should be discontinued one week prior to surgi-

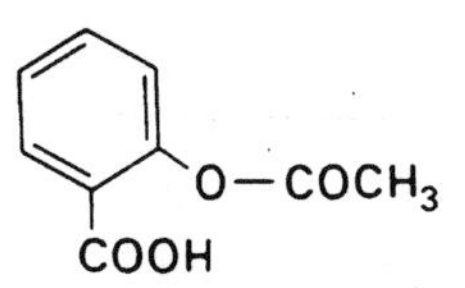

Figure 23-1. Acetylsalicylic acid structure. (*From Csáky TZ: Cutting's Handbook of Pharmacology, 6th ed, 1979. Courtesy of Appleton-Century-Crofts.*)

cal procedures, whenever this is possible. In routine extractions, patients have frequently taken a considerable amount of aspirin prior to their appointment, but prolonged time for clot formation may be avoided by careful attention to local measures for hemorrhage control. Although precautions are advised, the problem of postoperative aspirin therapy causing bleeding appears to be minimal. The use of aspirin following routine surgical procedures does not appear to cause significant postoperative bleeding, which may be due to the fact that the blood clot has formed prior to the development of a significant blood level of aspirin in the patient.

Respiratory stimulation. This is **not** ordinarily a significant effect, although it results in significant alterations of acid-base balance in cases of overdose and may contraindicate the use of aspirin in asthmatics, depending on the severity of their disease.

Allergy. Allergic reactions to aspirin are not unusual and can occur at any dose level. Allergic reactions may vary in severity, but they always contraindicate further use of the drug. Patients should be cautioned that preparations containing relatively small amounts of aspirin will **not** avoid the occurrence of an allergic reaction. Patients with a history of bronchial asthma or nasal polyps should not receive aspirin. These patients, although not truly allergic to aspirin, may have a high incidence of allergy-like reactions not only to aspirin but also to many other NSAIA. There appears to be no immunologic basis for this reaction, and when it occurs, it is often difficult to treat.

Hyperuricemia. Analgesic doses of aspirin can elevate serum uric acid levels by inhibiting its tubular secretion. This contraindicates the use of aspirin in patients with gout, in spite of the uricosuric action produced by high doses.

Uricosuria. This action results in an increased urinary excretion of uric acid but requires extremely high doses of aspirin. At normal doses, uric acid excretion is actually decreased, and the serum urate level is elevated. Thus, the use of aspirin for analgesia in patients with gout is contraindicated. Aspirin is not used at high doses for gout therapy because side effects are often encountered.

Toxicity and Lethality

Objective 23.C.4. Describe the symptoms and treatment of aspirin toxicity.

Objective 23.C.5. State the lethal dose of aspirin in adults and children.

The toxic effects of aspirin overdose are important, since many patients may self-prescribe excessive doses or excessive duration of therapy, and many children are poisoned each year by acute ingestion of toxic amounts of aspirin.

Salicylism. This is the term applied to a syndrome resulting from mild, chronic salicylate intoxication. It is characterized by the following signs and symptoms in various combinations: headache, dizziness, tinnitus, mental confusion, drowsiness, lassitude, sweating, thirst, hyperventilation, nausea, and vomiting.

At higher doses, taken acutely, the above effects may be seen and may then proceed to delirium, hallucinations, convulsions, coma, and death.

The treatment of salicylate toxicity is symp-

tomatic and usually involves taking a blood sample for determination of blood levels of the drug, followed by induction of emesis, intravenous fluid therapy, induction of alkaline diuresis, and dialysis. Salicylate intoxication is an acute medical emergency and should be treated in the hospital. The adult lethal dose of aspirin is 20 gm, or approximately 67 5-grain tablets. In children, about 5 gm, or 15 tablets, may cause lethal effects.

Alternate Forms of Salicylates

Objective 23.C.6. Describe some alternate forms of salicylates and describe clinical usefulness.

Chewable tablets. These are flavored and useful for children.

Timed-release capsules. A timed-release capsule contains many different small tablets which dissolve at different rates, thus providing aspirin for a longer period of time. This may be useful before bedtime to provide a constant dosage during sleep, but the half-time for salicylate excretion is so long that it is doubtful whether timed-release is needed.

Sodium salicylate. This liberates free salicylic acid in the stomach. This may be more irritating to gastric mucosa. However, the drug may be useful in patients with allergic-type reactions to aspirin and other NSAIA, although acetaminophen might be considered the drug of choice.

Buffered aspirin. Patients who consider aspirin irritating will often be able to take buffered aspirin. The buffering effect may be temporarily soothing, but there is probably no advantage in therapy because faster absorption is followed by faster excretion. Psychologic factors may be involved in better patient tolerance of buffered aspirin. When aspirin is given with sodium bicarbonate (*Alka-Seltzer*) a similar result occurs—rapid absorption, rapid excretion, and possibly better tolerance.

Enteric-coated capsules. These allow the aspirin to pass through the stomach and be absorbed in the intestinal tract. Although gastric distress is avoided, intestinal irritation may occur. Absorption of the ionized form in the intestinal tract may be slow and incomplete.

Salicylamide. This compound is not cross-allergenic, as it is not converted to aspirin. Its potency is reduced compared to aspirin, and it is rapidly excreted. A better choice for aspirin-allergic patients is acetaminophen.

D. ACETAMINOPHEN

Objective 23.D.1. List four major differences between aspirin and acetaminophen in actions and side effects.

Acetaminophen (also known as APAP and having many trade names, such as *Tylenol*) is a para-aminophenolic compound which is soluble in water. Acetaminophen is one of the metabolites of a related analgesic, phenacetin. Acetaminophen is a satisfactory, mild analgesic in patients who cannot tolerate aspirin, either because of gastrointestinal intolerance or allergy. Acetaminophen possesses two actions similar to aspirin, analgesia and antipyresis. In comparison with aspirin, acetaminophen exhibits:

1. no anti-inflammatory action (not considered to be an NSAIA)
2. no increase in occult gastrointestinal bleeding
3. no inhibition of blood clotting processes
4. no cross-allergenicity with aspirin

Objective 23.D.2. List the side effects and toxic effects of acetaminophen.

The side effects of acetaminophen include nausea and vomiting and, rarely, allergy. There are two potentially fatal toxic effects of acetaminophen overdose: hepatic necrosis (acute) and renal damage (which may occur with long-term use). Acetaminophen intoxication, like aspirin intoxication, is life-threatening and must be treated in a hospital.

Additional Aniline Derivatives

Objective 23.D.3. Describe two other aniline derivatives, their relationships to acetaminophen, and their place in therapeutics.

Phenacetin. This drug is metabolized to acetaminophen and other products which appear to be toxic, causing its popularity to constantly diminish (see the following).

Acetanilid. This is an early form of the aniline, but it is toxic, causing blood dyscrasias, and is no longer used.

E. ABSORPTION, METABOLISM, AND EXCRETION OF ANTIPYRETIC-ANALGESICS

Objective 23.E.1. Describe absorption, metabolism, and excretion of salicylates and acetaminophen.

Salicylates are well absorbed from the GI tract, protein-bound (50% or more), and widely distributed throughout all body fluids. Metabolism of salicylates occurs mainly in the liver microsomes by conjugation. A total dose of salicylate can be recovered in the urine as metabolites and free salicylate (about 10%). Acetaminophen is also well absorbed and is less well bound to protein (25% bound) than are salicylates. Acetaminophen is also conjugated in the liver and excreted mostly as metabolites, with only 3% unchanged. An interesting feature is that acetaminophen and phenacetin are metabolized to toxic products, and this may be accentuated in patients with drug-induced microsomal enzyme activity and impaired renal function.

F. PROPIONIC ACID DERIVATIVES AND OTHER NSAIA

Objective 23.F.1. Recognize three recently introduced NSAIA derivatives related to propionic acid.

Objective 23.F.2. Describe the mechanism of action of NSAIA.

Objective 23.F.3. Describe indications, precautions, contraindications, and side effects associated with propionic acid derivatives.

Recently, several propionic acid derivatives have been introduced for the treatment of pain and inflammation. Three such compounds are ibuprofen (*Motrin*), zomepirac (*Zomax*), and naproxen (*Anaprox, Naprosyn*), which are **not** chemically related to aspirin or acetaminophen. Other NSAIA include mefenamic acid (part G following), pyrazolones (H, following) indenes (I, following), and other drugs (see Table 23–2). Propionic acid derivatives are the most promising new members of the NSAIA group; these drugs inhibit prostaglandin synthetase.

The PG synthetase inhibitors have been referred to as NSAIA to distinguish them from the corticosteroids, which are also anti-inflammatory. The latter are different chemically and cause their anti-inflammatory effect by a different mechanism. This difference is shown in Figure 23–2. It may be noted that cortisol inhibits membrane function not only at the plasma membrane but also by stabilization of lysosomes. However, NSAIA block a later step after arachidonic acid release, inhibiting cyclo-oxygenase (prostaglandin synthetase), resulting in lowered protaglandin (PG) levels. Further details of the NSAIA mechanism are presented later in this chapter and in Chapter 19.

While the presence of simple, mild pain should be treated in the dental office with aspirin or acetaminophen, pain associated with inflammatory conditions may be better treated with these newer compounds, especially when pain is refractory to the commonly used analgesics. Specifically, acute myositis associated with TMJ dysfunction or TMJ pain of osteoarthritic origin should be treated with one of these drugs. Some investigators (Cooper and Beaver, 1976) claim that these agents may also be effective in treating moderate (or even moderate-to-severe) pain associated with tooth extraction. Their studies have shown that the propionic acid derivatives are as effective as an aspirin-codeine combination (with less codeine-induced side effects) for relief of postoperative pain following

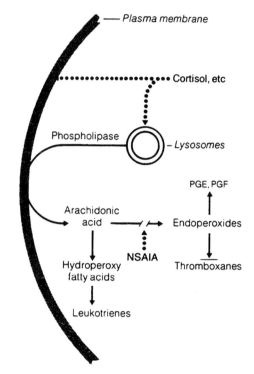

Figure 23–2. Mechanism of action of steroidal and nonsteroidal anti-inflammatory agents. (*From Weissman G: Prostaglandins and Inflammation, 1981. Courtesy of the Upjohn Company.*)

extraction of third molars. NSAIA have the following advantages over narcotic-analgesics: (1) anti-inflammatory, (2) not under DEA control, and (3) not causing drowsiness or drug dependence.

The side effects of these drugs appear to be relatively mild, although there are some situations in which the drugs are contraindicated or should be used with caution. Because NSAIA can cause prolonged bleeding time, they should be used only with caution in patients taking anticoagulants. Their use in combination with aspirin is not recommended, since aspirin tends to lower the blood levels of other NSAIAs. Because of a lack of experience with use in pregnant women, nursing mothers, or children, the NSAIA should be avoided or used only when necessary in such patients. The NSAIA should not be used in patients who exhibit bronchospastic, urticarial, or other allergic reactions to aspirin (Med Lett Drugs Ther, 1981).

Side effects include the following:

1. Gastrointestinal irritation is one of the more common side effects of these drugs, and, like aspirin, these drugs should not be used in patients with ulcers.
2. Visual disturbances, including scotomas and blurring, while relatively rare, have occurred.
3. Inhibition of platelet aggregation, resulting in prolongation of bleeding time.
4. Allergy occurs in various degrees of severity, and there appears to be cross-allergy with aspirin.
5. Edema contraindicates the use of these compounds in patients with compromised cardiovascular function.

G. FENAMIC ACID DERIVATIVE (MEFENAMIC ACID, *Ponstel*)

Objective 23.G.1. List advantages and disadvantages of mefenamic acid compared to aspirin.

Introduced in 1967, mefenamic acid has only restricted use as an alternate analgesic to aspirin. It provides analgesia similar to aspirin but has more side effects. If chosen as an aspirin substitute, it should be used for a maximum of seven days only. Side effects include frequent diarrhea, gastric ulceration and bleeding, serious blood alterations, nausea, vomiting, nervousness, headache, and possible enhancement of oral anticoagulants. In short, it is advertised to dentists but is not recommended by the authors. It should not be used in children or women of childbearing age.

H. PYRAZOLONES

Objective 23.H.1. List three pyrazolones and their place in medicine.

Aminopyrine and antipyrine are older analgesics that have been abandoned because of blood dyscrasia induction. **Phenylbutazone** was introduced more recently as a powerful uricosuric drug (for gout) and for rheumatoid arthritis. Cases of agranulocytosis (as found in the parent drugs) have been found, so phenylbutazone should be only rarely used, and careful blood studies should be performed if it is selected. It has been largely replaced by indomethacin for NSAIA activity and by probenecid for gout. Phenylbutazone is not recommended in dentistry because dentists generally do not treat rheumatoid arthritis. It is also not recommended for routine use in medicine, although it may be prescribed by some physicians.

I. INDENE DERIVATIVES

Objective 23.I.1. List the most important member of this group and describe its usefulness.

Indomethacin is a strong anti-inflammatory agent used in rheumatoid arthritis. It is also a prostaglandin synthetase inhibitor as is aspirin, but it has too many side effects to be useful as an NSAIA in dentistry.

Indomethacin is not popular in dentistry because dentists generally do not treat rheumatoid arthritis, but it may be prescribed medically.

J. COMBINATIONS

Both aspirin and acetaminophen continue to be marketed in combination with other analgesics, e.g., phenacetin, caffeine, sedatives, antacids, decongestants, and antihistamines. While some of these ingredients may be beneficial in certain conditions in which mild pain plays a part, e.g., the common cold, it is doubtful that they add any significant pain-relieving action. An exception to this, of course, is the combination of aspirin or acetaminophen with codeine, which is discussed under narcotic-analgesic combinations for mild-to-moderate pain.

Objective 23.J.1. List four specific drugs used in combination with aspirin and acetaminophen in OTC and prescription preparations.

Objective 23.J.2. Describe the therapeutic benefits and disadvantages of each of these adjunctive agents.

Phenacetin

Phenacetin is an effective analgesic, which is partially metabolized to acetaminophen by the body. When used as an APC combination (aspirin-phenacetin-caffeine), the dose of aspirin is concomitantly reduced, so that there is not a significant change in the analgesic efficacy of the preparation. Furthermore, phenacetin has been implicated in the renal damage that can occur with chronic and high-dose use of this combination. In addition, a reduction in aspirin content in such preparations does not reduce the likelihood of an allergic reaction in sensitive patients, and the combination is not better tolerated in patients with bleeding tendencies or ulcers.

Caffeine

There is no evidence that caffeine increases the analgesic efficacy of the mild analgesics, especially at the low doses used in APC combinations. It is equally doubtful that such doses exert a significant mood elevating effect, since a single cup of coffee usually contains 85 mg of caffeine, and there are 32 mg in most combination preparations.

Barbiturates

Barbiturates, e.g., butalbital, are added to analgesic combinations for the treatment of painful conditions associated with nervous tension. Barbiturates are not recommended for treating simple dental pain, unless a sedative action is required.

Combinations with Codeine

These are rational combinations because the two drugs act by different mechanisms to cause pain relief. The result of adding codeine to either aspirin or acetaminophen is to provide therapy for relief of moderate pain. The combination is usually not effective in severe pain, but it may be tried, if in doubt. The pharmacology of codeine is discussed in Chapter 24. Codeine is added to 325 mg tablets of aspirin or acetaminophen in the following amounts:

1. ⅛ grain codeine (7.5 to 8 mg)
2. ¼ grain codeine (15 to 16 mg)
3. ½ grain codeine (30 to 32 mg)
4. 1 grain codeine (60 to 65 mg)

Although these combinations are convenient and used by many dentists, some flexibility is lost when prescribing any combination, as compared to prescription of the drugs separately. For example, prescribing codeine and aspirin separately would allow the patient to add codeine only when absolutely necessary. Pure codeine should be avoided, however, in patients suspected of, or known to be involved with, abuse of narcotic-analgesics or other types of drugs.

Use of pure codeine requires Schedule II guidelines, whereas the combinations are Schedule III. This has led many dentists to prefer use of the combinations in spite of the more rational approach of separate prescriptions.

K. DRUG INTERACTIONS

Objective 23.K.1. Describe six drug interactions of aspirin, acetaminophen, and NSAIA.

The interactions of these drugs fall into six categories.

Interactions with Anticoagulants

Because these drugs (except acetaminophen) prolong clotting time, they can potentiate the action of oral anticoagulants (coumarin). In addition, they can also adversely prolong bleeding time in patients with bleeding tendencies, such as thrombocytopenia and liver disease.

Interactions at Serum Albumin

These agents have a high affinity for serum albumin and may, therefore, displace other protein-bound drugs from this reservoir, resulting in increased blood levels and toxicity of the latter. Such drugs include oral anticoagulants, oral hypoglycemic agents, and phenytoin.

Interactions with Aspirin

NSAIA can increase the incidence and severity of gastrointestinal irritation and other side effects of aspirin, presumably because of an additive effect. In addition to this, aspirin taken concurrently with NSAIA can actually lower blood levels of NSAIA through a mechanism that is, as yet, unestablished.

At present, there is no rationale for simultaneously administering aspirin and NSAIA. Although adverse reactions do not necessarily occur from the combined use of these drugs, there is no therapeutic advantage to the practice.

Food

Food does not appear to appreciably alter the effectiveness of most of the aspirin alternatives, except in the case of fenoprofen (another propionic acid derivative), whose absorption is significantly impaired by food. Fenoprofen should be given with food only if it causes intolerable gastrointestinal irritation. Neither food nor gastric antacids alter the bioavailability of the other aspirin alternatives.

Alcohol

The ulcerogenic effect of aspirin and other NSAIAs is increased by alcohol. Similarly, the hepatotoxicity of acetaminophen may be enhanced by alcohol.

Steroids

The ulcerogenic effect of aspirin and the NSAIAs is increased by the concurrent administration of steroid hormones.

REFERENCES

Cooper SA, Beaver WT: A model to evaluate mild analgesics in oral surgery outpatients. Clin Pharmacol Ther 20:241, 1976

Med Lett Drug Ther 23:2, 1981

Weissman G: Prostaglandins and Inflammation. Kalamazoo, MI, Upjohn, 1981

Csáky TZ: Cutting's Handbook of Pharmacology, 6th ed. New York, Appleton-Century-Crofts, 1979, p 540

BIBLIOGRAPHY

Beaver WT, Lasagna L (eds): Zomepirac: A New Narcotic Analgesic (Proceedings of the Symposium). J Clin Pharmacol 20:213, 1980

Gilman AG, Goodman LS, Gilman A (eds): Goodman and Gilman's The Pharmacological Basis of Therapeutics, 6th ed. New York, Macmillan, 1980, Ch 22, 29

QUESTIONS

1. **T F** Analgesia may be obtained by raising the pain threshold as well as by alteration of pain interpretation.

2. Which one of the following agents is properly classified as an antipyretic-analgesic?

   A. Codeine

   B. Aspirin

   C. Morphine

   D. None of the above

3. Chemically, aspirin is considered to be: (Select one.)

   A. An ester of benzoic acid

   B. An aniline derivative

   C. A pyrazolone

   D. A fenamic acid derivative

4. **T F** Aspirin has no therapeutic actions other than reduction of pain and inflammation.

5. Aspirin may exacerbate blood loss by which of the following mechanisms? (Select one.)

   A. Irritation of the gastrointestinal mucosa

   B. Inhibition of vitamin K absorption

   C. Inhibition of platelet aggregation

   D. All of the above

   E. A and C above

6. Which one of the following measures is used in the treatment of aspirin toxicity?

   A. Administration of naloxone

   B. Induction of acid diuresis

   C. Administration of a central stimulant

   D. Induction of alkaline diuresis

7. **T F** The adult lethal dose of aspirin is 20 tablets (100 grains).

8. **T F** Buffered aspirin preparations provide a therapeutic advantage in delaying the renal excretion of the drug.

9. Which one of the following side effects of aspirin is also characteristic of acetaminophen?

   A. Gastrointestinal bleeding
   B. Prolongation of clotting time
   C. Both of the above
   D. Neither of the above

10. The acute toxicity of acetaminophen usually results in which one of the following?

    A. Convulsions
    B. Cardiac arrest
    C. Hepatic necrosis
    D. None of the above

11. **T F** Acetaminophen is metabolized to phenacetin, accounting for its high incidence of renal toxicity.

12. Salicylate metabolism is accomplished primarily by which one of the following mechanisms?

    A. Conjugation
    B. Hydrolysis
    C. Acylation
    D. None of the above

13. **T F** Naproxen is a derivative of propionic acid.

14. **T F** NSAIA inhibit inflammation by stabilization of lysosomes.

15. **T F** Unlike aspirin, ibuprofen and other propionic acid derivatives do not increase bleeding time.

16. **T F** Compared to aspirin, mefenamic acid has fewer side effects.

17. Pyrazolones are primarily reserved for use in which one of the following conditions?

    A. Rheumatoid arthritis
    B. Mild pain of dental origin
    C. Moderate pain of dental origin
    D. None of the above

18. Which one of the following drugs is chemically classified as an indene?

    A. zomepirac
    B. mefenamic acid
    C. phenylbutazone
    D. indomethacin

19. **T F** Barbiturates are marketed in combination with analgesics.

20. **T F** The reduction of aspirin content in analgesic combinations containing phenacetin allows their use in aspirin-allergic individuals.

21. Which one of the following agents may increase the ulcerogenic effect of aspirin?

    A. Alcohol
    B. Steroids
    C. Both of the above
    D. Neither of the above

24
Narcotic-Analgesics

Opium, an extract of the poppy plant, is one of the oldest remedies. Its beneficial effects in control of pain were noted thousands of years ago. Its dependence potential and respiratory depressant effect were also noted, but society was willing to take these risks in order to overcome pain. After morphine was isolated from opium extracts (about 1800) there was a tremendous interest, which still persists today, in chemical modification for production of new derivatives having pain control potential and fewer side effects. Interestingly, almost every new derivative introduced (heroin and meperidine included) was claimed to be without dependence potential. Although some advances have been made, the dependence potential and respiratory depression seem to remain with drugs related to morphine and other narcotic analgesics.

In this chapter, we will study morphine and some related drugs, most of which have dependence potential. Morphine will be considered the prototype and studied thoroughly, while the differences from morphine will be emphasized for other drugs in the group.

A. CLASSIFICATION OF NARCOTIC-ANALGESICS

Objective 24.A.1. Recognize the classification of narcotic-analgesics: opium, opium alkaloids, opiates, and opioids.

It is important to remember names of compounds set in bold type.

Opium

1. dried juice of the poppy (*Papaver somniferum*)
2. crude extracts
3. **paregoric** (camphorated tincture of opium)—used for control of diarrhea

Natural Opium Alkaloids (Purified from Opium)

1. **morphine** (9% of crude extract)
2. **codeine** (0.5% of crude extract)
3. papaverine (a smooth muscle relaxant which is nonaddictive and not a pain control agent)
4. others

Opiates *Semisynthetic*

These are semisynthetic compounds made from morphine or codeine.

1. **heroin**—acetylated morphine
2. **hydromorphone** (*Dilaudid*)—made by oxidation
3. **oxymorphone**—oxidized morphine (further oxidation than hydromorphone)
4. **codeine**—methylated morphine
5. **hydrocodone** (*Dicodid, Hycodan*)
6. **oxycodone** (*Percodan*)—oxidized codeine
7. **dextromethorphan**—codeine related, sold OTC as a cough suppressant
8. **apomorphine**—used as an emetic

Opioids *synthetic*

Opioids are synthetic chemicals with a different structure from the morphine series but with similar pharmacologic actions.

1. Meperidine and its derivatives
   a. **meperidine** (*Demerol*)
   b. alphaprodine (*Nisentil*)
   c. anileridine (*Leritine*)
   d. **fentanyl** (*Sublimaze*)
   e. ethoheptazine (*Zactane*)
2. Methadone and its derivatives
   a. **methadone** (*Dolophine, Adanon*)
   b. **propoxyphene** (*Darvon*)
3. Others

Narcotic-Antagonists

1. **nalorphine** (*Nalline*)—chemically, N-allyl normorphine
2. **naloxone** (*Narcan*)
3. **pentazocine** (*Talwin*)
4. **butorphanol** (*Stadol*)
5. **nalbuphine** (*Nubain*)

B. ACTIONS OF MORPHINE

Therapeutic Effects

Objective 24.B.1. Recognize the therapeutic actions of morphine.

Analgesic. Morphine is a potent analgesic which modifies both the perception (sensory) component and reaction component of pain. Morphine's actions are central and are not well understood, but there is a definite increase in the pain threshold, as well as changes of mood, emotional status, and sedation.

CNS behavioral changes. The patient sometimes experiences dysphoria (especially during first-time use in a pain-free subject), but usually there is euphoria associated with pain relief. Calming and sedation are usually evident. The doctor may use euphoria and sedation as favorable adjunctive properties in his pain control regimen.

Cough suppression (antitussive). Morphine causes a direct suppression of the cough center in the medulla, although it is not usually used for this purpose because codeine has a better therapeutic index (comparing the dose that causes respiratory depression to the dose that causes cough suppression).

Vomiting. A good number of patients vomit when first taking morphine, due to a direct stimulation of the chemoreceptor trigger zone (CTZ) in the medulla. Morphine stimulation may also sensitize the vestibular component of vomiting. A specific CTZ stimulant, apomorphine, has been developed for induction of vomiting.

Side Effects

Objective 24.B.2. Recognize the side effects of morphine. (Depending upon the condition being treated, a side effect may become a therapeutic effect.)

Consideration of morphine's side effects should include the following:

Nausea and vomiting. (see above)

Constipation. Morphine increases GI tone but decreases GI tract motility, with a resultant spastic paralysis, causing constipation. (Paregoric is the preferred agent for causing spastic paralysis in controlling diarrhea.) Diphenoxylate, a meperidine analog, is also used to reduce GI motility (Chapter 33).

Orthostatic hypotension. This is due to a depressed vasomotor center. Morphine also releases histamine, which causes vasodilation, tending to lower blood pressure.

Respiratory depression. The respiratory center of the medulla is depressed and less responsive to increased plasma CO_2. Respiratory depression is the major cause of death due to morphine overdose, and some embarrassment of respiration may be noted when analgesic doses are being used.

Miosis. The pupillary constrictive effect of morphine results in pinpoint pupils, which remain constricted in the dark. Tolerance to this effect does not develop, which may help in diagnosing narcotic dependence.

Other CNS effects. Most nondependent patients taking morphine in a hospital setting will have mental clouding followed by drowsiness due to sedation. There is also suppression of REM sleep. Hypothalamic activity of morphine results in hypothermia, activation of sympathetic centers, and endocrine effects (release of ADH, decreased release of ACTH, LH, FSH, and TSH). Convulsions can occur at high doses.

Smooth muscle activity. This is generally increased, resulting in biliary tract spasms, increased bladder tone (urinary urgency), increased bladder sphincter tone (urinary difficulty), some bronchoconstriction, and decreased gastrointestinal motility due to spastic paralysis. The uterus is not affected.

Dependence potential.

Objective 24.B.3. Recognize morphine's tolerance and dependence potential.

Morphine causes a rapid development of tolerance. The euphoric effect, which accompanies pain relief or follows repeated use, causes the patient to seek out the drug, which may be reinforced by peer pressure. Due to tolerance, the dose needs to be constantly increased. There is a rapid development of psychic dependence (habit) and withdrawal syndrome (physical illness when the drug is withdrawn); the latter reinforces the need to continue the drug. A further discussion of drug dependence and abuse occurs in Appendix III.

Contraindications

Objective 24.B.4. Recognize contraindications to the use of morphine.

Allergy. As with any drug, allergy to morphine is a contraindication.

Susceptibility to Respiratory Depressants. Morphine should not be used in the following cases, where there would be increased susceptibility to the respiratory depressant action:

1. Fetus—avoid use in pregnancy during the late prenatal period
2. Newborn and elderly—more susceptible
3. Patients with decreased respiratory reserve (e.g., emphysema) or airway obstruction of any etiology

Head Injuries. Increased intracranial pressure may result. This is an important consideration in oral surgery after head injury. Since the injury may also cause increased intracranial pressure, there would be an additive effect, and the cranial injury may be difficult to diagnose.

Myxedema. Patients with myxedema (thyroid deficiency) are more susceptible to the CNS depressant activity of morphine.

Patients in Whom Pain may be Relieved but the Condition Worsened. This includes patients with prostatic hypertrophy, urinary problems, and biliary colic in whom these conditions are aggravated due to sphincter spasticity.

Drug Interactions

Objective 24.B.5. Recognize drug interactions of morphine.

Morphine interacts with other CNS depressants, resulting in exaggerated and prolonged activity. This includes all **CNS depressants, phenothiazines, MAO inhibitors,** and **tricyclic antidepressants.** Administration of a **narcotic-antagonist,** such as naloxone or pentazocine, can precipitate a withdrawal syndrome in patients dependent on narcotics.

Metabolism

Objective 24.B.6. Recognize absorption, distribution, metabolism, and excretion of morphine.

Morphine is rapidly metabolized in its first-pass effect through the liver and is, therefore, given parenterally. Even after parenteral injection, only small quantities of morphine are found in the CNS, but much drug is found in the liver, kidney, lung, and other organs. The major pathway of metabolism is by conjugation. Excretion of metabolites occurs by the kidneys.

C. DRUG DEVELOPMENT

Objective 24.C.1. Describe the goal of drug development in narcotic-analgesics and how some drugs have met these and other goals.

Many attempts have been made to modify morphine and to synthesize related drugs. The basic idea is to obtain drugs that have a better therapeutic ratio (toxic dose/therapeutic dose). Attempts to increase the potency of morphine have not been fruitful, since any increased potency generally results in increased respiratory depression and dependence potential (heroin is an example). Similarly, attempts to reduce toxicity have usually led to reduced potency. The structural formula for morphine and its relation to codeine are shown in Figure 24–1. Variations in the morphine structure or production of opioids result in the following compounds.

Codeine. Codeine is methylated morphine (Fig. 24–1). It was a significant breakthrough because it has a better therapeutic index for cough suppression and because it has less dependence potential. However, it can be used for only moderate pain because codeine cannot achieve the full analgesic effect of morphine. One advantage of codeine is its higher oral parenteral efficacy ratio compared to morphine. This is related to a lower rate of metabolism of codeine compared to morphine, during the first pass through the liver after oral absorption.

Meperidine. Meperidine (Fig. 24–1) is an opioid which is not chemically related to morphine, although the drug may fit the morphine receptor. It was developed in a search for a better spasmolytic, and its powerful pain control action was discovered by accident. Meperidine was at first regarded as a major breakthrough and was highly advertised as nonaddictive. However, its dependence potential rapidly became evident, and it must, therefore, be used cautiously. Many health practitioners themselves became addicted to meperidine because they were lulled by the popular opinion that this "easy fix" would be nonaddictive. Most pharmacologists now realize that meperidine was greatly overrated and that it has only limited usefulness, with no particular advantage, in most cases, over morphine.

Methadone. Methadone (Fig. 24–1) is also an opioid; its relation to morphine is shown by rearrangement of the molecule. Methadone has become the favorite of the narcotic substitution programs because of its long duration of action and mildness of withdrawal symptoms. Recently, methadone (*Dolophine*) was approved by the FDA for use in severe pain.

Nonnarcotic analgesics. Further chemical synthesis of opioids produced many analogs of meperidine and methadone in a program to develop nonnarcotic analgesics. As a result, ethoheptazine (*Zactane*) and propoxyphene (*Darvon*) were introduced. Although ethoheptazine was not well accepted, propoxyphene was marketed intensely as a codeine substitute for

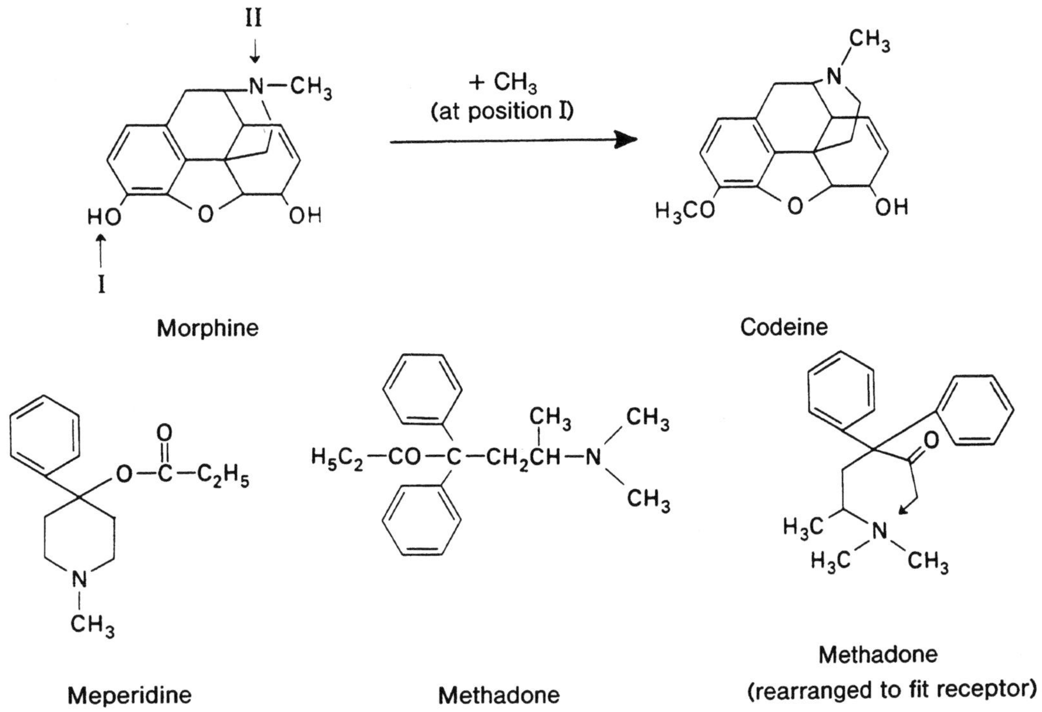

Figure 24–1. Chemical structure of morphine and related drugs. (*From Csáky TZ: Cutting's Handbook of Pharmacology, 6th ed, 1979. Courtesy of Appleton-Century-Crofts.*) Position I and II are major sites of chemical synthesis.

moderate pain. Recent experiments indicate that propoxyphene is equal to a placebo, but with significant side effects. Its analgesic action is probably related to placebo effects and its combination with aspirin or acetaminophen. Nevertheless, many patients and physicians consider propoxyphene an alternative to codeine. Although *Darvon* was not a scheduled narcotic for many years, recent cases of abuse of the drug, with dependence development, led the DEA to classify *Darvon* in Schedule IV. In addition, a lethal interaction of *Darvon* with alcohol abuse has been reported.

Narcotic antagonists. An interesting development in morphine analog development was the discovery that introduction of an allyl group on the N-atom (position II in Fig. 24–1) resulted in the narcotic antagonist, N-allyl normorphine, later officially named nalorphine (*Nalline*). This antagonist was found to induce morphine with-

drawal in animals and to reverse morphine's respiratory depressant activity. Nalorphine was used in detection of dependence by induction of withdrawal in addicts and for reversal of respiratory depression, in cases of morphine poisoning.

Several developments arose from studies of narcotic antagonists:

1. Further study of morphine's SAR, especially the conversion of agonist to antagonist by the N-allyl substitution, led to the concept that a specific morphine receptor exists. The N-allyl substituted compound is thought to displace morphine and other narcotics from this receptor, which then induces withdrawal or relieves toxic symptoms (as though the narcotic-analgesic were not present).

   Further study of morphine receptors led to the recent discovery of enkephalins and endorphins, molecules which are naturally occurring polypeptides having pain-relieving activity. Enkephalins are pentapeptides having leucine (leu-enkephalin) or methionine (met-enkephalin) in the terminal portion.

Endorphins are larger proteins that contain pentapeptide sequences similar to enkephalin sequences. Endorphins may be storage forms, acting as substrates for release of enkephalins after activation of proteolytic enzymes. An example of an endorphin is β-endorphin, a large polypeptide which contains a met-enkephalin sequence. Enkephalins are thought to react with the same receptor as morphine, since they are competitively antagonized by naloxone. Present theory considers that some mechanisms of pain reduction (e.g., central inhibition, acupuncture, yoga, peripheral nerve stimulation) may be due to enkephalin release at the appropriate synapses. Pharmacologists and neurophysiologists are now very interested in enkephalins and their role in controlling CNS functions, especially pain.

2. Since nalorphine was long-acting and also had mixed agonist and antagonistic effects, the pure antagonist naloxone (*Narcan*) was developed. It has the advantage of being a pure antagonist, with no agonist action, but it has a short duration of action. *Narcan* is now the drug of choice for treatment of toxicity of morphine (or narcotic-analgesics). As with all drugs, adequate CPR must be used in cases of severe respiratory depression in addition to drug treatment with *Narcan*.

3. Quite accidentally, it was discovered that nalorphine also had analgesic activity. This was noted in a study which combined nalorphine and morphine, attempting to counteract development of dependence. It was found that patients taking both drugs, or nalorphine alone, had a tendency to develop many side effects, but both groups showed significantly better analgesia than did controls. This experiment led to a flurry of activity in development of narcotic-antagonist derivatives having analgesic activity but lacking nalorphine's side effects. The N-allyl substitution of many morphine derivatives led to pentazocine (*Talwin*), which is a fairly potent analgesic. Pentazocine has less dependence potential than morphine and fewer side effects

than nalorphine. However, pentazocine's lack of dependence potential was grossly overrated, as there have been cases of dependence reported. Because of this dependence potential, pentazocine was recently placed into DEA Schedule IV. As with all new drugs, side effects eventually become evident; pentazocine has been reported to cause hallucinatory effects, as well as respiratory depression, especially when used by IV injection.

Recently, some new narcotic antagonist analgesics have entered the market. Again, the drug houses were trying to find competitive drugs that are better than pentazocine, morphine, codeine, and so on. Butorphanol (*Stadol*) and nalbuphine (*Nubain*) are probably the most hopeful of this group, but so far their use in postoperative pain control in dentistry has not been defined, and only parenteral forms are available.

D. OTHER NARCOTIC-ANALGESICS

Objective 24.D.1. Compare differences of opiate and opioids, narcotic-analgesics to morphine, and recognize the importance of these differences in pharmacotherapeutics.

Heroin
This is more potent than morphine and has higher drug abuse potential. It is not used medically in the United States, and is classified in DEA Schedule I.

Morphine Derivatives
Hydromorphone and oxymorphone are two examples of potent drugs which have toxicity and drug abuse potential equal to those of morphine. Like morphine, they are classified in DEA Schedule II. They have no particular advantage over morphine. These drugs are equally well substituted by morphine addicts; thus, they have high abuse potential.

Codeine
This is a useful narcotic-analgesic for moderate pain. It does not have the full agonist activity of morphine and, thus, cannot be used for severe pain. Codeine is equally effective by the oral or

parenteral route because its metabolism in the liver is slower than that of morphine, resulting in a minimal first-pass effect. Codeine has less tendency to produce drowsiness, euphoria, and dependence. Although codeine will satisfy a narcotic-dependent subject, it is not a preferred drug for this purpose. The following actions of morphine are found in codeine therapy but to a lesser degree:

1. respiratory depression (slight at clinical doses)
2. pupillary constriction
3. orthostatic hypotension

The following effects of morphine are quite evident with codeine:

1. constipation
2. antitussive (codeine has a better therapeutic ratio)
3. nausea and vomiting
4. allergic potential
5. tolerance

Codeine is often combined with aspirin or acetaminophen, and the combinations are frequently used by dentists for moderate dental pain (see Chapter 23 for available combinations with ASA and APAP).

Codeine, in combination, is a Schedule III compound, but when codeine is prescribed separately, it is in Schedule II. Some codeine products for cough suppression are in Schedule IV.

Codeine Analogs

The drug **oxycodone** (*Percodan*) has a greater potency and effectiveness than morphine. Along with the increased potency goes an increase in toxicity, so that its therapeutic index is the same as is morphine's but lower than codeine's. In recognition of oxycodone's high dependence potential, it is classified in DEA Schedule II, even in the combinations available (Chapter 6). Therefore, oxycodone offers no advantage over morphine. Dihydrocodone (*Hycodan*) remains about the same in potency and toxicity as codeine and is classified as Schedule III.

Meperidine (*Demerol*)

This synthetic opioid has similar CNS effects and mechanism to morphine. It was thought to be spasmolytic, but it can cause morphinelike changes in smooth muscle (e.g., biliary spasms). Nevertheless, meperidine has little or no constipating effect.

Actions similar to morphine include:

1. analgesia (full agonist)
2. not well absorbed orally
3. respiratory depression
4. sedation, euphoria, high dependence potential
5. most other side effects (except constipation)

Actions different than morphine include:

1. less miosis with mydriasis at higher doses
2. not antitussive
3. causes dry mouth (atropinic)
4. less cardiovascular effect
5. not constipating

Meperidine is in DEA Schedule II. Many dentists like to use meperidine when codeine and aspirin will not suffice. This may be used cautiously for moderate-to-severe pain. Parenteral injection is more effective for severe pain because of first-pass liver metabolism after oral use. However, nausea and vomiting occur more frequently (as with morphine) after injection, so that patients taking strong narcotic-analgesics should be confined to rest. Thus, it appears that meperidine has no particular advantage over morphine (Chapter 6).

Methadone

Like morphine, methadone produces strong analgesia and has all of morphine's side effects. Unlike morphine, methadone is active orally and its withdrawal symptoms develop more slowly in morphine addicts. Methadone also has a longer duration of action when compared with meperidine.

The basis for methadone substitution in addicts is that no injection is required and the withdrawal is mild compared to morphine. Recently, the DEA approved methadone as a Schedule II drug for pain (previously it was reserved for the withdrawal program). Thus, methadone may be cautiously used by the oral route for severe pain, and the authors believe that it is the drug of choice for oral use in patients with severe dental pain.

Propoxyphene (*Darvon*)

This derivative of methadone was widely hailed as a nonaddictive narcotic with analgesic potency equivalent to codeine. It is sold mainly in combination with aspirin and more recently with acetaminophen. Recent clinical trials indicate that it is equal to placebo in relieving pain when used alone. When in combination with aspirin, propoxyphene is equal in potency to aspirin alone. It produces significant side effects, such as nausea, vomiting, gastrointestinal irritation, headache, and rash. Recently, the DEA recognized its abuse potential and classified it in Schedule IV.

Meperidine Derivatives

Alphaprodine (*Nisentil*) and anileridine (*Leritine*) are similar to meperidine. Both are in Schedule II, recognizing the care that must be used in prescribing these drugs. Alphaprodine is slightly shorter in duration than meperidine, and anileridine is twice as potent as meperidine. Fentanyl (*Sublimaze*) is a short-acting meperidine derivative being used by some dentists as an IV analgesic when combined with sedatives. A recent study (Dionne, 1981) indicates that fentanyl, in IV sedation, added no significant beneficial properties but caused more side effects than diazepam alone. *Innovar* is a combination of fentanyl and droperidol, a neuroleptic drug related to antipsychotic drugs. The combination can cause many side effects and appears to be irrational; fentanyl is short-acting and droperidol is long-acting (Med Lett Drugs Ther, 1974). This emphasizes the difficulty of mixing drugs and administering a fixed combination. One may wish more analgesia, but an increased dose of the combination provides effects of both drugs. As a result, dangerous side effects can be produced. As with all IV drug use, the average dentist is not well advised to use more than one drug to achieve his effect. Before getting into more complex therapy, additional training and care are required (Chapter 35).

Ethoheptazine (*Zactane* or *Zactirin*)

Ethoheptazine is supposedly nonaddicting, but its analgesic properties do not appear to be very prominent. It seems to be very similar to *Dar-*von, but the latter is much more widely promoted.

Narcotic Antagonist Analgesics

Pentazocine (*Talwin*) is a weak narcotic antagonist showing about the same potency as codeine when given orally. When given parenterally, it is probably more potent than codeine but less potent than morphine. It has recently been added to Schedule IV by the DEA, recognizing its possible (albeit low) abuse potential. Pentazocine must be avoided in narcotic drug abusers because it can precipitate withdrawal. Like all drugs in the group, pentazocine causes side effects, such as dizziness, distortion of visual perception, and hallucinations.

Butorphanol and nalbuphine are newer narcotic antagonist analgesics similar in many respects to pentazocine. Though they are presently approved for parenteral use only, an oral preparation may be available soon. It is too early to tell how useful these compounds will become in clinical practice. All of the narcotic antagonist analgesics may precipitate withdrawal when given to a subject who is dependent on narcotics.

REFERENCES

Dionne R: Personal communication, 1981
Med Lett Drugs Ther 16:42, 1974
Med Lett Drugs Ther 19:27, 1977
Med Lett Drugs Ther 23:74, 1981

BIBLIOGRAPHY

Csáky TZ: Cutting's Handbook of Pharmacology, 6th ed. New York, Appleton-Century-Crofts, 1979, Ch 50
Gilman AG, Goodman LS, Gilman A (eds): In Goodman and Gilman's The Pharmacological Basis of Therapeutics, 6th ed. New York, Macmillan 1980, Ch 22
Goldstein A, Aronow L, Kalman S: Principles of Drug Action, 2nd ed. New York, Wiley, 1974, Ch 1
Zimmerman E: The opiate receptor, neuropeptides, and pain. In Nelson TE, Bourgault PC (eds): Current Concepts of Analgesic Action. The Fourth

Symposium of the Pharmacology, Toxicology and Therapeutics Group, International Association for Dental Research, Las Vegas, 1978, Vol 4

QUESTIONS

1. All are examples of natural opium alkaloids *except:*

   A. morphine
   B. heroin
   C. codeine
   D. papaverine

2. All of the following are opiates *except:*

   A. heroin
   B. hydromorphone
   C. oxycodone
   D. dextromethorphan
   E. propoxyphene

3. Paregoric is used for the control of:

   A. vomiting
   B. cough suppression
   C. diarrhea
   D. none of the above

4. Meperidine, alphaprodine, and fentanyl are all examples of:

   A. narcotic antagonists
   B. opioids
   C. opiates
   D. none of the above

5. **T F** Methadone and propoxyphene are related drugs and are opiates.

6. **T F** Morphine effectively blocks the reactive component of pain, as well as having an anti-inflammatory effect.

7. **T F** One of the expected behavioral effects of morphine is dysphoria in a pain-free individual taking morphine for the first time.

8. **T F** Stimulation of the chemoreceptor trigger zone by morphine results in nausea and vomiting.

9. **T F** Morphine acts as an analgesic because of its sedative effect.

10-13. The CNS effects of morphine include:

   10. **T F** Increased biliary tract pressure

   11. **T F** Orthostatic hypotension

   12. **T F** Depression of respiration

   13. **T F** Diminished or abolished peristalsis

14. Morphine's postural (orthostatic) hypotensive effect is due to:

   A. Depression of the vasomotor center
   B. Spastic paralysis of smooth muscle
   C. Both A and B are correct
   D. Neither A nor B is correct

15. Morphine's constipating effect is due to:

   A. Diminished or abolished peristalsis
   B. Increased sphincter tone
   C. Both A and B are correct
   D. Neither A nor B is correct

16. **T F** Morphine has a marked depressant effect on the respiratory center's response to CO_2.

17. **T F** Morphine is an effective anticonvulsant because it produces sedation.

18. The following are characteristic of morphine's tolerance and dependence potential:

   A. Psychic dependence
   B. Prominent euphoria

C. Both A and B are correct
D. Neither A nor B is correct

19. **T F** It is dangerous to use narcotic analgesics in a patient with a head injury.

20. **T F** Patients who have a history of hypothyroidism are generally more susceptible to the effects of morphine.

21. **T F** Use of morphine in a patient with prostatic hypertrophy would be contraindicated.

22. Morphine's sedative effect will be exaggerated if the patient also ingests any of the following *except:*

A. Phenothiazines
B. MAO inhibitors
C. tricyclic antidepressants
D. aspirin

23. **T F** Administration of a narcotic antagonist, such as naloxone or pentazocine, can cause withdrawal syndrome in patients with narcotic dependence.

24. **T F** The major pathway of metabolism of morphine is by conjugation.

25. **T F** Excretion of metabolites of morphine occurs mainly via the biliary system.

26. **T F** Pentazocine is not a drug which causes dependence.

27. **T F** Meperidine rarely produces tolerance, psychic dependence, or physical dependence.

28. **T F** Patients receiving chronic high dosages of methadone should receive pentazocine as an analgesic.

29. **T F** Nalorphine is capable of antagonizing (reversing) all of the effects of narcotic analgesics.

30. **T F** All of the following are true about enkephalins *except:*

A. they are polypeptides which have morphinelike activity
B. they may be derived from endorphins
C. they are derived from opium
D. they react with the opiate receptor

31. Codeine produces:

A. dependence to a lesser extent than oxycodone
B. minimal respiratory depression at normal therapeutic doses
C. both A and B are correct
D. neither A nor B is correct

32. **T F** The respiratory depressant effect of meperidine limits the amount of drug that should be administered.

33. **T F** Meperidine is useful for the treatment of diarrhea.

34. **T F** Meperidine is an excellent agent for the blockade of the cough reflex.

35. **T F** Patients who take an overdose of meperidine will usually have mydriasis due to the drug's anticholinergic effects.

36. **T F** The hallucinogenic effects of pentazocine are more exaggerated compared to morphine.

37–42. When codeine is administered at therapeutic doses, it produces:

37. **T F** significant antitussive effects

38. **T F** less dependence potential than morphine

39. **T F** marked drowsiness

40. **T F** minimal euphoria

41. **T F** pupillary constriction

42. **T F** effects on the cardiovascular system equal to morphine

43. Codeine alone, in full therapeutic dose, produces:

    A. more analgesia in combination with aspirin than does aspirin alone
    B. less analgesia than oxycodone
    C. both A and B are correct
    D. neither A nor B is correct

44. Codeine has:

    A. low enough abuse potential so that analgesic tablets are in Schedule IV
    B. minimal respiratory depression at normal therapeutic doses
    C. both A and B are correct
    D. neither A nor B is correct

45. Given a one-half grain codeine/aspirin combination tablet, approximately how many mg of codeine will the patient receive?

    A. 15 to 16 mg
    B. 30 to 32 mg
    C. 60 to 65 mg
    D. 300 to 325 mg

25

Principles in Use of Antimicrobials

A. HISTORY

The first successful attempt at treating an infection with a chemical that could be administered systemically can be attributed to Paul Ehrlich. While searching for a cure for syphilis, Ehrlich ultimately discovered that arsphenamine or salvarsan, the 606th organic arsenical compound he tested, inhibited *Treponema pallidum.* Ehrlich's work took place in the early 1900s, inaugurating chemotherapy of infection.

The modern era of chemotherapy of infection began in the 1930s, with the discovery of sulfa drugs, and continued into the early 1940s, with the introduction of penicillin. Some further details on the history of these agents appears in each appropriate chapter.

Considering the very long history of man, this important breakthrough in treatment of infection is really quite recent. The tremendous impact of the introduction of chemotherapy for infection is often overlooked. Prior to the late 1930s and early 1940s, many persons died of infection. The only agents available prior to that period were antiseptics—agents that are quite effective for topical (external) use but very toxic when used systemically.

B. DEFINITIONS

Objective 25.B.1. Recognize the definition of the following terms: antibiotic, antimicrobial, spectrum, gram-positive spectrum, gram-negative spectrum, broad spectrum, bactericidal, bacteriostatic, true selectivity, relative selectivity, sensitivity, natural resistance, acquired resistance, and cross-resistance.

Objective 25.B.2. Recognize five general mechanisms of acquired resistance.

Objective 25.B.3. Recognize four specific mechanisms of acquired resistance.

Antibiotic: a chemical substance, produced by or derived from living organisms, which in very dilute concentrations, inhibits or prevents the growth, reproduction, metabolism, or pathogenicity of other organisms. Antibiotics form the cornerstone of modern chemotherapy for infection. However, chemicals not formed by microbes are also important. **Antimicrobial** is a broader term, indicating any agent used to combat microbial infection, including antibiotics and synthetic chemicals (Table 25–1).

Spectrum: the types or actual list of microor-

239

TABLE 25–1. IMPORTANT FEATURES OF SOME ANTIMICROBIAL AGENTS

Agent	Mechanism of Action	Activity	Spectrum
aminoglycosides	inhibit protein synthesis	bacteriostatic	broad
amphotericin B	disrupt cell membranes	fungistatic	narrow (fungi)
bacitracin	inhibit cell wall synthesis	bactericidal	primarily gram positive
cephalosporins	inhibit cell wall synthesis	bactericidal	primarily gram positive[a]
chloramphenicol	inhibit protein synthesis	bacteriostatic	broad
erythromycin	inhibit protein synthesis	bacteriostatic	primarily gram positive
lincomycins	inhibit protein synthesis	bacteriostatic	primarily gram positive
nystatin	disrupt cell membranes	fungistatic	narrow (fungi)
penicillins	inhibit cell wall synthesis	bactericidal	primarily gram positive[b]
polymyxin B	disrupt cell membranes	bactericidal	primarily gram negative
sulfonamides	inhibit intermediary metabolism	bacteriostatic	broad
trimethoprim	inhibit intermediary metabolism	bacteriostatic	broad
vancomycin	inhibit cell wall synthesis	bactericidal	primarily gram positive

[a] Spectrum is approximately equal to the extended spectrum penicillins, such as ampicillin. Some newer cephalosporins are considered to have a modified spectrum of activity (e.g., cefamandole and cefoxitin).

[b] Penicillinase-resistant agents are thought to have a very narrow spectrum, e.g., staphylococci producing penicillinase. Other penicillins have an extended spectrum, e.g., ampicillin.

ganisms against which an antimicrobial is effective.

Gram-positive spectrum: effective primarily, but not exclusively, against many, but not all, gram-positive staining organisms.

Gram-negative spectrum: effective primarily, but not exclusively, against many, but not all, gram-negative organisms.

Broad spectrum: equally effective against certain gram-positive and gram-negative microorganisms. (NOTE: "broad" is not necessarily "good," since the organism may be outside of the spectrum or, in some cases, may require a higher than normal concentration.)

Bacteriostatic: an agent that, at optimal concentration, usually **inhibits** the growth, reproduction, or pathogenic capacity of the organism against which it is effective.

Bactericidal: an agent that, at optimal concentration, usually **kills** the organism against which it is effective.

True selectivity: affecting a biochemical mechanism of the invading organism and not of the host. An example is penicillin.

Relative selectivity: affecting a biochemical mechanism which is relatively common in both host and invader. The slight differences between the biochemical mechanisms of host and invader help to confer some degree of selectivity against the invader. Selectivity occurs secondarily because of rapid proliferation of invader cells in comparison to host cells. An example is tetracycline.

Sensitivity: generally refers to microorganism sensitivity. Sensitivity means susceptibility to a specific antimicrobial. The degree of sensitivity is concentration related.

Natural resistance: a type of microorganism that is not and never has been in the spectrum of activity of an antimicrobial drug.

Acquired resistance: the microorganism has acquired a mechanism to bypass or destroy the antimicrobial agent. The basis of the mechanism is generally genetic, and can include mutation, transduction, transformation, translocation, or conjugation. Actual mechanisms are usually (1) elaboration of drug-metabolizing enzymes, such as penicillinase or cephalosporinase (more recently acetylation, adenylation, and phosphorylation enzymes have also been described), (2) blockade of drug entry, resulting in alteration of the bacterial cell's permeability, (3) activation of a bacterial cell's natural (endogenous) antagonistic substance, and (4) alteration of drug receptor characteristics or receptor number on the bacterial cell membrane. The development of resistance to antimicrobials is one of many possible reasons for treatment failure.

Cross-resistance: in the presence of bacterial resistance to a drug (by whatever means), the microbe is often resistant to drugs that are chemically similar. In general, the more similar the chemical agents, the greater the chance for cross-resistance. An example of this phenomenon is cross-resistance to different tetracyclines. However, there are exceptions to this rule, e.g., a microorganism may become resistant to erythromycin and also show resistance to lincomycins, although these agents are dissimilar chemically.

C. MECHANISMS OF ACTION

Objective 25.C.1. Describe five possible mechanisms of action of antimicrobial agents. Be able to cite at least one example of each type of mechanism including subdivisions, such as agents binding to 30S and 50S subunits.

Inhibition of Cell Wall Synthesis

Most bacterial cells possess a cell wall, external to the cell membrane. When present, the cell wall confers rigidity and shape to the bacterium. In addition, it protects the bacterial cell from the environment, since the cells maintain a high internal osmotic pressure.

The backbone of the cell wall is a peptidoglycan chain that completely encircles the bacterial cells, is cross-linked between chains, and is linked between layers of peptidoglycan. Gram-positive bacteria possess more peptidoglycan than do gram-negative bacteria. In addition, gram-negative bacteria generally have lipopolysaccharide layers external to the peptidoglycan coat (Strominger, 1973). Several antibiotics interfere with cell wall synthesis at one or more of the above sites, resulting in incomplete cell wall formation and making the bacterial cell susceptible to osmotic forces.

The penicillins and cephalosporins prevent a cross-linking of a pentapeptide between pepti-

doglycan chains, an action that takes place entirely within the cell wall itself. (There is very good evidence that these agents also inhibit a number of other cell wall synthesizing steps, but these sites will not be discussed here.)

Bacitracin inhibits the regeneration of a cell membrane lipid carrier which carries synthesized peptidoglycan units from the cell cytoplasm to the external surface of the cell membrane, where final stages of cell wall assembly take place. Vancomycin inhibits the actual transfer of the peptidoglycan units from the cell membrane of the external surface.

Cycloserine inhibits the addition of one or both D-alanine residues to a peptidoglycan unit. This occurs in the cytoplasm of the bacterial cells and is the final synthetic step in the cytoplasm. All of these agents exhibit true selectivity and are considered to be bactericidal.

Inhibition of Bacterial Protein Synthesis

The aminoglycosides (e.g., streptomycin), tetracyclines, erythromycins, lincomycins (lincomycin and clindamycin), and chloramphenicol have been shown to inhibit protein synthesis.

Bacterial and mammalian protein syntheses are sufficiently different so that these agents can be safely used in mammals (bacteria have 70S ribosomes, while mammals have 80S ribosomes). However, with high enough doses and especially when used for a long duration, toxic effects are likely to occur due to eventual inhibition of mammalian protein synthesis. A second mechanism of inhibition is that the invader cells are rapidly proliferating while host cells are not (relative selectivity).

A general subclassification can be made according to whether the antimicrobial binds to the bacterial 30S or the 50S ribosomal subunit.

Agents binding to a 30S subunit. The aminoglycosides bind to the 30S subunit, blocking the initiation complex. This causes misreading of mRNA, which leads to synthesis of defective proteins. The aminoglycosides appear to rupture polysomes, producing monosomes. The end result is that these agents are most often bactericidal. (This is somewhat unusual, since most antimicrobials that inhibit protein synthesis generally are bacteriostatic at usual therapeutic doses.)

Tetracyclines bind to the 30S subunit and prevent the attachment of aminoacyl-tRNA.

Agents binding to a 50S subunit. Chloramphenicol binds to the 50S subunit, and it inhibits the enzyme peptidyltransferase. Ultimately, protein synthesis is inhibited due to blockade of transfer of the amino acid from the tRNA on the aminoacyl site to the tRNA on the peptidy site of the ribosome.

Erythromycin binds to the 50S subunit, resulting in inhibition of the initiation complex, and/or it may interfere with aminoacyl translocation.

Lincomycins bind to the 50S subunit, and the mechanism of inhibition of protein synthesis is thought to be the same as for erythromycin. There is clinical evidence that erythromycin and lincomycins are antagonistic. Their mutual competition for a common binding site on the 50S subunit may be the reason for the antagonism.

Disruption of Cell Membranes

Amphotericin B, colistin (also known as polymyxin E), nystatin, and polymyxin B are agents that disrupt or disturb the permeability of microbial cell membranes. Colistin probably does not have a use in dentistry, and, therefore, it will not be discussed further.

Polymyxin B is antibacterial; its action is much like a cationic detergent, causing disruption of the cell membrane and loss of cell contents. The action of polymyxin B is more specific for bacterial cells than for mammalian cells.

Amphotericin B and nystatin are antifungal agents that bind to a sterol in fungal cell membranes. Bacteria lack sterols in their membranes, which provides a reason for these two agents being specific for fungi. Even though mammalian cells possess sterols in their membranes, the effects of amphotericin B and nystatin are more specific for fungal cell membranes, and thus, these two agents are considered to possess relative selectivity.

Interference with Bacterial Intermediary Metabolism

Sulfonamides and trimethoprim are the primary agents acting on intermediary metabolism. Isoniazid, ethambutol, and *p*-aminosalicylic acid probably also act by metabolic interferences, but they will not be discussed, since they have no use in dentistry and are primarily used for the treatment of tuberculosis.

All sulfa drugs compete with *p*-aminobenzoic acid (PABA) for the synthesis of folic acid. Many bacterial cells cannot use preformed folic acid but must synthesize it; one component of folic acid is PABA. Mammalian cells cannot synthesize folic acid but must ingest the preformed substance. Sulfa drugs are, therefore, thought to have true selectivity.

Trimethoprim is also an inhibitor of the folic acid metabolic pathway. The active form of folic acid is tetrahydrofolic acid. Trimethoprim inhibits the enzyme that converts dihydrofolic acid to tetrahydrofolic acid. Mammalian cells also have this enzyme, and the enzymatic step is needed to generate the active fraction. However, it has been estimated that the bacterial enzyme is about 50,000 times more sensitive to the effect of trimethoprim than is the mammalian enzyme. Therefore, there is a wide margin of safety for the use of this agent in humans because relative selectivity occurs.

Inhibition of Nucleic Acid Synthesis

There is limited use of nucleic acid synthesis inhibitors in dentistry. Idoxuridine and vidarabine, two antiviral agents that fit this category, can be used in dentistry, and they are discussed in Chapter 30. Amantadine, although not useful in dentistry, is also discussed in the same chapter. Other drugs include rifampin, griseofulvin, nalidixic acid, and a number of antibiotics used solely as anticancer drugs.

D. ANTIMICROBIAL COMBINATIONS

Objective 25.D.1. Describe four reasons for using antimicrobial combinations.

Objective 25.D.2. Describe three reasons for not using antimicrobial combinations.

Objective 25.D.3. Recognize the three general rules for indicating (or contraindicating) antimicrobial combinations on a rational basis.

Treatment of infections with a combination of antimicrobial drugs is, in general, not recommended. Certain exceptions include:

1. mixed infections requiring more than one drug
2. known synergistic combinations or for specific uses (e.g., sulfa and trimethoprim, penicillin G and streptomycin)
3. delaying the emergence of resistant strains (this has found practical usefulness in the treatment of tuberculosis)
4. severe life-threatening infections in which the specific etiology is unknown

Reasons against the use of combinations include:

1. exposing the patient to adverse effects of each drug
2. increased incidence of supra-infections (supra-infection is an infection caused by the overgrowth of a resistant organism(s) as the result of antibiotic suppression of the susceptible normal flora)
3. possible antimicrobial antagonism

Some **general** rules for the use of antimicrobial combinations (other than known synergistic combinations, such as sulfa and trimethoprim) have been devised (Weinstein, 1975) and are described below:

1. Combining an antimicrobial that inhibits cell wall synthesis with one that inhibits protein synthesis will result in antagonism.
2. Combining two antimicrobials that inhibit cell wall synthesis will not be antagonistic.
3. Combining one antimicrobial that inhibits cell wall synthesis with another antimicrobial that disrupts cell membranes will not be antagonistic.

Another set of general rules is simpler, but less accurate, and includes merely the compatibility of antimicrobials of the same activity (e.g., static–static) and the incompatibility of antimicrobials of opposite activity (e.g., static–cidal).

E. SUPRA-INFECTION

Objective 25.E.1. Recognize three factors that may contribute to the increased incidence of supra-infection.

Objective 25.E.2. Recognize five microorganisms or groups of microorganisms that most often cause suprainfection.

Factors that contribute to increased incidence of supra-infection include:

1. patient under 3 years old
2. presence of acute or chronic pulmonary disease, except tuberculosis
3. the use of broad-spectrum antimicrobials (apparently, the broader the spectrum, the greater the potential for increased incidence)

Microorganisms that most often cause supra-infections include the following:

1. *Candida albicans* and other fungi
2. Staphylococci
3. *Pseudomonas* and *Proteus* strains

F. PROPERTIES OF AN IDEAL ANTIMICROBIAL AGENT

Objective 25.F.1. Recognize 12 properties of an ideal antimicrobial agent.

The ideal antimicrobial agent:

1. has selective activity
2. has a useful spectrum of activity
3. is bactericidal rather than bacteriostatic
4. does not induce bacterial resistance
5. has low side effects of highest useful doses
6. is nonallergenic
7. is active in the presence of body fluids, exudates, proteins, and tissue enzymes
8. is water soluble and stable in solution at room temperature
9. is effective by the oral route
10. reaches an antibacterial blood level rapidly and is of long duration
11. is an active drug in the presence of body fluids (e.g., urine, saliva, cerebrospinal fluid)
12. has a reasonable cost

G. CLINICAL USE OF ANTIMICROBIALS

Objective 25.G.1. Recognize 10 general guidelines involved in the clinical use of antimicrobials.

Guidelines for the clinical use of antimicrobials are summarized below:

1. Ascertain that antimicrobial therapy is indicated.
2. Use adequate dosage for adequate duration.
3. Mixed infections (in contrast to pure infections) may occur in the oral cavity, so higher than recommended dosage may be required for treatment of oral infections.
4. Systemic administration is preferred to topical administration, and parenteral administration is preferred to oral, especially in the presence of a severe infection.
5. If an infection does not show signs of abating in 48 to 72 hours, question your diagnosis and/or choice of antibiotic.
6. When possible, culture infected exudates to identify an organism and its sensitivities.
7. Fixed combinations should be avoided unless a single agent would not be effective and the combination is specifically indicated by culture and sensitivity testing. Single antimicrobials in adequate dosages are usually as effective as or more effective than combinations.
8. No antibiotic are effective against filterable viruses.
9. Static antimicrobials, when they are to be administered orally in four divided doses in 24 hours, must be taken every 6 hours in the 24-hour period. Conversely, if cidal antimicrobials are prescribed in four divided doses in 24 hours, they may be taken either every 6 hours or four times daily during waking hours.
10. Duration of treatment of dental infections with antimicrobials should be 5 to 10 days, or the antimicrobial should be taken for at least 48 hours after the cessation of all clinical signs and symptoms. Generally, streptococcal infections require 10 full days of treatment.

H. USES OF ANTIMICROBIALS IN DENTISTRY

Objective 25.H.1. Recognize eight specific uses for antimicrobials in dentistry.

The list below decribes specific uses for antimicrobials in dentistry.

1. Postextraction infections
2. Postsurgical infections
3. Pericoronitis
4. Dentoalveolar abscess
5. Osteomyelitis
6. Cellulitis
7. Acute necrotizing ulcerative gingivitis
8. Periodontitis

I. PROPHYLACTIC INDICATIONS FOR ANTIMICROBIALS

Objective 25.I.1. Recognize six prophylactic indications.

Objective 25.I.2. Recognize six bacteremia-producing situations which may require prophylaxis.

Prophylactic indications are:

1. before extensive extractions in an acutely infected field
2. before extraction of an impacted third molar with acute pericoronitis
3. before extensive, traumatic surgical procedures (plastic surgery, removal of neoplasm)
4. before surgical intervention in acute infections of oral structures (acute dentoalveolar abscess, cellulitis, severe periodontal disease)
5. to control acute phase of necrotizing gingivitis, prior to scaling
6. before manipulative procedures producing transient bacteremia in patients at risk.

Patients at risk from bacteremia requiring prophylactic include those with:

1. rheumatic, congenital, or valvular heart disease, especially with a heart valve prosthesis (**Note: accurate medical history is most important; failure to use adequate premedica-**

tion in such patients could result in medico-legal action.)

2. uncontrolled diabetes mellitus
3. glomerulonephritis
4. nephrosis
5. prosthetic joint replacement
6. marked debility due to advanced age, leukemia, long-term corticosteroid or antimetabolic therapy

J. FACTORS INFLUENCING EFFECTIVENESS

Objective 25.J.1. Recognize four factors that may influence the effectiveness of antimicrobials.

State of Activity of Infection
Antimicrobials are effective against organisms actively growing and reproducing (logarithmic growth phase), therefore, against acute infections and not usually against chronic infections.

Extent of Infection
The greater the extent of infection (tissue involvement) and relative resistance of the pathogens, the higher the dose required to combat organisms. Severe infections are more difficult to treat than are mild infections.

Concentration of Antimicrobial in Body Tissues and Fluids

1. Concentration of an antimicrobial in body tissues and fluids will vary according to dosage administered. Absorption, vascularity of the affected tissue, distribution of the antimicrobial in body fluids, and possible protein binding also affect the concentration of active antimicrobial that affects the pathogen.
2. Many bactericidal antimicrobials are bacteriostatic at low doses (concentrations).

Host Factors

1. Bacteriostatic agents require host defense mechanisms for destruction of organisms. Intact host defense mechanisms are also required to rid the body of dead organisms and their products following the use of bactericidal antimicrobials.
2. Host defense mechanisms are synergistic with bactericidal agents.
3. Host defense mechanisms can be compromised by age, genetic factors, pregnancy, concurrent disease, and the use of other drugs (e.g., corticosteroids).
4. Toxicity of antimicrobials may be increased by the presence of atopic allergies, depressed hepatic function, depressed renal function, and debilitating diseases.

K. COMPLICATIONS OF ANTIMICROBIAL THERAPY

Objective 25.K.1. Recognize the possible complications of antimicrobial therapy.

Toxic reactions that may occur include the types listed below:

1. Local chemical irritation of tissues at site of administration—topically or at an injection site
2. Local irritation at site of GI absorption, producing nausea, vomiting, and diarrhea
3. Local irritation at site of elimination (colon, rectum, and kidney)
4. Systemic, resulting in neurotoxicity, nephrotoxicity, hepatotoxicity, or hemopoietic depression

Allergic reactions (antigen-antibody reaction) are listed below:

1. Local application causes stomatitis venenata or contact dermatitis
2. Systemic administration causes:
   a. Immediate types
      (1) anaphylaxis
      (2) urticaria and angioneurotic edema
      (3) serum-type reactions (similar to reaction to horse serum). (*Note:* these are serious, causing pain, fear, and debilitation; symptoms include joint pain, headache, lymphadenopathy, general malaise, and fever.)
      (4) drug fever
      (5) asthma and rhinitis
      (6) vasculitis

b. Delayed types
   (1) cutaneous (not serious, but annoying, often expressed as rashes and itching)
   (2) agranulocytosis
   (3) aplastic anemia
3. Cross-allergenicity of agents. If a patient is allergic to one antimicrobial, he may also be allergic to others. This is especially true when the two antimicrobials are chemically related. For instance, all penicillins are thought to exhibit complete cross-allergenicity with each other, as do lincomycin and clindamycin. Conversely, there is virtually no cross-allergenicity between penicillin and lincomycin or erythromycin. The practitioner must take a good medical history to reduce or eliminate this potential reaction.

L. CAUSES OF FAILURE OF ANTIMICROBIAL THERAPY

Objective 25.L.1. Recognize 10 causes of failure of antimicrobial therapy.

1. Incomplete clinical or bacteriologic diagnosis
2. Improper selection of drugs
3. Improper method of administration with inadequate absorption
4. Inadequate dose—either too low or poorly spaced
5. Inadequate duration of therapy
6. Inaccessible lesion
7. Development of resistant strain
8. Alteration of bacterial flora and suprainfection

9. Drug toxicity and hypersensitivity
10. Deficiency of host defenses

Host Factors in Failure of Antimicrobial Therapy

Objective 25.L.2. Describe two important host factors that could alter the dosage of an antimicrobial drug.

There are two very important host factors that should be considered prior to initiating antimicrobial therapy: hepatic and renal function. Since all antimicrobials depend on the liver and/or kidney for elimination, the status of liver and kidney function is most important. A number of other pharmacology textbooks present a simplified table of how the practitioner might adjust dosage in the presence of hepatotoxicity or nephrotoxicity. In addition, most or all package inserts of the various products offer similar information. This information is not reproduced here; rather, the practitioner is urged to consult the appropriate reference sources (Weinstein, 1975) prior to treating patients with hepatic or renal dysfunction.

M. ANTIMICROBIAL DRUGS OF CHOICE

Table 25–2 is included as a reference source and may be used to choose antimicrobials for appropriate dental conditions when the organism is known. No objective is given because the table is **not** to be memorized and should be used, as intended, for reference.

TABLE 25–2. ANTIMICROBIAL DRUGS OF CHOICE IN DENTISTRY

Infecting Organism	Drug of Choice	Alternative Drugs
Gram-positive Cocci		
Streptococcus pyogenes groups A, B, C, and G	a penicillin	an erythromycin, a cephalosporin
Viridans group of *Streptococcus*[a]	a penicillin with or without streptomycin	cephalosporin, vancomycin
Enterococcus[a]	ampicillin or penicillin G[b] with streptomycin	vancomycin with or without streptomycin

(continued)

TABLE 25–2. (Continued)

Infecting Organism	Drug of Choice	Alternative Drugs
Gram-positive Cocci		
Streptococcus anaerobius[a]	penicillin G (P)	clindamycin, tetracycline, erythromycin
Streptococcus pneumoniae[a] (formerly *D. pneumoniae*)	a penicillin	an erythromycin, cephalosporin
Staphylococcus aureus[a] nonpenicillinase-producing	a penicillin	cephalosporin, clindamycin, vancomycin
penicillinase-producing	a penicillinase-resistant penicillin	clindamycin, cephalosporin, vancomycin
Gram-negative Cocci		
Neisseria gonorrhoeae[a]	a penicillin or tetracycline	ampicillin, spectinomycin, cefoxitin
Gram-positive Bacilli		
Bacillus anthracis (anthrax)	a penicillin	an erythromycin, a tetracycline
Listeria monocytogenes[a]	ampicillin with or without streptomycin	tetracycline, chloramphenicol
Bacillus perfringans[a] (*Clostridium welchii*, gas gangrene)	penicillin G (P)	chloramphenicol, clindamycin, tetracycline
Clostridium tetani[a]	penicillin G (P)	a tetracycline (P), cephalosporin
Corynebacterium diphtheriae	an erythromycin	a penicillin
Gram-negative Bacilli		
Salmonella[a]	ampicillin	chloramphenicol
Escherichia coli[a] enteropathogenic sepsis	gentamicin or tobramycin	ampicillin, a tetracycline, kanamycin (P), a polymyxin (P), a tetracycline (P), carbenicillin
Enterobacter (Aerobacter)[a]	gentamicin or tobramycin	carbenicillin or ticarcillin, cefamandole
Klebsiella pneumoniae[a]	gentamicin or tobramycin	a cephalosporin, kanamycin (P)
Pseudomonas aeruginosa[a]	gentamicin or tobramycin with carbenicillin or ticarcillin	amikacin with carbenicillin or ticarcillin
Brucella[a] (brucellosis)	a tetracycline with or without streptomycin	chloramphenicol, trimethoprim-sulfamethoxazole
Francisella tularensis (*Pasteurella*)[a] (tularemia)	streptomycin	a tetracycline, chloramphenicol
Haemophilus influenzae respiratory infections	ampicillin or amoxicillin	a tetracycline, trimethoprim-sulfamethoxazole
meningitis[a]	chloramphenicol	ampicillin
Bacteroides[a]	penicillin	clindamycin, erythromycin
Haemophilus ducreyi (chancroid)	trisulfapyrimidines	tetracycline
Bordetella (*Haemophilus*) *pertussis* (whooping cough)	erythromycin	—
Mima, Herellea[a]	gentamycin or tobramycin	kanamycin, amikacin

(*continued*)

TABLE 25–2. (Continued)

Infecting Organism	Drug of Choice	Alternative Drugs
Gram-negative Bacilli		
Fusobacterium nucleatum (formerly *F. fusiforme*) (Vincent's infection)	a penicillin	a tetracycline, an erythromycin
Fusobacterium plauti	a penicillin	a tetracycline, an erythromycin
Calymmatobacterium granulomatis (granuloma inguinale)	a tetracycline	streptomycin
Acid-fast Bacilli		
Mycobacterium tuberculosis[a]	isoniazid combined with ethambutol with or without rifampin	Streptomycin, PAS, pyrazinamide, cycloserine, ethionamide, viomycin, kanamycin (P), capreomycin
Atypical mycobacteria[a]	isoniazid combined with rifampin, with or without ethambutol	streptomycin, ethionamide, pyrazinamide, cycloserine, viomycin, kanamycin (P), capreomycin
Mycobacterium leprae (leprosy)	dapsone with or without rifampin	acedapsone, rifampin
Spirochetes		
Borrelia recurrentis (relapsing fever)	a tetracycline	a penicillin
Treponema vincenti (Vincent's infection)	penicillin G	an erythromycin, a tetracycline
Treponema pallidum (syphilis)	penicillin G (P)	a tetracycline (P), an erythromycin (P)
Treponema pertenue (yaws)	penicillin G (P)	a tetracycline (P)
Leptospira	a penicillin	a tetracycline
Actinomycetes		
Actinomyces israelii[a] (actinomycosis)	a penicillin	a tetracycline
Nocardia[a]	trisulfapyrimadines	trimethoprim-sulfamethoxazole, trisulfapyrimadines with minocycline or ampicillin or erythromycin
Rickettsia		
Rocky Mountain spotted fever, endemic typhus, Q fever	a tetracycline	chloramphenicol
Viruses, Filterable Agents		
Mycoplasma (all species)	an erythromycin	a tetracycline
Agent of psittacosis (ornithosis)	a tetracycline	chloramphenicol
Herpes simplex (keratitis)	vidarabine (topical)	idoxuridine (topical)

(continued)

TABLE 25–2. (Continued)

Infecting Organism	Drug of Choice	Alternative Drugs
Fungi		
Histoplasma capsulatum	amphotericin B	no dependable alternative
Candida albicans	nystatin (oral or topical)	amphotericin B
Cryptococcus neoformans	amphotericin B	no dependable alternative
Mucor	amphotericin B	no dependable alternative
Coccidioides immitis	amphotericin B	miconazole
Blastomyces dermatitidis (North America)	amphotericin B	2-hydroxystilbamidine
Blastomyces brasiliensis (South America)	amphotericin B	a sulfonamide
Sporotrichum schenckii	an iodide	amphotericin B
Fonsecaea (chromoblastomycosis)	amphotericin B	no dependable alternative

Adapted from Med Lett Drugs Ther 22:5, 1980. Courtesy of the Medical Letter.
[a] Because resistance may be a problem, susceptibility tests must be performed.
[b] Although both parenteral and oral formulations are available, parenteral administration is preferred for this infection.

REFERENCES

Strominger JL: The actions of penicillin and other antibiotics on bacterial cell wall synthesis. Johns Hopkins Med J 133:63, 1973

Weinstein L: Chemotherapy of microbial diseases. In Goodman LS and Gilman A (eds): The Pharmacological Basis of Therapeutics, 5th ed. New York, Macmillan, 1975, pp 1095, 1108–1109

BIBLIOGRAPHY

Accepted Dental Therapeutics, 38th ed. Chicago, American Dental Association, 1979

Bevan JA (ed): Essentials of Pharmacology, 2nd ed. Hagerstown, MD, Harper & Row, 1976

Gilman AG, Goodman LS, Gilman A (eds): Goodman and Gilman's The Pharmacological Basis of Therapeutics, 6th ed. New York, Macmillan, 1980

Goth A: Medical Pharmacology, 10th ed. St. Louis, Mosby, 1981

Melmon KL, Morelli HF (eds): Clinical Pharmacology: Basic Principles in Therapeutics, 2nd ed. New York, Macmillan, 1978

Meyers FH, Jawetz E, Goldfien A: Review of Medical Pharmacology, 7th ed. Los Altos, CA, Lange, 1980

QUESTIONS

1. **T** F The spectrum of a drug refers to the actual list of microorganisms against which an antibiotic is effective.

2. T **F** A bacteriostatic drug is an agent which at optimal dose usually kills the organism against which it is effective.

3. **T** F If an antibiotic possesses true selectivity, the drug affects a biochemical mechanism of the invading organism and not the host.

4. Specific mechanisms of acquired resistance include:

   A. conjugation
   B. elaboration of drug-metabolizing enzymes
   C. mutation
   D. transduction
   E. all of the above are correct
   F. none of the above is correct

5. All of the following agents inhibit cell wall synthesis *except:*

   A. bacitracin
   B. cephalosporins
   C. chloramphenicol *inhibits protein synthesis*
   D. penicillin
   E. vancomycin

6. Reasons for the rational use of antibiotic combinations include all of the following *except:*

   A. delaying emergence of resistant strains
   B. exposing the patient to adverse effects of each drug
   C. treating mixed infections
   D. treating severe life-threatening infections

7. General acceptable rules for using antibiotic combinations include:

   A. combining two cell wall synthesis inhibitors
   B. combining two static antibiotics
   C. combining a cell wall synthesis inhibitor with a cell wall disruptor
   D. all of the above are correct
   E. none of the above is correct

8. **T** F A patient with a history of chronic pulmonary disease (except tuberculosis) may show an increased incidence of supra-infection.

9. **T** F Supra-infections are often caused by *Candida albicans.*

10. All of the following are properties of an ideal chemotherapeutic agent *except:*

    A. bacteriostatic preferred over bactericidal
    B. efficacy by the oral route

    C. low side effects at highest useful doses
    D. selective activity
    E. useful spectrum of activity

11. General guidelines in the use of antibiotics include all of the following *except:*

    A. duration of treatment of dental infections with antibiotics is generally five days or less
    B. if an infection does not show signs of abating in 48 to 72 hours, question your diagnosis and/or choice of antibiotic
    C. single antibiotics in adequate dosage are usually as effective as or more effective than combinations
    D. when possible, culture infected exudates to identify organisms and their sensitivities.

12. All of the following are specific uses of antibiotics in dentistry *except:*

    A. cellulitis
    B. chronic necrotizing ulcerative gingivitis
    C. osteomyelitis
    D. pericoronitis
    E. postextraction infections

13. The prophylactic use of antibiotics may be indicated when patients present with:

    A. marked debility due to antimetabolite therapy
    B. uncontrolled diabetes mellitus
    C. valvular heart disease
    D. all of the above are correct
    E. none of the above is correct

14. Factors that may influence the effectiveness of antibiotics include:

    A. concentration of antibiotic in tissues and fluids

B. extent of infection
C. host factors
D. all of the above are correct
E. none of the above is correct

15. **T** F Complications resulting from antibiotic therapy can include the presence of toxic reactions, including both local and systemic types.

16. Possible causes of failure of antibiotic therapy include:

A. alteration of bacterial flora and suprainfection
B. development of resistant strains
C. drug toxicity and hypersensitivity
D. inaccessible lesion
E. all of the above are correct
F. none of the above is correct

26
Penicillin

A. HISTORY

In 1928, Sir Alexander Fleming observed that a mold had contaminated his staphylococcus cultures, causing lysis of staphylococcus colonies. Since the mold was of the genus *Penicillium*, he named the lysing substance "penicillin." Fleming and other investigators could not isolate the lytic substance, and when the sulfa drugs were discovered in the 1930s, attention was diverted away from penicillin. In 1939, Florey and Chain of Oxford University resumed the investigation of penicillin. The mold was grown almost everywhere in and around Oxford, including the bedpans of the hospital. Sufficient crude material was collected in 1940 to test it in mice, and the crude material was quite effective against streptococcus-induced infections. In 1941, the first human treatment with penicillin took place. An Oxford policeman was very ill with a mixed staphylococcal and streptococcal infection. He was cured by the use of the crude culture material (thought to contain about 10% penicillin) and a much purer penicillin derived from his urine and the urine of other patients. In fact, one Oxford professor referred to penicillin as "a remarkable substance grown in bedpans and purified by passage through the Oxford Police Force." Further and more extensive culturing of penicillin shifted from Great Britain to the United States, where the pressures of World War II were much less. With mass production, the "wonder drug" became a reality. Later, in 1957, Chain, Rolinson, and Batchelor isolated 6-aminopenicillanic acid, which initiated the development of a large series of semisynthetic penicillins.

B. CHEMISTRY AND SPECTRUM

Objective 26.B.1. Recognize the basic chemical nucleus of penicillins.

Objective 26.B.2. Recognize the sites of enzyme activity of β-lactamase and amidase on the penicillin molecule.

Objective 26.B.3. Recognize the spectrum of activity of the various penicillins.

Objective 26.B.4. Recognize the names of penicillins set in bold type in Table 26–1.

253

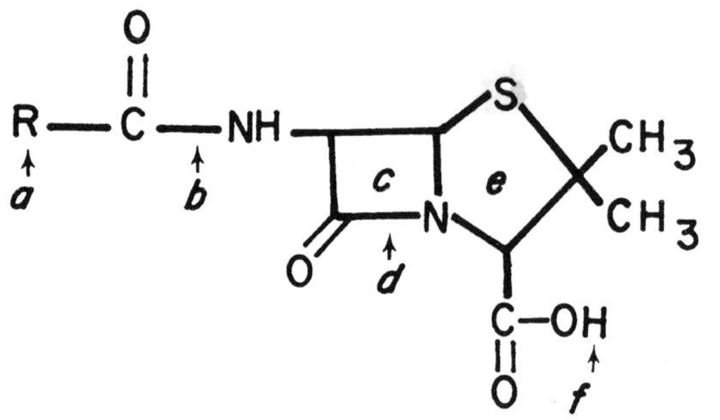

Figure 26–1. Features of the penicillin molecule. a, R, side chains; b, site of action of amidase; c, β-lactam ring; d, site of action of β-lactamases (penicillinases); e, thiazolidine ring; f, ionizable hydrogen.

Penicillin G (benzylpenicillin) was the compound eventually chosen for therapeutic use. It had the best efficacy when compared to other penicillins isolated previously (F, K, O, X, and so on).

All of the presently marketed penicillins are β-lactam thiazolidines; the chemical structure is shown in Figure 26–1. The legend describes the features of the molecule, and these are explained below.

Penicillin G (benzyl group at R) is considered to possess primarily (but not exclusively), a gram-positive spectrum of activity, with some effect against certain gram-negative organisms, including *Neisseria gonorrhoeae.*

Penicillin V (phenoxymethyl at R) and phenethicillin (phenoxyethyl at R) tend to be less potent, and increased blood levels are necessary to combat infections produced by susceptible organisms. The spectrum of activity of these analogs is virtually identical to that of penicillin G.

Ampicillin, amoxicillin, carbenicillin, and ticarcillin are extended-spectrum penicillins with different chemical groups at R. These agents are often erroneously referred to as "broad-spectrum" penicillins, which implies a spectrum of activity much like tetracycline. These penicillins are probably more correctly referred to as extended-spectrum penicillins and are effective against the gram-negative organisms *Escherichia coli, Proteus mirabilis, Haemophilus influenzae,* salmonellae, shigellae, and enterococci.

Methicillin, nafcillin, and isoxazolyl derivatives (oxacillin, cloxacillin, and dicloxacillin) were synthesized so as to substitute R groups which would protect the β-lactam ring. These agents are penicillinase resistant and are used specifically for the treatment of infections caused by staphylococci that produce penicillinase. These agents have no activity against gram-negative bacteria and their activity is poor against other gram-positive bacteria (Table 26–1).

TABLE 26–1. FEATURES OF PENICILLINS

Agent	Spectrum	Penicillinase	Preparations
penicillin G	primarily gram positive	susceptible	peroral and parenteral
penicillin V	primarily gram positive	susceptible	peroral
phenethicillin	primarily gram positive	susceptible	peroral
ampicillin	extended spectrum	susceptible	peroral and parenteral
amoxicillin	extended spectrum	susceptible	peroral
carbenicillin	extended spectrum	susceptible	peroral and parenteral
cyclacillin	extended spectrum	susceptible	peroral
ticarcillin	extended spectrum	susceptible	parenteral
methicillin	penicillinase-producing staphylococci	resistant	parenteral
nafcillin	penicillinase-producing staphylococci	resistant	peroral and parenteral
oxacillin	penicillinase-producing staphylococci	resistant	peroral and parenteral
cloxacillin	penicillinase-producing staphylococci	resistant	peroral
dicloxacillin[a]	penicillinase-producing staphylococci	resistant	peroral

[a] Considered equivalent to cloxacillin; dicloxacillin is more potent and less drug is usually used.

The penicillin molecule also shows the features described below:

1. Bond *b* is the site of amidase activity; cleavage here results in 6-aminopenicillanic acid, an important starting chemical for further synthesis of new analogs (R-group substitution).
2. Ring *c* is the β-lactam ring. This four-membered ring is unusual in biology and is thought to be the reason for its specificity.
3. Site *d* indicates the site of β-lactamase activity.
4. Ring *e* is the thiazolidine ring. Modification of ring *e* to a six-membered ring results in a cephalosporin (Chapter 27).
5. The hydrogen atom at *f* is acidic and can easily ionize. This is a site of formation of the various penicillin salts, e.g., if penicillin is substituted with Na^+, K^+, or procaine and is subsequently crystallized, the respective salts formed are penicillin G sodium, penicillin G potassium, and procaine penicillin G.

C. MECHANISM OF ACTION

Objective 26.C.1. Describe the mechanism of action of penicillins.

Objective 26.C.2. Recognize whether penicillins are bactericidal or bacteriostatic.

Objective 26.C.3. Recognize the type of selectivity of penicillins (true or relative).

The mechanism of action of the penicillins is by interference with the cross-linking of the peptidoglycan units of the bacterial cell wall (i.e., by inhibiting bacterial cell wall synthesis). The result is an organism with an incompletely formed cell wall (spheroplast) that is osmotically sensitive in the presence of body fluids because of a higher intracellular osmotic pressure maintained by bacteria. The spheroplasts absorb water, swell, and burst. For this reason, pharmacologists refer to the penicillins as bactericidal agents, even though these drugs do not cause cell death directly. Nonetheless, cell death does occur. Because this mechanism operates only on certain bacteria and not on mammalian cells, penicillins exhibit true selectivity.

D. ABSORPTION

Objective 26.D.1. Be able to convert units of penicillin to milligrams.

Objective 26.D.2. Recognize and contrast the absorption of the various salts of penicillin G, both perorally and intramuscularly.

Objective 26.D.3. Recognize factors that can inhibit the absorption of oral penicillin G and penicillin V.

Objective 26.D.4. Recognize the definition of the term depot form (or repository form).

Objective 26.D.5. Describe the dental use of extended-spectrum penicillins and penicillinase-resistant penicillins.

Since approximately 1600 units of penicillin G equals 1.0 mg, a patient receiving a 250 mg tablet would receive 400,000 units.

Penicillin should never be administered topically because of a high rate of induction of allergy. Penicillin G can be administered perorally, but absorption is relatively poor and erratic. Gastric acid hydrolyzes penicillin G, and the presence of food can also inhibit absorption. Hence, penicillin G must be administered either 30 minutes before or 1½ to 2 hours after meals. Figures 26–2 and 26–3 demonstrate, for fasting and nonfasting subjects respectively, some of the absorption characteristics of penicillin G in comparison to other forms.

Crystalline (or aqueous or soluble) penicillin G, as the sodium or potassium salt, may be administered IM or IV. This agent is rarely given IM by itself because its duration is too short, and it would require frequent injections (approximately every two to three hours). If sodium or potassium is replaced by a procaine molecule (procaine penicillin G), IM administration has a much longer duration (approximately 24 hours). This is referred to as a "repository (depot)" form. The crystalline and procaine salt forms of

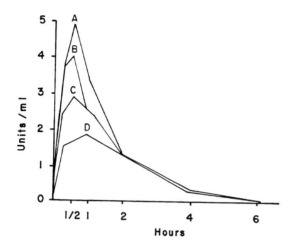

Figure 26–2. Average levels of penicillin (dose: 400,000 units) in the plasma of 10 fasting subjects. A, potassium penicillin V; B, calcium penicillin V; C, penicillin V (acid); D, sodium penicillin G. (*After Juncher H, Raaschou F: Antibiot Med 4:497, 1957.*)

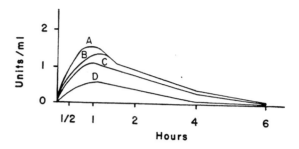

Figure 26–3. Average levels of penicillin (dose: 400,000 units) in the plasma of 10 nonfasting subjects. A, potassium penicillin V; B, calcium penicillin V; C, penicillin V (acid); D, sodium penicillin G. (*After Juncher H, Raaschou F: Antibiot Med 4:497, 1957.*)

the drug are often given in combination as the first injection because aqueous penicillin G provides a high blood level with rapid onset (approximately 15 minutes or less), and procaine penicillin G, though slower in onset, provides adequate blood levels for about 24 hours. The mixture is also called a "repository" form. Procaine penicillin G can be suspended in oil; this repository form has an even longer duration of action, which is extended to 48 to 72 hours.

One other preparation will be briefly discussed at this time and not again because it has no current use in dentistry. Benzathine penicillin G (do not confuse with benzylpenicillin G) is a repository form producing very low blood levels of 28 to 30 days duration after IM administration (the level is often too low to treat most acute infections). The repository preparations (benzathine penicillin G and procaine penicillin G) are poorly soluble salts. As they slowly dissolve in muscle tissue fluids, the various components are absorbed into the bloodstream. The only currently approved uses for benzathine penicillin G are (1) long-term rheumatic fever prophylaxis, (2) during the incubation period of syphilis, and (3) treatment of strep throat. The

repository forms of penicillin G **must not** be injected IV because they may cause multiple pulmonary infarcts.

Penicillin V and phenethicillin are marketed solely as oral forms. These agents are less likely to be destroyed by gastric acid, but the presence of food does inhibit absorption. Blood levels in the fasting state may be as much as three times the blood level when the drugs are taken in the presence of food (compare Figs. 26–2 and 26–3). Actually, all the oral forms of the many different penicillins should be taken on an empty stomach. Figures 26–2 and 26–3 demonstrate that penicillin V potassium is more completely absorbed than is penicillin V sodium or the free acid (Root et al., 1978).

The extended-spectrum penicillins (ampicillin, amoxicillin, carbenicillin, cyclacillin, and ticarcillin) are available for both oral and parenteral use. Amoxicillin, when ingested orally, produces blood levels that are much higher than the levels produced by the same dose of oral ampicillin. However, the increased cost of the former agent tends to negate this advantage in absorption. The extended-spectrum penicillins have little use in dentistry. Carbenicillin and ticarcillin should not be used routinely in dentistry, since their use should be reserved for treatment of infections caused by *Pseudomonas* and indole-positive *Proteus* species, which uncommonly cause dental infections. The only use for this group of penicillins is if culture and sensitivity tests suggest that one of the agents be used. However, some cardiologists are suggesting that ampicillin may be useful for antibiotic prophylaxis in patients with a heart valve prosthesis because this agent is very active against enterococci. Enterococci are potential causative organisms of bacterial endocarditis in patients with a heart valve prosthesis. When enterococci are frequent causative agents of bacteremia (as in gastrointestinal and urogenital tract manipulations), ampicillin may be useful, but oral manipulations usually do not require the extended-spectrum penicillins.

Of the penicillinase-resistant penicillins, methicillin in available only as a parenteral form, and cloxacillin and dicloxacillin are available only as oral forms. Nafcillin and oxacillin are marketed as either oral or parenteral forms. Cloxacillin and dicloxacillin are the best oral forms because they are most resistant to breakdown by gastric acid.

E. DISTRIBUTION

Objective 26.E.1. Describe the distribution of penicillins.

The penicillins, depending on the type, are 40 to 98% bound to plasma protein. Once adequate blood levels of free drug are reached, protein binding has no clinical significance because both the free drug (pharmacologically active) and bound drug are maintained by proper doses at the proper time intervals. In addition, there is no evidence in the literature that displacement of penicillin from its protein binding site by other drugs results in an adverse drug interaction.

The penicillins penetrate most tissues, including pericardial, pleural, and peritoneal cavities, the eye, and the joints. Penicillins do not penetrate the blood-brain barrier, but sufficient amounts will penetrate in the presence of meningeal inflammation. Significant penetration into the brain can result in convulsions. Penicillins do not readily penetrate into abscesses.

F. METABOLISM

Objective 26.F.1. Describe the metabolism of penicillins and relate the metabolism to various metabolites.

Little or no metabolism of most of the penicillins occurs in the body because the drugs are so readily excreted unchanged by the kidney. However, small amounts of 6-aminopenicillanic acid have been detected in the urine of patients ingesting penicillin by the oral route. Enteric bacteria are believed to be responsible for the appearance of the metabolite. The metabolite is thought to be absorbed and subsequently excreted by the kidney.

Oral forms of penicillins, especially penicillin G, can be hydrolyzed by gastric acid.

Bacterial penicillinase (β-lactamase) produced by some staphylococci or certain gram-negative strains is capable of splitting the lactam ring, forming penicilloic acid.

G. EXCRETION

Objective 26.G.1. Describe the major route of excretion of penicillins and other secondary routes of excretion.

Objective 26.G.2. Describe the mechanism of action of probenecid.

Sixty to ninety percent of the total amount of penicillin G that is absorbed is rapidly excreted unchanged in the urine (Fig. 26–4). Of the total amount excreted unchanged in the urine, the major route is by active tubular secretion (90%) and a secondary route by glomerular filtration (10%). Penicillin that is bound to plasma protein is not protected from active tubular secretion. The other penicillins are excreted by similar routes, except for nafcillin and the isoxazolyl analogs (e.g., dicloxacillin), which are primarily excreted in the bile and/or metabolized by the liver. Thus, the use of nafcillin or dicloxacillin in patients with renal failure does not generally require reduced dosages, although at times the dose may be slightly reduced.

Nafcillin & isoxazole — Liver

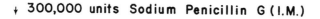

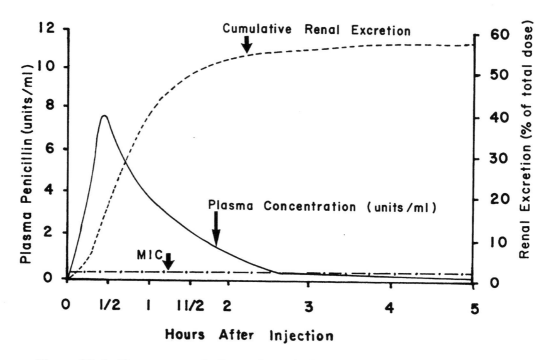

Figure 26–4. Plasma concentration and renal elimination of sodium penicillin G in healthy adults with normal renal function. The rapid decline of plasma concentration after a peak of 8 units/ml is the result of the rapid excretion of penicillin G and is due to glomerular filtration and active secretion by the kidney tubules. By the end of the five-hour period shown in the figure, nearly 60%, or 180,000 units, of the administered dose has been eliminated in the urine.

The minimum inhibitory concentration (MIC) (0.3 units/ml), noted on the figure, is an average MIC for the viridans group of streptococci, an example of a common oral streptococcus. The lack of persistence of effective blood levels after injection of aqueous solutions of soluble penicillin G salts is a major reason why repository preparations of the antibiotic are so commonly employed. (*After Mandell GL, Sande MA: In Gilman AG, Goodman LS, Gilman A (eds): Goodman and Gilman's The Pharmacological Basis of Therapeutics, 6th ed, 1980. Courtesy of Macmillan Publishing Company.*)

Active tubular secretion of penicillins can be blocked by the drug probenecid, resulting in an approximate doubling of usual blood levels. This regimen of penicillin and probenecid can be of value in maintaining high blood levels for an extended duration. Probenecid may be used with penicillin in the treatment of gonorrhea.

Smaller amounts are excreted in milk, saliva, and sweat. For example, it has been found that penicillin levels in milk are about 3 to 15% of the plasma level. However, this low level may be sufficient to induce allergy in the baby of a nursing patient.

H. PHARMACOLOGIC EFFECTS

Objective 26.H.1. Describe the pharmacologic effects of penicillins.

The penicillins, especially penicillin G, have essentially no pharmacologic effects in mammals at usual and recommended therapeutic doses. The reason is a reflection of the mechanism of action on the bacterial cell wall; mammalian cells have no cell wall. In fact, only after huge doses, i.e., 40 to 80 million units per day IV, do patients with normal body function begin to show signs of toxicity. Even then, the toxic effects are mostly due to the cations (sodium and potassium) in the solution rather than to the drug itself. A lethal dose for penicillin G in man is unknown.

I. ADVERSE EFFECTS

Objective 26.I.1. Describe adverse effects of penicillins, including allergies.

Objective 26.I.2. Be able to compare and contrast potential cross-allergenicity between different penicillins and between penicillin and other agents.

As cited previously, the penicillins are remarkably free of toxicity. Intravenous and intramuscular injections may cause local irritation and pain. Accidental injection into a nerve could cause degeneration of the nerve fiber, and IV administration can result in thrombophlebitis.

Stomach upset with nausea, vomiting, and diarrhea can occur with ingestion of all forms of penicillin via the oral route. Penicillin taken by this route can also result in overgrowth of resistant organisms in the GI tract and induction of enteritis. Supra-infection can also occur, but this is less likely to happen with the penicillins than with antibiotics having a wider spectrum of activity.

The induction of an allergic reaction is the most dangerous side effect, and the penicillins account for the highest incidence of drug allergy. In allergic subjects, the full range of allergic reactions can be observed (Chapter 25, p. 245). Skin rashes are often seen when allergy is first induced, and acute anaphylactic reactions are observed both with and without a history of

previous reactions. Oral allergic manifestations can occur and include acute glossitis, severe stomatitis, brown or black hairy tongue, and angular cheilosis.

A history of an allergic reaction to penicillin contraindicates its use again because a second exposure to the drug often results in a more severe reaction. Patients with atopic allergies present an increased risk of an allergic reaction even when the patient has no history of prior exposure to the drug. The life-threatening anaphylactic reactions to penicillin are most often noted after parenteral dosing, but they have also followed oral ingestion and even intradermal injection of extremely small doses (as in allergy testing).

The penicillins should be assumed to exhibit complete cross-allergenicity, i.e., if a patient is allergic to one penicillin, it should be assumed that allergy will occur with other forms. There is good evidence that some degree of cross-allergenicity occurs between penicillins and the cephalosporins, agents that are similar chemically (Chapter 27). However, the degree of cross-allergenicity between the two classes of antibiotics is quite controversial. The early literature suggested that as high as 30% of penicillin-allergic subjects would also be allergic to the cephalosporins. Conversely, one expert more recently claimed that cross-allergenicity between groups is uncommon in his experience (Weinstein, 1975), and another group claimed that 8% of the patients who have a history of allergy to penicillin will also react to the cephalosporins (Moellering, Swartz, 1976). Moreover, these authors have suggested that patients with a history of an immediate reaction to penicillin (p. 245) should **not** receive one of the cephalosporins. Conversely, cephalosporins may be used (with caution) in patients with a history of delayed allergic reaction to penicillin.

Methicillin, nafcillin, and isoxazolyl analogs (dicloxacillin) can produce granulocytopenia, especially in children. Methicillin and nafcillin have been associated with nephritis. Carbenicillin can increase bleeding time, and ampicillin can produce a skin rash that is not of allergic origin.

J. DRUG INTERACTIONS

Objective 26.J.1. Describe important drug interactions, both favorable and unfavorable, involving penicillins.

A number of mild and/or minor drug interactions have been described in the literature. These will not be discussed because they apparently have no clinical significance.

Parenteral administration of one of the penicillins with one of the aminoglycosides (e.g. streptomycin) results in a synergistic effect due to broadening of the spectrum of activity, a possibly increased cidal activity, and no apparent unfavorable interaction between these classes of drugs. However, the concomitant administration of a penicillin with chloramphenicol or tetracycline can result in antagonism of penicillin's effect. Some sulfa drugs have been shown to inhibit the oral absorption of oxacillin, and oral neomycin can inhibit the oral absorption of penicillin V or G. Probenecid causes high and prolonged blood levels, especially when combined with penicillin G, penicillin V, and the extended-spectrum penicillins.

K. CONTRAINDICATIONS

Objective 26.K.1. Describe contraindications to the use of penicillins.

A history of an allergic reaction (even a mild rash) to penicillin contraindicates its use again. In patients with reduced renal function, the dosage should be adjusted downward, especially for penicillin G, penicillin V, and the extended-spectrum penicillins.

L. THERAPEUTIC USE, BASIS FOR SELECTION, AND IMPLICATIONS FOR DENTISTRY

Objective 26.L.1. Recognize seven factors that aid in success of therapy and that should be considered prior to selection of penicillins.

Objective 26.L.2. Recognize the importance of culture and antibiotic sensitivity testing.

Objective 26.L.3. Recognize four reasons why penicillin is the antibiotic drug of choice for dental infections.

Objective 26.L.4. Recognize the antibiotic drug of choice in patients allergic to penicillin.

Seven factors that aid in success of therapy follow:

1. The dentist must first establish that an antibiotic is needed. Most oral infections will respond to penicillin, although other choices might be considered.
2. A good medical history must be taken (or updated) to aid in selection. For penicillin, a history of allergy and decreased renal function are the most significant patient factors.
3. The dentist must incise and drain an abscess which is accessible and sufficiently developed (pointing). In the case of a dentoalveolar abscess, the tooth's pulp chamber should be opened for establishment of drainage. Antibiotic therapy alone is often inadequate for resolution of infection in the presence of an acute dentoalveolar abscess. Sometimes, the first one or two days of therapy with the antimicrobial agent will aid in the pointing process.
4. The dentist must, when possible, take a sample of the infected exudate for culture and sensitivity testing. In vitro activity of an antibiotic does not guarantee in vivo activity, but culturing must be done, because if a therapeutic failure occurs (a) the lack of a culture may evoke medicolegal questions, and (b) choosing the second-guess antibiotic is very difficult. For example, if the patient does not improve on oral penicillin V, the therapeutic failure could be due to (a) lack of patient compliance or drug of substandard quality, (b) drug not reaching the site of active infection (bioavailability) after absorption, (c) drug not being absorbed, resulting in low blood levels (parenteral penicillin G may have been a better choice), (d) the infection being caused by penicillinase-producing staphylococci (a culture would now indicate a switch to cloxacillin or dicloxacillin), (e) the infection being caused by a gram-negative

microorganism that is not in the spectrum of penicillin V, (f) the microorganism being out of the spectrum of all penicillins, and perhaps another class of antibiotics is needed, (g) the organism being a resistant anaerobe, and the drug that should be used is clindamycin, and so on. Obviously, attempting to choose the second-guess antibiotic is a potential nightmare, and if that fails, further guesses are extremely difficult.

5. If the patient does not have a history of allergy to penicillins, a penicillin is the drug of "first choice by best guess" for most oral infections. A regimen of penicillin is started **pending culture and sensitivity tests.** Penicillin is the drug of choice for the usual dental infection because (a) bacterial invaders from the oral cavity are the usual causative agents of dental infection, and these invaders are generally susceptible to penicillin G or penicillin V, (b) penicillin has true selectivity, (c) penicillin has a wide margin of safety (this is related to b), and (d) penicillin is bactericidal.

For adult patients, and when the infection is severe, parenteral penicillin G may be best. A typical regimen is 600,000 to 1,000,000 units aqueous penicillin G combined with 300,000 to 600,000 units procaine penicillin G IM. This combination is repeated daily for 5 to 10 days. An alternative is one injection of the above combination of penicillin salts, followed 24 hours later by 500 mg penicillin V PO every six hours for 4 to 9 days. If the infection is severe but good drainage is obtained, or if the infection is less severe, oral penicillin V may be used without the injection. A typical course of therapy is 1 gm stat (immediately), then 500 mg every six hours for 5 to 10 days. Penicillin V, 500 mg stat followed by 250 mg every six hours, is suitable only for mild infections. Oral penicillin G may be used but is absorbed less reliably. Therefore, the dose is doubled, and patient compliance is absolutely necessary when prescribing oral penicillin G.

If the patient is allergic to penicillin, erythromycin is the first-guess drug to be used (erythromycin is discussed in Chapter 27).

6. The extended spectrum penicillins should not be used as the drugs of "first choice by best guess." If culture and sensitivity tests suggest these agents should be used, the dentist should switch to them. However, there is one situation where ampicillin might be chosen first; in a patient with a heart valve prosthesis and with a healthy mouth, ampicillin (alone) may be suitable to prevent bacterial endocarditis (p. 257).

7. The penicillinase-resistant penicillins are of value only for treatment of infections caused by penicillinase-producing staphylococci and, thus, are not the "first choice by best guess." Staphylococcal resistance develops rapidly and persists. Among the outpatient population, at least 15 to 20% of staphylococci are penicillin-resistant. In hospital employees and inpatients, 90 to 95% of staphylococci are penicillin resistant (Weinstein, 1975). More recently, Mandell and Sande (1980) claim that more than 50% of staphylococci are penicillin resistant in the outpatient population. Only two possibly acceptable reasons have been found for starting with a penicillinase-resistant penicillin: (1) one textbook (*Accepted Dental Therapeutics*, 1979) advocates starting with both a penicillinase-sensitive and a penicillinase-resistant agent and then withdrawing one or the other pending sensitivity tests, (2) still another textbook (Meyers et al., 1978) suggests that penicillin G or V should be combined with a penicillinase-resistant drug for treatment of infection caused by penicillinase-producing staphylococci because the penicillinase-resistant agent (they suggest methicillin, cloxacillin, or cephalosporins) will bind penicillinase and allow penicillin G or V to have its usual cidal effect.

M. PREVENTION OF BACTERIAL ENDOCARDITIS (BE)

Objective 26.M.1. Describe seven important and useful facts concerning BE.

Objective 26.M.2. Recognize eight different kinds of patients who may require prophylactic antibiotic coverage.

Objective 26.M.3. Describe the recommended antibiotic regimen available for use.

Although prevention of this serious disease involves the potential use of several different antibiotics, the penicillins are most often used. Therefore, this subject will be dealt with in some depth at this time.

Some useful facts concerning this disease (BE) are:

1. BE is one of the most serious complications of cardiac disease.
2. Mortality of BE is high once it is induced, but prophylaxis results in a very low incidence. (*Note:* the incidence is low, not completely prevented, and, therefore, patients must be closely followed after treatment.) Health professionals cannot do much about prophylactic failures, since no treatment known ever guarantees 100% cure or prevention of any disease. However, the dentist must provide coverage whenever needed, not only on ethical grounds but also because of moral considerations. In addition, failure to provide coverage can result in medicolegal action.
3. BE can occur in patients with **structural abnormalities of the heart and great vessels** (aorta, pulmonary artery, and vein and superior and inferior vena cava).
4. Manipulation of oral tissues, especially infected tissues, results in a high bacteremia. Since mastication can cause bacteremia in patients with periodontal diseases, continuous good oral hygiene must be encouraged.
5. Any procedure that causes bleeding can result in bacteremia, with possible initiation of BE. Two exceptions appear to be bleeding in association with the shedding of deciduous teeth and the simple adjustment of orthodontic appliances; there is no evidence that these can cause BE.
6. Local gingival degerming immediately before a procedure may protect a patient, but

degerming with irrigating devices may be dangerous because they have been shown to produce bacteremia (Kaplan et al., 1977).
7. Absolute indications; patients requiring prophylaxis include those with:
   a. Evidence of valvular heart damage. A history of rheumatic fever or scarlet fever makes the subject extremely suspect as a candidate for prophylaxis
   b. A previous episode of BE even in the absence of clinically detectable heart disease
   c. Structural abnormalities of the great vessels, including congenital heart disease and vascular grafts
   d. Heart valve prosthesis
8. Relative indications (consultation with physician is required):
   a. Indwelling, transvenous cardiac pacemakers
   b. Patient with implanted arteriovenous shunt appliance for dialysis
   c. Brain-to-heart shunts (ventriculoatrial) in patients with a history of hydrocephalus
   d. Patients with prosthetic joint replacements (induction of infection does not result in BE but, rather, a potential loss of the prosthetic joint)

Table 26–2 presents the recommended regimens for prophylaxis of BE.

N. ADDITIONAL INFORMATION CONCERNING BE

Objective 26.N.1. Describe additional information concerning BE that may be useful to the practice of dentistry.

1. The Committee on Prevention of Rheumatic Fever and Bacterial Endocarditis of the American Heart Association recommends parenteral administration when possible.
2. Patients who are taking low dose penicillin regularly to prevent recurrence of rheumatic fever can usually be successfully covered for BE prophylaxis by using the penicillin regimen outlined in Table 26-2 (increased dos-

TABLE 26-2. RECOMMENDED REGIMENS FOR PROPHYLAXIS OF BACTERIAL ENDOCARDITIS

Regimen A (for most patients)

Penicillin

1. *Parenteral-oral*
   Adults: 1,000,000 units aqueous penicillin G plus 600,000 units procaine penicillin G IM ½ to 1 hour before the procedure, then 500 mg penicillin V every 6 hours for 8 doses.
   Children: 30,000 units/kg aqueous penicillin G plus 600,000 units procaine penicillin G IM. Timing is the same as for adults. Oral penicillin V doses are also the same, except that children weighing less than 60 pounds should receive 250 mg doses.
2. *Oral (alternate therapy when compliance is assured)*
   Adults: 2 grams penicillin V PO ½ to 1 hour before the procedure, then 500 mg penicillin V every 6 hours for 8 doses.
   Children: Timing is the same as for adults. Penicillin V doses are also the same except that children weighing less than 60 pounds should receive 1 gm initially, and then 250 mg every 6 hours for 8 doses.

Erythromycin (for patients allergic to penicillin)

Adults: 1 gm PO 1½ to 2 hours before the procedure, then 500 mg every 6 hours for 8 doses.
Children: 20 mg/kg erythromycin, by mouth, then 10 mg/kg every 6 hours. Timing is the same as for adults.

Regimen B (for patients with heart valve prosthesis and as alternative to Regimen A)

Penicillin and streptomycin

Adults: 1,000,000 units aqueous penicillin G plus 600,000 units procaine penicillin G IM plus at another site, 1 gm streptomycin IM; both agents are given ½ to 1 hour before the procedure, then 500 mg penicillin V PO every 6 hours for 8 doses.
Children: 30,000 units/kg aqueous penicillin G plus 600,000 units procaine penicillin G IM; plus at another IM site, 20 mg/kg streptomycin. Timing is the same as for adults. Oral penicillin doses are also the same except that children weighing less than 60 pounds should receive 250 mg doses.

Vancomycin (for patients allergic to penicillin)

Adults: 1 gm vancomycin IV given over a ½ to 1 hour period by IV infusion. Start infusion ½ to 1 hour before the procedure, then 500 mg erythromycin orally every 6 hours for 8 doses.
Children: 20 mg/kg vancomycin IV. Oral erythromycin dose is 10 mg/kg. Timing is the same as for adults.

age). However, the dentist may choose to use the erythromycin regimen, which is also acceptable (the patient should probably stop the low dose penicillin while taking erythromycin). Another alternative is Regimen B, Table 26–2.

3. If healing is delayed, continued therapy may be necessary by extending the number of doses.
4. If the patient needs multiple appointments, the AHA recommends:

a. Use the usual penicillin regimen and schedule the appointments at least one week apart, OR
b. Alternate the penicillin regimen with the erythromycin regimen, without overlapping the drugs.

5. The authors suggest efficient use of appointment time during the period of coverage.

All practitioners are strongly urged to read the full committee report of the American

Heart Association (Kaplan et al., 1977) and the valuable additional information in the Journal of the American Dental Association (1978), which represents the responses of a committee of the American Heart Association to a number of inquiries submitted by several dentists.

REFERENCES

Accepted Dental Therapeutics, 38th ed. Chicago, American Dental Association, 1979, p 192

Juncher H, Raaschou F: The Solubility of oral preparations of penicillin V. Antibiot Med 4:497, 1957

Kaplan EL, Anthony BF, Bisno A, et al.: Prevention of bacterial endocarditis: A committee report of the American Heart Association. J Am Dent Assoc 95:600, 1977

Letter, J Am Dent Assoc 96:27, 1978

Mandell GL, Sande MA: Antimicrobial agents. In Gilman AG, Goodman LS, Gilman A (eds): Goodman and Gilman's The Pharmacological Basis of Therapeutics, 6th ed. New York, Macmillan, 1980, p 1132

Meyers FH, Jawetz E, Goldfien A: Review of Medical Pharmacology, 6th ed. Los Altos, CA, Lange Medical Publications, 1978, p 603

Moellering RD Jr, Swartz MN: Drug therapy: The newer cephalosporins. N Engl J Med 294:24, 1976

Root RK, Hierholzer WJ Jr: Infectious disease. In Melmon KL, Morelli HF (eds): Clinical Pharmacology: Basic Principals in Therapeutics, 2nd ed. New York, Macmillan, 1978, p 745

Weinstein L: Penicillins and cephalosporins. In Goodman LS, Gilman A (eds): The Pharmacological Basis of Therapeutics, 5th ed. New York, Macmillan, 1975, pp 1135, 1163

BIBLIOGRAPHY

Accepted Dental Therapeutics, 38th ed. Chicago, American Dental Association, 1979

Bevan JA (ed): Essentials of Pharmacology, 2nd ed. Hagerstown, MD, Harper & Row, 1976

Gilman AG, Goodman LS, Gilman A (eds): Goodman and Gilman's The Pharmacological Basis of Therapeutics, 6th ed. New York, Macmillan, 1980

Goth A: Medical Pharmacology, 10th ed. St. Louis, Mosby, 1981

Melmon KL, Morelli HF (eds): Clinical Pharmacology: Basic Principles in Therapeutics, 2nd ed. New York, Macmillan, 1978

Meyers FH, Jawetz E, Goldfien A: Review of Medical Pharmacology, 7th ed. Los Altos, CA, Lange Medical Publications, 1980

QUESTIONS

1. Penicillin G can be metabolized by:

    A. β-Lactamase
    B. amidase
    C. A and B are correct
    D. neither A nor B is correct

2. Penicillin V has a spectrum of activity that is best described as:

    A. broad spectrum
    B. entirely antifungal
    C. primarily gram negative
    D. primarily gram positive

3. The mechanism of action of penicillin is:

    A. disruption of cell membranes
    B. inhibition of bacterial protein synthesis
    C. inhibition of cell wall synthesis
    D. inhibition of nucleic acid synthesis

4. T F Ampicillin is considered to be a bacteriostatic antibiotic.

5. T F Dicloxacillin is thought to possess true selectivity against susceptible organisms.

6. T F Oral penicillin G is absorbed more completely in the presence of food than on an empty stomach.

7. T F Procaine penicillin G is a repository form of penicillin.

8. T F Penicillin V is generally absorbed more completely from the gastrointestinal tract than is penicillin G.

9. The drug of choice for the treatment of an infection caused by staphylococci that produce penicillinase is:

   A. ampicillin
   B. cloxacillin
   C. penicillin V
   D. ticarcillin

10. T F Penicillins reach adequate levels in the central nervous system but only in the presence of inflamed meninges.

11. T F All penicillins are extensively metabolized by the liver

12. T F Penicillin G is excreted primarily by glomerular filtration in the kidney.

13. T F Five hundred milligrams of penicillin G is approximately equal to 800,000 units.

14. Potential adverse effects of penicillins include:

   A. enteritis (supra-infection)
   B. nausea, vomiting, diarrhea
   C. supra-infection
   D. all of the above are correct
   E. none of the above is correct

15. T F The most dangerous potential side effect of penicillin G is an allergic reaction.

16. Oral allergic manifestations of penicillin therapy can include:

   A. furry tongue
   B. cheilosis
   C. stomatitis + glossitis
   D. all of the above are correct
   E. none of the above is correct

17. T F If a patient is allergic to penicillin V, he probably is not allergic to ampicillin.

18. T F Ampicillin can produce a skin rash that is not allergic in origin.

19. Other drugs that may interact with penicillin include:

   A. any aminoglycoside (strepto)
   B. probenecid
   C. tetracycline
   D. all of the above are correct
   E. none of the above is correct

20. T F Probenecid administration results in prolonged blood levels of penicillin G when they are given concomitantly.

21. T F A past history of allergic reaction to penicillin absolutely contraindicates its use again in the patient.

22. T F The dosage of penicillin G should be reduced in the presence of renal dysfunction.

23. T F Penicillin V therapy is all that is ever necessary to bring about cure of a dentoalveolar abscess that is susceptible to penicillins.

24. T F Culture and antibiotic sensitivity testing is not necessary, and the dentist only needs to begin penicillin therapy.

25. Penicillin G or penicillin V is the drug of choice to treat a dental infection, pending sensitivity tests because:

   A. bacterial invaders from the oral cavity are generally susceptible
   B. the agent has true selectivity
   C. the agent is bactericidal
   D. all of the above are correct
   E. none of the above is correct

26. T F When a patient reports a history of anaphylaxis to penicillin, one of the cephalosporins becomes the drug of choice pending culture and sensitivity tests.

27. T **F** All patients with a history of rheumatic fever or scarlet fever require antibiotic prophylaxis prior to a dental procedure.

28. **T** F Except for adjustment of orthodontic appliances, antibiotic prophylaxis is required prior to any dental procedure that may produce gingival bleeding.

29. T **F** Edentulous patients with valvular heart damage are free from risk of BE.

30. Patients who may require prophylaxis include those with:

    A. an indwelling, transvenous cardiac pacemaker

    B. a previous episode of BE in the absence of clinically detectable heart disease

    C. renal dialysis patients with implanted arteriovenous shunt appliances

    D. the presence of valvular heart damage

    E. all of the above are correct

    F. none of the above is correct

31. Other patients who may require prophylaxis include:

    A. a patient with an aortic graft

    B. hydrocephalic patients with a ventriculoatrial shunt

    C. a patient with a heart valve prosthesis

    D. a patient with a prosthetic joint replacement

    E. all of the above are correct

    F. none of the above is correct

32. T **F** When erythromycin is used for prophylaxis, it is usually given ½ to 1 hour before the procedure. *(1 ½ to 2 h)*

33. T F Oral vancomycin may be used in patients allergic to penicillin for BE prophylaxis.

34. T F Oral penicillin V is adequate for antibiotic prophylaxis in patients with a heart valve prosthesis.

35. Patients taking low dose penicillin therapy to prevent the occurrence of rheumatic fever may be adequately covered to prevent BE by the use of:

    A. regimen B

    B. the erythromycin regimen

    C. the usual penicillin regimen

    D. any one of the above is correct

    E. none of the above is correct

36. If a patient needs multiple appointments and the patient requires antibiotic prophylaxis, the dentist may:

    A. alternate the penicillin and erythromycin regimen

    B. use the usual penicillin regimen and schedule appointments at least one week apart

    C. either of the above is correct

    D. none of the above is correct

27

Alternatives to Penicillin

A. INTRODUCTION: PENICILLIN ALTERNATIVES

Objective 27.A.1. Recognize antimicrobial drugs that can be used as alternatives to penicillin.

This chapter will consider the pharmacology of alternatives to penicillin and will include discussions of erythromycins, cephalosporins, clindamycin, lincomycin, streptomycins, vancomycin, and chloramphenicol. There are two other possible alternatives to penicillin that will not be discussed in this chapter: (1) tetracyclines are presented in Chapter 28, and (2) sulfonamides and trimethoprim are discussed in Chapter 29. At the end of this chapter, we describe implications in dentistry and basis for selection, including all the alternative agents cited above.

B. ERYTHROMYCIN: SOURCE AND SPECTRUM OF ACTIVITY

Objective 27.B.1. Recognize source and spectrum of erythromycins.

Erythromycin is derived from *Streptomyces erythreus*. It has a primarily gram-positive spectrum of activity, much like penicillin G.

C. MECHANISMS OF ACTION AND RESISTANCE

Objective 27.C.1. Describe the mechanism of action of erythromycin.

Objective 27.C.2. Recognize whether erythromycin is a static or cidal antibiotic.

Objective 27.C.3. Recognize bacterial resistance and cross-resistance with erythromycin.

Erythromycin inhibits bacterial protein synthesis by binding to the 50S subunit of the ribosome. Erythromycin is considered to be a bacteriostatic antibiotic.

Bacteria become resistant to erythromycin relatively rapidly. This is one reason why erythromycin is usually not the drug of choice for the treatment of dental infections. (Can you think of another reason?) There is evidence of cross-resistance between lincomycins and erythromycin involving some strains of the *viridans* group of streptococci. There is complete cross-resistance between erythromycin and troleandomycin. Troleandomycin is not described further in this chapter; its pharmacology is very similar to erythromycin, and it is a less desirable agent than erythromycin.

D. ABSORPTION, DISTRIBUTION, METABOLISM, AND EXCRETION

Objective 27.D.1. Describe the absorption, distribution, metabolism, and excretion of erythromycin.

Peroral and parenteral forms are marketed. Erythromycin IM is quite painful and is, therefore, generally avoided, though the preparation is available. If parenteral therapy is necessary, IV administration is preferred.

Oral forms of the drug are marketed as the nonesterified form and as stearate, ethylsuccinate, or estolate esters. The different PO forms vary in absorption from the GI tract. For example, the presence of food tends to inhibit the absorption of the free base form of the drug, and gastric acid tends to destroy it. Absorption of the estolate or stearate esters or the acid-resistant, enterically coated preparations are not appreciably inhibited by food, and they are less likely to be destroyed by stomach acid. The presence of food inhibits the absorption of the ethylsuccinate ester, and this form is somewhat resistant to breakdown by gastric acid. Except for the estolate, the preparations are best administered on an empty stomach. Only the ethylsuccinate and estolate esters are available in pediatric formulations. Recent evidence has shown that the stearate or free base (nonesterified form) achieves higher blood levels of active drug even though the estolate was reported to be better absorbed (FDA Drug Bull, 1979). The higher blood levels of estolate ester are misleading because that form is less inactive. Moreover, the FDA (1979) proposed to start proceedings to ban the estolate from the marketplace be-

cause of the induction of cholestatic jaundice in some patients. Later, this proposal was rescinded (FDA, 1982), but the authors still believe that the estolate ester should not be used in dental practice because of the danger of cholestatic jaundice.

Erythromycin is distributed to all tissues and fluids. Except for the brain, tissue concentrations are higher than plasma concentrations.

Orally administered erythromycin is concentrated in the liver and secreted by the bile into the GI tract. Some drug is reabsorbed, but most is excreted in the feces (about 95%). Approximately 5% is excreted in the urine. Little or no metabolism takes place.

E. ADVERSE EFFECTS

Objective 27.E.1. Describe adverse effects of erythromycin.

1. **Allergic reactions,** including fever, eosinophilia, and skin eruptions. The estolate can produce a cholestatic hepatitis that has an allergic basis. The onset of hepatitis occurs in 10 to 20 days, regresses when erythromycin estolate is withdrawn and, of course, recurs with an additional challenge of the drug.
2. **Epigastric distress** is a prominent side effect of oral erythromycin. When it occurs, the practitioner should advise the patient to take the drug closer to mealtimes, with a light snack, such as tea and crackers, with milk, or as an enteric-coated preparation.
   (*Note:* these recommendations are also usually useful when patients are taking other drugs on an empty stomach and require adjustment because of gastrointestinal distress.)
3. **Thrombophlebitis** frequently occurs with IV administration of the drug.
4. **Ototoxicity** occurs with high IV doses but is reversible. In addition, large oral doses of the estolate derivative have produced a transient ototoxic effect. A with streptomycins, high-frequency tones are lost initially. Audiometric studies are advised when using high IV dosages.
5. **Supra-infections** can occur, but they are uncommon.

F. CONTRAINDICATIONS AND DRUG INTERACTIONS

Objective 27.F.1. Recognize two contraindications to erythromycin therapy.

Contraindications include the following:

1. Erythromycin, especially the estolate, is contraindicated in patients with liver dysfunction. No precautions are necessary when treating patients with renal dysfunction.
2. Erythromycin is contraindicated in those patients who are allergic to the drug.

Objective 27.F.2. Recognize drugs that may interact with erythromycin.

Drug interactions include the following:

1. Lincomycin, clindamycin, or chloramphenicol may be mutually antagonistic with erythromycin.
2. Effects of penicillin or cephalosporins will be antagonized with the concurrent use of erythromycin.
3. Erythromycin can cause increased blood levels of theophylline, probably by inhibiting theophylline's metabolism. (Theophylline is sometimes used for patients with bronchial asthma.)

G. CEPHALOSPORINS: CHEMISTRY, SOURCE, AND SPECTRUM OF ACTIVITY

Objective 27.G.1. Describe the chemistry, source, and spectrum of activity of cephalosporins.

The basic structure of the cephalosporins is quite similar to the penicillins (Fig. 27–1). Both contain a β-lactam ring, which for cephalosporins is attached to a six-sided sulfur-containing ring (penicillins have a five-sided sulfur-containing ring). An amide linkage is also present, connecting the β-lactam ring to R groups. By referring to Figure 26–1 (p. 254) and comparing this to the structure of cephalothin sodium (Fig.

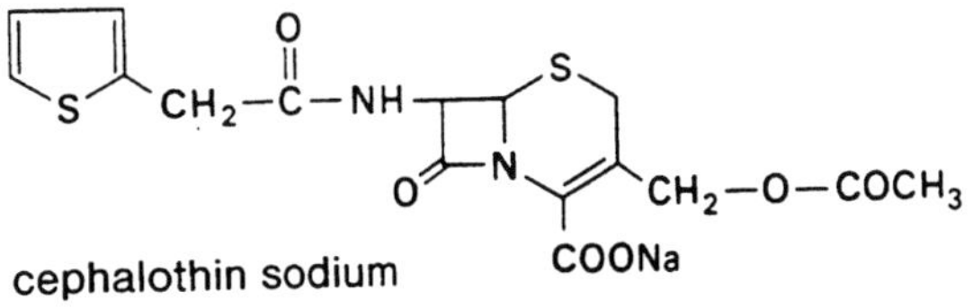

cephalothin sodium

Figure 27–1. Chemical structure of cephalothin sodium. (*From Csáky TZ: Cutting's Handbook of Pharmacology, 6th ed, 1979. Courtesy of Appleton-Century-Crofts.*)

27–1), the chemical similarities and differences can be visualized and remembered.

The first agent to be marketed was cephalothin sodium, and Table 27–1 compares some features of most of the currently available cephalosporin derivatives.

Cephalosporium acremonium was the initial source of cephalosporins. All the marketed agents are semisynthetic derivatives of a subunit of cephalosporin C, which was originally isolated.

Except for enterococci, the older cephalosporins have a spectrum of activity that is approximately equal to that of extended-spectrum penicillins, e.g., ampicillin. There are some minor differences between agents, but the differences are not too important in clinical dentistry. **Cefamandole**, cefotaxime, and cefoxitin (this is not technically a cephalosporin, but its pharmacology is similar to that of cephalosporins) are unique in that they (1) have significantly more activity in the gram-negative spectrum and (2) are resistant to breakdown by all β-lactamases, both penicillinases and cephalosporinases. The three agents are available for parenteral use only and should be reserved for the two special properties just cited.

H. MECHANISM OF ACTION AND RESISTANCE

Objective 27.H.1. Recognize the mechanism of action of cephalosporins.

Objective 27.H.2. Recognize whether cephalosporins are static or cidal.

Erythromycin
Interactions - Penicillin Lincomycin Clindamycin Chloramphenicol Cephalosporin Theophilline

TABLE 27-1. FEATURES OF CEPHALOSPORINS

Agent	Spectrum	Route of Administration	β-lactamase Activity
cephalothin (*Keflin*) *	extended	IV	susceptible
cefazolin (*Ancef, Kefzol*)	extended	IM; IV	susceptible
cephapirin (*Cefadyl*)	extended	IV	susceptible
cephaloridine (*Loridine*)	extended	IM; IV	susceptible
cephalexin (*Keflex*)	extended	peroral	susceptible
cephradine (*Velosef, Anspor*)	extended	peroral	susceptible
cephaloglycin (*Kafocin*)	extended	peroral	susceptible
cefamandole (*Mandol*)	broad	IM; IV	resistant
cefotaxime (*Claforan*)	broad	IM; IV	resistant
cefoxitin (*Mefoxin*)	broad	IM; IV	resistant
cefaclor (*Ceclor*)	extended	peroral	susceptible
cefadroxil (*Duricef*)	extended	peroral	susceptible

* In this and the following table of Chapter 27, only the drugs set in boldface should be memorized. The others are presented for reference purposes.

Objective 27.H.3. Recognize the theory of bacterial resistance to cephalosporins.

All cephalosporins act by inhibiting bacterial cell wall synthesis as do the penicillins. See Chapter 25 for a more complete description. Cephalosporins are considered to have bactericidal activity.

Resistance to the drug does occur. One of the primary reasons is the elaboration of β-lactamases, which split the β-lactam ring. Cephalosporinases tend to effectively split all cephalosporin β-lactam rings (except for cefamandole, cefotaxime, and cefoxitin), and some, but not all, penicillinases are also active. Resistance when it does occur seems to develop more often in gram-negative strains or staphylococci.

I. ABSORPTION, DISTRIBUTION, METABOLISM, AND EXCRETION

Objective 27.I.1. Recognize the absorption, distribution, metabolism, and excretion of cephalosporins.

Cephalothin, cephaloridine, and cefamandole are poorly absorbed from the GI tract because they are all acid-labile. Conversely, cephalexin is acid-stable and well absorbed from the GI tract, and, therefore, it is often used in dentistry. Table 27–1 will serve as a reference concerning features of other cephalosporins if another is chosen.

The agents penetrate most tissues and fluids (except for the eye and cerebrospinal fluid) about as well as do the penicillins. Therefore, although an organism isolated from CSF may be susceptible in vitro to a cephalosporin, in vivo there will be no effect because of lack of penetration, even in the presence of inflamed meninges.

Not much is known about the metabolism of these agents. Apparently some metabolism takes place in the liver.

All the drugs are excreted primarily by the kidney, much as are the penicillins, and dosage reductions are required in the presence of renal failure. As with the penicillins, probenecid blocks the excretion of cephalosporins.

J. ADVERSE EFFECTS

Objective 27.J.1. Recognize adverse effects of the cephalosporins.

1. Cephaloridine can be nephrotoxic, as can cephalothin but to a lesser degree. However, when any cephalosporin is combined with any one of the nephrotoxic aminoglycoside antibiotics, there may be an increased incidence and degree of nephrotoxicity. This

synergistic effect can also occur in the presence of polymyxin B or colistin, in the presence of vancomycin, or when the potent diuretics furosemide or ethacrynic acid are combined with cephalosporins.

2. Granulocytopenia has been recorded, and an occasional case of hemolysis of red cells associated with a positive Coombs' test.
3. Local pain and induration at the site of an IM injection and phlebitis after IV administration have occurred.
4. Peroral preparations occasionally produce nausea, vomiting, and diarrhea.
5. Supra-infections (generally gram-negative) can occur. The frequency is probably more than with penicillin G but less than that found with the use of the broad-spectrum agents.
6. A full range of allergic reactions has been recorded, much like the penicillins, but few data are available. Cross-allergenicity between cephalosporins and penicillins is somewhat controversial. This is discussed quite thoroughly in Chapter 26 (p. 259), and the reader is urged to review this important topic at this time.

K. CONTRAINDICATIONS AND DRUG INTERACTIONS

Objective 27.K.1. Describe contraindications and drug interactions of cephalosporins.

Contraindications include the following:

1. Cephalosporins should not be administered to patients with a prior history of allergy to these drugs.
2. Dosages may have to be reduced in those patients with renal failure.
3. A nephrotoxic effect can more readily occur in patients with renal damage, and it can occur when these drugs are taken concurrently with vancomycin, aminoglycosides, polymyxin B, or colistin, or the potent diuretics, furosemide and ethacrynic acid.

Drug interactions include the following:

1. Probenecid inhibits the renal excretion of cephalosporins.
2. Cephalosporins probably would be antago-

nized when combined with erythromycin, lincomycins, tetracyclines, and chloramphenicol.

L. LINCOMYCINS: SOURCE AND SPECTRUM OF ACTIVITY

Objective 27.L.1. Recognize the source and spectrum of activity of lincomycins.

Lincomycin was isolated from *Streptomyces lincolnensis.*

The spectrum of activity of lincomycin or clindamycin is very similar to erythromycin, i.e., primarily gram-positive. However, clindamycin is a more active drug, and its spectrum also includes primarily gram positive anaerobes. Of the two drugs, clindamycin is considered more useful in dentistry. Thus, clindamycin is discussed primarily, and lincomycin is mentioned only for comparison.

M. MECHANISM OF ACTION

Objective 27.M.1. Recognize the mechanism of action of clindamycin.

Objective 27.M.2. Recognize whether clindamycin is a static or cidal antibiotic.

Clindamycin inhibits bacterial protein synthesis by binding to the bacterial 50S subunit of the ribosome.

Clindamycin is considered to be a bacteriostatic antibiotic, but cidal activity can be achieved at high dosages.

N. ABSORPTION, DISTRIBUTION, METABOLISM, AND EXCRETION

Objective 27.N.1. Recognize the absorption, distribution, metabolism, and excretion of clindamycin.

Clindamycin is well absorbed when administered PO, and the presence of food has little effect on absorption. Lincomycin should normally be given by injection because of less gastrointestinal absorption.

Clindamycin is distributed to most tissues and fluids of the body, including bone, although little drug makes its way to cerebrospinal fluid, even in the presence of inflamed meninges.

The liver participates in the metabolism of clindamycin, and antibacterial metabolites are produced, including an N-demethylated derivative. Metabolites are excreted via the urine and feces.

About 10% of a dose of clindamycin is excreted unaltered in the urine. The presence of renal dysfunction does not require adjustment of dosage, but severe hepatic failure can result in marked accumulation of the drug.

O. ADVERSE EFFECTS

Objective 27.O.1. Describe adverse effects that can occur with the use of clindamycin.

1. About 10% of treated individuals report a skin rash that has an allergic basis.
2. Other allergic reactions that can occur (though rarely) include angioedema, serum sickness, and anaphylactic shock.
3. Nausea and diarrhea are frequent problems.
4. The incidence of supra-infection is low but greater than that produced by erythromycin.
5. Uncommon reactions include exudative erythema multiforme, granulocytopenia, and thrombopenia.
6. Thrombophlebitis often occurs with IV administration.
7. Cardiovascular collapse can occur with rapid IV infusion of lincomycin.
8. The lincomycins can produce a neuromuscular blockade, especially in conjunction with neuromuscular blocking agents.
9. The induction of pseudomembranous colitis is a dangerous effect that can occur with the use of lincomycins [perhaps this should be called simply "colitis" because the adverse effect can occur with or without pseudomembranes (Med Lett Drugs Ther, 1979)]. The successful management of this problem has been difficult. Because of the life-threatening nature of the problem, we describe, chronologically, some attempts to manage or prevent this side effect.

a. The incidence of pseudomembranous colitis with the use of clindamycin was thought to be low compared to the incidence with lincomycin. More recent evidence suggests the exact opposite (Med Lett Drugs Ther, 1979).
b. At the first sign of severe diarrhea, if the drug is withdrawn, most, if not all, patients will revert toward normal and not progress to colitis. This statement by George et al. (1979a) is probably correct.
c. The concurrent use of most antidiarrheal agents with lincomycin or clindamycin is dangerous. Some examples of antidiarrheal preparations are paregoric, loperamide (*Imodium*), diphenoxylate plus atropine (*Lomotil*).
d. At least one source (Kreutzer and Milligan, 1978) has suggested that PO cholestyramine may be useful in reducing diarrhea and colitis by binding a bacterial exotoxin.
e. Information from at least one laboratory (Tedesco et al., 1978) suggests that the colitis is caused by an exotoxin produced by strains of *Clostridium difficile* that are resistant to lincomycins. They recommend that PO vancomycin, administered every six hours for seven days, will inhibit the resistant microorganisms and solve the problem. One advantage of vancomycin therapy is that the drug is not absorbed when given PO, and, therefore, side effects are avoided.
f. More recent evidence in laboratory animals suggests that upon withdrawal of vancomycin therapy, colitis may recur. Similar results have occurred in humans, but a second course of vancomycin therapy has been successful (George et al., 1979b).

P. CONTRAINDICATIONS AND DRUG INTERACTIONS

Objective 27.P.1. Describe contraindications to lincomycins.

Objective 27.P.2. Recognize potential drug interactions.

Contraindications include the following:

1. Patients with a history of allergy to either clindamycin or lincomycin.
2. Reduced dosage or decreased frequency of administration is necessary in the presence of severe hepatic failure.

Drug interactions include the following:

1. Erythromycin and chloramphenicol may be mutually antagonistic with the lincomycins.
2. Cyclamates cause a decreased absorption of lincomycin and possibly clindamycin.
3. Kaolin-pectin preparations decrease the absorption of lincomycin and possibly clindamycin.
4. An enhanced neuromuscular blocking effect can occur when the lincomycins are used concurrently with neuromuscular blocking agents, certain general anesthetics, aminoglycosides, polymyxin B, and colistin.

Q. STREPTOMYCINS: SOURCE AND SPECTRUM OF ACTIVITY

Objective 27.Q.1. Recognize the chemical group name, source, spectrum, and type of activity of streptomycins.

Streptomycin is an aminoglycoside containing three units: (1) a sugar (streptose), (2) a base (streptidine), and (3) an aminosaccharide (N-methyl-l-glucosamine). Streptomycin is the prototype agent and is described. Effects and side effects of the other aminoglycosides are essentially the same. Streptomycins are considered cidal agents. Streptomycin was originally isolated from *Streptomyces griseus*.

Streptomycin's spectrum of activity is considered to be broad and includes the tubercle bacillus. The other aminoglycosides have a similar spectrum of activity. Often, when a new aminoglycoside was introduced, it was capable of inhibiting a microorganism(s) that became resistant to a previously marketed agent. However, with increased use of the new agent, resistance developed. The knowledge of the exact spectrum of each agent probably is not very useful in dentistry, where these agents have very limited usefulness.

TABLE 27–2. PREPARATIONS OF AMINOGLYCOSIDES

Official Name	Trade Name
amikacin	Amikin
gentamicin	Garamycin
kanamycin	Kantrex
neomycin	Various manufacturers
paromomycin	Humatin
streptomycin	Various manufacturers
tobramycin	Nebcin

When streptomycins are combined with penicillins or cephalosporins, a synergistic effect occurs. Apparently, the latter agents allow not only broadening of the spectrum but also more easy entry of streptomycins into bacterial cells, resulting in increased cidal activity. However, there is one disadvantage of one type of combination: when streptomycins are combined with cephalosporins, enterococci remain out of the spectrum of activity. Table 27–2 lists the names of available aminoglycosides.

R. MECHANISM OF ACTION AND RESISTANCE

Objective 27.R.1. Describe the mechanism of action of streptomycins.

Objective 27.R.2. Recognize whether streptomycin is a static or cidal antibiotic.

Objective 27.R.3. Describe the theory of bacterial resistance to streptomycin.

Streptomycin binds to 30S subunits of bacterial ribosomes and inhibits protein synthesis. A misreading of the genetic code can occur, and some bacteria, instead of being inhibited, become dependent on the presence of streptomycin. However, this property is of no value clinically, because once the drug is withdrawn, the microorganisms readapt and no longer require the drug.

At low concentrations, the drug is bacteriostatic, but at the higher concentrations usually employed, the drug is bactericidal.

Resistance to the drug can occur, and sometimes it occurs quite readily. Resistance occurs by three mechanisms: (1) prevention of entrance of the drug into the cell, (2) blockade of binding of the drug on the ribosome, and (3) production of metabolizing enzymes that result in phosphorylation, adenylation, or acetylation of the aminoglycoside. Amikacin is resistant to phosphorylation and adenylation.

S. ABSORPTION, DISTRIBUTION, METABOLISM, AND EXCRETION

Objective 27.S.1. Recognize the absorption, distribution, metabolism, and excretion of streptomycin.

Streptomycins (and other aminoglycosides) are not absorbed from the GI tract because of their highly charged, polycationic structure. Therefore, the aminoglycosides must be administered parenterally. Deep IM injections are used, with the use of different injection sites on alternate days. The drugs are occasionally administered PO in an attempt to sterilize the GI tract prior to GI tract surgery. Streptomycin gains access to most extracellular fluids, but access to the CNS is considered to be poor.

Some metabolism may occur because, when the agent is administered, 10 to 30% of the drug is not accounted for in excretory material. However, there are no data available outlining the metabolism of streptomycin.

Streptomycin is excreted primarily by the kidney and almost entirely by glomerular filtration.

T. ADVERSE EFFECTS

Objective 27.T.1. Recognize adverse effects of streptomycin.

1. Although uncommon, a full range of allergic reactions has been recorded with the use of this drug.
2. Pain at the site of IM injection frequently occurs, as well as formation of sterile abscesses that are often accompanied by fever.
3. Damage to the eighth cranial nerve can occur (ototoxicity), including both the auditory and vestibular portions. The vestibular division is apparently more susceptible. The damage is usually reversible, but irreversible damage has been recorded occasionally. Damage consists of disruption of ability to maintain one's balance and loss of hearing. The high-pitched tones are the first to be lost, and, for that reason, most patients are unable to detect the loss. Frequent audiometric measurements are strongly recommended with long-term treatment, i.e., more than one week in duration.
4. Peripheral neuritis and paresthesia may occur.
5. Streptomycin is capable of producing neuromuscular junction blockade, and the probability of a dangerous blockade increases with the concurrent use of neuromuscular junction blocking drugs and certain general anesthetics that have this same property. Patients with myasthenia gravis or chronic obstructive pulmonary disease are particularly at risk.
6. Nephrotoxicity can occur, and the incidence and severity are increased in the presence of prior renal damage or when streptomycins are used with other nephrotoxic agents (see the following). The nephrotoxic reaction is hastened in the presence of acidic urine, and alkalinization of the urine may afford some protection.

U. CONTRAINDICATIONS AND DRUG INTERACTIONS

Objective 27.U.1. Recognize contraindications and drug interactions of streptomycin.

1. Aminoglycosides are contraindicated in patients with a prior history of allergy. Although there are no data to support cross-allergenicity between agents, cross-allergenicity is very possible because of their chemical similarity.
2. The drugs should be used with caution in patients with myasthenia gravis.

3. Streptomycins should be used with caution in patients with a history of renal damage. There may be an increased nephrotoxic effect when streptomycin is used concurrently with other aminoglycosides, furosemide or ethacrynic acid, cephalosporins, polymyxin B or colistin, and vancomycin. *neomycin*

4. There may be an increased ototoxic effect with the concurrent use of streptomycin and other aminoglycosides, with the potent diuretics furosemide and ethacrynic acid, with high doses of erythromycin, or with the use of vancomycin. *neomycin*

5. There may be an increased neuromuscular blocking effect when streptomycin is combined with other aminoglycosides, lincomycins, polymyxin B, colistin, neuromuscular blocking agents, or general anesthetics.

6. Anticholinergic drugs or antihistamines that are used to treat motion sickness may mask vestibular damage caused by the streptomycins.

7. Aminoglycosides and tetracyclines may be mutually antagonistic because they bind at the same site on the ribosome.

V. VANCOMYCIN

Objective 27.V.1. Describe the mechanism of action and spectrum of activity of vancomycin.

Objective 27.V.2. Recognize the absorption, distribution, and excretion of vancomycin.

Objective 27.V.3. Recognize adverse effects and potential drug interactions.

Vancomycin inhibits bacterial cell wall synthesis. For a more complete discussion of this topic, see Chapter 25. The drug is considered to have bactericidal activity. Vancomycin's spectrum of activity is primarily gram-positive organisms.

With PO administration, little or no drug is absorbed. This agent should be administered IV. Its distribution is much like that of penicillin, and vancomycin will appear in CSF when the meninges are inflamed.

The drug is excreted in urine by the kidney, and the presence of renal dysfunction results in very high blood levels.

Known adverse effects include:

1. allergy, virtually every type, from rash to anaphylaxis
2. phlebitis and pain at the injection site
3. a shocklike state during an IV infusion
4. ototoxicity, mostly auditory
5. nephrotoxicity

Potential drug interactions include the following:

1. increased ototoxicity when combined with aminoglycosides, potent diuretics, and very high dosages of erythromycin
2. increased nephrotoxicity when combined with aminoglycosides, potent diuretics, cephalosporins, and polymyxin B or colistin

W. CHLORAMPHENICOL

Objective 27.W.1. Describe the mechanism of action and spectrum of activity of chloramphenicol.

Objective 27.W.2. Recognize the absorption, distribution, metabolism, and excretion of chloramphenicol.

Objective 27.W.3. Recognize adverse effects and drug interactions.

Chloramphenicol produces its inhibitory effect on bacteria by inhibiting bacterial protein synthesis. The drug binds to the 50S ribosomal subunit, much like lincomycin and erythromycin. Chloramphenicol is considered to be a bacteriostatic antibiotic.

Chloramphenicol has a broad spectrum of activity including inhibitory effects on rickettsiae.

Absorption of chloramphenicol from the GI tract is considered to be rapid, and it penetrates virtually all tissues and fluids, including brain and CSF.

Liver metabolism occurs, producing hydrolysis products and glucuronide conjugates. When administered PO, about 5 to 10% of the drug is excreted by the kidney in an unchanged form, and the remaining portions in the urine are metabolites.

Adverse effects include the following:

1. allergic reactions, including
   a. skin rashes
   b. fever
   c. angioedema
   d. spontaneous hemorrhage of skin and mucosal linings, including the oral cavity
   e. atrophic glossitis
   f. Herxheimer reaction
   g. pancytopenia, leukopenia, thrombopenia, and aplastic anemia (potentially lethal)
2. nausea, vomiting, diarrhea, unpleasant taste
3. blurred vision
4. digital paresthesias
5. supra-infection, including oropharyngeal candidiasis and staphylococcal enterocolitis
6. inhibition of liver microsomal enzymes

Potential drug interactions include the following:

1. Erythromycin or lincomycin may be mutually antagonistic with chloramphenicol.
2. Chloramphenicol may antagonize the effect of penicillins or cephalosporins.
3. Increased anticoagulant effects may occur when oral anticoagulants are combined with chloramphenicol.
4. There may be an enhanced hypoglycemic response when used concurrently with oral antidiabetic drugs.
5. Chloramphenicol may inhibit the metabolism of phenytoin.

X. IMPLICATIONS IN DENTISTRY AND BASIS FOR SELECTION

Objective 27.X.1. Describe implications in dentistry and basis for selection of alternative antibiotics.

1. Erythromycin is the drug of choice for dental infections in patients who are allegic to penicillin. It is also the secondary drug to prevent bacterial endocarditis (BE) in penicillin-aller-

gic patients. Adults should be given either the free base or stearate ester; pediatric patients should be given the ethylsuccinate ester.

Reasons for not selecting erythromycin as the drug of choice instead of penicillin are:
   a. the drug does not possess true selectivity (Chapter 25).
   b. erythromycin is considered to be a bacteriostatic drug.
   c. many microorganisms rapidly become resistant to the drug. Nevertheless, erythromycin is an excellent drug which is useful to the dentist. However, except in patients allergic to penicillin, this and other antibiotics should not be used as the drugs of choice unless culture and sensitivity testing suggest one of them as the best agent.

2. If a patient is allergic to both penicillin and erythromycin, the choice of drug is a difficult decision to make on a clinical basis prior to results of culture and sensitivity testing. Presently, we believe one of the cephalosporins should be used. However, the choice does not include cefamandole, cefotaxime, or cefoxitin. These three agents should be reserved for special cases that require the unique properties of the drugs (e.g., resistance to β-lactamases and significant gram-negative spectrum) and when sensitivity testing suggests that they are the agents to be used. The authors recommend cephalexin because it is one of the better PO forms, and it currently has the lowest price. At one time, clindamycin was recommended, but because of its toxicity, this choice can no longer be supported.

Tetracycline might be considered the drug of choice in patients allergic to penicillin and erythromycin, especially if the use of cephalosporin is contraindicated (pp. 259 and 271). Tetracyclines are discussed in Chapter 28.

Recently, the authors have noted an increased number of recommendations by cardiologists for the use of sulfamethoxazole plus trimethoprim (*Bactrim, Septra*) for prophylaxis of BE in those patients who are allergic to both penicillin and erythromycin and require coverage. The authors believe that, in addition to the latter use, these agents may also be considered (Cawson and Spector, 1975) as drugs of choice for the treatment of dental infections in patients with similar allergic histories, pending culture and sensitivity tests. This is further discussed in Chapter 29.

3. Tetracycline could become the drug of choice for dental infections, pending sensitivity tests, for the following reasons:
   a. opening into the maxillary sinus
   b. compound fracture of the jaws
   c. traumatic injuries
   d. for certain periodontal patients whose disease does not respond to scaling and curettage alone

   The rationale for these recommendations is based on the possibility that the infection may be caused by bacteria that are not ordinarily found in most other dental infections (which are usually caused by gram-positive organisms).

4. Streptomycin has a special use in dentistry; it is given along with one of the penicillins to prevent BE in dental patients who have a heart valve prosthesis. Otherwise, streptomycin should be reserved for the treatment of tuberculosis.

   Despite streptomycin's toxic effects (neuromuscular junction blockade, nephrotoxicity, and ototoxicity), there is very little risk when it is used according to the regimen recommended in Table 26–2 and along with the cautions given on page 274.

5. Vancomycin also has a special use in dentistry. It is used IV as an alternative to penicillin-streptomycin in those patients who are allergic to penicillin.

   In Chapter 26 (Table 26–2), the use of vancomycin to prevent BE was discussed. The regimen for use of vancomycin IV includes a dose of 1.0 gm given as an infusion over a ½ to 1 hour period. According to Krogstad et al. (1980), a dose of that magnitude may not be well tolerated. Their data suggest that adequate blood levels are achieved with 500 mg. Higher doses, 700 to 1000 mg, produced numerous toxic effects in two subjects, while those given 500 mg reported no side effects. At 1000 mg, side effects included tachycardia, pruritis at the site of injection, and generalized flushing (these are probably due to a histamine reaction). At 700 mg, the subjects experienced nausea, palpitations, substernal pressure, and lightheadedness.

6. Clindamycin or choramphenicol, both of which can produce dangerous toxic effects, should be used only when indicated by microbial sensitivity testing. These drugs should never be used pending the results of such tests.

   Clindamycin and chloramphenicol may be the only useful antibiotics for some infections caused by anaerobes, especailly *Bacteroides fragilis*. A third agent, metronidazole (a synthetic antimicrobial drug, Chapter 29), is also a possible choice for the treatment of anaerobic infections, including colitis.

   The authors believe that clindamycin therapy can be managed by the dentist. As soon as significant diarrhea occurs (more than five stools per day), clindamycin therapy should be discontinued, thereby avoiding the development of colitis, which may be lethal (George et al., 1979a). Clindamycin may be chosen for therapy of osteomyelitis based not only on results of sensitivity testing but also on clindamycin's ability to concentrate in bone.

   The use of chloramphenicol requires close medical monitoring of both blood cytology and chemistry before, during, and after therapy. For that reason, chloramphenicol should probably be administered by the patient's physician.

REFERENCES

Cawson RA, Spector RG: Clinical Pharmacology in Dentistry. Edinburgh, Churchill Livingstone, 1975, p 29

Csáky TZ: Cutting's Handbook of Pharmacology, 6th ed. New York, Appleton-Century-Crofts, 1979, p 18

FDA Drug Bull 9:26, 1979

George WL, Rolfe RD, Mulligan ME, Finegold SM: Infectious diseases 1979—Antimicrobial agents-induced colitis: an update. J Infect Dis 140:266, 1979a

George WL, Volpicelli NA, Stiner DB, et al.: Relapse of pseudomembranous colitis after vancomycin therapy. N Engl J Med 301:414, 1979b

Kreutzer EW, Milligan FD: Treatment of antibiotic-associated pseudomembranous colitis with cholestyramine resin. Johns Hopkins Med J 143:67, 1978

Krogstad DJ, Moellering RD Jr, Greenblatt DJ: Single-dose kinetics of intravenous vancomycin. J. Clin Pharmacol 20:197, 1980

Med Lett Drugs Ther 21:97, 1979

Moellering RC Jr, Swartz MN: Drug therapy: The newer cephalosporins. N Engl J Med 294:24, 1976

Tedesco F, Markham R, Gurwith M, Christie D, Bartlett JG: Oral vancomycin for antibiotic-associated pseudomembranous colitis. Lancet 2:226, 1978

Weinstein L: Penicllins and cephalosporins. In Goodman LS, and Gilman A (eds): The Pharmacological Basis of Therapeutics, 5th ed. New York, Macmillan, 1975, p 1163

BIBLIOGRAPHY

Accepted Dental Therapeutics, 38th ed. Chicago, American Dental Association, 1979, Sec II, Antimicrobial agents

Bevan JA (ed): Essentials of Pharmacology, 2nd ed. Hagerstown, MD, Harper & Row, 1976, Ch 55, 56, 57, 58

Gilman AG, Goodman LS, Gilman A (eds): Goodman and Gilman's The Pharmacological Basis of Therapeutics, 6th ed. New York, Macmillan, 1980, Ch 50, 51, 52, 54

Goth A: Medical Pharmacology, 10th ed. St. Louis, Mosby, 1981, Ch 53

Melmon KL, Morelli HF (eds): Clinical Pharmacology: Basic Principles in Therapeutics, 2nd ed. New York, Macmillan, 1978, Ch 14

Meyers FH, Jawetz E, Goldfien A: Review of Medical Pharmacology, 7th ed. Los Altos, CA, Lange, 1980, Ch 49, 50, 51, 54

QUESTIONS

1. Under certain conditions, all of the following drugs can be used as possible alternates to penicillin *except:*

   A. a cephalosporin
   B. erythromycin
   C. chloramphenicol
   D. tetracycline
   E. vidarabine

2. **T** F Erythromycin is an antibiotic with a spectrum of activity that is similar to that of penicillin G.

3. T **F** Erythromycin's mechanism of action is inhibition of cell wall synthesis.

4. T **F** Erythromycin is a cidal antibiotic.

5. **T** F Bacteria become resistant to erythromycin relatively rapidly.

6. **T** F Erythromycin (base) and the stearate ester are best absorbed from the GI tract.

7. T **F** Erythromycin is excreted primarily by the kidneys.

8. Adverse effects of erythromycin include:

   A. allergic reactions
   B. epigastric distress
   C. ototoxicity, with high dosages
   D. all of the above are correct
   E. none of the above is correct

9. **T** F Erythromycin estolate is contraindicated in patients with liver dysfunction.

10. **T** F Lincomycin, clindamycin, and chloramphenicol may be mutually antagonistic.

11. T **F** The spectrum of activity of cephalosporins is essentially the same as cloxacillin.

12. T **F** Cephalosporins are thought to inhibit bacterial protein synthesis.

13. **T** F Cephalosporins are classified as bactericidal agents.

14. **T** F With regard to cephalosporins, the elaboration of bacterial β-lactamases is thought to be the major cause of development of resistant strains.

15. **T F** All cephalosporins are absorbed from the GI. tract and are excreted mainly in the feces.

16. Adverse effects of cephalosporins consist of:

   A. allergy
   B. nausea and vomiting
   C. granulocytopenia
   D. all of the above are correct
   E. none of the above is correct

17. **T F** If patients have renal failure, the dosage of cephalosporins must be reduced.

18. **T F** Cephalosporins will probably be antagonized with the concurrent use of tetracyclines.

19. **T F** Lincomycin has a spectrum of activity that is similar to penicillin G.

20. **T F** Clindamycin inhibits bacterial protein synthesis and is generally considered to be a static antibiotic.

21. **T F** The liver participates in the metabolism of clindamycin, and an active N-demethylated derivative is often formed.

22. **T F** Lincomycin is capable of producing neuromuscular junction blockade.

23. **T F** The most feared toxic effect of lincomycin or clindamycin is colitis.

24. **T F** Reduced dosages of clindamycin are required in patients with severe hepatic failure.

25. **T F** Kaolin-pectin preparations decrease the absorption of lincomycin.

26. **T F** Streptomycin is a broad-spectrum antibiotic.

27. **T F** Streptomycin inhibits bacterial protein synthesis, yet the drug is considered to be bactericidal.

28. **T F** Streptomycin is rapidly and completely absorbed from the gastrointestinal tract.

29. **T F** Streptomycin's excretion is almost entirely by the kidneys.

30. Streptomycin's adverse effects include:

   A. nephrotoxicity
   B. neuromuscular junction blockade
   C. ototoxicity
   D. all of the above are correct
   E. none of the above is correct

31. **T F** Streptomycin is contraindicated in patients with myasthenia gravis.

32. **T F** Scopolamine or diphenhydramine could mask vestibular damage caused by streptomycin.

33. **T F** Vancomycin inhibits cell wall synthesis.

34. **T F** Little or no vancomycin is absorbed from the gastrointestinal tract.

35. Adverse effects of vancomycin include:

   A. allergy
   B. nephrotoxicity
   C. ototoxicity
   D. all of the above are correct
   E. none of the above is correct

36. **T F** When vancomycin is combined with erythromycin, an increased nephrotoxicity can occur.

37. **T F** Chloramphenicol inhibits bacterial protein synthesis, and the drug has a narrow spectrum of activity.

38. **T F** Chloramphenicol is rapidly absorbed from the gastrointestinal tract.

39. All of the following are adverse effects of chloramphenicol *except:*

    A. aplastic anemia
    B. leukocytosis
    C. pancytopenia
    D. thrombocytopenia

40. **T F** Increased anticoagulant effects may occur when oral anticoagulants are combined with chloramphenicol.

41. **T F** Erythromycin stearate is a possible drug of choice to treat dental infections in patients who are allergic to penicillin.

42. **T F** If a patient is allergic to both penicillin and erythromycin, the drug of choice (pending sensitivity tests) is clindamycin.

43. Tetracycline may become the drug of choice when patients:

    A. are allergic to both penicillin and erythromycin
    B. have a compound fracture of the jaw
    C. have oral infections encroaching on the maxillary sinus.
    D. have traumatic injuries
    E. all of the above are correct
    F. none of the above is correct

44. **T F** Streptomycin and vancomycin are used exclusively in dentistry to prevent BE in patients with a heart valve prosthesis

45. **T F** Due to their toxic effects, both clindamycin and chloramphenicol are used only when absolutely necessary.

28
Tetracycline

A. INTRODUCTION

Following the introduction of penicillin and streptomycin, tetracyclines were the third class of antibiotics introduced as antimicrobial agents. Chlortetracycline was the first derivative that was isolated and marketed, and six other preparations followed (Table 28–1).

Since the pharmacology of all the agents is so similar, we will discuss tetracycline as the prototype and cite important differences where applicable. Major differences are due to absorption and elimination, which influence the duration of action and dosage chosen.

B. CHEMISTRY AND SPECTRUM OF ACTIVITY

Objective 28.B.1. Recognize the chemistry of tetracycline.

Objective 28.B.2. Recognize the spectrum of activity of tetracycline.

Tetracyclines contain four fused 6-sided rings (a hydronaphthalene skeleton) as a basic unit,

with various side groups attached (See Figure 28–1 for the structure of tetracycline.)

Tetracyclines have a broad spectrum of activity, including many gram-positive and gram-negative organisms. The spectrum also includes rickettsiae and amebae.

C. MECHANISM OF ACTION AND RESISTANCE

Objective 28.C.1. Describe the mechanism of action of tetracyclines.

Objective 28.C.2. Describe whether tetracyclines are static or cidal antibiotics.

Objective 28.C.3. Describe the theory of resistance to tetracyclines.

Tetracyclines inhibit bacterial protein synthesis by binding to the 30S subunit of the ribosome, similar to streptomycin (see Chapter 25 for a more complete discussion of this mechanism).

In general, tetracyclines are considered as

TABLE 28–1. SOME FEATURES OF TETRACYCLINES

Agent	Major Elimination	t½ (hours)	Dosage Range
chlortetracycline HCl (*Aureomycin*)*	renal	6–9	250–500 mg q6h
demeclocycline HCl (*Declomycin*)	renal	16	150–300 mg q6h
doxycycline hyclate (*Vibramycin*)	hepatic	17–20	100 mg q12h first day, then 100 mg/day or q12h
methacycline HCl (*Rondomycin*)	renal	16	150 mg q6h or 300 mg q12h
minocycline HCl (*Minocin, Vectrin*)	hepatic/renal	17–20	200 mg stat, then 100 mg q12h
oxytetracycline HCl (*Terramycin*)	renal	6–9	250–500 mg q6h
tetracycline HCl (various manufacturers)	renal	6–9	250–500 mg q6h

* Memorize drugs set in bold type.

bacteriostatic antibiotics. However, cidal effects can occur against certain organisms at higher therapeutic dosages.

Microorganisms that become resistant to one tetracycline are often (but not always) resistant to another derivative, demonstrating a high degree of cross-resistance between drugs. Organisms involved are frequently gram-negative strains. The resistance is apparently carried by an R factor and ultimately results in exclusion of the drug from the bacterial cell. Gram-positive organisms have also become resistant to tetracyclines.

D. PHARMACOKINETICS

Objective 28.D.1. Recognize the absorption, distribution, metabolism, and excretion of tetracyclines.

Tetracyclines are usually given PO but are poorly absorbed by this route. Two exceptions are doxycycline, which is absorbed about as well orally as parenterally, and minocycline, which is almost completely absorbed from the GI tract. The only other method of administration recommended is the IV route.

With the exception of doxycycline, and to a degree with minocycline, the presence of food inhibits the absorption of all other tetracycline derivatives, and the presence of divalent or trivalent cations markedly inhibits the absorption

of all derivatives due to chelation. Examples of cations most often cited are aluminum, iron, calcium, and magnesium, but generally all divalent and trivalent cations are involved. Substances containing cations, such as antacids, milk, other dairy products, laxatives, and mineral preparations, should be avoided when taking tetracyclines. In addition, sodium bicarbonate interferes with absorption by increasing stomach pH, causing precipitation of the agents.

Tetracyclines are distributed to essentially all tissues and body fluids, including teeth and bones, and, with the exception of doxycycline and minocycline, apparently are excreted unchanged.

Excretion of chlortetracycline, demeclocycline, methacycline, oxytetracycline, and tetracycline is mostly by the kidney, despite the fact

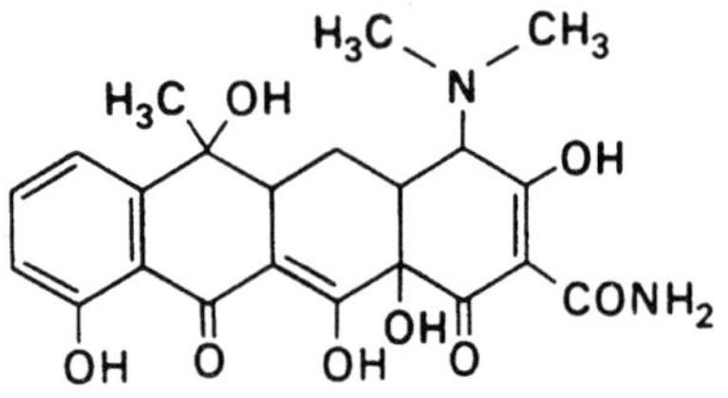

Figure 28–1. Chemical structure of tetracycline. (*From Csáky TZ: Cutting's Handbook of Pharmacology, 6th ed, 1979. Courtesy of Appleton-Century-Crofts.*)

that the liver tends to concentrate all the derivatives. Doxycycline is excreted mostly in feces via the liver and bile, whereas minocycline excretion is somewhere between the two extremes.

Elimination rate (t½) is different for each agent, this results in categorization into three groups (see Table 28–1). Agents with a half-life of 6 to 9 hours include chlortetracycline, oxy-tetracycline, and tetracycline. Demeclocycline and methacycline have a half-life of about 16 hours, while doxycycline and minocycline have half-lives of 17 to 20 hours.

E. ADVERSE EFFECTS

Objective 28.E.1. Recognize adverse effects of tetracyclines.

Adverse effects include the following:

1. A full range of allergic reactions including dermatologic reactions, black hairy tongue, cheilosis, glossitis, serum sickness, and anaphylaxis. Cross-allergenicity between agents is thought to occur.
2. Gastric irritation and diarrhea; colitis may occur but apparently at a much lower frequency than with clindamycin therapy.
3. Thrombophlebitis following IV use.
4. With long-term use, leukocytosis, atypical lymphocytes, granulation of granulocytes, and thrombocytopenic purpura.
5. Phototoxicity (a sunburnlike reaction when patients taking the drug are exposed to sunlight), although uncommon, has been reported mostly with the use of demeclocycline but also with oxytetracycline and, to a lesser degree, with tetracycline.
6. Hepatotoxicity can occur with high doses, especially during pregnancy. There is less hepatotoxicity with oxytetracycline and tetracycline.
7. Worsening of existing renal disease, with the exception of doxycycline.
8. Increased excretion of riboflavin, folic acid, and amino acids with a negative nitrogen balance. This effect is thought to be antian-

abolic and is probably an extension of the mechanism of action.
9. The appearance of Fanconi syndrome, including renal damage, with the use of outdated drug.
10. Reversibe increased intracranial pressure.
11. Induction of vestibular toxicity by minocycline.
12. Increased incidence of supra-infection due to the broad spectrum of activity. Three types of supra-infection predominantly reported are:
    a. candidiasis,
    b. staphylococcal infection, and
    c. gram-negative microbial infection.
13. Delay of blood coagulation, possibly due to tetracycline forming a calcium chelate in blood.
14. Effects on teeth and bones. These have been extensively reported and studied. Tetracyclines deposit on developing and remodeling bone, producing a fluorescent product that can be used as a tag or label during bone growth. A similar complex (probably a calcium orthophosphate complex) forms when tetracyclines interact with developing teeth. The reaction produces permanent staining of teeth that may be yellow to brown or gray to black with fluorescence under ultraviolet light. There is evidence that these teeth have increased caries susceptibility. Some recent techniques have been published in an attempt to rid tooth structure of the stain. To our knowledge, all are considered temporary treatments, though some newer methods may achieve longer durations. Full crown coverage can be performed, but much sound tooth structure is often destroyed. Laminate veneers have recently been introduced which may be applied with acid-etch techniques.

In addition to increased caries susceptibility, the esthetic damage to enamel can be severe. For this reason, tetracycline therapy should be avoided during the last trimester of pregnancy and in infancy and childhood to at least 8 years old. Many authors recommend the drugs be avoided until the age of 12.

F. CONTRAINDICATIONS AND PRECAUTIONS

Objective 28.F.1. Recognize contraindications and precautions of tetracyclines.

1. Tetracyclines should not be administered during pregnancy.
2. They should be avoided in children 8 to 12 years old and younger (unless they are the **only** agents indicated).
3. Except for doxycycline, the tetracyclines should be avoided in the presence of renal disease.
4. Caution is advised when using tetracyclines for prophylactic reasons (Sande and Mandell, 1980).
5. Outdated tetracyclines should be destroyed, as breakdown products may cause Fanconi's syndrome.
6. Caution is advised when performing surgical procedures on patients taking tetracyclines because of increased anticoagulant effects.

G. DRUG INTERACTIONS

Objective 28.G.1. Recognize drug interactions of the tetracyclines.

1. Tetracyclines may antagonize penicillins and cephalosporins.
2. Sodium bicarbonate inhibits absorption.
3. All divalent and trivalent cations inhibit absorption. Substances that contain significant levels of these cations include milk, dairy products, antacids, laxatives, and vitamin-mineral or mineral preparations. If these preparations must be used, tetracyclines should be administered 1 to 2 hours before the cationic preparation.
4. Chronic ethanol ingestion causes increased metabolism of doxycycline.
5. Oxytetracycline may enhance the effect of antidiabetic drugs.

6. Barbiturates, many nonbarbiturate sedative-hypnotics, carbamazepine, and phenytoin may increase the metabolism of doxycycline.
7. Tetracyclines should be avoided in patients taking diuretics.
8. When tetracycline is combined with corticosteroids, a severe supra-infection may occur.
9. Tetracyclines plus oral anticoagulant drugs may cause an increased anticoagulant effect. Tetracycline by itself may increase bleeding time, due to Ca^{++} chelation in blood and/or inhibition of vitamin K-producing enteric bacteria.

H. BASIS FOR SELECTION AND USE

Objective 28.H.1. Recognize the basis for selection and use of tetracyclines.

1. In general, when a tetracycline drug is needed, we recommend the use of tetracycline hydrochloride because it is lower in price than other derivatives. Tetracycline hydrochloride should be taken four times a day, which is a disadvantage in patients who do not comply. For such patients, one of the longer-acting derivatives, such as doxycycline, may be a better choice (see Table 28–1).
2. If a tetracycline is needed in a patient with kidney dysfunction, doxycycline should be used (see item 3, Section 28.F.1.).
3. Tetracycline may be considered a possible drug of choice in a patient allergic to both penicillin and erythromycin, pending sensitivity tests (see the discussion at the end of Chapter 27, p. 276).
4. Tetracycline may be used as the drug of choice, pending sensitivity tests, in patients with infections caused by organisms that are ordinarily foreign to the oral cavity because of:
   a. opening into the maxillary sinus
   b. compound fracture of the jaws
   c. traumatic injuries
5. Tetracycline is being recommended for use more frequently for the treatment of certain

types of periodontal disease. Rationale for use is based on positive results in some clinical studies, i.e., treatment outcomes (using only tetracycline) that are comparable to scaling and prophylaxis with no drug treatment (Listgarten et al.: 1978). However, according to Genco (1981), tetracycline therapy is recommended in adults with refractory periodontal disease, i.e., little or no response to conventional periodontal therapy, in patients with juvenile periodontitis (periodontosis), and in patients with a systemic disease which may contribute to the worsening of periodontal disease (e.g., diabetes mellitus).

REFERENCES

Csáky TZ: Cutting's Handbook of Pharmacology, 6th ed. New York, Appleton-Century-Crofts, 1979, p 29

Genco RJ: Antibiotics in the treatment of human periodontal disease. J Periodontol 53:545, 1981

Listgarten MA, Lindhe J, Hellden L: Effect of tetracycline and/or scaling on human periodontal disease. J Clin Periodontol 5:246, 1978

Sande MA, Mandell GL: Tetracyclines and chloramphenicol. In Gilman AG, Goodman LS and Gilman A (eds): Goodman and Gilman's The Pharmacological Basis of Therapeutics, 6th ed. New York, Macmillan, 1980, p 1189

BIBLIOGRAPHY

Accepted Dental Therapeutics, 38th ed. Chicago, American Dental Association, 1979, Sec II, Antimicrobial agents

Bevan JA (ed): Essentials of Pharmacology, 2nd ed. Hagerstown, MD, Harper & Row, 1976, Ch 57

Gilman AG, Goodman LS, Gilman A (eds): Goodman and Gilman's The Pharmacological Basis of Therapeutics, 6th ed. New York, Macmillan, 1980, Ch 52

Goth A: Medical Pharmacology, 10th ed. St. Louis, Mosby, 1981, Ch 53

Melmon KL, Morelli HF (eds): Clinical Pharmacology: Basic Principles in Therapeutics, 2nd ed. New York, Macmillan, 1978, Ch 14

Meyers FH, Jawetz E, Goldfien A: Review of Medical Pharmacology, 7th ed. Los Altos, CA, Lange, 1980, Ch 50

QUESTIONS

1. **T F** Tetracyclines (hydronaphthalenes) are thought to possess a broad spectrum of activity.

2. Tetracyclines are thought to:
   A. disrupt cell membranes
   B. inhibit bacterial protein synthesis
   C. inhibit cell wall synthesis
   D. inhibit nucleic acid synthesis
   E. interfere with intermediary metabolism

3. **T F** Tetracyclines are, in general, thought to be bactericidal agents.

4. **T F** Resistance to tetracyclines occurs exclusively with gram-negative bacteria.

5. **T F** All tetracyclines are rapidly and completely absorbed.

6. Factors that may interfere with the absorption of tetracycline include:
   A. antacids
   B. dairy products
   C. laxatives
   D. all of the above are correct
   E. none of the above is correct

7. **T F** Tetracyclines are excreted primarily by the kidney, except doxycycline, which appears primarily in feces.

8. **T F** Minocycline is capable of inducing vestibular toxicity.

9. **T F** Tetracyclines should be avoided during pregnancy and in children up to 8 to 12 years old to prevent permanent tooth stains.

10. The tetracycline that produces the highest incidence of phototoxicity is:

   A. chlortetracycline
   B. demeclocycline
   C. doxycycline
   D. minocycline
   E. tetracycline

11. T F Dental patients taking tetracycline may experience a delay of blood coagulation during oral surgery.

12. T F Except for doxycycline, tetracyclines should be avoided in the presence of renal disease.

13. T F A synergistic antibacterial effect occurs when a combination of penicillin and tetracycline is used.

14. Increased metabolism of doxycyline may occur if the patient also ingests:

   A. alcohol, chronically
   B. carbamazepine
   C. pentobarbital
   D. phenytoin
   E. all of the above are correct
   F. none of the above is correct

15. T F Tetracycline may be an acceptable drug to treat certain patients with periodontal disease.

29

Sulfonamides and Other Synthetic Antimicrobials

A. INTRODUCTION

The sulfonamides (sulfa drugs) were the first really useful antimicrobials introduced into medicine. The first human treated with a sulfa drug was an infant, and the treatment took place in 1933. The child was treated with *Prontosil*, an azo dye, which later was found to be inactive in vitro. The active component of *Prontosil* is sulfanilamide, and it is generated by liver metabolism. A French group from the Pasteur Institute (1935) was responsible for this research, and, in 1936, they demonstrated that the newly synthesized metabolite (sulfanilamide) was as effective as *Prontosil* in vivo in addition to being active in vitro. Many derivatives have been synthesized since that time, especially during the decade following this discovery.

B. CHEMISTRY AND SPECTRUM OF ACTIVITY

Objective 29.B.1. Recognize the chemistry and spectrum of activity of the sulfa drugs.

Sulfanilamide (*p*-aminobenzenesulfonamide) contains an aromatic ring with an SO_2NH_2 attached and an NH_2 group in the *para* position. As stated previously, sulfanilamide is an active metabolite of *Prontosil*, and it is derived from liver azo-reduction, as shown in Figure 29–1. All other congeners are derivatives of sulfanilamide.

The sulfa drugs are considered to have a broad spectrum of activity.

C. MECHANISM OF ACTION AND RESISTANCE

Objective 29.C.1. Recognize the mechanism of action of sulfa drugs.

Objective 29.C.2. Recognize whether the sulfa drugs are static or cidal antibiotics.

Objective 29.C.3. Recognize the theory of development of resistance.

The sulfa drugs inhibit bacteria by competing with *p*-aminobenzoic acid (PABA) for the synthesis of folic acid. Many, but not all, bacteria

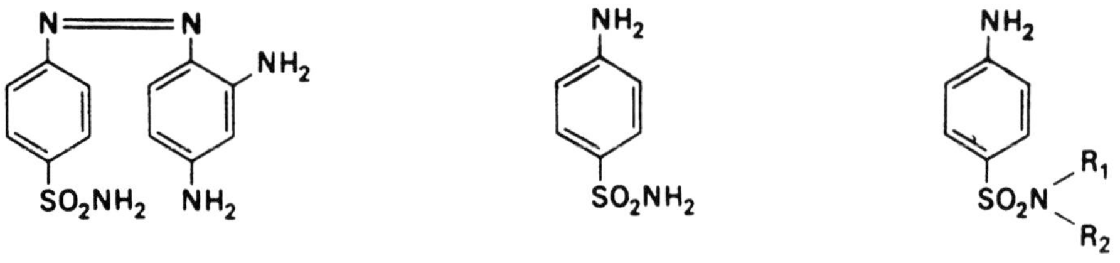

Prontosil   sulfanilamide   derivatives

Figure 29–1. Structure of antibacterial sulfonamides. (*From Csáky TZ: Cutting's Handbook of Pharmacology, 6th ed, 1979. Courtesy of Appleton-Century-Crofts.*)

must synthesize folic acid, which is needed as an intermediate in important biosynthetic reactions. The drugs are, therefore, more selective against microorganisms than humans, which require preformed folic acid. For comparison of the structure of sulfanilamide with that of PABA, see Figure 29–2.

The sulfa drugs are considered to be bacteriostatic agents. Bacteria have become resistant to the drugs, either by bacterial production of large amounts of PABA or by destruction of the sulfa.

D. PHARMACOKINETICS

Objective 29.D.1. Recognize the absorption, distribution, metabolism, and excretion of sulfa drugs.

Sulfa drugs are used almost exclusively as PO agents. They have some topical indications and occasionally are used IV.

Sulfasalazine and phthalylsulfathiazole are poorly absorbed from the GI tract and are used either to treat GI tract infections or to attempt sterilization of the tract prior to bowel surgery (Table 29–1). All other agents are rapidly absorbed.

The drugs, when absorbed, are distributed to all tissues and fluids, including the CNS. However, blood, pus, and tissue breakdown products of wounds tend to inhibit the action of sulfa drugs because they are rich in PABA. The degree of protein binding varies with each agent and is in the range of 20 to 90%.

Both acetylation and oxidation of the sulfa drugs take place in the liver. There is some evidence that many toxic effects, including allergic effects, may be due to the oxidation products. However, in most cases, the acetylated derivatives are the major metabolic products, and they are more likely than the oxidation products to produce crystalluria. (NOTE: the active drug can also produce crystalluria.)

The sulfa drugs, when absorbed, are excreted almost entirely by the kidney. Glomerular filtration is the primary mechanism, but some active secretion also occurs, depending on the drug. There is a varying rate of excretion of sulfa drugs (Table 29–1), which accounts for their differences in duration.

E. ADVERSE EFFECTS

Objective 29.E.1. Recognize adverse effects of sulfa drugs.

1. Acute hemolytic anemia (which occurs when glucose-6-phosphate dehydrogenase is absent

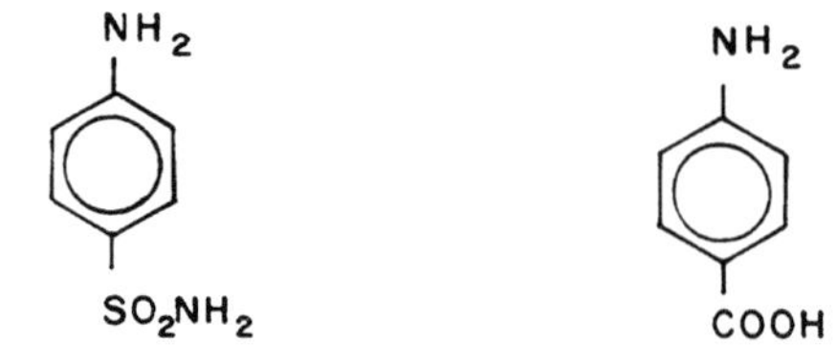

sulfanilamide   PABA

Figure 29–2. Chemical structures of sulfanilamide and PABA.

TABLE 29–1. SOME FEATURES OF SULFA DRUGS

Feature	Preparation
Short acting rapid absorption, rapid excretion	**sulfadiazine** sulfacytine sulfamethizole **sulfisoxazole** (*Gantrisin* and others)
Intermediate acting rapid absorption, more slowly excreted	**sulfamethoxazole** (*Gantanol*)
Long acting rapid absorption, slowly excreted	sulfameter* sulfamethoxypyridazine*
Poorly absorbed	phthalylsulfathiazole (*Sulfathalidine*) sulfasalazine (*Azulfidine* and others)
Topical preparations	mafenide (*Sulfamylon Cream*) for burns silver sulfadiazine (*Silvadene*) for burns sulfacetamide (*Bleph* and others), ophthalmic

* No longer available in the United States.

from red cells), agranulocytosis, aplastic anemia, thrombocytopenia, and eosinophilia.

2. Crystalluria and renal damage can be much reduced or avoided by using the more soluble sulfa derivatives, by increasing fluid intake to produce a daily urine volume of at least 1200 ml, by alkalinizing the urine, thus favoring solubility of the agents within the genitourinary tract, and by using triple sulfa preparations. Trisulfapyrimidine USP, containing sulfadiazine, sulfamerazine, and sulfamethazine, is an example of a triple sulfa. The rationale for use of triple sulfa therapy to prevent crystalluria is that each agent is independently soluble in urine, yet the low dose of each agent allows a therapeutic dose (by addition or summation) and development of adequate blood levels.

3. Allergic reactions can occur, and, in fact, the sulfa drugs rank second to penicillins in frequency of production of allergies. Reactions

reported include skin and mucous membrane lesions, vascular lesions, including lesions in the heart, serum sickness, drug fever, and anaphylaxis. There is some cross-allergenicity between agents. An increased frequency of allergic reactions occurs with the use of long-acting agents, and, therefore, they should be avoided.

4. Hepatitis, hypothyroidism with or without goiter, arthritis, neuropsychiatric disturbances, and peripheral neuritis.

5. Anorexia, nausea, and vomiting.

F. CONTRAINDICATIONS AND PRECAUTIONS

Objective 29.F.1. Recognize contraindications and precautions for sulfa drugs.

1. Resistant organisms
2. History of allergy

G. DRUG INTERACTIONS

Objective 29.G.1. Recognize drug interactions.

1. PABA local anesthetics (e.g., procaine) may antagonize the sulfa effect.
2. Sulfa may increase the anticoagulant effect of oral anticoagulants.
3. Enhanced hypoglycemia occurs when used with antidiabetic drugs (which are sulfa derivatives).
4. Sulfas may reduce the bioavailability of digoxin.
5. Methenamine compounds increase the incidence of crystalluria.
6. Sulfa drugs may displace methotrexate from plasma protein binding sites.
7. Sulfa drugs may inhibit the oral absorption of oxacillin.
8. There may be an increased phenytoin effect when combined with sulfa drugs.
9. There is a markedly potentiated inhibitory effect on bacteria when sulfamethoxazole is combined with trimethoprim.

$$\text{Dihydropteridine + PABA} \xrightarrow{\text{sulfa}} \text{dihydropteroic acid + glutamate} \longrightarrow$$

$$\text{folic acid} \longrightarrow \text{dihydrofolic acid} \xrightarrow{\text{trimethoprim}} \text{tetrahydrofolic acid}$$

(the active component)

Scheme 29–1.

H. SULFAMETHOXAZOLE PLUS TRIMETHOPRIM (*Bactrim, Septra*)

This is also referred to as co-trimoxazole.

Objective 29.H.1. Recognize the pharmacology of sulfamethoxazole plus trimethoprim.

Synergistic activity against susceptible microorganisms occurs when these two drugs are administered concurrently. They act as sequential enzyme inhibitors in the same metabolic pathway in bacteria. Trimethoprim is thought to be about 20 times more potent than the sulfa derivative with regard to inhibition of the pathway. The enzyme affected by trimethoprim is dihydrofolate reductase, and it is thought that the bacterial enzyme is 50,000 times more sensitive to trimethoprim than is the human enzyme (see Scheme 29–1).

When 400 mg of sulfamethoxazole is combined with 80 mg of trimethoprim, the resultant blood level is about 20 and 1 μg/ml respectively, the optimal ratio of drug in plasma (remember, trimethoprim is 20 times more potent than sulfamethoxazole). Although the drugs are absorbed and excreted at slightly different rates, after the first dose and with constant dosing, the 20:1 ratio is essentially maintained.

Most of the adverse effects produced by the combination are due to the sulfa derivative. Exceptions include (1) the possibility of folate deficiency occurring with the combination, (2) increase in frequency of skin reactions, (3) increased risk of thrombocytopenia in patients taking diuretics, and (4) permanent renal function impairment in patients with renal disease.

Ingestion of adequate amounts of water is advised when this combination is used (see above).

I. IMPLICATIONS FOR DENTISTRY

Objective 29.I.1. Recognize implications of sulfa drug use in dentistry.

There are three possible uses of the sulfa drugs in dentistry, and, in all cases, the combination of sulfamethoxazole plus trimethoprim is preferred (Cawson and Spector, 1975).

1. Prophylactically, to prevent BE in patients allergic to both penicillin and erythromycin
2. When the results of culture and sensitivity testing suggest sulfamethoxazole plus trimethoprim be used and especially when alternative antibiotics may be more toxic
3. As a possible drug of choice (behind penicillin and erythromycin) to treat dental infections in patients allergic to both penicillin and erythromycin, pending results of sensitivity tests

J. METRONIDAZOLE (*Flagyl*)

Metronidazole is a chemical that was used primarily in the United States for the treatment of trichomonal vaginitis.

In Europe, the drug is used also for acute necrotizing ulcerative gingivitis (Cawson and Spector, 1975) and for the treatment of clindamycin- or chloramphenicol-resistant anaerobic infections. Concerning the latter indication, metronidazole was tested in the US and recently approved by the FDA for use because tests have shown that it is effective (Med Lett Drugs Ther, 1979). These reports are encouraging because there might be instances in which metronidazole may be needed to control certain dental infections, especially those caused by penicillin-resistant strains of *Bacteroides fragilis.*

One major disadvantage of using metronidazole is its carcinogenicity in mice. Furthermore, the urine of patients containing the excreted drug is capable of causing genetic changes in bacteria (Med Lett Drugs Ther, 1979). Therefore, metronidazole should be used only when necessary and with the lowest dose and shortest duration possible.

REFERENCES

Cawson RA, Spector RG: Clinical Pharmacology in Dentistry. Edinburgh, Churchill Livingstone, 1975, pp 29–30

Csáky TZ: Cutting's Handbook of Pharmacology, 6th ed. New York, Appleton-Century-Crofts, 1979, p 2

Med Lett Drugs Ther 21:89, 1979

BIBLIOGRAPHY

Bevan JA (ed): Essentials of Pharmacology, 2nd ed. Hagerstown, MD, Harper & Row, 1976

Gilman AG, Goodman LS, Gilman A (eds): Goodman and Gilman's The Pharmacological Basis of Therapeutics, 6th ed. New York, Macmillan, 1980

Goth A: Medical Pharmacology, 10th ed. St. Louis, Mosby, 1981

Melmon KL, Morelli HF (eds): Clinical Pharmacology: Basic Principles in Therapeutics, 2nd ed. New York, Macmillan, 1978

Meyers FH, Jawetz E, Goldfien A: Review of Medical Pharmacology, 7th ed. Los Altos, CA, Lange, 1980

QUESTIONS

1. **T F** The sulfa drugs are thought to have a broad spectrum of activity.

2. **T F** Sulfa drugs inhibit bacteria by competing with *p*-aminobenzoic acid for the synthesis of folic acid.

3. **T F** Blood, pus, and tissue breakdown products tend to inhibit the action of sulfa drugs.

4. Most allergenic manifestations of sulfa drugs are produced by:

    A. acetylated sulfa derivatives

    B. oxidation products of sulfa

    C. sulfa itself

    D. all of the above are correct

    E. none of the above is correct

5. **Adverse effects of sulfa drugs include:**

    A. acute hemolytic anemia

    B. allergy

    C. crystalluria

    D. all of the above are correct

    E. none of the above is correct

6. **T F** One contraindication to the use of sulfa drugs is the presence of resistant strains.

7. **T F** PABA may antagonize sulfa's antibacterial effect.

8. **T F** Methenamine tends to increase sulfa's crystalluric effect.

9. **T F** Synergism results from the use of a combination of sulfamethoxazole and trimethoprin, because both drugs act on the same metabolic pathway in bacteria.

10. **T F** It is possible and rational to use sulfamethoxazole plus trimethoprim prophylactically to prevent BE in patients allergic to both penicillin and erythromycin.

30

Topical Antibiotics, Antifungals, and Antivirals

A. INTRODUCTION TO TOPICAL ANTIBIOTICS

Objective 30.A.1. Describe potential uses of topical antibiotics in dentistry.

Objective 30.A.2. Recognize two topical antibiotics that may be useful in dentistry.

Objective 30.A.3. Recognize two topical antibiotics that should not be used in dentistry.

Topical antibiotics (antibacterials) often are available alone or in combination, and may have some utility during the course of dental practice. However, such use has been questioned.

Potential indications or uses may be (1) necrotizing ulcerating gingivitis, (2) following deep scaling and curettage, (3) infected traumatic ulcers, (4) intraoral burns, (5) pericoronitis, and (6) alveolitis.

The most frequently used topical antibiotics are **bacitracin, polymyxin B,** neomycin, and tyrothricin. All are either poorly absorbed or not absorbed after oral administration, and all are fairly toxic when administered parenterally.

The first two agents (bacitracin and polymyxin B) are extremely poorly absorbed, including from mucous membranes. The latter two agents (neomycin and tyrothricin) can reach significant blood levels from mucous membranes, especially if the membranes are inflamed or if a recent surgical procedure has been done. When the latter agents are absorbed, hemolysis can occur with tyrothricin and ototoxicity and nephrotoxicity with neomycin. For these reasons, tyrothricin and neomycin are not further discussed in this chapter; the dentist is urged not to employ them topically.

B. CHEMISTRY AND SPECTRUM OF ACTIVITY

Objective 30.B.1. Recognize the general chemical structure of bacitracin and polymyxin B.

Objective 30.B.2. Recognize the spectrum of activity of bacitracin and polymyxin B.

Bacitracin is a polypeptide antibiotic and it is marketed as the zinc salt or free base. There is some evidence that the presence of zinc in-

TABLE 30–1. TOPICAL ANTIBACTERIAL AGENTS

Drugs	Spectrum	Mechanism of Action	Possible Uses in Dentistry
bacitracin	primarily gram positive	inhibits cell wall synthesis	necrotizing ulcerative gingivitis, following deep scaling and curettage, infected traumatic ulcers, intraoral burns, pericoronitis or alveolitis
polymyxin B	primarily gram negative	disrupts bacterial cell membranes	

creases the bactericidal activity of this antibiotic. Bacitracin has a spectrum of activity that is primarily gram positive.

Polymyxin B is one of a number of polymyxin antibiotics and is related chemically to colistin (polymyxin E). Polymyxin B is a peptide antibiotic, and its spectrum of activity is primarily gram negative.

C. MECHANISM OF ACTION

Objective 30.C.1. Describe the mechanism of action of bacitracin and polymyxin B.

Objective 30.C.2. Recognize whether bacitracin and polymyxin B are static or cidal agents.

Bacitracin inhibits cell wall synthesis by a different mechanism than penicillins (Chapter 25). Bacitracin is a bactericidal antibiotic.

Polymyxin B is a cationic detergent, and the agent disrupts bacterial cell membranes, resulting in increased permeability of the cell membrane. Polymyxin B is considered to be a bactericidal antibiotic (Table 30–1).

D. ABSORPTION AND EXCRETION

Objective 30.D.1. Recognize the absorption and excretion of bacitracin and polymyxin B.

Negligible absorption of bacitracin and polymyxin B takes place when either agent is applied to oral mucous membranes, and they are poorly absorbed even when swallowed. Both agents are excreted in the feces when given PO.

E. ADVERSE EFFECTS

Objective 30.E.1. Recognize adverse effects of bacitracin and polymyxin B.

Bacitracin has essentially no adverse effects because of almost complete lack of absorption of the agent when applied topically. Only hypersensitivity reactions have been infrequently reported.

Similarly, polymyxin B has essentially no adverse effects because of the almost complete lack of absorption when applied topically. Hypersensitivity reactions have been uncommonly reported, but nausea, vomiting, and diarrhea can occur if high doses are taken perorally. However, when either agent is administered systemically, a number of toxic effects occur (e.g., bacitracin: nephrotoxicity; polymyxin B: nephrotoxicity and NMJ blockade). Since the authors do not believe that either agent should be used parenterally in dentistry, the numerous untoward effects when these agents are given parenterally will not be considered.

F. THERAPEUTIC USE, BASIS FOR SELECTION, AND IMPLICATIONS FOR DENTISTRY

Objective 30.F.1. Describe dental implications for bacitracin and polymyxin B.

As cited previously, the use of topical antibiotics in dentistry has been questioned. If topical antibacterial therapy is used, it should be limited to bacitracin and polymyxin B alone or in combination. Combination products often also

TABLE 30-2. ANTIFUNGAL AGENTS

Drugs	Spectrum	Mechanism of Action	Uses in Dentistry
nystatin	fungi, yeasts, no bacteria	disrupts fungal cell membranes	drug of choice, topically, for oral candidiasis
amphotericin B	fungi, yeasts, no bacteria	disrupts fungal cell membranes	alternate drug for topical treatment of oral candidiasis

contain neomycin and/or tyrothricin (and possibly others). The latter agents should be avoided. Possible uses were described earlier.

Both bacitracin and polymyxin B are available for topical use, the former as an ointment (500 units/gm), the latter as a solution (20,000 units/ml).

G. INTRODUCTION TO ANTIFUNGAL DRUGS

Objective 30.G.1. Describe three factors that may predispose to oral candidiasis.

The single most important fungal infection of the oral cavity is candidiasis (thrush), caused by *Candida albicans*. There are intestinal and systemic forms of the disease, but in these cases, the patient should be referred to a physician. These forms of the disease can be very serious, especially systemic infection.

The following factors may predispose to the onset of oral candidiasis: (1) alteration of normal oral flora by previous antibiotic therapy, (2) decreased resistance to disease (e.g., in diabetes) or drugs (e.g., corticosteroids or anticancer agents), and (3) malnutrition.

H. CHEMISTRY AND SPECTRUM OF ACTIVITY

Objective 30.H.1. Recognize the proposed chemical structure of nystatin and amphotericin B.

Objective 30.H.2. Recognize the spectrum of activity.

Both **nystatin** and **amphotericin B**, the two most useful antifungal drugs in dentistry, are

polyene antibiotics. Their exact chemical structure is as yet unknown. Nystatin is the drug of choice for the treatment of oral candidiasis (Table 30-2).

Nystatin and amphotericin B inhibit many, but not all, fungi. Bacteria and viruses are completely out of their spectrum of activity. In dentistry, the agents are used primarily for infections caused by *Candida*. *Candida albicans* continues to be susceptible to both agents, and there is no evidence of development of resistant strains.

I. MECHANISM OF ACTION

Objective 30.I.1. Describe the mechanism of action of nystatin and amphotericin B.

Objective 30.I.2. Recognize whether nystatin and amphotericin B are static or cidal agents.

Both nystatin and amphotericin B bind to a sterol molecule in the cell membrane of fungi, resulting in leakage or increased permeability of the cell membrane. In general terms, disruption of a cell membrane by a drug is a cidal action, but in this case, the action is considered static and the agents are referred to as fungistatic drugs. However, in high concentrations, the drugs are fungicidal.

J. ABSORPTION AND EXCRETION

Objective 30.J.1. Recognize the absorption and excretion of nystatin and amphotericin B.

When nystatin or amphotericin B is applied to oral structures and swallowed, little or no drug is absorbed into the systemic circulation.

This is most fortunate since both drugs are toxic when given IV, especially nystatin. In fact, nystatin should never be used systemically. In the presence of systemic fungal infection, amphotericin B is used and is administered IV.

Both drugs are excreted in the feces.

K. ADVERSE EFFECTS

Objective 30.K.1. Describe adverse effects and contraindications for use of nystatin and amphotericin B.

Adverse effects of topical nystatin or amphotericin B are considered to be uncommon. Occasional reports of nausea, vomiting, and diarrhea have occurred, as have irritation of oral mucous membranes. Amphotericin B has an unpleasant taste when used topically. Candidal resistance to the drugs, induction of allergy, and production of supra-infections have never been reported after topical application. Similarly, there are no known drug interactions when the agents are used for treatment of oral candidiasis, nor are there any known contraindications. However, if a history of allergic reaction to either agent is encountered, the agent should be withdrawn and is contraindicated for future use.

When amphotericin B is used IV for treatment of systemic fungal infections, there is a long list of adverse effects. Since this agent will probably not be used IV in dentistry, these adverse effects will not be presented. Any practitioner interested in side effects with systemic administration should refer to package inserts.

L. THERAPEUTIC USE, BASIS FOR SELECTION, AND IMPLICATIONS FOR DENTISTRY

Objective 30.L.1. Recognize the drug of choice for the treatment of oral candidiasis.

Objective 30.L.2. Recognize the usual dosage of nystatin for children, adults, and infants.

Objective 30.L.3. Recognize potentially useful dosage forms of nystatin and how each form may be used.

Oral candidiasis can often be tentatively diagnosed by observation of the typical lesions produced. However, as with all infections, a sample should be taken to positively identify the organism.

Nystatin (the drug of choice) therapy should be started while awaiting fungal analysis. Therapy should continue for 48 to 72 hours after disappearance of all clinical symptoms. If unresponsive, the fungal analysis will be useful.

Nystatin may be administered in an oral suspension; the usual adult and child's dosage is 400,000 to 600,000 units four times a day. The agent should be swished (to reach all parts of the oral cavity), held in the mouth as long as possible (for increased contact time with lesions), and swallowed (not expectorated). The agent is swallowed because lesions are sometimes present on the soft palate and pharynx. The dosage for infants is 200,000 units four times a day.

Nystatin oral tablets (500,000 units) can be used in the mouth by dissolution, or by chewing and dissolution.

Nystatin vaginal tablets are also marketed, and they have been recommended for use in the oral cavity. One problem is that the agent is marketed in 100,000 or 200,000 unit tablets, and this dosage may be too low for children and adults (see earlier).

Nystatin cream and ointment are also available; these dosage forms can be conveniently applied to a denture tissue surface, provided the lesion contacts the denture. However, the denture itself may be the source of reinfection, and many prosthodontists and microbiologists advise that the denture be destroyed.

Amphotericin B for topical use is available only as a cream, lotion, or ointment. These dosage forms have an unpleasant taste, and they may not be desirable for use in the mouth.

M. INTRODUCTION TO ANTIVIRAL DRUGS

Until recently, there were no agents known that inhibited viruses in vivo. Normally in chemotherapeutics, one attempts to specifically inhibit the parasite without altering the host cells.

Since the virus takes over the host's genetic and reproductive mechanisms, it has been difficult to find agents which have any specificity. Nevertheless, the search for drugs with antiviral properties continues, and this is now one of the great frontiers for developing new drugs.

Scientists are now studying viral reproduction intensely to find mechanisms for attacking viral disease. This approach is promising but so far only modestly successful. In the last 15 years, several new drugs that are considered antiviral have been introduced, and there is a great interest in finding others.

N. VIRAL REPRODUCTION MECHANISMS

Objective 30.N.1. State seven phases of the viral cycle and describe viral inhibition by drugs at these phases.

Objective 30.N.2. Recognize five useful antiviral drugs (set in bold type) and state their chemistry, site of action in the viral cycle, therapeutic usefulness, and disadvantages.

Stages of the viral cycle are as follows:

1. Virus Travels from Cell to Cell

Nonspecific agents, such as UV and x-ray irradiation or radiomimetic drugs, may act on the virus in the extracellular fluids. Specific antibodies may neutralize viruses at this phase. Many clinicians have advocated use of ether and other nonspecific drugs in the hope of inactivating the viruses, but this approach has not been fruitful (Guinan et al., 1980). There was a great deal of interest in photodynamic inactivation (Melnikoff, 1972). The lesion was painted with a dye that reacts with the viral DNA, and the DNA was inactivated in the presence of incandescent light. This works in vitro, but it was recently proven to be no better than placebo in vivo (Meyers et al., 1975). Furthermore, photodynamic inactivation is a dangerous approach because mammalian cells show cancerous changes in the presence of virus, dye, and light in vitro. Such altered cells form tumors when implanted

in vivo (Rapp and Duff, 1973). For these reasons, photodynamic inactivation should never be used by the dentist.

2. Adsorption of Virus to Cell Surface

This step probably involves reaction of virus with cell receptors. Blocking receptors would seem to be a hopeful approach to viral chemotherapy, but not much is known about the viral-receptor interaction, and no drugs are currently available that block this step.

3. Penetration of Virus into Cell

Little is known about this mechanism, and blocking penetration is in the same status as blocking receptors.

4. Uncoating

The virus must lose its coat after getting into the cell. **Amantadine** is a drug that is thought to act on the early stages of the influenza A viral replication cycle. At first, amantadine was thought to prevent adsorption (phase 2) or penetration (phase 3). More recent evidence indicates that it interferes with uncoating (phase 4). The value of amantadine is limited to prophylaxis of influenza A. Amantadine may be active against rhinorrheal symptoms, which gave some medical scientists false hopes when it was first introduced as an antiviral. Nevertheless, its use in prophylaxis is well substantiated and accepted, but the patient must be treated before flu symptoms develop or at least within the first 24 hours. This may be useful, along with vaccines, in an epidemic of influenza A or for high-risk patients. Amantadine is not useful for other types of flu (e.g., influenza B). Amantadine is also used to treat Parkinson's disease (Chapter 40).

5. Transcription and Replication of Genome

The viral code must be read and new viral DNA formed (two phases). In order to block the latter of the two phases, researchers have introduced purine and pyrimidine, nucleoside analogs that block DNA (genome) formation. The best success in viral chemotherapy has been on DNA formation. **Idoxuridine**, **vidarabine** (Ara-A,

Vira-A) and acycloguanosine (**acyclovir** or *Zovirax*) have been used with some success.

Idoxuridine (iododeoxyuridine, IDU, *Stoxil, Dendrid, Herplex*). IDU is an analog of thymidine, an essential pyrimidine which is part of DNA. IDU inhibits all steps involved in thymidine incorporation into DNA. DNA is phosphorylated (like thymidine) and eventually incorporated into DNA. The result is that false DNA is formed, and the imperfect virus cannot reinfect another cell. One problem with this mechanism is nonspecificity, since IDU can incorporate into mammalian DNA. Nevertheless, Kaufman (1962) found that IDU is effective in corneal HSV-1 keratitis, the leading cause of blindness due to corneal disease.

IDU has been marketed as an ophthalmic solution and, more recently, as an ophthalmic ointment. The drug penetrates the cornea well, but it is useless to apply the ointment to skin because it does not penetrate. Nevertheless, many physicians and dentists are using the ointment on HSV-1 herpes oralabialis. We discourage this practice because it is believed that a small amount of the drug can encourage viral resistance.

Gangarosa and co-workers (1977) have proposed a method to increase antiviral drug penetration. By applying IDU to the active viral lesion by means of an electrical current (iontophoresis), the IDU reaches antiviral concentrations and arrests the disease, usually with one treatment (Gangarosa et al., 1979) (Appendix VII).

IDU has had a therapeutic trial by intravenous injection for herpes encephalitis, but it was unsuccessful because it causes myelosuppression and other serious side effects, and the cure is as bad as the disease. Recent studies (Boston Interhospital et al., 1975) showed that HSV encephalitis patients were not improved by IDU therapy and many cases developed significant problems due to IDU toxicity when the drug was used systemically.

Vidarabine (Ara-A; *Vira-A*) is a purine nucleoside analog of adenine riboside. In Ara-A, the ribose moiety is replaced by arabinose. Because of this similarity, Ara-A prevents certain key conversions of adenosine, thereby inhibiting DNA formation. Ara-A was found to be much less toxic than IDU both in vitro and in vivo. Because of this lowered toxicity, Ara-A is the drug of choice for HSV encephalitis. Ara-A has been useful in preventing morbidity in 80% of HSV encephalitis cases after intravenous injection (Whitley et al., 1977). Ara-A is also marketed as an ophthalmic solution and as an ointment. Either preparation may be indicated for IDU-resistant HSV keratitis, but penetration of the skin is poor.

One problem with Ara-A is that it is insoluble, and, therefore, large amounts of fluid must be infused during IV therapy for encephalitis. This creates electrolyte problems, especially in children. Therefore, the producers have introduced Ara-AMP (*Vira-AMP*), the monophosphate analog of Ara-A. This is ionic and highly water soluble and is now being investigated for IV use in HSV encephalitis and for herpes zoster. Skin penetration by Ara-AMP is poor.

Ara-AMP is highly negatively charged and is an ideal antiviral drug for iontophoresis (Park et al., 1977). It appears to be effective against both HSV-1 and HSV-2 in mice (Park et al., 1978; Kwon et al., 1979). It is now being used in humans by iontrophoresis under FDA approved studies by one of the authors (LPG).

Acycloguanosine (**acyclovir**) is a novel antiviral agent that appears to be even more specific for viral DNA replication than IDU or *Ara-A*. Although **acyclovir** is an analog of guanosine (a purine), it still acts by inhibiting a specific viral pyrimidine kinase, as well as a specific viral DNA polymerase. Because of these mechanisms, the drug is very specific, affecting only virally infected cells. It is the least toxic antiviral agent of this group (inhibitors of DNA) and may well become the preferred agent for IV use (encephalitis), for other systemic uses (it is absorbed after peroral administration), and for herpes keratitis (eye). Unfortunately, there is still an absorption problem after mucocutaneous application. Iontophoresis is now being used under the same studies (above) for increasing the penetration of **acyclovir**.

6. Translation of Protein Synthesis
The next phase involves viral direction of protein synthesis through RNA. Probably the drugs

described under (5) have the effect of blocking translation because of defective DNA formation. Since the virus uses the same protein synthesis mechanism as the host cell (mammalian protein synthesis), the antibiotics (e.g., tetracycline, chloramphenicol) which act on protein synthesis are not specific inhibitors and generally are considered inactive against most viruses, but a few large viruses may be in their spectrum.

Interferon. This polypeptide is produced by cells under viral attack or by certain inducers (poly I:C). It is effective against DNA and RNA viruses. It is thought to act on ribosomes by interfering with viral protein translation. Although specific, there are still several problems: (1) interferon is difficult to produce and expensive, (2) the interferon inducers have side effects, (3) interferon is species specific, and (4) quite unexpectedly, interferon has been found to have its own side effects. Most available interferon is being used in cancer chemotherapy trials, so that the amount available for localized herpes is not enough. It is hoped these problems will be overcome in the near future.

7. Assembly or Maturation

The virus must be reassembled in the cell before release. Drugs called thiosemicarbazides interfere with assembly by causing a defect in the assembly protein. These drugs are thought to be effective against pox viruses. Generally, the vaccination approach has been more successful in smallpox, and the need for these drugs is almost nonexistent, since smallpox is virtually nonexistent in the world today.

REFERENCES

Boston Interhospital Virus Study Group and the NIAID-Sponsored Cooperative Antiviral Clinical Study: Failure of high dose of 5-iodo-2'-deoxyuridine in the therapy of herpes simplex virus encephalitis. N. Engl J Med 292:599, 1975

Gangarosa LP, Park NH, Hill JM: Iontophoretic assistance of 5-iodo-2' deoxyuridine penetration into neonatal mouse skin and effects on DNA synthesis. Proc Soc Exp Biol Med 154:439, 1977

Gangarosa LP, Merchant HW, Park NH, Hill JM: Iontophoretic application of idoxuridine for recurrent herpes labialis: Report of preliminary trials. Methods Findings Exp Clin Pharmacol 1:105, 1979

Guinan ME, MacCalman J, Kern ER, et al.: Topical ether and herpes simplex labialis. JAMA 243:1059, 1980

Kaufman HE: Clinical cure of herpes simplex keratitis by 5-iodo-2-deoxyuridine. Proc Soc Exp Biol Med 109:251, 1962

Kwon BS, Hill JM, Wiggins CA, Tuggle C, Gangarosa LP: Iontophoretic application of adenine arabinoside monophosphate for the treatment of herpes simplex virus type 2 skin infections in hairless mice. J Infect Dis 140:1014, 1979

Melnikoff RM: Photodynamic inactivation of herpes simplex virus. Calif Med 116:51, 1972

Meyers MG, Oxman MN, Clark JE, Arndt KA: Failure of neutral-red photodynamic inactivation in recurrent herpes simplex virus infections. N Engl J Med 293:945, 1975

Park NH, Gangarosa LP, Hill JM: Iontophoretic application of ara-AMP (9-β-D-arabinofuranosyladenine-5'-monophosphate) in adult mouse skin. Proc Soc Exp Biol Med 156:326, 1977

Park NH, Gangarosa LP, Kwon BS, Hill JM: Iontophoretic application of adenine arabinoside monophosphate to herpes simplex virus type 1-infected hairless mouse skin. Antimicrob Agents Chemother 14:605, 1978

Rapp F, Duff R: Transformation of hamster embryo fibroblasts by herpes simplex viruses type 1 and 2. Cancer Res 33:1527, 1973

Whitley RJ, Soong S-J, Dolin R, et al., The Collaborative Study Group: Adenine arabinoside therapy of biopsy-proved herpes simplex encephalitis. NIAID Collaborative Antiviral Study. N Engl J Med 297:289, 1977

BIBLIOGRAPHY

Accepted Dental Therapeutics, 38th ed. Chicago, American Dental Association, 1979, Sec II, Antimicrobial agents

Bevan JA (ed): Essentials of Pharmacology, 2nd ed. Hagerstown, MD, Harper & Row, 1976, Ch 58, 66

Gilman AG, Goodman LS, Gilman A (eds): Goodman and Gilman's The Pharmacological Basis of Therapeutics, 6th ed. New York, Macmillan, 1980, Ch 54

Goth A: Medical Pharmacology, 10th ed. St. Louis, Mosby, 1981, Ch 53

Melmon KL, Morelli HF (eds): Clinical Pharmacology: Basic Principles in Therapeutics, 2nd ed. New York, Macmillan, 1978, Ch 14

Meyers FH, Jawetz E, Goldfien A: Review of Medical Pharmacology, 7th ed. Los Altos, CA, Lange, 1980, Ch 54, 55, 57

QUESTIONS

1. Potential indications for use of topical antibiotics in dentistry include:

   A. infected traumatic ulcers
   B. intraoral burns
   C. pericoronitis
   D. all of the above are correct
   E. none of the above is correct

2. One topical antibiotic that may be useful in dentistry is:

   A. gentamicin
   B. neomycin
   C. polymyxin B
   D. tyrothricin

3. T F Both bacitracin and polymyxin B are polypeptide antibiotics, and they both have a primarily gram-positive spectrum of activity.

4. Bacitracin's mechanism of action is:

   A. disrupts cell membranes
   B. inhibits bacterial protein synthesis
   C. inhibits cell wall synthesis
   D. all of the above are correct
   E. none of the above is correct

5. T F Both bacitracin and polymyxin B are considered to be bactericidal agents.

6. T F Both bacitracin and polymyxin B are in general poorly absorbed from topical sites, but they can be adequately absorbed in the presence of gingival inflammation.

7. T F Both bacitracin and polymyxin B have essentially no adverse effects when applied topically.

8. T F The use of topical antibiotics in dentistry could include the combination of bacitracin and polymyxin B.

9. Factors that may predispose to the onset of oral candidiasis include:

   A. alteration of normal flora due to antibiotic therapy
   B. decreased resistance due to presence of disease
   C. decreased resistance due to use of certain drugs
   D. malnutrition
   E. all of the above are correct

10. T F Both nystatin and amphotericin B are polyene antibiotics that inhibit fungi.

11. T F Antifungal agents inhibit cell wall synthesis. (disrupt cell membrane)

12. T F Antifungal drugs are thought to be fungistatic when used at the usual therapeutic dosages.

13. T F Nystatin is rapidly absorbed from the GI tract and excreted by the kidneys.

14. T F There are no known drug interactions nor contraindications to the topical use of nystatin.

15. T F Amphotericin B is the drug of choice to treat oral candidiasis.

16. The usual dosage of nystatin oral suspension for adults and children is:

    A. 100,000 units
    B. 100,000 to 200,000 units
    C. 300,000 units

Infant 200,000

D. 400,000 to 600,000 units

E. 800,000 units

17. **T** **F** Nystatin oral suspension should always be taken in the mouth and swished, *Swallowed* then expectorated to avoid systemic absorption from the GI tract.

18. Phases of a viral cycle include:

    A. adsorption of virus to cell surface

    B. assembly or maturation

    C. uncoating

    D. all of the above are correct

    E. none of the above is correct

19. Amantadine is thought to act by interference with:

    A. viral uncoating

    B. penetration of virus into the cell

    C. both A and B are correct

    D. neither A nor B is correct

20. Useful antiviral drugs include:

    A. thymidine

    B. vidarabine

    C. both A and B are correct

    D. neither A nor B is correct

21. **T** **F** Interferon is an agent that may interfere with translation.

22. Which of the following drugs blocks adsorption of virus to the cell surface?

    A. interferon

    B. idoxuridine

    C. vidarabine

    D. Poly I:C

    E. none of the above is correct

23. All of the following are useful antiviral drugs *except*:

    A. vidarabine

    B. idoxuridine

    C. acyclovir

    D. tetracycline

    E. interferon

24. **T** **F** Photodynamic inactivation is a useful method of treating viral lesions in the dental office.

SECTION THREE
MEDICAL DRUGS IMPORTANT TO
DENTISTRY (SELF-STUDY)

31
Cardiovascular System Drugs

The dental practitioner is currently faced with an increasing number of patients who are undergoing medical treatment for cardiovascular disease. This increase is indicative of the improved diagnosis of such disorders and an increasing awareness on the part of the public of the dangers of untreated cardiovascular disease. The dentist is often encouraged to participate in the recognition of such disorders by routinely measuring the patients' blood pressure and by taking a detailed health history. With respect to rendering dental care to patients with cardiovascular disease, the dentist must be familiar with (1) the underlying disease processes, (2) how these alter dental treatment, and (3) the pharmacology of the drugs used to treat cardiovascular disease. The latter can alter the patient's behavior, the condition of the oral cavity, and the activity of other drugs which the dentist administers or prescribes.

While it is not within the scope of this textbook to detail all treatments for the various types of cardiovascular disease, the basic characteristics of cardiovascular diseases will be presented, along with the pharmacology of drugs used to treat them.

A. CARDIAC GLYCOSIDES AND CONGESTIVE HEART FAILURE

Objective 31.A.1. List three factors which can cause the reduction in cardiac output associated with congestive failure of the circulation.

Congestive failure of the circulation, perhaps better known as congestive heart failure, is a complex, chronic syndrome rather than some specific, singular defect in the circulation. The characteristic etiologic factor in congestive failure is inadequate cardiac output, which can be attributed, in a simplified manner, to three basic factors:

1. **Increased work load** on the heart. This could be due to hypertension (increased vascular resistance), excessive volume work (as in the case of a leaky heart valve), or increased demands on myocardial function (as in anemia).
2. **Impaired contractility** of the heart. This could be associated with a deficient myocardial blood supply, inflammation or infection of the heart, or cardiac arrhythmias of various etiologies.

3. **Impedance to cardiac inflow,** as in cases of A-V valvular stenosis (constriction) or pressure around the myocardium (e.g., cardiac tamponade, where fluids fill the pericardial space).

Keep in mind that these precipitating factors can and frequently do occur together in the same patient.

Because the heart is unable to pump blood from the venous side back into the arterial side, venous congestion is manifested mainly by the symptom of edema, which occurs in the abdominal viscera, the lungs, and other tissues; hence, the term "congestive" failure.

Objective 31.A.2. List three cardiac and two extracardiac compensatory mechanisms that occur in patients with congestive failure of the circulation.

Inadequate cardiac output is, of course, detrimental to physiologic function, and the body attempts to compensate for the defect. In congestive failure of the circulation, three cardiac compensatory mechanisms come into play:

1. **tachycardia** (through increased sympathetic discharge to the heart)
2. **cardiac hypertrophy** (increased size of myocardial fibers)
3. **cardiac dilatation** (increased ventricular volume results in an increased myocardial contractility through increased initial fiber length, in accordance with the Frank-Starling law)

Consider the Frank-Starling curve in Figure 31–1, which relates cardiac contractility to the initial myocardial fiber length. Figure 31–1 illustrates the relationship between initial ventricular fiber length (end-diastolic pressure) and the force of ventricular contraction (stroke work). In curve A (normal heart), increased end-diastolic pressure is compensated by increased stroke work. In curve B (heart failure), cardiac performance is depressed throughout the range of end-diastolic pressures. This demonstrates that in heart failure, the heart is less able to effectively deliver a cardiac output when end-

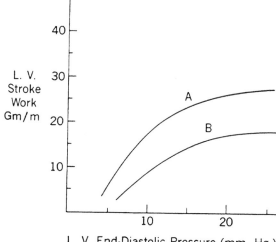

Figure 31–1. Frank-Starling ventricular function curves. (*From Conn HL Jr: In Conn HL, Horowitz O (eds): Cardiac and Vascular Diseases, 1971. Courtesy of Lea & Febiger.*)

diastolic volumes increase. Cardiac dilatation, therefore, can compensate for a decreased cardiac output associated with increasing end-diastolic volumes, but after a certain end-diastolic pressure (not shown in Fig. 31–1), left ventricular stroke work actually decreases with increasing end-diastolic pressures, forcing the heart into a state of decompensation.

In addition to these cardiac compensatory mechanisms, two extracardiac compensatory mechanisms become involved:

1. **renal retention of salt and water** (which expands plasma volume)
2. **increased tissue extraction of arterial O_2** (increased A-V O_2 differences)

In summary, when the cardiac output is diminished because of one of the aforementioned factors, compensatory mechanisms come into play in an attempt to restore tissue blood flow. In some cases, compensation may be successful. In others, where the inadequate cardiac output persists, frank congestive failure develops with symptoms that depend to a great extent on the side of the heart which is affected (see the following).

Objective 31.A.3. Recognize the symptoms of left ventricular failure.

In left ventricular failure, blood accumulates in the pulmonary vascular bed, and **signs and symptoms** include:

1. dyspnea, cough, and other respiratory abnormalities
2. pulmonary edema (the lungs become engorged with blood)
3. enlargement of the heart (the left ventricle dilates)
4. abnormal cardiac rhythms
5. weakness and fatigue

Objective 31.A.4. Recognize the symptoms of right ventricular failure.

In right ventricular failure, blood accumulates in the systemic veins, and the **signs and symptoms** include:

1. distention of veins (e.g., the neck veins may bulge)
2. venous congestion of the viscera, with possible hepatomegaly and occasional splenomegaly
3. enlargement of the heart (the right ventricle dilates)
4. generalized edema (e.g., swollen ankles)

In the diagnosis of congestive failure of the circulation, ECG and radiographic changes in the heart and a variety of nonspecific clinical laboratory tests help to verify a case suspected on the basis of the above signs and symptoms.

Objective 31.A.5. Recognize five medical measures used in the treatment of congestive failure of the circulation.

The cardiac glycosides form the backbone of modern therapy of congestive heart failure. By increasing cardiac output, these drugs directly reverse the underlying cause of the disease. They do not, however, cure the disease by permanently correcting myocardial pathology but, when combined with the measures described below, offer satisfactory relief for the patient and allow him to pursue a relatively normal life. The **additional treatment modalities** include:

1. correction of etiologic factors (this may involve treatment of associated pathologies, including cardiac surgery to correct valve disorders)
2. supportive measures (oxygen administration and bed rest)
3. diet (usually a low-salt diet)
4. diuretics (used for the mobilization of edema fluid)
5. drugs that reduce peripheral resistance (reducing cardiac work)

Objective 31.A.6. List the sources and pharmacologic (therapeutic) actions of the cardiac glycosides.

The term **digitalis** refers to the entire group of **cardiac glycosides**, and they have the general composition:

sugar(s)–steroid nucleus–lactone

The structures of digitoxin and digoxin are shown in Figure 31–2. There are a number of

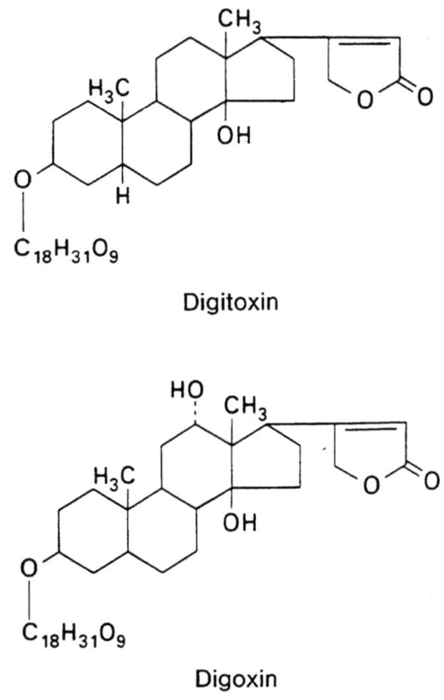

Digitoxin

Digoxin

Figure 31–2. Chemical structures of digitoxin and digoxin. (*From Csáky TZ: Cutting's Handbook of Pharmacology, 6th ed, 1979. Courtesy of Appleton-Century-Crofts.*)

TABLE 31-1. CHARACTERISTICS OF SOME CARDIAC GLYCOSIDES

Name	Source	% Absorption[a]	Onset[a]	Duration
digitalis[b]	*Digitalis purpurea*	0.1	medium	long
digitoxin	*Digitalis purpurea*	90	slow	long
acetyldigitoxin	*Digitalis lanata*	75	medium	medium
digoxin	*Digitalis lanata*	65	fast	medium
deslanoside	*Digitalis lanata*	40	fast	medium
ouabain	*Strophant hus gratus*	0	fast	short

After Cutting: Handbook of Pharmacology, 5th ed., 1972. Courtesy of Appleton-Century-Crofts.
[a] After oral administration (except ouabain, a water-soluble, injectable form).
[b] Digitalis is a plant material containing a mixture of various glycosides.

cardiac glycosides which are used in medicine. Various glycoside preparations are shown in Table 31-1, along with their respective plant sources and pharmacokinetic information. The most commonly prescribed cardiac glycoside currently is **digoxin** (Fig. 31-2).

Therapeutic effects (cardiovascular) of cardiac glycosides include the following:

1. **Positive inotropic effect** (or increased contractility) resulting in:
   a. decreased duration of systole
   b. increased ventricular filling time
   c. shortened ventricular ejection with more complete emptying
   d. increased cardiac output

The cardiac glycosides probably exert their effect through an inhibition of Na^+,K^+-ATPase, the enzyme which provides energy to the so-called sodium pump. Inhibition of this enzyme results in an increase in intracellular sodium ions. These sodium ions can then exchange for extracellular calcium ions, resulting in an increase in intracellular calcium and a correlative increase in the contractility of the heart.

2. **Negative chronotropic effect** (decreased heart rate) by:
   a. vagal stimulation (vagomimetic)
   b. direct depressant effect
3. **Peripheral vascular effects,** including:
   a. vasoconstriction (both arteriolar and venular)
   b. increased renal blood flow (a probable indirect effect), resulting in diuresis

Objective 31.A.7. Recognize the important side effects of the cardiac glycosides.

The therapeutic index for the glycosides is low, and all of the following **side effects** may occur at therapeutic dose levels:

1. cardiac arrhythmias (wide variety)
2. nausea and vomiting
3. headache, vertigo, delirium
4. visual alterations, including scotomas, blurring, and color changes

Objective 31.A.8. Recognize other indications for the cardiac glycosides.

The cardiac glycosides can be used for the **treatment of other disorders of** the cardiovascular system, including:

1. atrial fibrillation
2. atrial flutter
3. paroxysmal atrial tachycardia

(*Note:* disturbances of rhythm are described in other parts of this chapter.)

Objective 31.A.9. List the interactions that may occur between the cardiac glycosides and other drugs.

The cardiac glycosides interact with numerous drugs in many varied ways. The interactions described below are those interactions limited to drugs commonly used in dentistry.

1. Barbiturates and most nonbarbiturate sedative-hypnotics accelerate the rate of hepatic

degradation of numerous drugs, and digitoxin is no exception. Concurrent administration of barbiturates may decrease blood levels of digitoxin and, therefore, its therapeutic action. While the clinical significance of this reduction may not be great, these agents should be used with caution or avoided in such patients. This interaction does not appear to be significant for the other cardiac glycosides.

2. Propantheline. By reducing gastrointestinal motility, the absorption of slowly dissolving preparations of digoxin is increased, with concomitantly elevated blood levels and a greater chance for the occurrence of toxicity. Apparently, this is not a problem with *Lanoxin*, a rapidly dissolving form of digoxin, but the patient's physician should be consulted whenever the dentist is considering the use of an antisialogog in a patient taking digoxin. Another potential interaction between these agents may result in production of a cardiac arrhythmia, since the cardiac glycosides produce a vagomimetic effect on the heart, while the anticholinergic, antisialogogs produce vagolytic effects.

3. Sympathomimetic amines. Because of the inherent arrhythmogenic activity of the sympathomimetic amines (e.g., epinephrine) and the cardiac glycosides, the use of these agents together constitutes a potentially dangerous situation. In patients taking cardiac glycosides, it may be best to use local anesthetic solutions without vasoconstrictors or to use precautions (reduced concentrations) when such local anesthetic additives are deemed necessary.

4. Phenylbutazone. This anti-inflammatory agent (rarely used in dentistry, Chapter 23) can increase the hepatic metabolism of digitoxin and also can promote renal sodium retention. Therefore, this drug should be avoided or used only with caution in patients taking cardiac glycosides.

5. Carbamazepine (*Tegretol*). This drug, used in the treatment of trigeminal and glossopharyngeal neuralgias, has been shown to rarely interact with cardiac glycosides to produce bradycardia. The significance of this interaction is not clear.

Objective 31.A.10. Describe the special precautions to be taken when treating a dental patient undergoing therapy for congestive heart failure.

A history of congestive heart failure or the use of cardiac glycosides should alert the dentist to the necessity for further information and for taking precautions. The following should be observed:

1. Consult the patient's physician to determine the severity of the disease and whether the patient can receive dental treatment.
2. Determine whether the patient should receive prophylactic antibiotic therapy (history of cardiac surgery or congenital heart problem associated with the congestive failure).
3. Avoid stress and the potential for impaired respiratory function during dental treatment.
4. Be prepared to handle potential emergencies associated with this type of patient, including hypotension, hypertension, acute pulmonary edema, cardiac arrhythmias, nausea and vomiting, and so on (Appendix I).
5. You should be sure that the patient is under adequate medical control and that he is complying completely with his prescribed drug regimen. Patients who do not continue to take their medication present a potential emergency situation. (NOTE: In some cases, the swelling which may ensue may involve the oral cavity to the extent that the fit of partial and complete dentures is compromised, and impressions may be inaccurate.)

The following questions should be asked during the health history assessment to screen all patients for possible congestive failure of the circulation:

1. Do you tire easily or experience shortness of breath after mild exercise?
2. Do your ankles swell?
3. Do you require extra pillows for sleep, or do you have to sleep while sitting up?

Affirmative responses to any of the above questions would indicate the need for further investigation by a physician.

B. ANTIARRHYTHMIC AGENTS

Objective 31.B.1. Recognize seven types of cardiac arrhythmias.

A cardiac arrhythmia is defined as an abnormality of rate, regularity, or site of origin of the cardiac impulse that alters the activity of the atria and/or ventricles. Arrhythmias may be due to natural alterations of the automaticity and/or conductivity of heart tissues, which may also be caused by drug side effects or drug interactions.

In addition to classifying arrhythmias into atrial or ventricular types (discussion follows), they can also be classified as tachyarrhythmias (accelerations of heart rate) or bradyarrhythmias (reductions of heart rate). The former generally respond to drug treatment, while the latter do not. In addition, most tachyarrhythmias respond favorably to cardioversion, and drug therapy is often not needed.

In general, ventricular tachyarrhythmias are more dangerous because they may lead to ventricular fibrillation. Conversely, atrial arrhythmias by themselves are not dangerous; the heart functions efficiently with or without atrial contractions. The potentially dangerous aspect of atrial tachyarrhythmias is that with a rapid atrial rate, an increasing number of impulses cross the A-V node, resulting in increasing ventricular rate, which may then reduce the pumping efficiency of the heart or even lead to ventricular fibrillation. Therefore, both atrial and ventricular tachyarrhythmias usually require treatment.

The following list summarizes several of the various types of cardiac arrhythmias. All are tachyarrhythmias except Stokes-Adams syndrome, which is a bradyarrhythmia that is usually treated with a pacemaker.

a. Atrial Fibrillation. This is the irregular and uncoordinated contractions of large numbers of atrial muscle fibers.

b. Atrial Flutter. This is a condition of extremely rapid atrial contractions (180 to 400/min), which are rhythmic and uniform. As a result, the ventricles are bombarded with excessive impulses, and a partial or complete A-V block occurs, with the sinoatrial node no longer able to control the rate of cardiac contractions.

c. Paroxysmal Atrial Tachycardia. In this type of arrhythmia, sudden attacks of excessively high rates of atrial contractions occur and terminate abruptly.

d. Premature Ventricular Contractions (PVCs). In this condition, the ventricles contract prematurely, i.e., before a normal wave of impulses has passed from the atria to the ventricles and before adequate filling of the ventricles has occurred. If these occur frequently, they can lead to a decreased output, which may be severe or even life-threatening.

e. Ventricular Tachycardia. This condition is characterized by an excessively rapid rate of ventricular contractions, usually greater than 100/min.

f. Ventricular Fibrillation. This is the same type of disruption of contractions as described under atrial fibrillation, except that it is immediately life-threatening, since ejection of blood from the ventricles cannot occur. In atrial fibrillation, ventricle filling can still occur so that cardiac output usually continues.

g. Stokes-Adams Syndrome. This condition is characterized by sudden attacks of unconsciousness, sometimes with convulsions, due to acute onset of heart block (in which electrical impulses cannot travel from the atria to the ventricles).

Obviously, this list is not a complete description of all known arrhythmias. (For further information, see References.)

Objective 31.B.2. Define the three properties of myocardial impulses that are involved in the occurrence of cardiac arrhythmias.

Objective 31.B.3. Describe the mechanisms by which cardiac arrhythmias can occur.

The three **properties of myocardial impulses** involved in the generation of cardiac arrhythmias are listed below.

1. Automaticity. This refers to the spontaneous depolarizations that occur in the sinoatrial node and the cardiac conducting system (Purkinje fibers, bundle of His). Increases or decreases in automaticity would then be manifested as increased or decreased rates of spontaneous depolarizations at impulse-generating sites.

2. Refractory Period. This refers to the period during which a previously activated part of the cardiac conduction system cannot be further excited (absolute or functional refractory period) or during which increased degrees of stimulation are required for excitation (relative refractory period).

3. Conduction Velocity. This refers to the rate (expressed in meters/second) at which impulses travel through the cardiac conduction system.

In terms of the above cardiac properties involved in impulse generation and conduction, **cardiac arrhythmias** appear to develop in one of the following manners.

Changes in Automaticity. When the rate of spontaneous depolarizations increases, the rate of atrial and/or ventricular contractions increases, resulting in the tachyarrhythmias described above. In the case of atrial flutter, this increase in the number of impulses can result in partial or complete A-V block, accompanied by a loss of control of heart rate by the sinoatrial node.

Reentry Phenomenon. In this situation (illustrated in Fig. 31–3), blockade of some part of the normal impulse pathway (slowing of the rate of impulse conduction) and/or shortening of the refractory period occurs. Therefore, when an impulse travels in a normally conducting branch near the Purkinje fiber branch which is blocked, the impulse can travel retrograde (assuming that retrograde conduction can still occur in the blocked branch) toward the unblocked branch, resulting in a second excitation of the unblocked branch. Such an impulse path is appropriately termed "circus movement."

Objective 31.B.4. Recognize the pharmacologic properties of quinidine.

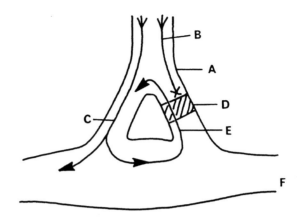

Figure 31–3. Diagram illustrating circus movement in a bundle-branch block. A, Purkinje fiber; B, blocked impulse; C, normal impulse; D, site of unidirectional block; E, reentrant impulse; F, cardiac muscle fiber. (*Adapted from Hoffman BF: Prog Cardiovasc Dis 8:319, 1966.*)

Quinidine is one of the oldest drugs used to treat abnormal cardiac rhythms.

Cardiac Effects. Quinidine produces a general depressant effect on the myocardium. This results in the following **cardiac actions:**

1. decreased myocardial contractility
2. decreased excitability
3. decreased conduction velocity
4. decreased automaticity
5. prolongation of refractory period
6. blockade of the cardiac vagus

Mechanism of Action. Cardiac depression probably occurs at the level of the cell membrane in conductile and contractile tissues due to a decreased membrane permeability with decreased inward flux of Na^+ and decreased outward flux of K^+.

Side Effects. These include the following:

1. xerostomia
2. hypotension and postural hypotension
3. fatigue
4. thrombocytopenic purpura
5. **cinchonism** (a syndrome characteristic of drugs obtained from cinchona bark, including nausea, vomiting, diarrhea, and tinnitus)

6. production of **other cardiac arrhythmias** (paradoxical ventricular tachycardia)

Objective 31.B.5. Recognize the features of lidocaine as an antiarrhythmic agent.

Lidocaine (without epinephrine), a local anesthetic widely used in dentistry, is also an effective antiarrhythmic drug. Lidocaine is now used as a prophylactic measure against ventricular fibrillation following the occurrence of a myocardial infarction.

Cardiac Effects. These include:

1. decreased automaticity
2. shortening of the refractory period
3. conduction velocity may be unaffected or may be increased
4. myocardial contractility and excitability are not affected

Mechanism of Action. Lidocaine increases the outward current of K^+ ion, which counteracts inward depolarizing currents, thus stabilizing the membrane. (This action occurs at low concentrations and is different from the type of membrane stabilization that causes nerve fiber block and depends upon blocking inward movement of sodium; Chapter 15.)

Side Effects. These include:

1. hyperexcitability
2. convulsions
3. respiratory depression
4. hypotension
5. sedation
6. ventricular arrhythmias (including cardiac arrest)

Objective 31.B.6. Recognize the pharmacologic properties of procainamide.

Procainamide is similar to the local anesthetic, procaine, except that an amide linkage has been substituted for the ester linkage of the procaine molecule (Fig. 31–4). This chemical modification results in a molecule that is not as

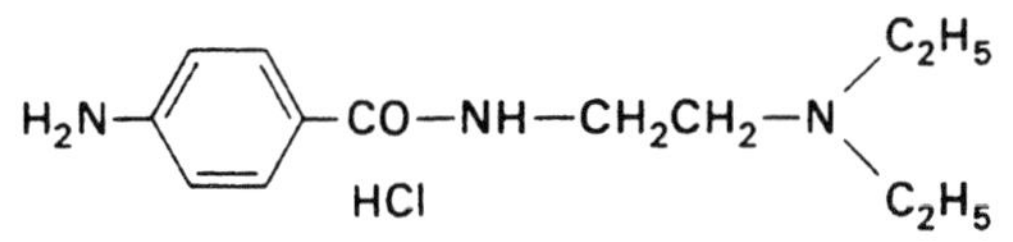

Figure 31–4. Chemical structure of procainamide HCl. (*Figures 31-4, 31-5, 31-6, and 31-7 are from Csáky TZ: Cutting's Handbook of Pharmacology, 6th ed, 1979. Courtesy of Appleton-Century-Crofts.*)

rapidly metabolized as procaine, so as to be effective as an antiarrhythmic agent.

Cardiac Effects. These are termed "quinidine-like" and include the same as those listed above for quinidine.

Mechanisms of Action. These are similar to quinidine.

Side Effects. These include:

1. xerostomia
2. hyperexcitability
3. convulsions (at high doses)
4. respiratory depression
5. hypotension and postural hypotension
6. ventricular arrhythmias
7. nausea
8. mental confusion
9. hallucinations
10. chills
11. fever
12. agranulocytosis
13. lupus erythematosus-like syndrome (this is reversible and includes arthralgia, pericarditis, pleuropneumonia, and hepatomegaly)

Objective 31.B.7. Recognize the pharmacologic properties of propranolol as an antiarrhythmic agent (do not include noncardiac, autonomic actions).

Propranolol, along with some other beta adrenergic blocking agents (e.g., atenolol and metoprolol, Chapter 18), is an effective antiarrhythmic agent as a result of its ability to block sympathetic input to the heart. Beta blockers are generally used <u>only for atrial arrhythmias</u>, hypertension, and angina pectoris.

Cardiac Effects. These include:

1. decreased myocardial contractility
2. decreased conduction velocity
3. decreased automaticity
4. shortening of the refractory period
5. blockade of sympathetic beta$_1$ (cardiac) receptors

Mechanism of Action. Beta blockers prevent sympathetic-mediated increases in the spontaneous firing rate of the S-A node and also increase the effective refractory period of the A-V node.

Side Effects. These include:

1. cardiac depression
2. other arrhythmias (A-V block, asystole)
3. hypotension
4. clinically significant increases in airway resistance in asthmatic patients

Objective 31.B.8. List the pharmacologic properties of phenytoin when used as an antiarrhythmic agent.

Phenytoin (*Dilantin*) is best known as an antiepileptic drug. However, it is used to treat cardiac arrhythmias and <u>may be the most useful</u> agent in counteracting <u>digitalis-induced arrhythmias.</u>

Cardiac Effects. These are essentially the same as for lidocaine.

Mechanism of Action. This is the same as for lidocaine.

Side Effects. These include:

1. drowsiness
2. nystagmus
3. vertigo
4. nausea
5. ataxia
6. allergic reactions

Other side effects associated with chronic use are described in Chapter 38.

Objective 31.B.9. Recognize an alternate drug for quinidine and describe its pharmacologic properties.

Disopyramide (*Norpace*) has cardiac actions that are very similar to those described for quinidine (p. 309) and may be used as an alternate agent for some ventricular arrhythmias.

Objective 31.B.10. Recognize the cardiac effects, indications, and side effects of verapamil.

Verapamil (*Calan, Isoptin*) is a drug that belongs to a relatively new group of agents known as "calcium channel antagonists." They interfere with the movement of calcium ions in cardiac tissue, slowing the rate of impulse generation. A summary of verapamil follows.

Cardiac Effects. Verapamil depresses the rate at which the sinoatrial node depolarizes and slows atrioventricular conduction.

Indications. Verapamil is used to treat supraventricular tachycardias. It is not used in the treatment of ventricular arrhythmias.

Side Effects. Side effects of verapamil include hypotension, A-V block, ventricular fibrillation, ventricular asystole (which is aggravated by beta blockers), and bradycardia. Verapamil can also cause or worsen cardiac failure.

Objective 31.B.11. List the implications for dental treatment of patients using antiarrhythmic drugs.

Because of the side effects and drug interactions of the antiarrhythmic drugs, the use of these drugs by dental patients may **influence dental care** as follows:

1. Such patients have a cardiovascular disease which dictates a careful pretreatment evaluation and medical consultation.
2. Xerostomia may be prominent in patients taking quinidine, procainamide, or disopyra-

TABLE 31–2. SUMMARY OF ANTIARRHYTHMIC DRUGS

Drug	Action/Mechanism	Toxicity	Indications	Trade Name
quinidine	general depression of heart, primarily increase in refractory period	cinchonism, thrombocytopenia	ventricular tachycardia, atrial fibrillation	*Cardioquin*
procainamide	same action as quinidine	hypotension, arrhythmias, CNS stimulation followed by depression	same indication as quinidine	*Pronestyl*
lidocaine	primarily decreased refractory period, decreased automaticity	hypotension, CNS stimulation (also depression)	ventricular arrhythmias, especially post-MI	*Xylocaine*
phenytoin	same action as lidocaine	CNS depression, sensitivity, other chronic effects	atrial tachycardia, ventricular arrhythmias (digitalis-induced)	*Dilantin*
propranolol	sympathetic β blockade	cardiovascular depression	atrial arrhythmias (adrenergically-induced)	*Inderal*

Adapted from Csáky TZ: Cutting's Handbook of Pharmacology, 6th ed, 1979. Courtesy of Appleton-Century-Crofts.

mide; for proper management, see Appendix V.

3. Postural hypotension may easily occur in patients taking quinidine or procainamide.
4. Many physicians prefer that local anesthetics without vasoconstrictors be used in patients taking antiarrhythmic drugs (Chapter 2).

Summary

Table 31–2 is presented as a summary of the pharmacologic characteristics of the antiarrhythmic drugs.

C. DRUGS AFFECTING BLOOD COAGULATION

The dentist must constantly deal with the problem of control of localized bleeding which can occur as a result of many dental procedures, from cavity preparation to oral surgery. Also, the dentist is occasionally called upon to provide dental services to patients whose blood coagulation mechanisms have been chemically altered as a therapeutic measure. This section will present a brief review of the coagulation process and a survey of drugs used to alter local bleeding in the oral cavity and those used medically to inhibit blood clotting.

Objective 31.C.1. Recognize the 12 clotting factors that are involved in the process of blood coagulation.

Table 31–3 lists 12 factors necessary for blood clot formation (please review).

TABLE 31–3. BLOOD CLOTTING FACTORS

Factor	Common Name
I	fibrinogen
II	prothrombin
III	thromboplastin
IV	Ca^{++}
V	accelerator globulin
VII	proconvertin (autoprothrombin I)
VIII	antihemophilic globulin
IX	Christmas factor (autoprothrombin II)
X	Stuart factor (autoprothrombin III)
XI	PTA (plasma thromboplastin antecedent)
XII	Hageman factor
XIII	fibrin-stabilizing factor

tissue damage → thromboplastin

prothrombin → thrombin

fibrinogen → fibrin (clot)

profibrinolysin → fibrinolysin - - - -

→ polypeptides

Figure 31–5. Blood coagulation mechanism. (From Csáky.)

Objective 31.C.2. Recognize the sequence by which blood clotting occurs.

The blood clotting sequence is shown schematically in Figure 31–5.

When tissue damage occurs, thromboplastin is released from the tissues, which then converts prothrombin to thrombin (in the presence of Factors IV and V). Thrombin then changes fibrinogen to fibrin (also requiring Factor IV), and the fibrin deposition then gives rise to the actual clot. It should be noted that platelet plugging also occurs to stem the flow of blood, since platelets become adherent to one another in damaged tissue areas.

As mentioned above, physicians frequently use drugs to inhibit the blood coagulation system in patients with cardiovascular disease. Such patients are constantly balanced near the hemorrhagic state, so that consultation with the patient's physician prior to undertaking dental procedures and a thorough knowledge of such drugs are imperative for the dentist.

Objective 31.C.3. List the mechanisms of action of heparin, its major side effects, the method of its antagonism, and its drug interactions.

Heparin is a naturally occurring anticoagulant which, along with endogenous factors that promote blood clotting, helps to maintain a balanced coagulability of the blood. It is stored in mast cells and is a high-molecular-weight mucopolysaccharide. The chemical structure of heparin is shown in Figure 31–6.

Heparin is isolated from cattle lung tissue or porcine intestinal mucosa (which contains many mast cells). Heparin must be administered by

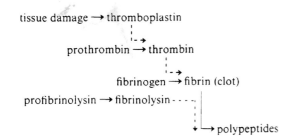

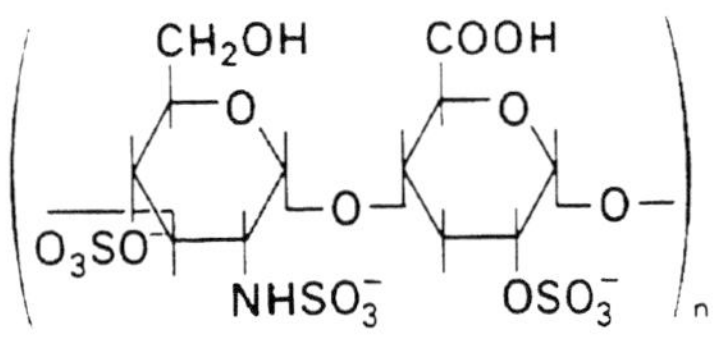

heparin (polymeric unit)

Figure 31–6. Chemical structure of heparin. (From Csáky.)

the parenteral route (usually IV) and is usually used in a hospital setting. The anticoagulant effect of heparin is immediate because it acts within the blood. Heparin is useful as an anticoagulant in vitro, such as in test tubes of blood samples, whereas the oral anticoagulants are not. The duration of action of heparin ranges from 3 hr (by the IV route) to as long as 6 hr (by the subcutaneous route). It is metabolized by the liver, although much of an administered dose is inactivated by other methods, especially protein binding. Twenty-five percent of the dose is excreted in the urine as uroheparin.

The mechanisms of heparin's anticoagulant effect are as follows:

1. interference with conversion of prothrombin to thrombin
2. antagonism of the action of thrombin on fibrinogen
3. reduction of platelet aggregation

Other mechanisms have been proposed, and probably contribute to its actions.

The major side effects of heparin are:

1. hemorrhage (especially from previously unsuspected sites, e.g., ulcerative GI tract lesions)
2. hypersensitivity reactions
3. thrombocytopenia

Heparin is antagonized by highly basic compounds which bind to and inactivate the negatively charged groups of the heparin molecule. The most widely used heparin antagonist is protamine sulfate. The onset of action of protamine sulfate in neutralizing heparin is immediate. The antagonism of heparin should be compared with that described for the coumarin-type anticoagulants.

TABLE 31-4. ORAL ANTICOAGULANTS

Official Name	Trade Name
I. Coumarin Derivatives	
dicumarol	none
acenocoumarol	Sintrom
phenprocoumon	Liquamar
ethylbiscoumacetate	Tromexan
warfarin	Coumadin
II. Indandione Derivatives[a]	
anisindione	Miradon
bromindione	Halinone
diphenadione	Dipaxin
phenindione	Danilone, Indon

[a] These compounds are pharmacologically similar to the coumarin agents, with a longer duration of action. Because of their greater toxicity, they are generally reserved for use in patients sensitive to coumarins.

Objective 31.C.4. List the mechanisms of action, the major side effects, the methods of antagonism, and the dental drug interactions for the coumarin-type anticoagulants.

Dicumarol (a coumarin) was originally discovered as a toxic component of sweet clover, the ingestion of which caused death in cattle. Since that time, the structure of this drug has been established, and it is closely related to the structure of vitamin K. Of these agents (Table 31-4), **warfarin** is the most frequently used. Because of the close structural similarity with vitamin K, coumarin and related anticoagulant compounds act as vitamin K antagonists to inhibit blood coagulation through the following mechanisms:

1. reduction of circulating prothrombin (by inhibition of hepatic synthesis)
2. reduction of hepatic synthesis of Factors VII, IX, and X

Unlike heparin, the coumarin anticoagulants have a relatively slow onset and long duration. Because the mechanism of action of these drugs involves an absolute reduction in circulating clotting factors, antagonism of the anticoagulant effect involves one or more of the following:

1. blood transfusions (administration of whole blood)

2. administration of vitamin K_1 (phytonadione)
3. administration of concentrated Factor IX

The major side effects of the coumarin-type anticoagulants include:

1. hemorrhage
2. nausea, vomiting, and diarrhea
3. anorexia

Because the coumarin anticoagulants are extensively protein bound and because they are metabolized by the liver, they can interact with other drugs in many ways. Although drug interactions are presented in Appendix II of this book, the interactions of the coumarin anticoagulants are presented here (Table 31-5) because of their potentially lethal outcome and for review at this time.

Objective 31.C.5. Recognize other factors which can alter oral anticoagulant activity.

In addition to drug interactions, pathologic and other patient factors (listed below) can increase the patient's response to the oral anticoagulants:

1. Hepatic function (liver disease can seriously enhance the activity of this group of drugs by reducing the rate of their biodegradation and by further reducing natural clotting factor synthesis)
2. Renal function
3. Fever
4. Genetic factors
5. Newborn or fetal age (reduced drug-handling capacity)

Objective 31.C.6. Recognize drugs belonging to the oral anticoagulant class.

The term "oral anticoagulants" refers to the group of drugs which, unlike heparin, can be used on an outpatient basis by the oral route for a number of cardiovascular conditions (e.g., patients who have had a myocardial infarction, rheumatic heart disease, cerebrovascular disease, venous thrombosis, pulmonary embolism, and disseminated intravascular clotting). For this reason, the dentist is likely to encounter patients taking oral anticoagulants. Table 31-4

TABLE 31–5. DRUG INTERACTIONS OF ORAL ANTICOAGULANTS

Drugs that Diminish Response

Inhibition
    griseofulvin
    cholestyramine
    laxatives
    clofibrate[a]
Induction of hepatic microsomal enzymes
    barbiturates[b]
    ethchlorvynol
    glutethimide
    griseofulvin
    carbamazepine
    phenytoin
    meprobamate[a]
    haloperidol[a]
Stimulation of synthesis of clotting factors
    vitamin K
    glucocorticoids[a]
    estrogens[a] (including oral contraceptives)

Drugs that Enhance the Anticoagulants' Response

Displacement of drug from albumin-binding sites
    chloral hydrate
    clofibrate
    mefenamic acid
    phenylbutazone
    tolbutamide
    phenytoin[b]
    diazoxide[a]
    ethacrynic acid[a]
    nalidixic acid[a]
    sulfinpyrazine[a]
    sulfonamides[a] (long acting)
    indomethacin[a]
    salicylates[a]
Increased affinity for the receptor
    d-thyroxine
Inhibition of hepatic microsomal enzymes
    chloramphenicol
    clofibrate
    allopurinol[a]
    disulfiram[a]
    mercaptopurine[a]
    methylphenidate[a]
    nortriptyline[a]
Reduction in availability of vitamin K
    anabolic steroids
    clofibrate
    d-thyroxine
    broad-spectrum antibiotics

(continued)

TABLE 31–5. (Continued)

Drugs that Enhance the Anticoagulants' Response

Inhibition of synthesis of clotting factors
    anabolic steroids
    glucagon
    quinidine
    salicylates
    acetaminophen[a]
    mercaptopurine[a]
    PAS[a]
Increase in clotting factor catabolism
    anabolic steroids
    d-thyroxine

Adapted from Levine WG: In Goodman LS, Gilman A (eds): The Pharmacological Basis of Therapeutics, 5th ed, 1975. Courtesy of Macmillan, Inc.
[a] Clinical significance is minor *or* has not been firmly established.
[b] Drugs set in bold type are dental drugs that should be memorized to meet the objective.

will alert the dentist to the various names of available oral anticoagulant preparations.

Objective 31.C.7. Describe the precautions needed for dental patients undergoing anticoagulant therapy.

Guidelines for dental management of patients taking anticoagulants are listed below.

1. Data accumulated thus far indicate that, in the majority of such cases, anticoagulant therapy does not need to be interrupted for routine dental care.
2. If a dental patient requires some form of surgery, the dentist must not interrupt anticoagulant therapy. The patient's primary care practitioner is the only person who should alter the patient's anticoagulant treatment.
3. When surgical treatment proceeds without interruption of anticoagulant therapy, the dentist should increase use of local measures for hemorrhage control. For example, sutures, topical hemostatics, pressure dressings, ice packs, and soft diet.
4. The dentist should consult and work closely with the patient's physician throughout dental treatment.

Objective 31.C.8. Describe several types of topical hemostatics used in dentistry and their mechanism of action.

Topical hemostatics are agents that are applied to localized areas for the purpose of arresting minor hemorrhagic problems. In dentistry, several different types of agents are used. Sometimes these agents are used in addition to pressure, which is often sufficient by itself to arrest bleeding.

Aluminum Chloride. $AlCl_3$ is both a hemostatic and an astringent (shrinks tissues by coagulation of surface proteins). Concentrations of 5 to 10% (which are not locally corrosive) are usually used for both a hemostatic and astringent effect in gingival retraction cord (*Hemodent*).

Absorbable Sponge Materials. There are three types of materials in this group: absorbable gelatin (*Gelfoam*), oxidized cellulose (*Novocell, Oxycel*), and oxidized, regenerated cellulose (*Surgicel*). These agents act as artificial clots, serving as matrices for deposition of blood components. They are generally used to control mild-to-moderate bleeding (capillary) when suturing is impractical, e.g., in extraction sockets. They are naturally absorbed by the body tissues in four to six weeks.

Epinephrine. Like aluminum chloride, epinephrine has found widespread use as a retraction cord additive. It can also be applied at a 1:500 dilution for control of arteriolar or capillary oozing. However, significant absorption of epinephrine occurs from the gingival crevice, as well as from surgically or traumatically denuded surfaces, and thus contraindicated for patients with cardiovascular disease because of systemic side effects. The concentration of epinephrine used in retraction cord (8%) may also be locally corrosive by inducing a severe, prolonged local ischemia (Chapter 2).

Thrombin. This is prepared from bovine prothrombin and acts topically by directly inducing fibrin formation from fibrinogen.

D. ANTIANGINAL DRUGS

Objective 31.D.1. Recognize the definition of angina pectoris, including its symptoms and factors which precipitate its occurrence.

Angina pectoris is defined as a paroxysmal chest pain due most often to myocardial hypoxia or ischemia and precipitated by effort or excitement. The impairment of myocardial oxygen supply is usually due to an inadequate flow of blood in the coronary vessels, which in turn may be associated with coronary arteriosclerosis or even spasms of the coronary vessels (known as Prinzmetal's angina). Anginal pain, which frequently radiates to the left shoulder and arm, results when compromised coronary blood flow is no longer able to keep up with myocardial oxygen demand, that is, when there is discrepancy between the supply of O_2 and the consumption of O_2. Conditions under which the oxygen demands of the heart increase and which may precipitate anginal attacks are listed below.

1. Exercise
2. Emotional upset
3. After meals
4. Smoking
5. Severe temperature changes
6. During sleep (due to postural changes or dreams)

The pharmacotherapy of angina pectoris is directed at reduction of myocardial oxygen demands, as described below. Ultimately, the mechanism by which antianginal drugs produce their therapeutic effect involves a reduction in the work load on the heart, rather than by simply dilating coronary vessels (previously considered to relieve angina). However, each group of clinically effective antianginal drugs accomplishes this reduction in myocardial work through a different mechanism. For example, nitroglycerin decreases demand on the heart by dilating all peripheral vessels (not simply the coronaries), thereby reducing peripheral resistance, beta blockers depress resting cardiac function by blocking adrenergic drive to the heart, and a new group of antianginal drugs (**verapamil, nifedipine**) depress cardiac function by antagonizing calcium ion movements in the myocardial cells.

The dentist should be familiar with the symptoms described above and with the pharmacology of the agents described below, since he will be rendering dental care for the patient with angina pectoris and occasionally must deal with an anginal attack on an emergency basis.

Objective 31.D.2. List the nondrug treatments for angina pectoris.

In addition to the drugs described below, certain other measures can contribute to a reduction in the frequency and severity of anginal attacks. These measures include avoidance of exertion, excitement, and overeating, and avoiding excessive smoking.

Objective 31.D.3. List two classes of drugs used in the treatment of angina pectoris.

The two types of agents used to treat angina pectoris include the so-called **organic nitrates** (or nitrites, since the nitrates are apparently metabolized to active nitrite ions in the body tissues), and the **beta adrenergic blocking drugs.** The pharmacologic actions of these drugs in treating angina are described below.

Objective 31.D.4. Recognize the mechanisms of action of nitroglycerin, its side effects, and its emergency use in the dental office.

Nitroglycerin (Fig. 31–7), along with the other organic nitrates, is thought to relieve angina pectoris through the cardiovascular effects listed below.

a. Primary Effect. This is direct relaxation of all vascular smooth muscle, including that of the coronary vessels.

b. Secondary Effects. These are a result of the primary effect and include:

1. reduction of diastolic and systolic blood pressures
2. increased venous capacitance with a decreased venous return to the heart
3. decreased cardiac output

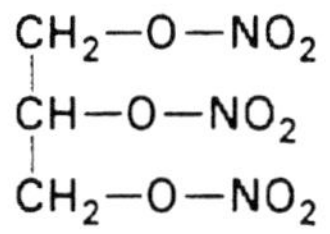

$$CH_2-O-NO_2$$
$$CH-O-NO_2$$
$$CH_2-O-NO_2$$

Figure 31–7. Chemical structure of nitroglycerin.

Apparently, the above actions all contribute to a reduction in oxygen demand on the heart, as well as to an improvement of myocardial blood flow.

The side effects of nitroglycerin that follow are also attributable to its cardiovascular actions:

1. Postural hypotension, syncope
2. Reflex tachycardia
3. Headache
4. Vertigo
5. Weakness
6. Formation of methemoglobin (by nitrite ions, at high doses)

Nitroglycerin, or one of its related compounds, should be kept in the dental office for the emergency treatment of anginal attacks. The treatment considerations described below should be used in this emergency therapy.

Objective 31.D.5. Describe treatment considerations for dental patients with angina pectoris.

1. When indicated, nitroglycerin is administered sublingually at a dose of 0.3 mg, which should relieve the symptoms in 3 minutes. The patient should be moved to a reclining position to prevent syncope, which may result from drug administration.
2. When more than three tablets taken over a 15-minute time period do not produce relief, an alternative diagnosis of myocardial infarction should be assumed, and appropriate emergency measures must be instituted promptly.
3. Nitroglycerin is unstable and must be kept tightly sealed in a dark glass container without a plastic plug. The emergency supply of nitroglycerin should be replaced at yearly intervals, if unopened.
4. Avoid conditions that may predispose the

TABLE 31-6. SUMMARY OF ANTIANGINAL DRUGS

Official Name[a]	Route of Administration	Dose	Onset	Duration
nitroglycerin	sublingual	0.15–0.6 mg	rapid	short
	ointment	2 inches	rapid	medium
amyl nitrite	inhalation	0.18–0.3 ml	rapid	short
isosorbide dinitrate	sublingual	2.5–10 mg	rapid	medium
	oral	5–30 mg	slow	long
erythrityl tetranitrate	sublingual	5–15 mg	slow	long
	oral	30 mg	slow	long
mannitol hexanitrate	oral	15–60 mg	slow	long
pentaerythritol tetranitrate	oral	10–20 mg	slow	long

[a] These drugs are available under many trade names.

patient to an attack, such as inadequate local anesthesia or excitement.

5. If the patient has not been previously diagnosed as having angina, he should be referred to a physician if an attack occurs in your office.

Objective 31.D.6. Recognize other organic nitrates available for the treatment of angina and their differences in comparison to nitroglycerin.

There are several alternatives to nitroglycerin in treating angina pectoris, although all of them share the same basic mechanism of action and side efects. These preparations differ primarily in route of administration, onset, and duration as described in Table 31-6.

Objective 31.D.7. Recognize the mechanism of action and side effects of the beta blocking drugs in the treatment of angina pectoris.

The pharmacology of the beta adrenergic blocking agents has already been described elsewhere (Chapters 16 and 18). Two such agents (propranolol and nadolol) are used in the treatment of angina; they probably relieve anginal attacks by the following actions:

1. blockade of sympathetic nervous activity at the heart, resulting in decreased heart rate, decreased force of myocardial contraction, with decreased cardiac output and protection against reflex tachycardia
2. reduction of systemic blood pressure

The side effects of these drugs include:

1. bronchoconstriction
2. precipitation of heart failure
3. hypotension

The β blocking drugs are of little value in treating angina of an acute nature. Moreover, the use of beta blocking drugs may not prevent completely the occurrence of occasional attacks of angina pectoris, and such patients must also be prepared to use nitroglycerin as an adjunct when such attacks occur.

E. ANTIHYPERTENSIVES

Introductory Comments

Objective 31.E.1. Describe the different forms and degrees of hypertension and its relation to dental therapy.

Probably the most common cardiovascular disease with which the dentist must deal (15% incidence in the general population), hypertension is frequently unrecognized by the patient because of its lack of symptoms. Hypertension simply defined is a consistent elevation of blood pressure above normal levels, with diastolic pressure readings of 90 to 105 mm Hg considered to be "mild," and diastolic pressures of greater than 105 mm Hg being termed "moderate-to-severe." If the disease is left undetected and untreated, related disorders can result, in-

Methyl dopa   Hydralazine   ┌ Prazosin
Clonidine   Minoxidil   × ┤ Pargyline (MAO I)
Reserpine   Diazoxide.   └ Phentolamine ┤ Adrenergic
*   Guanethidine*

TABLE 31–7. SITE OF ACTION OF ANTIHYPERTENSIVE DRUGS

Drugs	Primary Site	Secondary Site
thiazides	kidney	arteriolar smooth muscle
hydralazine	arteriolar smooth muscle	—
prazosin	α adrenergic receptors	arteriolar and venular smooth muscle
methyldopa	vasomotor center	adrenergic nerve endings
clonidine	vasomotor center	α adrenergic receptors
guanethidine	adrenergic nerve endings	—
reserpine	vasomotor center	adrenergic nerve endings
β blockers[a]	β adrenergic receptors	[a]
diazoxide	arteriolar smooth muscle	—
minoxidil	arteriolar smooth muscle	—
phentolamine	α adrenergic receptors	—
pargyline (MAOI)	adrenergic nerve endings	vasomotor center
captopril	renin-angiotensin system	—
ganglionic blockers	sympathetic ganglionic receptors	—

[a] The mechanism by which some β blockers are thought to act in the CNS is unknown.

cluding congestive heart failure, kidney failure, cerebral hemorrhage, visual changes, and aneurysms. Risk factors known to increase the likelihood of a patient's developing hypertension include smoking, elevated serum cholesterol, diabetes, and obesity. The dentist is now being called upon to monitor his patients' blood pressures, and he should enthusiastically undertake this charge to serve the patient as well as to be better equipped to properly treat the patient. While blood pressure should be routinely measured in all dental patients, a history of cardiovascular disease in the patient's family, obesity, stress, or changes in renal function (edema, reduced urine flow) should alert the dentist to the possibility of hypertension. Although one reading certainly does not establish a diagnosis of hypertension (especially when the stress of a dental appointment may raise the blood pressure), an elevated reading should be made known to the patient with the recommendation that further readings be made by a physician.

Hypertension may be broadly classified into three categories, based upon the etiologic characteristics of the disease. Essential hypertension is the term for hypertension that cannot be associated with a specific abnormality, that is, it is an idiopathic form of the disease. Secondary hypertension is an elevation of blood pressure which is due to an identifiable abnormality, for example, a tumor of catecholamine-secreting tissues (pheochromocytoma), renal arterial stenosis, and so on. Finally, hypertensive crisis refers to the clinical syndrome in which blood pressure becomes acutely elevated to very high, sustained, and life-threatening levels. This form of the disease includes malignant hypertension, hypertensive encephalopathy, eclampsia, overdoses of vasopressor drugs, and interactions of vasoactive amines with MAO-inhibiting drugs.

Drugs used in the management of hypertension vary in their sites and mechanisms of action, from sedative effects in the cerebral cortex to dilation of peripheral arterioles. The agents are not curative; generally, patients must continue the therapy indefinitely. Table 31–7 presents an overview of the various types of antihypertensive drugs and their sites of action.

Generally, multiple-drug therapy is used (two or three drugs) because lower doses of each drug are more effective when combined than in single-drug therapy. Most cases of hypertension (even severe) can be controlled, and the reduced dosages cause fewer or less intense side effects compared to those encountered with large doses of a single, potent agent.

The dentist should understand the pharmacology of the drugs used to treat hypertension, as side effects caused by these agents may affect dental treatment and drugs prescribed by the dentist may interact with antihypertensive drugs.

Before discussing each drug separately, the following general statements will serve as guidelines.

1. A thiazide diuretic, which is often effective by itself in treating mild hypertension, is used in the treatment of most cases of hypertension, as most of the other antihypertensive drugs result in a retention of salt and water.
2. Since most antihypertensive drugs block adrenergic function, side effects often include parasympathetic predominance, especially bradycardia.
3. Some degree of postural hypotension will occur with the use of most antihypertensive agents, especially with guanethidine.
4. Some degree of impotence occurs with the use of most antihypertensives, especially with guanethidine.
5. Caution should be observed when using vasoconstrictors in patients taking most antihypertensive drugs, especially with guanethidine.

Thiazides

Objective 31.E.2. Recognize the mechanism of action, major effects, toxicity, routes of administration, and drug interactions of thiazide diuretics in the treatment of hypertension.

The diuretic action of the thiazides is described in detail in Chapter 32. In addition to their renal actions of promoting an increase in urinary loss of sodium and chloride, the thiazides (and a related group of drugs, the phthalimidines, e.g., chlorthalidone) produce a decrease in peripheral vascular resistance, which persists beyond the duration of their reduction in plasma volume. Therefore, thiazide diuretics cause reduction in blood pressure by two distinct mechanisms: (1) acutely, by increasing renal excretion of salt and water, which then decreases plasma volume, venous return, and cardiac output, and (2) chronically, by a direct relaxation of vascular smooth muscle. They appear to be most useful either as the sole agent in mild hypertension or used in combination with more efficacious drugs in moderate-to-severe hypertension.

Mechanism of Action. Peripheral arterial relaxation occurs secondary to a reduction in plasma volume.

Related Cardiovascular Effects. These include decreased peripheral resistance, initial decrease in cardiac output and plasma volume (which returns to normal after initiation of therapy), increased aldosterone and renin levels, and decreased plasma volume (returns to normal after initiation of therapy).

Adverse Effects. These include hypokalemia, hyperglycemia, hyperuricemia, orthostatic hypotension, xerostomia, thirst, and lethargy. Allergy to the drugs can occur, and they may aggravate renal or hepatic insufficiency.

Route of Administration. Oral

Drug Interactions. The thiazides can aggravate the hypokalemia and associated cardiac changes produced by digitalis glycosides, can aggravate gout or precipitate an acute attack, and increase the incidence of orthostatic hypotension when used with other antihypertensive drugs. Some preparations are listed below:

1. bendroflumethiazide (*Naturetin*)
2. benzthiazide (*Exna*)
3. **chlorothiazide** (*Diuril*)
4. cyclothiazide (*Anhydron*)
5. flumethiazide (*Ademol*)
6. **hydrochlorothiazide** (*Esidrix, Hydrodiuril*)
7. methyclothiazide (*Enduron*)
8. quinethazone (*Hydromox*)

This list is not complete, nor does it include preparations consisting of thiazide diuretics in combination with other antihypertensive agents. Some of these combinations are listed in 31.E.3. (Preparations of hydralazine).

Other Diuretics. In patients whose hypertension is complicated by edema, other, more potent diuretics may be used. The reader is referred to Chapter 32 for a discussion of these agents.

Hydralazine

Objective 31.E.3. Recognize the mechanism of action, related cardiovascular effects, and drug interactions of hydralazine.

Mechanism of Action. Hydralazine acts by directly relaxing vascular smooth muscle.

Related Cardiovascular Effects. Hydralazine results in an increased heart rate and cardiac output by sympathetic reflex and by a direct action on the heart. While renal blood flow is increased, urine output is diminished, resulting in salt and water retention.

Adverse Effects. In order of decreasing incidence, these include headache, palpitations, loss of appetite, postural hypotension, nausea, dizziness, sweating, nasal congestion, flushing, lacrimation, conjunctivitis, parethesias, edema, tremors, muscle cramps, drug fever, urticaria, skin rash, polyneuritis, gastrointestinal hemorrhage, anemia, pancytopenia, acute rheumatoid state, and a lupus erythematosus-like state.

Route of Administration. In addition to being available in oral form, hydralazine is available for parenteral use.

Drug Interactions. Hydralazine can interact with any other drug which lowers blood pressure to produce postural hypotension and, in some cases, severe depression of blood pressure.

Preparations of Hydralazine. Some combinations are listed below:

1. *Apresoline*
2. *Apresazide* (combined with hydrochlorothiazide)
3. *Apresoline-Esidrix* (combined with hydrochlorothiazide)
4. *Dralserp* (combined with reserpine)
5. *Ser-Ap-Es* (combined with reserpine and hydrochlorothiazide)
6. *Serpasil-Apresoline* (combined with reserpine)
7. *Unipres* (combined with reserpine and hydrochlorothiazide)

Prazosin

Objective 31.E.4. Recognize the mechanism of action, related cardiovascular effects, adverse effects, and drug interactions of prazosin.

Mechanism of Action. Alpha$_1$ adrenergic receptor blockade (Chapter 18).

Related Cardiovascular Effects. The antihypertensive effect of prazosin is not accompanied by significant changes in cardiac output, heart rate, or renal blood flow.

Adverse Effects. These include (most commonly) postural hypotension and syncope, dizziness, headache, drowsiness, lack of energy and weakness, nausea, and palpitations. Less frequently, prazosin can cause gastrointestinal upset, with nausea and vomiting.

Route of Administration. Oral

Drug Interactions. There is enhanced hypotension (possibly producing syncope) when prazosin is used with other antihypertensives.

Preparation. Minipress.

Methyldopa

Objective 31.E.5. Recognize the mechanisms of action, related cardiovascular effects, adverse effects, and drug interactions of methyldopa.

Mechanisms of Action. Noradrenergic brain neurons convert methyldopa to methylnorepinephrine. When released in the medulla oblongata, this potently combines with central alpha receptors to inhibit sympathetic vasomotor outflow. In the peripheral vessels, methyldopa may further inhibit vascular tone by acting as a weak adrenergic neurotransmitter (false transmitter, Chapters 16 and 18) or by directly inhibiting vascular smooth muscle tone.

Related Cardiovascular Effects. These include bradycardia, decrease in total peripheral resistance, decreased cardiac output, decrease in plasma renin level (slight), and minimal postural hypotension (sympathetic reflexes intact).

Adverse Effects. These include sedation (common), vertigo, extrapyramidal signs, postural hypotension (minor problem, see above), edema (due to salt and water retention), impotence, drug fever (chills and high, spiking temperature), hepatic dysfunction, hemolytic anemia, lactation (in either sex), and rebound hypertension. Xerostomia has also been reported.

Drug Interactions. These include potential enhancement of CNS depressants, enhanced hypotension (if given with other antihypertensives), possibly *increased* blood pressure if given with amphetamines, tricyclic antidepressants, phenothiazines, or sympathomimetics, hallucinations if given with MAO inhibitors, and reduction of efficacy of levodopa (antiparkinson agent).

Preparations of methyldopa include *Aldomet* and *Aldoclor* (combined with chlorothiazide).

Clonidine

Objective 31.E.6. Recognize the mechanism of action, related cardiovascular effects, adverse effects, and drug interactions of clonidine.

Mechanism of Action. Clonidine inhibits sympathetic outflow in the medulla oblongata by stimulation of central alpha adrenergic receptors (essentially the same as methyldopa, see 31.E.5.).

Related Cardiovascular Effects. These include peripheral alpha adrenergic blockade, peripheral impairment of norepinephrine release, decreased cardiac output, bradycardia, decrease in plasma renin levels, renal sodium retention with decreased urine output, and minimal postural hypotension (cardiovascular reflexes intact).

Adverse Effects. These include sedation, dry mouth, impotence, hypertensive crisis (if drug is suddenly withdrawn), postural hypotension, and allergic skin reactions (rashes, pruritus, urticaria).

Drug Interactions. These include sedation enhanced by other CNS depressants, and blood pressure increased by tricyclic antidepressants.

Preparation. Clonidine (*Catapres*).

Guanethidine

Objective 31.E.7. Recognize the mechanisms of action, related cardiovascular effects, adverse effects, and drug interactions of guanethidine.

Mechanisms of Action. (1) Guanethidine blocks the release of norepinephrine, either through reduction of the amount of norepinephrine synthesized or by interference with the release mechanism. (2) Guanethidine also depletes noradrenergic neurons of their norepinephrine content (Chapters 16 and 18).

Related Cardiovascular Effects. Rapid IV infusion results in an initial response that is triphasic (rapid fall in BP, then hypertension occurs for several hours, then a progressive decrease in BP). Other effects include bradycardia, decreased pulse pressure, decreased cardiac output, sodium and water retention, and prominent postural hypotension (cardiovascular reflexes inhibited).

Adverse Effects. These include orthostatic hypotension, edema (may require concurrent diuretic therapy), diarrhea, and inhibiton of ejaculation.

Drug Interactions. These include:

1. antagonism of hypotensive effect by chlorpromazine, tricyclic antidepressants, haloperidol, and thioxanthines
2. acute hypertensive crisis if given with sympathomimetic amines, including phenylephrine, levonordefrin, norepinephrine, epinephrine, and mephentermine
3. antagonism of hypotensive effect by amphetamine, diethylpropion, ephedrine, hydoxyamphetamine, and methylphenidate

4. antagonism of hypotensive effect by MAO inhibitors
5. exaggerated hypotensive effect if given with methotrimeprazine or levodopa

Preparations. Guanethidine (*Ismelin*).

Reserpine

Objective 31.E.8. Describe the mechanisms of action, related cardiovascular effects, adverse effects, and drug interactions of reserpine.

Mechanisms of Action. Reserpine acts by depleting noradrenergic neurons of their catecholamine stores and also blocks the reuptake of norepinephrine into the storage vesicles of these same neurons.

Related Cardiovascular Effects. These include bradycardia, decrease in plasma renin levels, sodium retention and decreased urine volume, and minimal postural hypotension (except at high doses).

Adverse Effects. These include sedation, psychic depression, nightmares, development of suicidal tendencies, gastrointestinal distress (cramps, increased acidity, diarrhea), nasal congestion, decreased sex drive, and breast cancer (possibly in females only).

Drug Interactions. These include antagonism of ephedrine and levodopa, potentiation of the central effects of LSD, antagonism by MAO inhibitors, potentiation by methotrimeprazine, and potentiation of CNS depressants.

Preparations. These include:

reserpine (*Rau-Sed*)
SK-Reserpine
Sandril
Serpasil

Other commercial preparations in which reserpine is combined with a diuretic or other antihypertensive agent:

Demi-Regroton	*Naquival*
Diupres	*Hydromox R*
Diutensen-R	*Hydropres*
Hydrotensin	*Salutensin*
Metatensin	*Ser-Ap-Es*
Exna-R	*Dralserp*
Renese-R	*Regroton*

Beta Adrenergic Blocking Drugs

Objective 31.E.9. Recognize the mechanism of action, related cardiovascular effects, adverse effects, and drug interactions of the beta blockers.

Mechanism of Action. Beta adrenergic blockade results in decreased cardiac output, blockade of catecholamine actions, and decreased renin secretion by the kidney.

Related Cardiovascular Effects. These include bradycardia, decreased plasma renin levels, sodium retention, and decreased urine output.

Adverse Effects. These include precipitation of heart failure in individuals with preexisting cardiac deficits, cardiac arrest in the presence of heart block, aggravation of asthmatic conditions by increased airway resistance, gastrointestinal upset (nausea, vomiting, constipation, or diarrhea), CNS disturbances (nightmares, hallucinations, insomnia, depression), infrequent allergic reactions (rash, fever, purpura).

Drug Interactions. These include aminophylline antagonism of beta adrenergic antagonists, potentiation of sulfonylurea oral antidiabetic agents, enhanced myocardial depression by chloroform, phenytoin, quinidine, and ether, possible cardiac arrest with digitalis, enhancement of insulin activity, epinephrine reversal (marked bradycardia and/or hypertension), intense vasoconstriction and elevated BP with ergot alkaloids, hypertensive episode with methyldopa or MAO inhibitors, enhancement of hypotension with phenothiazines, additive beta blockade with reserpine, and prolongation of the action of tubocurarine.

Preparations. These, listed with type of blockade, include:

propranolol (*Inderal*)	β_1 and β_2
metoprolol (*Lopressor*)	β_1
nadolol (*Corgard*)	β_1 and β_2

atenolol (*Tenormin*) β_1
timolol (*Blocadren*) β_1 and β_2

Secondary Agents

Objective 31.E.10. Recognize other antihypertensive drugs that have previously been employed or have only limited application in the treatment of hypertension.

Secondary antihypertensive agents are those agents reserved only for the treatment of special cases of elevated blood pressure (cases refractory to other conventional agents or agents to lower the patient's blood pressure during surgery). Some of these agents are no longer used clinically. A list of these agents with a brief description follows.

1. **Minoxidil** (*Loniten*) is a recently introduced, potent antihypertensive agent reserved for use in severe hypertension. It apparently acts by directly relaxing arteriolar smooth muscle. Minoxidil can produce side effects similar to those of hydralazine and can also produce a dangerous condition known as "pericardial effusion." Minoxidil is usually used in combination with a beta blocking drug and a diuretic to reduce its dosage and, hence its side effects.

2. **Captopril** (*Capoten*) blocks the conversion of angiotensin I to angiotensin II, the latter being the active, vasoconstricting form of the endogenous peptide. This makes the drug useful in treating hypertension associated with high activity of the renin-angiotensin system, as in renovascular hypertension. However, the drug appears to be useful in other forms of hypertension as well. Side effects include increases in plasma potassium and renin, tachycardia, fever, rash, alteration of taste, and proteinuria (Chapter 19).

3. Ganglionic blocking drugs (e.g., mecamylamine)

4. Monoamine oxidase inhibitors (e.g., pargyline)

5. Veratrum alkaloids

The pharmacology of the ganglionic blocking agents and the MAO inhibitors is discussed in Chapters 16 and 17.

Objective 31.E.11. Recognize emergency antihypertensive drugs.

The following drugs are those which can be used in cases of emergency hypertensive crises (e.g., malignant hypertension); they are usually administered parenterally. The use of diazoxide is presented in Appendix I; the others are considered to be medical emergency drugs.

1. **diazoxide**
2. sodium nitroprusside
3. trimethaphan
4. phenotolamine
5. furosemide
6. hydralazine

Objective 31.E.12. Recognize the potential complications in dental patients taking specific antihypertensive medications.

The following is a summary of potential dental treatment complications associated with the use of specific antihypertensive drugs.

Thiazide Diuretics. These may be associated with postural hypotension, xerostomia, and hyperuricemia. The latter effect may be a consideration in the dental patient with temporomandibular joint dysfunction associated with gout.

Prazosin. This drug may induce postural hypotension.

Methyldopa. This drug may cause postural hypotension or xerostomia and may enhance CNS depression when given with other CNS depressants. Precautions should be taken with the use of vasoconstrictors in patients taking methyldopa (reduce dosages of vasoconstrictors).

Guanethidine. Postural hypotension is frequently encountered with guanethidine. Antipsychotic drugs, such as chlorpromazine, should be avoided in patients taking guanethidine. Vasoconstrictors should be used with caution in these patients (avoid vasoconstrictor if possible or use reduced dose if considered necessary).

Reserpine. Patients taking reserpine may experience psychic depression, and the sedation produced by this drug can result in an enhancement of the effect of CNS depressants administered by the dentist. Postural hypotension can also be a problem in patients taking this drug.

Beta Blockers. These agents may occasionally produce psychic depression, with resultant implications for dental therapy.

Clonidine. This drug has similar implications as methyldopa (see discussion above).

REFERENCES

Conn HL Jr: Congestive heart failure. In Conn HL Jr, Horowitz O (eds): Cardiac and Vascular Diseases. Philadelphia, Lea & Febiger, 1971, Vol I, p 433
Csáky TZ: Cutting's Handbook of Pharmacology, 6th ed. New York, Appleton-Century-Crofts, 1979, pp 171, 173, 178, 181–182, 242, 273
Hoffman BF: The genesis of cardiac arrhythmias. Prog Cardiovasc Dis 8:319, 1966
Levine WG: Anticoagulant, antithrombotic, and thrombolytic drugs. In Goodman LS, Gilman A (eds): The Pharmacological Basis of Therapeutics, 5th ed. New York, Macmillan, 1975, p 1357

BIBLIOGRAPHY

Gilman AG, Goodman LS, and Gilman A (eds): Goodman and Gilman's The Pharmacological Basis of Therapeutics, 6th ed. New York, Macmillan, 1980, Ch 27, 30, 31, 32, 33

QUESTIONS

1. In addition to impedance to cardiac inflow and impaired contractility of the heart, which one of the following can result in congestive heart failure?

   A. Increased work load on the heart
   B. Lowering of pulmonary vascular resistance
   C. Hyperuricemia
   D. None of the above

2. **T F** In patients with congestive circulatory failure, the heart may compensate by an increased heart rate, by cardiac dilatation (increased contractility), and by cardiac hypertrophy.

3. Congestive failure of the left ventricle results in symptoms primarily associated with which one of the following?

   A. Gastrointestinal system
   B. Pulmonary system
   C. Musculoskeletal system
   D. All of the above

4. Congestive failure of the right ventricle results in symptoms primarily associated with which one of the following?

   A. Abdominal viscera
   B. Pulmonary system
   C. Central nervous system
   D. All of the above.

5. In addition to cardiac glycosides, patients with congestive heart failure may also be treated by (*select one answer*):

   A. Peripheral vasodilators
   B. Controlled diet
   C. Diuretic drugs
   D. All of the above
   E. None of the above

6. Digitalis, a common cardiac glycoside, is isolated from which one of the following sources?

   A. *Digitalis lanata*
   B. *Digitalis purpurea*
   C. *Strophanthus gratus*
   D. None of the above

7. At therapeutic doses, cardiac glycosides produce all of the following actions *except:* (*select one*)

A. Positive inotropic effect

B. Positive chronotropic effect

C. Peripheral vasoconstriction

D. Increased renal blood flow

8. **T F** Side effects of cardiac glycosides include nausea and cardiac arrhythmias.

9. **T F** Cardiac glycosides are useful in the treatment of atrial flutter.

10. **T F** Epinephrine, at levels used in local anesthetic solutions, does not interact with the cardiac glycosides to produce any adverse effects.

11. **T F** Medical consultation and possible antibiotic prophylaxis may be necessary in patients with congestive heart failure.

12. **T F** Atrial fibrillation is an immediately life-threatening situation.

13. **T F** Automaticity refers to the period following activation of the cardiac conduction system.

14. **T F** In the reentry phenomenon, a cardiac arrhythmia results from an increased rate of spontaneous depolarization of the SA node.

15. **T F** Quinidine results in an increased conduction velocity in the heart.

16. **T F** Lidocaine exerts an antiarrhythmic effect by decreasing automaticity.

17. **T F** Procainamide closely resembles quinidine in its pharmacologic actions.

18. In addition to blocking cardiac adrenergic impulses, propranolol acts as an antiarrhythmic drug by which one of the following mechanisms?

A. Increased A-V refractory period

B. Increased firing rate of the sinoatrial node

C. Arresting atrial contractions

D. None of the above

19. Phenytoin most closely resembles which one of the following in its antiarrhythmic actions?

A. Procainamide

B. Quinidine

C. Lidocaine

D. Propranolol

20. The pharmacologic properties of disopyramide most closely resemble those of which one of the following antiarrhythmic drugs?

A. Phenytoin

B. Lidocaine

C. Digitalis

D. Quinidine

21. Verapamil is indicated in which one of the following types of cardiac arrhythmias?

A. Ventricular fibrillation

B. Ventricular tachycardia

C. A-V block

D. Supraventricular tachycardia

22. In patients taking quinidine or procainamide, the condition of the oral cavity may be characterized by which one of the following?

A. Excessive salivation

B. Gingival hyperplasia

C. Xerostomia

D. None of the above

23. Clotting Factor IV is (*select one*):

A. Thromboplastin

B. Calcium

C. Prothrombin

D. Fibrinogen

24. In the process of blood clot formation, which one of the following is the material which forms the structure of the actual clot?

A. Fibrinogen
B. Thrombin
C. Globulin
D. None of the above

25. The action of heparin can be antagonized by which one of the following?

A. Vitamin C
B. Vitamin K
C. Protamine sulfate
D. Calcium

26. Barbiturates may reduce the effectiveness of the oral anticoagulants by which one of the following mechanisms?

A. Increased protein binding of the anticoagulant
B. Stimulation of the synthesis of natural clotting factors
C. Induction of hepatic degradation of the anticoagulant
D. Direct complexing of the barbiturate and the anticoagulant in the blood

27. In patients with liver disease, the activity of the oral anticoagulants would most likely be affected in which one of the following ways?

A. Anticoagulant activity would be decreased
B. Anticoagulant activity would be increased
C. Liver function would not affect anticoagulant activity

28. T F Diphenadione is classified as a parenteral-only anticoagulant.

29. T F Prior to beginning dental treatment of a patient taking anticoagulants, a consultation with the patient's physician is not necessary.

30. T F Gelatin-based topical hemostatics act by precipitation of blood proteins.

31. T F Angina pectoris may be precipitated by stress associated with a dental visit.

32. T F Avoidance of smoking and overeating may be nondrug treatments for angina pectoris.

33. T F The two types of drugs used in the treatment of angina are beta blockers and antiarrhythmics.

34. Nitroglycerin and other antianginals produce all of the following therapeutic actions *except* (*select one*):

A. Relaxation of coronary vascular smooth muscle
B. Decreased cardiac output
C. Decreased venous return
D. Increased systolic blood pressure

35. T F The usual emergency dose of nitroglycerin is 0.3 mg sublingually.

36. Amyl nitrite differs from nitroglycerin in which one of the following ways?

A. It does not relax vascular smooth muscle
B. It has a rapid onset of action
C. It is administered by inhalation
D. It does not reduce cardiac output

37. In addition to reducing cardiac contractility and heart rate, beta blocking drugs are useful in treating angina because of which one of the following actions?

A. Increased venous return
B. Reduction of systemic blood pressure
C. Increased oxygenation of arterial blood
D. None of the above

38. The etiology of essential hypertension is associated with:

A. Renal arteriosclerosis
B. Central aberration of the vasomotor center

C. Elevated cardiac output

D. Unknown factors

39. Which one of the following side effects is not characteristic of the thiazide diuretics?

A. Hypertension

B. Hypokalemia

C. Hyperuricemia

D. Xerostomia

40. Hydralazine exerts its antihypertensive effect through which one of the following mechanisms?

A. Increased renal excretion of salt and water

B. Inhibition of renal renin output

C. Direct relaxation of vascular smooth muscle

D. Blockade of beta adrenergic receptors

41. **T F** Prazosin acts by blockade of alpha adrenergic receptors.

42. When given along with amphetamines or tricyclic antidepressants, methyldopa may produce which one of the following adverse effects?

A. Cardiac arrest

B. Severe hypotension

C. Hypertension

D. None of the above

43. Clonidine acts at which one of the following sites?

A. Medulla oblongata

B. Sympathetic autonomic ganglia

C. Smooth muscle cell membrane

D. None of the above

44. Guanethidine is especially prone to produce which one of the following adverse effects?

A. Depletion of plasma volume by rapid renal excretion of water

B. Orthostatic hypotension

C. Tachycardia

D. None of the above

45. **T F** Reserpine acts by blocking cholinergic receptors in sympathetic ganglia.

46. **T F** Propranolol may produce marked bradycardia when given with epinephrine.

47. **T F** Ganglionic blocking drugs are secondary antihypertensive agents for patients refractory to conventional drugs.

48. **T F** Sodium nitroprusside is considered to be an antihypertensive drug used in emergency situations only.

49. In addition to postural hypotension, reserpine can complicate dental therapy in which one of the following ways?

A. Potentiation of CNS depressants administered by the dentist

B. Paradoxical hypertension

C. Antagonism of CNS depressants administered by the dentist

D. None of the above

32

Diuretics

A. INTRODUCTION

Diuretics are drugs that act directly on the kidney to increase the rate of formation of urine by increasing the rate at which the kidneys excrete salt and water. The diuretic drugs exert their action specifically by inhibiting the renal reabsorption of ions and water.

The diuretics are primarily used to treat hypertension and to treat edema associated with cirrhosis of the liver, congestive heart failure, and in steroid therapy. They have other applications, which will be dealt with in the discussion of individual agents.

B. NORMAL KIDNEY FUNCTION

Objective 32.B.1. Recognize the normal reabsorptive processes in the proximal, distal, and collecting tubules and the loop of Henle which can be altered by diuretic drugs.

Before the therapeutic actions and side effects of the diuretics can be fully appreciated, it will be necessary to briefly review renal function

(Fig. 32–1). The functions reviewed here are those pertinent to diuretic action; it should be remembered that many other processes are accomplished by the kidney. The process of urine formation begins with glomerular filtration. In this process, the hydrostatic pressure in glomerular capillaries drives an ultrafiltrate of the blood plasma (devoid of blood cells and protein) through the capillary walls, the glomerular basement membrane, and the glomerular epithelial cells into the proximal tubule (which is the beginning of the nephron proper). It should be recalled that the kidney is composed of many such nephrons with their associated glomeruli. Glomerular filtration rate is proportional to renal blood flow, which is autoregulated, and is normally 120 ml/min. The diuretic drugs discussed here do not act by increasing glomerular filtration rate, although some drugs (e.g., cardiac glycosides or xanthines) are capable of this action.

Process A (Fig. 32–1) occurs in the proximal tubule. A large fraction of the filtered Na^+ (70 to 80%) is actively reabsorbed, with Cl^- and H_2O following passively. Tubular and interstitial fluid are isosmotic here. Process B occurs in the

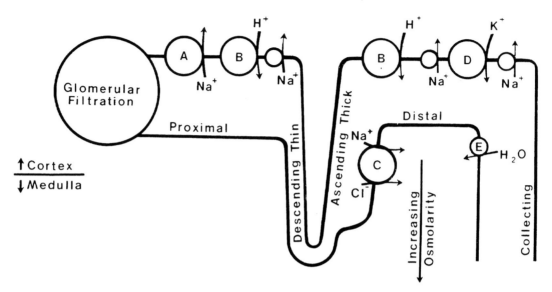

Figure 32-1. Physiologic processes in the renal nephron. Process A. Active reabsorption of Na$^+$ in proximal tubule. Process B. H$^+$ generation of secretion (proximal and distal). Process C. Active reabsorption of Cl$^-$ in ascending limb. Process D. K$^+$ exchange for Na$^+$ (distal tubule). Process E. Water reabsorption (collecting ducts). (*Adapted from Mudge GH: In Gilman AG, Goodman LS, Gilman A (eds): Goodman and Gilman's The Pharmacological Basis of Therapeutics, 6th ed, 1980. Courtesy of Macmillan.*)

proximal and distal tubules. H$^+$ ion is generated by carbonic anhydrase in tubular cells and actively secreted in exchange for Na$^+$, which accompanies the HCO$_3^-$ ion into the plasma. In this way, urinary bicarbonate is converted to H$_2$CO$_3$, which then breaks down into H$_2$O and CO$_2$. The CO$_2$ passes into the tubular cells to be converted into HCO$_3^-$ by carbonic anhydrase. In other words, urinary bicarbonate is first converted into CO$_2$, and plasma bicarbonate is then restored by the action of the kidney cells on CO$_2$. Process C occurs in the ascending, thick limb of the loop of Henle. Cl$^-$ is actively reabsorbed, with Na$^+$ following passively. This segment is impermeable to water, so that urine osmolarity is less than that of the surrounding interstitium (this is the so-called diluting segment of the kidney). The interstitial osmolarity progressively increases from the corticomedullary junction to the renal papillae due to a countercurrent multiplying effect of the loop of Henle. Process D occurs in the distal tubule. K$^+$ is actively secreted in exchange for Na$^+$. This process is stimulated by the mineralocorticoid

hormone, aldosterone. Process E occurs in the collecting tubule. Water may be passively reabsorbed under the influence of the hypertonic medullary interstitium, when antidiuretic hormone (ADH or vasopressin) is present (as in conditions of fluid depletion, when the plasma is excessively concentrated). When ADH is absent (as when fluid intake is excessive and the plasma is dilute), the collecting tubule is impermeable to water, and water is not reabsorbed here but is excreted.

C. OSMOTIC DIURETICS

Objective 32.C.1. Recognize the mechanism of action of the osmotic diuretics and their effects on blood and urine composition.

Objective 32.C.2. Recognize an osmotic diuretic drug and the reason for the diuretic effect of glucose.

Osmotic diuretics are substances which are pharmacologically inert, which are freely filtered at the glomerulus, and which are not appreciably reabsorbed by the tubules. When such an agent is given, it enters the proximal tubule, where it osmotically obligates water to remain within the tubule. This dilutes the Na^+ ion in the proximal tubule and thereby reduces its reabsorption. Osmotic diuretics also increase blood flow in the medulla of the kidney which washes out the hypertonicity of the medulla and reduces water reabsorption in the collecting tubule. Because tubular fluid volume is elevated, tubular flow rate is increased, which further reduces distal Na^+ reabsorption.

Mannitol is an osmotic diuretic and is used for the prophylactic treatment of acute renal failure and for reduction of cerebrospinal fluid pressure. Osmotic diuretics are not used to treat edema, because they expand extracellular fluid volume acutely. Glucose acts as an osmotic diuretic in diabetes mellitus because the rate at which it is filtered exceeds th, rate at which the kidney can reabsorb it.

Osmotic diuretics result in the formation of a dilute urine with a low salt concentration. They usually produce no adverse effects when given intravenously for their therapeutic action. The osmotic diuretic most widely used is mannitol (*Osmitrol*).

D. ORGANIC MERCURIALS

Objective 32.D.1. Recognize the mechanism of action of the organic mercurial diuretics and their effect on blood and urine composition.

Objective 32.D.2. Recognize two mercurial diuretics and their actions.

It was noted long ago that the use of calomel (mercurous chloride) as a component of drug mixtures resulted in a diuresis. Later, in searching for compounds with diuretic activity, organic mercurial compounds were developed and served as the mainstay of diuretic therapy until the advent of the more potent, orally effective diuretics (discussion follows).

The organic mercurials have the basic chemical structure shown in Figure 32–2. This struc-

$$O - CH_3$$
$$|$$
$$R - CH - CH_2 - Hg^+$$

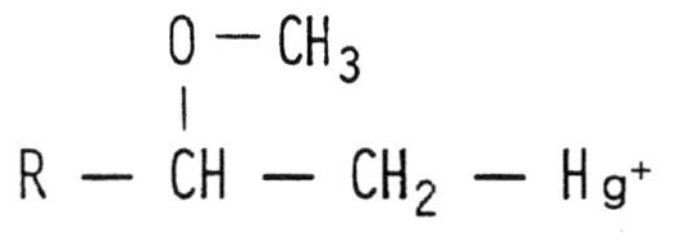

Figure 32–2. Structure of organic mercurials.

ture demonstrates an acid-labile bond between mercury and carbon. Apparently, in the presence of an acid medium (as when urinary pH is acidic), the organic mercurial compounds are concentrated in the kidney and release mercuric ion in the renal tissue. It is believed that this mercuric ion then complexes with components of renal metabolism (e.g., sulfhydryl groups on critical enzymes) to impair Na^+ transport. The organic mercurials do not impair the regeneration of bicarbonate, however, and the major anion that is excreted with Na^+ during the diuresis is Cl^-. This results in a hypochloremic or subtraction alkalosis. As the alkalosis develops, urinary pH rises and the effectiveness of the organic mercurial diuretics is diminished because less mercuric ion is released. The development of a refractory state within a few days and the poor oral absorption of the organic mercurials constitute their major disadvantages and account for their relatively rare use. The two organic mercurials currently in use are **mercaptomerin** (*Thiomerin*) and **meralluride** (*Mercuhydrin*).

E. THIAZIDES

Objective 32.E.1. Recognize the mechanism of action of the thiazide diuretics and their effect on blood and urine composition.

Objective 32.E.2. Be able to recognize the names chlorothiazide and hydrochlorothiazide.

The thiazides are sulfonamide derivatives that were discovered as a result of a search for new carbonic anhydrase inhibitors. The thiazides are widely used for both hypertension and edematous states. There are many different commercial preparations of thiazide diuretics, all of which share the same basic pharmacologic actions but vary in potency (dose) and in their duration of action (the latter is dependent on differences in protein binding).

The thiazides act by blocking active Na^+ reabsorption in the first part of the distal tubules. This results in an increased delivery of Na^+ in the tubular fluid to the major portion of the distal tubule, which results in a marked increase in Na^+–K^+ exchange. As a result of enhanced distal K^+ secretion, in an attempt by the kidney to conserve Na^+, a systemic hypokalemia results. This is a potentially dangerous side effect in individuals who are also taking cardiac glycosides, since the actions of the glycosides are potentiated by low serum K^+ levels. Such individuals usually receive K^+ supplements. There are currently many thiazide preparations in use, including methyclothiazide (*Enduron*), **chlorothiazide** (*Diuril*), bendroflumethiazide (*Naturetin*), **hydrochlorothiazide** (*Hydrodiuril*), and quinethazone (*Hydromox*).

F. FUROSEMIDE AND ETHACRYNIC ACID

Objective 32.F.1. Recognize the mechanism of action of furosemide and ethacrynic acid (high-ceiling diuretics) and their effect on blood and urine composition.

Objective 32.F.2. Recognize the names of two high-ceiling diuretics.

Furosemide and ethacrynic acid are chemically distinct diuretics which are characterized by (1) a very rapid onset of action (within 30 min.), (2) an action on active Cl^- transport in the ascending thick limb of the loop of Henle, (3) an action that is independent of acid-base balance, with (4) a high degree of efficacy (a high percentage inhibition of salt reabsorption) and a relatively great increase in effect per unit increase in dose (a relatively steep dose-response curve). Because of such characteristics, these agents are also known as "loop diuretics" and "high-ceiling" diuretics.

As with thiazides, ethacrynic acid and furosemide increase the delivery of Na^+ to the distal tubule with an increase in Na^+–K^+ exchange

and hypokalemia. Contributing to this increased Na^+–K^+ exchange is an increase in aldosterone secretion by the adrenal cortex, which results from an increase in angiotensin levels secondary to the reduction in circulating plasma volume. The commercially available **furosemide** preparation is *Lasix*, while the trade name for ethacrynic acid is *Edecrin*.

G. POTASSIUM-SPARING DIURETICS

Objective 32.G.1. Recognize the mechanism of action of potassium-sparing diuretics and their effect on blood and urine composition.

Objective 32.G.2. Recognize names of two potassium-sparing diuretics.

There are two agents in this category, **spironolactone** (*Aldactone*) and **triamterene** (*Dyrenium*). Spironolactone acts as a competitive inhibitor of aldosterone and inhibits the distal tubular Na^+–K^+ exchange mechanism by interfering with aldosterone's stimulation. Triamterene is not a competitive antagonist of aldosterone but appears to directly inhibit distal Na^+–K^+ exchange. Because of the relatively small amount of Na^+ that is reabsorbed distally (in comparison with the proximal tubule), spironolactone and triamterene are characterized by relatively low efficacy. However, they are useful adjuncts with K^+-depleting diuretics, such as thiazides and the high ceiling diuretics, because they reduce the amount of K^+ that is excreted.

H. CARBONIC ANHYDRASE INHIBITORS

Objective 32.H.1. Recognize the mechanism of action of the carbonic anhydrase inhibitors and their effect on blood and urine composition.

Objective 32.H.2. Be able to recognize the drug acetazolamide.

Carbonic anhydrase is an enzyme that is distributed throughout the body, including kidney, cortex, brain, GI tract, pancreas, eye, and red blood cells. This enzyme catalyzes step A of the following reaction.

$$CO_2 + H_2O \xrightleftharpoons{A} H_2CO_3 \xrightleftharpoons{B} H^+ + HCO_3^-$$

Step B of the reaction proceeds spontaneously.

The carbonic anhydrase inhibitors are sulfonamide derivatives which act by inhibiting the production of H^+, which is normally secreted in exchange for Na^+ in both the proximal and distal portions of the nephron. This results in an increased excretion of $NaHCO_3$ without concomitant loss of Cl^-. Since the K^+–Na^+ exchange mechanism is not affected, K^+ loss also occurs. The net effect of these diuretics is a hyperchloremic/hypokalemic acidosis, which then reduces the effectiveness of the drugs. Because $NaHCO_3$ is being excreted, the urine becomes alkaline. The carbonic anhydrase inhibitors are relatively weak diuretics. Because of their effects on blood pH and H^+ secretion, however, they are also used in grand mal and petit mal epilepsy, glaucoma, and conditions in which alkalinization of the urine is desirable, such as salicylate toxicity. Available drugs in this group include **acetazolamide** (*Diamox*), dichlorphenamide (*Daranide*), ethoxzolamide (*Cardrase*), and methazolamide (*Neptazane*).

I. SIDE EFFECTS OF DIURETICS

Objective 32.I.1. Recognize general side effects that may occur with specific classes of diuretic drugs.

Because the diuretics reduce circulating plasma volume, they can produce dry mouth, thirst, orthostatic hypotension, and tachycardia. Similarly, modification of serum electrolytes by diuretics can result in nausea, vomiting, and central nervous system aberrations, such as dizziness and headache. These side effects are general and may be produced by any of the diuretic agents discussed above. Likewise, allergy to any of these agents may occur, although this side effect is more likely with the sulfonamide derivatives.

In addition to these general side effects, some types of diuretic agents are associated with specific side effects, as follows:

1. hyperuricemia (thiazides, furosemide, ethacrynic acid)
2. cardiac arrhythmias (intravenously administered mercurials)
3. hypokalemia (thiazides, furosemide, ethacrynic acid)
4. ototoxicity (ethacrynic acid, furosemide)
5. hyperglycemia (thiazides, furosemide, ethacrynic acid)
6. paresthesias (acetazolamide, furosemide, ethacrynic acid)
7. oral lesions (mercurials)

J. CLINICAL IMPLICATIONS

Objective 32.J.1. Describe clinical implications for dental patients who are taking diuretic drugs.

The use of a diuretic agent by one of your patients should alert you to the presence of some systemic disease, especially a cardiovascular disorder, such as hypertension or congestive heart failure. As noted above, patients taking carbonic anhydrase inhibitors may be suffering from glaucoma or epilepsy.

The treatment of a dental patient who is taking diuretics may need to be altered, according to consultation with the patient's physician. It may be necessary to consider salt and water intake resulting from drugs or dietary regimens you may prescribe, and you should be aware that the side effects of the diuretics may affect dental care, e.g., dry mouth may reduce the retention of removable prostheses, and it may also increase the incidence of cervical caries. Orthostatic hypotension may predispose the patient to fainting, especially on rising from the dental chair. With respect to drug interactions, streptomycin and other aminoglycoside antibiotics should not be given to a patient taking one of the high-ceiling diuretics because of an increased risk of deafness. Finally, thiazides, furosemide, and ethacrynic acid may worsen gouty arthritis of the temporomandibular joint by elevating serum uric acid levels.

TABLE 32–1. DIURETICS

Classification	Drug Names	Major Mode of Action	Major Side Effect
osmotics	mannitol (*Osmitrol*)	osmotically obligates H_2O to remain in tubule	—
mercurials	mercaptomerin (*Thiomerin*) meralluride (*Mercuhydrin*)	block Na^+ reabsorption	hypochloremic alkalosis
thiazides	bendroflumethiazide (*Naturetin*) chlorothiazide (*Diuril*) hydrochlorothiazide (*Hydrodiuril*) methyclothiazide (*Enduron*) quinethazone (*Hydromox*)	block Na^+ reabsorption	hypokalemia
high-ceiling	furosemide (*Lasix*) ethacrynic acid (*Edecrin*)	block Cl^- reabsorption	hypokalemia
potassium-sparing	spironolactone (*Aldactone*) triamterene (*Dyrenium*)	competitively inhibits aldosterone inhibits distal Na^+–K^+ exchange	—
carbonic anhydrase inhibitors	acetazolamide (*Diamox*) methazolamide (*Neptazane*)	inhibits carbonic anhydrase	metabolic acidosis

K. SUMMARY OF DIURETICS

Table 32–1 is presented as a reference and aid in remembering the important diuretic agents.

REFERENCES

Mudge GH: Drugs affecting renal function and electrolyte metabolism. In Gilman AG, Goodman LS, Gilman A (eds): Goodman and Gilman's The Pharmacological Basis of Therapeutics, 6th ed. New York, Macmillan, 1980, p 887

BIBLIOGRAPHY

Csáky TZ: Cutting's Handbook of Pharmacology, 6th ed. New York, Appleton-Century-Crofts, 1979, Ch 20
Gilman, AG, Goodman LS, Gilman A (eds): Goodman and Gilman's The Pharmacological Basis of Therapeutics, 6th ed. New York, Macmillan, 1980, Ch 36
Pitts RH: Physiology of the Kidney and Body Fluids, 3rd ed. Chicago, Year Book, 1974

QUESTIONS

1. The largest fraction of sodium filtered through the glomerulus is reabsorbed in which one of the following segments of the nephron?

   A. proximal tubule
   B. descending thin limb of the loop of Henle
   C. distal tubule
   D. collecting tubule

2. In addition to diluting proximal tubular sodium concentration by retaining water, osmotic diuretics can increase urine output by which one of the following mechanisms?

   A. antagonism of aldosterone
   B. increased medullary blood flow
   C. increased glomerular filtration rate
   D. inhibition of carbonic anhydrase activity

3. Mercurial diuretics are believed to act by which one of the following mechanisms?

   A. inhibition of renin release from the juxtaglomerular apparatus
   B. inhibition of sulfhydryl groups on enzymes by release of mercuric ion
   C. blockade of the distal action of antidiuretic hormone
   D. none of the above

4. Because thiazides result in an increased distal delivery of sodium, they tend to produce (*select one*):

   A. hypochloremic alkalosis because of excess loss of chloride
   B. systemic hyperkalemia (excess K^+) due to inhibition of K^+ secretion
   C. systemic hypokalemia due to increased Na^+-K^+ exchange
   D. none of the above

5. Loop diuretics (ethacrynic acid and furosemide) increase urine output by which one of the following mechanisms?

   A. inhibition of carbonic anhydrase
   B. inhibition of proximal tubular sodium transport
   C. increased renal blood flow
   D. inhibition of active chloride transport in the loop of Henle

6. The diuretic action of spironolactone and triamterene can be classified as (*select one*):

   A. high-ceiling (very potent)
   B. transient (short duration)
   C. potassium-sparing
   D. rapid-acting.

7. **T F** Ethacrynic acid is classified as a thiazide diuretic.

8. Spironolactone acts as a diuretic by which one of the following mechanisms?

   A. inhibition of carbonic anhydrase
   B. inhibition of active chloride transport in the loop of Henle
   C. antagonism of the action of aldosterone
   D. none of the above

9. Diuresis caused by mercuhydrin and acetazolamide have which of the characteristics in common?

   A. both mercurial diuretics
   B. both inhibit carbonic anhydrase
   C. both lose activity on continued use
   D. both cause acidosis

10. Diuretics that inhibit carbonic anhydrase produce which one of the following combinations of body fluid pH alterations?

    A. urinary acidification and blood alkalinization
    B. urinary alkalinization and blood acidification
    C. urinary and blood acidification
    D. none of the above

11. **T F** Acetazolamide is a carbonic anhydrase inhibitor.

12. Ototoxicity is associated with the use of which one of the following diuretics?

    A. hydrochlorothiazide
    B. mercuhydrin
    C. triamterene
    D. ethacrynic acid

13. In addition to cardiovascular disease, the use of a carbonic anhydrase inhibitor may indicate the presence of which one of the following disorders in a dental patient?

    A. glaucoma
    B. cancer
    C. rheumatoid arthritis
    D. none of the above

33
Respiratory and GI Drugs

A. INTRODUCTION

In this chapter, a wide variety of drugs are discussed. In many instances, the drugs are more thoroughly reviewed in other chapters, and the appropriate chapter is identified. In addition, some drugs have an effect on the respiratory tract that is often considered to be a side effect but becomes the primary effect when that effect is desired. For instance, codeine is often used as an analgesic, and the antitussive effect is considered a side effect. However, when codeine is used as an antitussive, this becomes the primary effect.

B. OXYGEN

Objective 33.B.1. Recognize the methods of administration of oxygen.

Administration
Oxygen can be administered by tent, hood (head tent), nasal catheter, mask, endotracheal tube, and hyperbaric method. The first three are open systems and can produce concentrations of 20 to 80%; only closed systems can produce between 80 and 100%. Administration by mask or endotracheal tube is closed, allowing 80 to 100%. Hyperbaric oxygen is oxygen provided under increased atmospheric pressures, often as high as 3 atmospheres. Possible use of this method of oxygen administration is for carbon monoxide poisoning and gas gangrene. Except for emergency use, oxygen should be bubbled through water before delivery; this adds moisture and prevents drying of the respiratory tract.

Uses

Objective 33.B.2. Describe situations in which oxygen is needed.

Inadequate Ventilation. This is due to inadequacy of respiratory mechanisms. One example of this use is in patients who are afflicted with chronic obstructive pulmonary disease (asthma, bronchitis, emphysema) and are heavily dependent on hypoxic drive. A second example is in a patient who has received an excessive dosage of narcotic-analgesic or barbiturate or nonbarbiturate sedative-hypnotic; such patients may be functioning almost entirely on hypoxic drive.

A review of the three drives of respiration is probably in order. (1) Neurogenic drive is the inherent activity of the respiratory center in the medulla oblongata of the brain, resulting in the rhythmic production of inhalation and exhalation. (2) Chemical drive is due to P_{CO_2} in blood or cerebrospinal fluid which bathes the *respiratory center;* increased CO_2 tension causes stimulation, whereas decreased CO_2 tension causes inhibition of respiration. (3) Hypoxic drive occurs by action of P_{O_2} and P_{CO_2} at the *chemoreceptors of the aortic and carotid bodies.* Increased CO_2 or decreased O_2 tension in blood results in stimulation, whereas decreased CO_2 or increased O_2 tension results in respiratory inhibition.

Therefore, although oxygen may be needed and used in the above situations, care should be exercised when oxygen is applied to the patients because the increased oxygen tension in arterial blood may cause respiratory depression. Under these circumstances, assisted ventilation and CO_2 may also be necessary.

Interference with Diffusion. This is caused by pulmonary blockage, most often due to mucous plugs.

Anoxia. This is due to anemia, stagnation of blood, and toxic chemicals.

Adverse effects

Objective 33.B.3. Describe the adverse effects of oxygen.

1. Respiratory depression can occur by the action of oxygen on carotid and aortic bodies (see Objective 33.B.2.).
2. Respiratory tract irritation often occurs, resulting in substernal soreness and induction of cough. When concentrations of oxygen are maintained at 60% or less, respiratory irritation is not a problem.
3. Retrolental fibroplasia resulting in blindness can occur when oxygen is administered to infants, especially premature infants.

Implications in Dentistry

Objective 33.B.4. Recognize implications of the use of oxygen in dentistry.

Oxygen is useful in dentistry, both as an emergency agent and in combination with nitrous oxide when the latter is used as a psychosedative. Every dental office *must* have oxygen available. This agent can be safely administered during most emergencies. In some instances of cardiopulmonary embarrassment, oxygen may be life-saving, while in others, even though no specific benefit may be obtained, it is helpful to have the assurance that the patient is well oxygenated.

C. BRONCHODILATORS

Objective 33.C.1. Describe the mechanisms of action of bronchodilator drugs, including examples.

Bronchodilators are used most often on a chronic basis but sometimes acutely by patients with a history of bronchial asthma. These agents are useful as an emergency treatment to reverse bronchoconstriction due to any cause in a nonasthmatic patient.

Sympathomimetics. These are discussed in depth in Chapters 2, 16, and 18. Ideally, these agents should activate β_2 receptors (lung) and not β_1 receptors (heart), thereby decreasing unwanted cardiac side effects. In addition, when available, these agents are best administered by inhalation into the lungs. They are thus administered to the site of action and in a much lower dose than would be required if they were used systemically. However, in the presence of mucous plugs, systemic administration is necessary because the agents will not reach their site of action by inhalation.

1. **Epinephrine** may be administered by inhalation or parenterally. Epinephrine has prominent alpha and beta effects.
2. **Ephedrine** is often referred to as an indirect sympathomimetic and is most often adminis-

tered orally, but a parenteral preparation is available. Ephedrine activates both alpha and beta receptors, but it has a longer duration than does epinephrine.

3. **Isoproterenol** (*Isuprel*) is a pure beta agonist and can be administered orally, parenterally, and by inhalation.

4. **Metaproterenol** (*Alupent*) is thought to possess a more selective β_2 action, but higher than therapeutic doses result in activation of β_1 receptors. The agent may be administered by inhalation or by mouth.

5. **Terbutaline** (*Brethine, Bricanyl*) has activity much like that of metaproterenol, i.e., selective activation of β_2 receptors. The agent is available for oral and parenteral administration.

6. **Albuterol** (*Proventil, Ventolin*), known as salbutamol in other parts of the world, is newly marketed in this country. This long-anticipated agent is reported to have a more selective action on β_2 receptors (this is even more selective than either metaproterenol or terbutaline).

Xanthines. (See also Chapter 37 and, for emergency use, Chapter 2.)

The primary agent in this case is theophylline (many trade names) and its ethylenediamine salt, **aminophylline.** Caffeine and theobromine are too weak to be useful as bronchodilators. Theophylline is thought to produce its effect by inhibiting the enzyme, phosphodiesterase, thereby allowing the accumulation of cyclic AMP. (Other mechanisms have been proposed, Chapter 37.) Levels of intracellular cyclic AMP are also increased by β agonists, and this may be the common mechanism by which xanthines and sympathomimetics produce their effect. Other effects and side effects include nausea, vomiting, increased gastric acid secretion, CNS stimulation, and diuresis.

Implications for Dentistry

Objective 33.C.2. Describe the implications of bronchodilator use in dental practice.

The dentist should have on hand in his emergency kit such drugs as parenteral epinephrine, aminophylline, a corticosteroid, and an antihistamine, not only for anaphylactoid reactions but also for acute allergic and asthmatic reactions. Furthermore, if the patient is a known asthmatic, a supply of medications, which has been prescribed, should be on hand for use if needed at the time of dental treatment. The practitioner may choose to include an inhalation agent, such as metaproterenol or albuterol, in the emergency kit.

Patients with a history of bronchial asthma or emphysema (two groups of patients who often use bronchodilators) may exhibit an increased probability of development of a supra-infection when treated with antibiotics (Weinstein, 1975).

D. EXPECTORANTS AND MUCOLYTIC AGENTS

Objective 33.D.1. Recognize the mechanisms of action of expectorants and mucolytic agents, and cite examples of each.

Mucolytics

1. **Acetylcysteine** is thought to decrease the viscosity of mucus by depolymerizing mucopolysaccharides. The agent is administered by inhalation for this purpose.

2. **Terpin hydrate** is thought to act by stimulating bronchial secretory cells to increase secretion.

3. **Pancreatic dornase** hydrolyzes DNA.

Expectorants

These are listed according to decreasing potency.

1. **Potassium iodide**
2. **Ammonium chloride**
3. **Syrup of ipecac**
4. **Guaifenesin** (formerly known as glyceryl guaiacolate)

These agents are thought to stimulate bronchial secretions by reflex irritation of the stomach.

E. MISCELLANEOUS AGENTS

Objective 33.E.1. Recognize the mechanism of action and dental implications of cromolyn sodium, antibiotics, corticosteroids, anticholinergics, and antitussives.

Cromolyn Sodium. This is thought to prevent a bronchial asthmatic attack by increasing intracellular cyclic AMP and preventing the release of asthma-producing mediators. This agent is of no value for the treatment of an acute asthmatic attack; rather, it is used entirely prophylactically.

Antibiotics. These are taken by patients for the treatment of respiratory infections. Antibiotics are extensively discussed in Chapters 25 through 30.

Corticosteroids. These are often taken by the asthmatic patient. For example, they are often used chronically, taken either by the oral route or by inhalation. In the case of a patient who has developed a tolerance to sympathomimetics or in status asthmaticus, chronic steroid therapy may be required. **Beclomethasone** (*Vanceril*) is an inhalant preparation of particular value because low doses can be used, little drug is absorbed systemically, and the agent is applied directly to lung tissue. Disadvantages include possible systemic absorption, possible atrophy of the lining of the respiratory tract, and increased incidence of oral and/or pharyngeal infection, especially candidiasis. The dentist may frequently diagnose this infection in patients taking the drug.

Not only are these agents potent antiinflammatory drugs and antiimmune agents, but they also somehow potentiate the sympathetic nervous system. The agents, when taken systemically, are potentially dangerous, causing numerous side effects (Chapters 7 and 34).

Anticholinergics. These are potentially useful for the asthmatic patient (Chapter 17), although no agent is available as yet for this purpose. Preliminary trials with an inhalant preparation suggest these drugs may be useful (Ruffin et al, 1978).

Antitussives. These are agents used to suppress the cough reflex. Some narcotic-analgesics, especially **codeine,** may be useful. More recently, the narcotic derivative, **dextromethorphan,** was introduced as an agent that has little or no abuse potential. It is not a controlled substance, is not analgesic, and is sold OTC. Narcotic-analgesics and related drugs are cough suppressants by virtue of their depressant activity on the cough center of the medulla oblongata. Antitussives should not be used in the asthmatic patient or in any other patient with a productive cough, since the drugs will suppress the necessary movement of material from the bronchial tree.

One side effect of the narcotic-analgesics not usually seen with codeine is depression of respiration by an action on the respiratory center of the medulla oblongata. Narcotic-analgesics are discussed in detail in Chapters 6 and 24.

F. GI DRUGS

Objective 33.F.1. Recognize four reasons for the necessity of the dentist to be familiar with the actions of gastrointestinal agents.

This section deals with a group of drugs currently in widespread use. The GI drugs are, in many cases, self-prescribed by the layman and sometimes abused. When prescribed by a practitioner, GI drugs constitute important agents that can be indicated in a variety of gastroenterologic disorders. GI drugs are important to the dentist for four reasons: (1) they can alter dental therapy, because of both their therapeutic and side effects, (2) they can interact with drugs the dentist may prescribe, (3) they indicate the presence of some disorder, either major or minor, and (4) the dentist may wish to prescribe them.

G. GASTRIC ANTACIDS

Objective 33.G.1. Recognize two indications for gastric antacids.

Objective 33.G.2. Recognize the definition of two types of gastric antacids.

Objective 33.G.3. Name one systemic antacid and two nonsystemic antacids, comparing advantages and disadvantages of each.

Objective 33.G.4. Recognize side effects of the various gastric antacids.

Objective 33.G.5. Recognize the major interaction between dental drugs and the gastric antacids.

Indications

Antacids are available OTC and are used primarily for the **symptomatic relief of nonspecific stomach irritations,** such as heartburn, indigestion, and others which may be perceived as being due to an excessive amount of stomach acid. In the **rational therapy of peptic ulcer,** these agents are used to reduce stomach acidity, to alleviate symptoms, and to promote healing of the ulcer.

Classification

There are two types of gastric antacids.

Systemic. Systemic antacids are those which result in alkali absorption. The most commonly used systemic antacid is **sodium bicarbonate,** or baking soda. While an effective neutralizer, the use of sodium bicarbonate results in a systemic, metabolic alkalosis because of complete intestinal bicarbonate absorption. This type of antacid also results in a rebound hypersecretion of gastric acid, with an even greater need for further relief.

Nonsystemic. Nonsystemic antacids are those which are not absorbed to a significant degree and do not, therefore, cause a systemic pH imbalance. An example is **aluminum hydroxide.** In the stomach, the following reaction occurs:

$$Al(OH)_3 + 3\ HCl \rightarrow AlCl_3 + 3\ H_2O$$

In the intestine, the reaction is reversed, so that the antacid is excreted in the same form as it was administered, thus avoiding systemic effects. Nonsystemic antacids include many preparations of **aluminum, magnesium,** and calcium. Such preparations include dihydroxyaluminum aminoacetate, magnesium trisilicate, calcium carbonate, dihydroxyaluminum sodium carbonate, and magnesium oxide (or hydroxide) or various combinations of antacids.

Side Effects

The systemic alkalosis produced by sodium bicarbonate can result in weakness, disorientation, and other disturbances of a central nature. The chronic use of bicarbonate can result in kidney stones due to chronically elevated urinary pH. Calcium carbonate and aluminum hydroxide tend to be constipating, while the magnesium preparations can produce diarrhea. Aluminum hydroxide and magnesium trisilicate are frequently combined so that each compound counteracts the side effect of the other.

Drug Interaction

Gastric antacids can alter the absorption of a number of drugs. Drugs important in dentistry whose absorption is significantly impaired include tetracyclines, atropine, aspirin, and barbiturates (Appendix II).

H. DRUGS USED IN THE TREATMENT OF ULCERS

Objective 33.H.1. Recognize two categories of drugs used for treatment of ulcers (drugs set in bold type) and provide actions and side effects of each category.

There are currently two categories of drugs used to treat ulcers, as described below.

Anticholinergics

The actions of these drugs are described in detail in Chapter 17. They were widely employed in the treatment of ulcers of the GI tract because it was thought that they might reduce GI motility and gastric acid secretion. However, they tend to first reduce salivation, followed by blocking cholinergic functions of the eye (resulting in mydriasis and paralysis of accommodation), increased heart rate, decreased bladder function, and, finally, at high doses, reduced gastrointestinal motility and secretion. However, at the lower dosages, drugs in this category do provide relief of pain of ulcer (by some unknown mechanism), especially when used with a gastric antacid. Anticholinergics used to treat ulcers include **atropine, methantheline, propantheline, glycopyrrolate,** methscopolamine bromide, and clidinium bromide.

H₂ Antihistamines

Gastric acid secretion now appears to be controlled by histamine acting on the histamine H₂ receptor (Chapter 19). Recently, a new category of drugs which specifically block H₂ receptors was introduced. These drugs are chemical analogs of histamine; one of the drugs in this group, **cimetidine** (*Tagamet*), which is currently in widespread use, acts to block H₂ receptors and decreases both basal and stimulated rates of gastric acid secretion. The side effects of cimetidine are relatively mild and include diarrhea, muscle pain, dizziness, and rash.

I. LAXATIVES AND CATHARTICS

Objective 33.I.1. Recognize three types of laxatives and describe their respective mechanisms of action.

Objective 33.I.2. Recognize examples of each type of laxative.

Laxatives and cathartics include agents that function by different mechanisms. They are listed below by mechanism of action. These drugs are available OTC and are generally overused by the public, since most instances of constipation can be alleviated by proper diet or exercise. When prescribed, they are usually used to reduce defecation stress in hemorrhoidectomy or in heart patients.

Irritants (Stimulants)
These laxatives act by irritating the GI tract to increase motility.

1. Castor oil
2. Anthraquinones (cascara, senna, rhubarb, aloe, emodin)
3. **Phenolphthalein**
4. Bisacodyl

Bulk-Forming Agents
These agents act by osmotically swelling in the GI tract, distending and thereby stimulating the smooth muscle peristalsis.

1. Saline cathartics (**magnesium sulfate** or epsom salts, **citrate of magnesia,** and **milk of magnesia**)
2. Hydrophilic colloids (**bran,** agar, psyllium seed, **methylcellulose**)

Fecal Softeners
These act by softening or emulsifying the feces.

1. **Mineral oil**
2. **Glycerin suppositories**
3. **Dioctyl sodium sulfosuccinate**

Side Effects
The major problem associated with laxatives and cathartics is development of their habitual use, with disruption of normal defecation patterns. Additionally, these agents can cause gastrointestinal disturbances, such as spastic colitis and enterocolitis. Finally, fluid and electrolyte depletion, malnutrition, and avitaminosis may result from too vigorous cathartic therapy.

J. ANTIDIARRHEAL AGENTS

Objective 33.J.1. Recognize two types of antidiarrheal agents and describe their respective mechanisms of action.

Objective 33.J.2. Recognize two examples of each type of antidiarrheal agent.

As with other GI drugs, antidiarrheal agents tend to be overused by the public. The best treatment for diarrhea is careful diagnosis, followed by rational elimination of the cause, rather than simply alleviating the symptoms. While simple diarrhea may respond well to antidiarrheal agents, their use in other diarrheas is discouraged because they may mask symptoms of serious systemic disorders, such as pseudomembranous colitis. For this reason, the diarrhea that may accompany clindamycin therapy necessitates discontinuation of the drug followed by hospitalization of the patient without employing antidiarrheals. There are two general types of antidiarrheals as follows:

Adsorbents

These drugs act by adsorbing bacterial toxins and by forming a protective coating of the bowel. Like the antacids, these agents can impair the absorption of tetracyclines and other antibiotics and anticholinergics. The most frequently used adsorbents are **kaolin** (hydrated aluminum silicate) and **pectin** (a citrus carbohydrate). A trade name is *Kao-Pectate.*

Narcotic Derivatives

These drugs act on gastrointestinal smooth muscle to decrease peristaltic movements and to increase nonpropulsive movements and sphincter tone. The net result is spastic paralysis. The decreased bowel motility results in increased absorption of water from the feces. Drugs in this category (all compounds are scheduled narcotics) include **diphenoxylate** (a chemical relative of meperidine, marketed in combination with atropine as *Lomotil*), camphorated tincture of opium (*Paregoric*), and **loperamide HCl** (*Imodium*).

K. EMETICS

Objective 33.K.1. Recognize two examples of emetic drugs and two situations in which their use is contraindicated.

This group of drugs is used in the treatment of poisoning. Care must be exercised when using these drugs, however, since it is undesirable to produce vomiting in certain types of poisoning (e.g., petroleum distillates, strychnine, and corrosives) and in unconscious individuals. There are two drugs which are used as emetics, as described below.

1. **Ipecac syrup** acts by irritating the gastrointestinal tract and by stimulating the central vomiting center.
2. **Apomorphine hydrochloride** must be administered parenterally (by injection) and in-

duces emesis by stimulating the chemoreceptor trigger zone (CTZ). Since this drug is a narcotic, care must be exercised in its use to avoid excessive respiratory depression.

L. ANTIEMETICS

These are discussed as antihistamines in Chapters 7 and 19 and antipsychotics (phenothiazines) in Chapter 36.

REFERENCES

Ruffin RE, Wolff RK, Dolovich MB: Aerosol therapy with Sch 1000. Chest 73:501, 1978
Weinstein L: Antimicrobial agents. In Goodman LS, Gilman A (eds): The Pharmacological Basis of Therapeutics, 5th ed. New York, Macmillan, 1975, p 1106

BIBLIOGRAPHY

Gilman AG, Goodman LS, Gilman A (eds): Goodman and Gilman's The Pharmacological Basis of Therapeutics, 6th ed. New York, Macmillan 1980, Ch 42
Goth A: Medical Pharmacology, 10th ed. St. Louis, Mosby, 1981, Ch 40, 41
Meyers FH, Jawetz E, Goldfien A: Review of Medical Pharmacology, 7th ed. Los Altos, CA, Lange, 1980, Ch 31, 32

QUESTIONS

1. **T F** Oxygen is administered only by mask and endotracheal tube.

2. Oxygen is used in the presence of:

    A. inadequate respiratory mechanisms
    B. pulmonary blockage
    C. anoxia
    D. all of the above are correct
    E. none of the above is correct

3. **T F** Adverse effects of oxygen include induction of respiratory depression.

4. **T F** Oxygen is a useful dental emergency drug, except for local anesthetic-induced convulsions.

5. **T F** All sympathomimetics produce their bronchodilator effect by activation of beta receptors.

6. An example of a sympathomimetic is:

   A. theophylline
   B. caffeine
   C. metaproterenol
   D. theobromine

7. **T F** Patients with a history of asthma or emphysema may be more prone to supra-infections when treated with systemic antibiotics.

8. Mucolytics include:

   A. acetylcysteine
   B. terpin hydrate
   C. pancreatic dornase
   D. all of the above are correct
   E. none of the above is correct

9. **T F** Both potassium iodide and guaifenesin are expectorants.

10. **T F** Expectorants are thought to act by reflexly irritating the stomach.

11. **T F** Cromolyn sodium increases intracellular cyclic AMP.

12. **T F** Beclomethasone is frequently used by inhalation in the asthmatic patient.

13. **T F** Codeine's only action is an antitussive effect.

14. Which one of the following is not an indication for a gastric antacid?

   A. peptic ulcer associated with elevated stomach acidity

   B. mild gastrointestinal distress perceived to be heartburn
   C. diarrhea
   D. none of the above

15. The term "systemic antacid" refers to which one of the following?

   A. gastric antacid whose route of administration is parenteral
   B. gastric antacid with a wide range of systemic actions
   C. gastric antacid which is absorbed after exerting its neutralizing effect
   D. gastric antacid which has limited action on one organ system

16. Which one of the following can result from chronic use of sodium bicarbonate as a gastric antacid?

   A. constipation
   B. kidney stones
   C. osteoarthritis
   D. diarrhea

17. The absorption of which one of the following drugs is significantly impaired by gastric antacids?

   A. tetracyclines
   B. aspirin
   C. atropine
   D. all of the above

18. Cimetidine, an agent used to treat gastric ulcers, exerts its action through which one of the following mechanisms?

   A. blockade of cholinergic (vagal) impulses to the stomach
   B. blockade of histamine type 2 receptors
   C. neutralization of gastric acid
   D. formation of a protective coating on the stomach lining

19. Castor oil is classified as which one of the following types of laxatives?

    A. irritant
    B. bulk former
    C. saline cathartic
    D. fecal softener

20. One group of antidiarrheal agents is:

    A. emulsifiers
    B. saline cathartics
    C. carminatives
    D. narcotic derivatives

21. Which one of the following is an example of an adsorbent?

    A. pectin
    B. methylcellulose
    C. magnesium trisilicate
    D. none of the above

22. Apomorphine is contraindicated in which one of the following situations?

    A. controlled diabetes
    B. acute poisoning
    C. unconsciousness
    D. none of the above

34
Endocrine Pharmacology

A. INTRODUCTION

The subject of endocrine pharmacology is extensive and requires a broad understanding of the physiology of endocrine function and dysfunction. Endocrine physiology and pathophysiology are too broad for complete coverage in a textbook focusing on pharmacotherapeutics in dentistry. Therefore, we will proceed on the assumption that the reader already has a sound understanding of the subject and that a brief review will suffice for reinforcement of the basic facts. This will serve as a basis for further discussions of drugs used in endocrine therapy and how endocrine status influences dental therapy.

There are four chemical classes of endocrine hormones: (1) steroids, (2) proteins, (3) polypeptides, and (4) amino acid derivatives, and they are discussed in this chapter.

B. ENDOCRINE DRUGS

Definition

Objective 34.B.1. Define endocrine drugs.

Endocrine drugs may mimic the actions of hormones and may be used to achieve a physio-logic balance or for a therapeutic effect. Some endocrine drugs are used to block hormones.

Uses of Endocrine Drugs

Objective 34.B.2. Recognize three reasons for using an endocrine drug.

Endocrine drugs may be used:

1. To replace missing or deficient hormones in an attempt to achieve the normal physiologic level
2. As a diagnostic test for responsiveness of the target organ, often by using supraphysiologic blood levels
3. To treat disease or attain a new physiologic state (e.g., contraception) usually by using supraphysiologic levels.

Classification and Names of Hormones

Objective 34.B.3. Recognize four chemical classes of hormones and name the hormones in each class.

Classification of hormones into four chemical classes and of the specific hormones into each class follows:

1. Steroid hormones
   a. adrenocorticosteroids
   b. estrogens and progestins
   c. androgens and anabolic steroids
2. Protein hormones
   a. adenohypophyseal hormones (anterior pituitary)
      (1) growth hormone or somatotropin (STH)
      (2) adrenocorticotropic hormone (ACTH)
      (3) thyrotropic hormone (TSH)
      (4) luteinizing hormone (LH)
      (5) follicle-stimulating hormone (FSH)
      (6) prolactin
      (7) melanocyte-stimulating hormone (MSH)
   b. parathyroid hormone and calcitonin
   c. insulin and glucagon
3. Polypeptides
   a. hypothalamic factors which influence the adenohypophysis
   b. neurohypophyseal hormones (posterior pituitary)
      (1) oxytocin
      (2) vasopressin or antidiuretic hormone (ADH)
4. Amino acid derivatives
   a. thyroid hormones

C. STEROID HORMONES

Adrenocorticosteroids

Chemistry

Objective 34.C.1. Recognize the general chemical nature of adrenocorticosteroids.

Cells of the adrenal cortex have the capacity and enzymes to form a great number of steroids. The 18-carbon steroid nucleus is formed from acetate, which is converted to cholesterol and which then forms the adrenal steroid, pregnenolone. After further chemical conversion, pregnenolone may become one of the adrenocorticosteroids.

Types of Adrenocorticosteroids

Objective 34.C.2. Recognize the difference between glucocorticoids, mineralocorticoids, and androgenic steroids.

The main active adrenocorticosteroids formed are: the glucocorticoids, hydrocortisone and cortisol; the mineralocorticoids, aldosterone and desoxycorticosterone (DOC); and androgenic corticoids. Glucocorticoids are steroids which have an effect on gluconeogenesis, mineralocorticoids have an effect on retaining sodium, and androgens have a masculinizing effect.

Secretion of Adrenocorticosteroids

Objective 34.C.3. Describe the secretion of adrenocorticosteroids and how they are controlled.

The balance of steroids secreted depends upon the biochemical and physiologic status of the adrenocortical cells. ACTH from the adenohypophysis stimulates the adrenocortical cells via cyclic AMP to form mainly glucocorticoids, but other steroids, including DOC, androgens, and others, may be stimulated, depending upon physiologic or pathophysiologic state. The mineralocorticoid, aldosterone, is controlled partially by ACTH regulation of adrenal cells but mainly by the level of angiotensin II (Chapter 19, p. 182).

Deficiency and Excess Syndromes

Objective 34.C.4. Describe the effects of deficiency and excess of corticosteroids.

A deficiency of corticosteroid production may result in Addison's disease. The cells will not respond to ACTH, and both glucocorticoids and mineralocorticoids are absent in Addison's disease. Sometimes, the adrenal cells will continue to produce enough mineralocorticoids but not enough glucocorticoids. In this case, selective use of the proper steroid and in proper dosage must be the goal of therapy. However, the usual addisonian crisis occurs when there is not enough mineralocorticoid production, and, in this case, the mineralocorticoid can be life-saving.

An excess of glucocorticoids causes Cushing's syndrome, which can eventually lead to death. In cushingoid disease, the fat deposits change, with weight gain creating rounded facial features and humped back. There is also hypertension, glucose intolerance, and, in children, growth retardation. The excessive use of steroids in therapy can be dangerous and is the most frequent cause of suppression of ACTH, leading to atrophy of the adrenocortical cells. After atrophy, the cells cannot respond to further ACTH stimulation. The only recourse when the adrenal cells are nonfunctional is to supply steroids at a dosage consistent with the patient's physiologic status. This balance is difficult to achieve because more corticosteroids are required during stress. Sometimes the patient taking steroids notices CNS excitatory effects, which can be either pleasant (causing patient abuse of the drug) or unpleasant. Use in the relief of arthritic pain can also lead to patient overmedication. Sometimes the physician will overprescribe, attempting to achieve a certain effect, but side effects almost always limit the medication.

Determination of adrenal cellular response to ACTH is a diagnostic test for function. However, ACTH is seldom used as a therapeutic agent because it must be given parenterally and has only a short duration of action.

Mineralocorticoid therapy requires careful control, as excessive sodium retention may cause edema and hypertension. The patient should weigh himself daily. By following average daily weight, BP, and serum electrolytes, the physician can properly control the dosage.

Mechanism of Action

Objective 34.C.5. Describe the mechanism of action of glucocorticosteroids.

The mechanism of action of glucocorticoids is not well understood, although many actions of the drug have been studied. In inflammation, the glucocorticoids are believed to exert an anti-inflammatory effect by stabilizing lysosomal membranes. In addition, stabilization prevents release of phospholipase A_2 from plasma membranes, which is thought to release arachidonic acid and supply substrate for prostaglandin generation (Chapter 19, p. 183; Chapter 23, p. 222). Corticosteroids result in nuclear stimulation of mRNA, which stimulates protein synthesis. Another effect of corticosteroids is on intermediary metabolism, e.g., stimulation of gluconeogenesis, hyperglycemic stimulation of insulin release, glucose and insulin effects on fat metabolism and deposition, and other metabolic effects.

Major Effects

Objective 34.C.6. Recognize major effects of glucocorticoids.

The major effects of glucocorticoids are:

1. Glycogenesis and gluconeogenesis, which, during the fasting state, tend to maintain normal plasma glucose. If steroids are low, there is depletion of glycogen, hypoglycemia, and hyperresponsiveness to insulin. The opposite occurs during the hyper-state.
2. Redistribution of body fat. This causes "moon face" and "buffalo hump." Lipolytic effects (FFA release) synergize with those of the catecholamines.
3. Salt and water retention. This causes edema, mainly due to aldosterone and DOC, but most corticosteroids have this ability to some extent. Edema and sodium retention lead to increased blood pressure and blood volume. The hypo-state shows opposite effects.
4. Skeletal muscles. A weakness may occur in either the hypo- or hyper-state.
5. CNS effects. These occur in either the hypo-state (apathy, depression, irritability, psychosis, seizures) or the hyper-state (neurosis, psychosis, decreased brain excitability).
6. Blood system effects. In the hypo-state, normochromic, normocytic anemia, lymphocytosis, and lymphadenitis occur, and, in the hyper-state, polycythemia, lymphocytopenia, decreased lymph gland mass result.
7. Immune system. This is suppressed by excess

steroids. Also, inhibition of growth occurs with excess steroids.
8. Anti-inflammatory activity. This occurs by stabilization of lysosomal membranes and other membranes.

Pharmacokinetics

Objective 34.C.7. Briefly describe the pharmacokinetics of glucocorticoids.

The pharmacokinetics include:

1. well absorbed orally
2. bound to plasma globulin—90%
3. metabolized in the liver
4. excreted by the kidney, mainly as 17-hydroxysteroids

Toxicity Following Overdosage

Objective 34.C.8. Describe toxicity due to overdosage with corticosteroids.

Overdosage of glucocorticoids causes:

1. cushingoid syndrome—moon face, buffalo hump, edema, hypokalemia, increased blood pressure, and salt and water retention
2. metabolic effects—hyperglycemia, glycosuria, resistance to insulin
3. adrenocortical suppression lasting up to nine months or longer after withdrawal (this may be life threatening and requires supplementation or slow withdrawal)
4. increased susceptibility to infection due to immune system suppression
5. peptic ulcer induction or activation, with possible perforation
6. posterior subcapsular cataracts
7. osteoporosis, myopathy, CNS disturbances

Medical Uses

Objective 34.C.9. Describe medical uses of glucocorticoids.

Medical uses include:

1. addisonian syndrome (but mineralocorticoids, or both, may be needed, see below)
2. arthritis, for anti-inflammatory effect

3. allergic disorders, including bronchial asthma, rheumatic carditis, allergic nephritis, and collagen diseases
4. inflammation of eye
5. dermatopathology—used very often by the dermatologist for erythema multiforme, pemphigus, psoriasis, lichen planus, and so on
6. malignancies
7. shock
8. cerebral edema and increased cranial pressure
9. celiac sprue and chronic ulcerative colitis
10. some liver and kidney diseases

Glucocorticoids and Their Relative Potencies

Objective 34.C.10. Name six important glucocorticoids and recognize their relative potencies for anti-inflammatory effect and sodium retention.

In Table 34–1, corticosteroid compounds are described. Six compounds you should remember are set in bold type. Cortisol (hydrocortisone) is described as the prototype, thus its activity is considered the unit of measurement for the anti-inflammatory (AI) and sodium retention (SR) activities of other compounds. In therapy for anti-inflammatory effect, compounds with low salt retention (mineralcorticoid) activity should be selected.

Drug Interactions

Objective 34.C.11. Recognize drug interactions which would interfere with dental use of glucocorticoid therapy.

Dental drug interactions include:

1. amphotericin B (enhances K^+ depletion)
2. oral anticoagulants are antagonized
3. antidiabetic drugs are antagonized
4. liver enzyme inducers (e.g., sedative-hypnotic, barbiturates) increase metabolism of corticosteroids
5. diuretics enhance hypokalemia
6. estrogens enhance glucocorticoid activity
7. NSAIA (nonsteroidal anti-inflammatory agents) have ulcerogenic activity that is enhanced by corticosteroids

TABLE 34–1. COMMONLY USED CORTICOSTEROIDS AND THEIR ACTIVITIES

Glucocorticoids	AI[a]	SR[a]	Duration
cortisol (hydrocortisone)[b]	1	1	short
cortisone	0.8	0.8	short
prednisolone	4	0.3	short
methylprednisolone[b]	5	0	short
triamcinolone	5	0	intermediate
betamethasone	25–40	0	long
dexamethasone[c]	30	0	long
Mineralocorticoids			
desoxycorticosterone (DOC)	0	20	short
fludrocortisone	10	250	short

[a] AI, anti-inflammatory activity; SR, salt-retention activity.
[b] Hemisuccinate (*Solu-Cortef, Solu-Medrol*) available for IV injection.
[c] Sodium phosphate available for IV injection.

Dental Uses

Objective 34.C.12. Describe dental uses of glucocorticosteroids.

Dental uses include the following (when no infection is present):

1. systemic treatment of oral ulcerations—consult physician to ascertain desirability of therapy and lack of contraindications
2. treatment of TMJ arthritis—consult physician to ascertain desirability of therapy and lack of contraindications
3. topical treatment of oral ulcerations—topical preparations (ointments or gels) or by iontophoresis (Chapter 7)
4. emergency treatment of anaphylaxis after initial and successful epinephrine treatment (Chapters 2 and 7)
5. emergency treatment of hypotensive shock when the response to pressor drugs has failed
6. adrenocortical-deficient patient—consult physician, may require a temporary increase in dosage when faced with a stressful dental procedure
(*Note:* any patient taking steroids chronically, even if withdrawn up to three years earlier, may require this therapy)
7. in excessive edema

Contraindications

Objective 34.C.13. Describe containdications for glucocorticoid use.

Contraindications for use include the presence of:

1. viral, bacterial, or fungal infection
2. diabetes
3. peptic ulcer
4. hypertension

Uses of Mineralocorticoids

Objective 34.C.14. Recognize uses of mineralocorticoids.

Aldosterone is the major mineralocorticoid secreted in humans, although it is not available as a drug. The mechanism of secretion is related to angiotensin II formation due to sodium depletion, low blood volume, or low blood pressure in the kidney (See Chapter 19 for further discussion). Aldosterone has little glucocorticoid activity and is only partially influenced by ACTH.

In an addisonian crisis, it is important to administer a mineralocorticoid. The mineralocorticoid of choice is **fludrocortisone,** although the water-soluble sodium succinate salt of hydrocortisone (*Solu-Cortef*, Table 34–1) is needed for IV use in a crisis.

Principles of Glucocorticoid Use

Objective 34.C.15. State eight principles of glucocorticoid use.

1. Topical therapy is usually acceptable unless prolonged or if patient is already on steroid therapy.
2. Short course of systemic therapy is usually not harmful. High dose for a few days is very safe, and even 5 days of therapy produce no suppression. For 5 or more days of therapy, use high dose and gradually reduce it. Alternate day dosing is used for prolonged therapy. A full dose at 8 AM causes the least adrenocortical suppression.
3. Supplement patient on steroids for dental stress.
4. Contraindicated in viral, bacterial, or fungal infection, diabetes, peptic ulcer, hypertension.
5. Consult with physician when more than five days are needed or patient is on steroid medication.
6. Withdrawal after chronic use may unmask adrenocortical insufficiency. It is best to reduce the dose gradually over a period of days.
7. The anti-inflammatory steroids provide symptomatic relief but are not curative.
8. Toxicity with chronic use is very frequent.

Drugs That Block Steroid Actions

Objective 34.C.16. Recognize two drugs that block steroid actions.

Spironolactone blocks action of aldosterone and may be used in hyperaldosteronism. **Metyrapone** interferes with steroid synthesis and may be used in adrenocortical tumors (hyperglucocorticism). The use of these drugs must be carefully controlled by a physician and is only mentioned here to make the dentist aware of a medical problem related to dental care.

Estrogens, Progestins, and Oral Contraceptives

Endogenous Sex Steroids and Mechanism of Secretion

Objective 34.C.17. List three natural estrogens and one natural progestin and recognize the mechanism of their secretion.

Three natural estrogens are estradiol, estrone, and estriol. A natural progestin (or progestogen) is progesterone. Estrogens are secreted by developing ovarian follicles under the control of FSH. Estrogens may also be secreted by the placenta and, in limited amounts, by the adrenal cortex and by the testes. Progesterone is secreted from the corpus luteum during the second half of the menstrual cycle. Progestins are also secreted from the placenta and, in limited amount, from the adrenal cortex and testes. LH from the pituitary controls the maturation of the corpus luteum. By cyclical production of FSH and estrogens and of LH and progesterones, the female menstrual cycle is maintained.

Mechanism of Action

Objective 34.C.18. Recognize the cellular mechanism of action of estrogens and progestins.

Estrogens and progestins are thought to enter the nucleus and cause a marked increase in messenger RNA, resulting in protein synthesis.

Effects of Estrogens

Objective 34.C.19. Recognize the effects of estrogens on other organs and functions.

Effects of estrogens include:

1. promotes and maintains development of female organs (vagina, uterus, fallopian tubes, and breasts)
2. regulates female body contours and characteristics of hair growth
3. cooperates with GH to allow growth; excess

causes epiphyseal closure, arresting long bone growth

4. promotes feminine behavior
5. during follicular phase of menses, causes proliferation of uterine and vaginal mucosa, increased secretion of cervical glands, and promotes fullness of breasts
6. at the end of the cycle, decline of estrogen levels results in menstruation
7. triggers LH secretion at middle of cycle, but low or high levels inhibit LH secretion
8. some salt- and water-retaining activity
9. possible carcinogenic effect in high doses
10. excess may cause nausea, vomiting, diarrhea

Effects of Progesterone

Objective 34.C.20. Recognize effects of progesterone on other organs and functions.

Effects of progesterone include:

1. during luteal phase of menses, the secretory endometrium develops
2. major determinant of onset of menstruation
3. alters cervical gland secretion to scant mucus type
4. with aid of estrogen, causes proliferation of mammary acini (*Note:* lactation does not begin until estrogen and progestin influences are removed)
5. increases body temperature
6. blocks release of LH and FSH (dose dependent)

Pharmacokinetics

Objective 34.C.21. Recognize pharmacokinetic properties of estrogens and progestins.

Both estrogens and progestins are:

1. well absorbed orally
2. metabolized in the liver to water-soluble metabolites
3. excreted by the kidney as the metabolites

In addition, estrogens may be well absorbed by skin.

Uses of Estrogens

Objective 34.C.22. Recognize uses of estrogens.

Estrogens are used in:

1. oral contraceptives
2. menopause
3. senile or atrophic vaginitis
4. dysmenorrhea
5. failure of ovarian development
6. acne
7. osteoporosis
8. carcinoma of breast or prostate
9. combined with progestins, suppresses post-partum lactation

Uses of Progestins

Objective 34.C.23. Recognize uses of progestins.

Progestins are used in:

1. oral contraception
2. functional uterine bleeding
3. dysmenorrhea
4. premenstrual tension
5. prevention of abortion
6. combination with estrogens to suppress post-partum lactation
7. endometrial carcinoma

Antiestrogens

Objective 34.C.24. Recognize two antiestrogens, their uses and mechanisms.

Clomiphene is an antiestrogen used to increase fertility. It acts by blocking estrogen's feedback inhibition of LH, FSH, and the pituitary-releasing factors for LH and FSH. Use results in increased incidence of fertility, sometimes with multiple births. Side effects include increased incidence of ovarian cysts, gastric upset, rashes, and visual disturbances.

Tamoxifen is related to clomiphene but is used as an anticancer drug (Chapter 41).

Oral Contraceptive Ingredients and Mechanism of Action

Objective 34.C.25. Recognize the ingredients found in currently available oral contraceptive preparations and their mechanism of action.

Generally, oral contraceptives are hormone preparations that may contain a combination of estrogens and progestogens (progesterone analogs) or may contain only progestogens (the so-called mini-pill). Oral contraceptives are widely used because of their high degree of effectiveness in preventing pregnancy and because of their relative safety. Oral contraceptives act by at least two mechanisms:

1. Estrogen inhibits the secretion of follicle-stimulating hormone (FSH) and so prevents development of the graafian follicle.
2. Both progesterone and estrogen inhibit the secretion of luteinizing hormone (LH) and so block the stimulus (LH) required for release of the ovum from mature follicles. The progestin also ensures prompt, brief, and physiologic bleeding during the monthly withdrawal of the oral contraceptives.

Additionally, the oral contraceptives may reduce sperm penetration by alteration of the cervical mucus and by altering the endometrium in such a way as to inhibit implantation of the fertilized egg.

Because of their pharmacologic actions, oral contraceptives can be used for treating certain disorders, among them endometriosis, hypermenorrhea, and for the production of cyclical withdrawal bleeding.

Side Effects of Oral Contraceptives

Objective 34.C.26. Recognize the systemic side effects of the oral contraceptives.

Many of the systemic side effects of oral contraceptives are attributable to alterations in the cardiovascular system, including blood-clotting alterations. These effects may include:

1. Thromboembolism. This phenomenon may lead to idiopathic thromboembolic disease (2

to 11 times greater risk than in nonusers), hemorrhagic stroke (2 to 2.3 times greater risk), postsurgical thromboembolic complications (4 to 7 times greater risk), stroke (4 to 9.5 times greater risk), and myocardial infarction (2 to 12 times greater risk). Cardiovascular complications are known to be increased by smoking 15 or more cigarettes per day, as well as by age.

2. Hypertension. As many as 10% of women taking oral contraceptives may show elevations in blood pressure, and this side effect may be more prevalent or severe in patients with other contributing factors (family or racial history, kidney disease, poor diet, anxiety, and so forth).
3. Gallbladder disease. The use of oral contraceptives is known to increase the incidence of this adverse effect, and the likelihood of its development increases with prolonged use of these drugs.
4. Nausea, vomiting, and headache.
5. Alteration of mood. Many women taking oral contraceptives experience depression, which may alternate with periods of euphoria. Lack of initiative may also occur.
6. Increased fatigability.
7. Development of benign adenomas of the liver. A relationship may also exist between ingestion of oral contraceptives and other tumors, including malignancies, although this has not been confirmed.
8. Congenital defects. The use of oral contraceptives is associated with an increased incidence of birth defects in the offspring who are exposed to these drugs during pregnancy.

Side Effects of Oral Contraceptives in Relation to Dental Treatment

Objective 34.C.27. Describe the side effects of oral contraceptives that may occur in the mouth and associated structures and which may alter dental treatment and diagnosis.

It is well known that cyclical steroid levels in females can alter the condition of the gingival tissues, especially in pregnancy, and the oral contraceptives are·similarly related to such changes. The following changes in gingiva have been documented in women taking oral contraceptives:

1. swelling, redness, bleeding on mild stimulation (Lynn, 1967)
2. loss of gingival attachment independent of variations in plaque control (Knight and Wade, 1974)
3. gingival hyperplasia and "pregnancy tumors" (Kaufman, 1969)
4. increased gingival exudate in the maxillary anterior region (Lindhe and Bjorn, 1967)

Other changes in the oral cavity associated with the use of oral contraceptives include the following:

1. altered salivary composition (Magnusson et al., 1975)
2. increased incidence of alveolar osteitis (dry socket) after third molar extraction (Sweet and Butler, 1977)
3. increased radiopacity of the mandible, possibly due to an effect on parathyroid hormone activity (Darzenta and Giunta, 1977)

Dental Implications of Oral Contraceptive Use

Objective 34.C.28. Describe the precautions and diagnostic considerations to be taken when treating the dental patient who is taking oral contraceptives

The diagnosis and treatment of oral conditions in patients taking birth control pills require the following special considerations by the dentist.

1. Establishing that the female patient is definitely taking oral contraceptives. Patients frequently do not consider that such agents are drugs because they are taken regularly and are not associated with a disease. Therefore, it is important that the dentist inquire specifically about "birth control pills," rather than simply asking the patient if she is taking any "medications" or "drugs."
2. Emphasizing the importance of oral hygiene. While some alterations of gingival tissue occur independently of plaque accumulation,

there is no doubt that the gingival side effects of oral contraceptives are worsened by poor oral hygiene. Similarly, the effect of the medications must be considered in the diagnosis of periodontal disease and in establishing its etiology.
3. Screening for high blood pressure all patients taking oral contraceptives. Elevated blood pressure, along with an increased fibrinolysis associated with oral contraceptives, can increase postoperative bleeding and may alter the dentist's prescription of salicylate-analgesics and the use of vasoconstrictors in local anesthetic preparations.
4. Prepare for an increased risk of postextraction alveolar osteitis.
5. Consider oral contraceptives as a factor related to bony trabecular patterns in radiographs of female patients.

Androgenic Steroids

Natural Androgen and Mechanism of Secretion

Objective 34.C.29. Name a natural androgen and recognize its mechanism of secretion.

The most important natural androgen is testosterone, a steroid secreted mainly by the testes but also in small quantities by the ovaries. Testosterone and other anabolic steroids may also be secreted by the adrenal glands. In some situations, this becomes a significant source, resulting in overmasculinization of male and a masculinizing effect on the female. The testicular secretion is under the control of LH (ICSH), and, in turn, high levels of testosterone inhibit LH and FSH.

Mechanism of Action

Objective 34.C.30. Describe the cellular mechanism of action of testosterone.

The cellular mechanism of testosterone is similar to other steroids. The target organ DNA is stimulated to form mRNA, resulting in increased protein synthesis.

Pharmacokinetics

Objective 34.C.31. Recognize the pharmacokinetics of testosterone.

The pharmacokinetics of testosterone are similar to those described for estrogen. However, metabolism may result in activation, as dihydroxytestosterone has been described as the active form.

Effects

Objective 34.C.32. Recognize the effects of testosterone.

The effects of testosterone are:

1. growth and maintenance of testes, scrotum, penis, and male hair pattern
2. cooperates with GH, causing anabolic effects of rapid growth, including height, weight, skeletal and bony mass
3. causes loss of subcutaneous fat and prominence of veins
4. promotes aggressive and male sexual behavior
5. causes change of voice

Side Effects

Objective 34.C.33. Recognize side effects of androgen therapy.

Side effects of androgen therapy are:

1. use in women may result in masculinization
2. salt and water retention
3. cholestatic jaundice
4. hepatic carcinoma
5. steroid fever
6. prolonged treatment results in decreased spermatogenesis
7. initial treatment may result in sustained and painful penile erection

Uses of Androgens

Objective 34.C.34. List uses of androgen therapy.

The uses of androgen therapy are:

1. hypogonadism
2. hypopituitarism
3. acceleration of growth in childhood
4. osteoporosis
5. anemias
6. promotion of anabolism
7. suppression of lactation
8. breast carcinoma

Sex-Steroid Preparations

Objective 34.C.35. Name the sex steroids (set in bold type) from the list of preparations in Table 34–2.

Table 34–2 contains a list of important sex steroids, including estrogens, progestins, androgens, antiestrogens and anabolic steroids. The table should be used as a reference, but the drugs set in bold type should be familiar and memorized.

D. PROTEIN HORMONES

Growth Hormone (GH) or Somatotropin (STH)

GH is an adenohypophyseal, protein hormone which is species specific.

Effects of GH

Objective 34.D.1. Recognize the effects of GH.

The effects of GH are:

1. stimulation of protein synthesis and growth in all tissues
2. increased lipid synthesis and decreased lipolysis
3. retention of minerals in teeth and bones

TABLE 34-2. IMPORTANT SEX STEROIDS

Estrogens	Progestins	Androgens	Anabolic Steroids	Antiestrogens
diethylstilbestrol	**progesterone**	**testosterone**	dromostanolone	**clomiphene**
benzestrol	medroxyprogesterone	**methyltestosterone**	methandriol	**tamoxifen**
dienestrol	hydroxyprogesterone	fluoxymestrone	nandrolone	
methallenestril	megestrol	mesterolone	oxandrolone	
promethestrol	dydrogesterone		oxymethalone	
estradiol	**norethindrone**		stanozolol	
estrone	ethisterone		testolactone	
ethinyl estradiol			**methandrestenolone**	
conjugated estrogens				
esterified estrogens				
chlorotianisene				

4. increased amino acid and glucose uptake into cells

GH Secretion

Objective 34.D.2. Recognize characteristics of GH secretion.

The stimuli for secretion of GH are:

1. hypoglycemia
2. fasting

Secretion of growth hormone is inhibited by increased circulating free fatty acids and by feedback inhibition due to high levels of GH. GH secretion is also under the control of hypothalamic growth hormone releasing or inhibiting factors, which are currently the subject of much interest and research. Hypothalamic releasing and inhibitory factors are thought to be polypeptide hormones.

GH Deficiency and Excess Syndromes

Objective 34.D.3. Recognize the pathologic results of GH excess or deficiencies and the use of the hormone.

Excess GH causes gigantism in the child and acromegaly in the adult. In the child, a deficiency of GH causes dwarfism, and the hormone is used to correct this condition.

Luteinizing Hormone (LH)
This is also called, in males, **interstitial cell-stimulating hormone (ICSH)** and is an adenohypophyseal, glycoprotein hormone.

Effects of LH

Objective 34.D.4. Recognize effects of luteinizing hormone (LH).

The effects of LH in females are:

1. induces ovulation (LH surge), which peaks in midcycle
2. probably initiates progesterone secretion from ovary
3. probably aids in inducing follicular growth

In males, ICSH causes secretion of testosterone.

Secretion of LH

Objective 34.D.5. Recognize the mechanism of secretion of LH.

LH secretion is controlled by hypothalamic LH and FHS releasing- and/or inhibiting-factors. The hypothalamic factors are thought to be polypeptides. There is also feedback control from rising progesterone levels. During the menstrual cycle, the estrogen peak (approximately day 13) is thought to be responsible for the LH surge on day 14.

Uses of LH

Objective 34.D.6. Recognize uses of LH.

The uses of LH are:

1. with FSH, to induce ovulation in infertile women; (multiple births frequently occur)
2. with FSH, to treat cryptorchism

Follicle-stimulating Hormone (FSH)
FSH is an adenohypophyseal, glycoprotein hormone.

Effects of FSH

Objective 34.D.7. Recognize effects of follicle-stimulating hormone (FSH).

Effects of FSH include:

1. induces follicular growth in ovaries
2. influences formation of estrogen in follicles
3. stimulates spermatogenesis

FSH Secretion

Objective 34.D.8. Recognize characteristics of FSH secretion.

Secretion of FSH is characterized by the following:

1. peaks in midcycle along with LH
2. slight elevation early in the cycle to promote follicular growth
3. controlled by hypothalamic LH–FSH-releasing and inhibiting factors (polypeptide hormones)
4. feedback control from rising estrogen levels

Uses of FSH

Objective 34.D.9. Recognize uses of FSH.

Uses of FSH are listed below:

1. with LH, to induce ovulation in infertile women (multiple births frequently occur)
2. with LH, to treat cryptorchism

Thyrotropin (TSH)
TSH is an adenohypophyseal, glycoprotein hormone.

Effects of TSH

Objective 34.D.10. Recognize effects of TSH.

Effects of TSH include:

1. regulation of synthesis and release of thyroid hormones
2. stimulation of accumulation of iodine, amino acids, and glucose in thyroid gland

Secretion of TSH and Role of Protirelin

Objective 34.D.11. Recognize characteristics of TSH secretion and role of protirelin.

Secretion of TSH is under control of:

1. stimulation by hypothalamic TSH-releasing factor (TSH–RF, a polypeptide hormone)
2. negative feedback inhibition by thyroid hormones

Protirelin is a tripeptide identified as the TSH–RF.

Use of TSH

Objective 34.D.12. Recognize use of TSH.

The major use of TSH is as a diagnostic for thyroid function testing.

Adrenocorticotropic Hormone (ACTH)
ACTH is an adenohypophyseal, protein hormone.

Effects of ACTH

Objective 34.D.13. Recognize effects of ACTH.

Effects of ACTH include the following:

1. increases production of cortisol and, to some degree, aldosterone
2. stimulates growth of adrenal gland
3. mobilizes lipids from adipose tissue
4. causes hyperpigmentation of skin

ACTH Secretion

Objective 34.D.14. Recognize characteristics of ACTH secretion.

Secretion of ACTH is characterized below.

1. Hypothalamic corticotropin-releasing factor is thought to be the controlling factor.
2. Secretion is increased by stress, via CNS.
3. Negative feedback control occurs through cortisol excess in plasma.

Uses of ACTH

Objective 34.D.15. Recognize uses of ACTH.

Uses of ACTH include:

1. replacement for cortisol (but the protein hormone must be given parenterally so it is easier to administer cortisol)
2. occasional treatment of allergic phenomena
3. mainly as a test for adrenal function (see above)

Prolactin

This is an adenohypophyseal, protein hormone that regulates lactation.

Effects of Prolactin

Objective 34.D.16. Recognize the effects of prolactin.

The effects of prolactin are:

1. promotes proliferation of mammary ductal epithelium
2. induces synthesis of milk proteins and enzymes for lactose production

Prolactin Secretion

Objective 34.D.17. Recognize characteristics of prolactin secretion.

Secretion of prolactin increases due to:

1. pregnancy, with peak levels at term
2. nursing, stimulated by sucking or breast manipulation

3. other factors, including psychic and physical stress, insulin-induced hypoglycemia, and high levels of estrogens

Melanocyte-stimulating Hormone (MSH)

MSH is an adenohypophyseal, protein hormone.

Status of MSH

Objective 34.D.18. Recognize status of MSH in human physiology.

The exact function of MSH in humans is unknown. Excess of MSH causes hyperpigmentation of skin. Corticotropin (ACTH) is chemically related to MSH.

Parathyroid Hormone and Calcitonin

Parathyroid hormone (PTH), from the parathyroid gland, and calcitonin, from the thryoid gland, are both protein hormones that participate in cellular mechanisms which aid in maintaining calcium ion concentration at a constant level in the extracellular fluids (including blood).

Hypocalcemia and hypercalcemia

Objective 34.D.19. Describe symptoms of hypocalcemia and hypercalcemia.

Symptoms of hypocalcemia are:

1. increased excitability of nervous tissue
2. tetanic muscle contractions
3. convulsions
4. death

Symptoms of hypercalcemia are:

1. depression of nervous tissue and muscle
2. constipation, nausea, vomiting
3. diuresis
4. precipitation of calcium salts, especially into kidneys

Mechanisms of Action of Parathyroid Hormone (Parathormone or PTH)

Objective 34.D.20. Describe mechanisms of action of PTH.

Mechanisms of action include:

1. mobilization of calcium from bone
2. enhanced absorption of calcium from the GI tract
3. enhanced reabsorption of calcium from kidney tubules

Secretion of PTH

Objective 34.D.21. Describe the stimuli of secretion of PTH.

A stimulus for secretion is a falling level of ionized calcium in blood perfusing the parathyroid gland. With decreased calcium perfusing the gland, there is an increased release of PTH, with PTH causing an increased level of calcium. With an increased blood level of calcium, the reverse occurs.

Uses and Pharmacokinetics of PTH

Objective 34.D.22. Describe uses and pharmacokinetics of PTH.

Uses and pharmacokinetics of PTH are:

1. Currently, there are no therapeutic uses.
2. PTH is used as an aid in the diagnosis of pseudohypoparathyroidism.
3. PTH must be administered by injection. It is metabolized by the liver and partly excreted by the kidney.

Mechanisms of Action of Calcitonin. This is a protein hormone of the thyroid gland.

Objective 34.D.23. Describe mechanisms of action of calcitonin.

Mechanisms of action of calcitonin include:

1. inhibition of bone resorption
2. increased kidney excretion of calcium

These effects may occur through activation of cyclic AMP.

Secretion of Calcitonin

Objective 34.D.24. Describe the stimulus for calcitonin secretion.

The stimulus for secretion of calcitonin is the amount of ionized calcium perfusing the thyroid gland. When calcium concentration is high, the amount of calcitonin released is increased and results in a depression of serum calcium. With a decreased blood level of calcium, the reverse occurs.

Uses and Pharmacokinetics of Calcitonin

Objective 34.D.25. List the uses and pharmacokinetics of calcitonin.

Uses of calcitonin are:

1. hyperparathyroidism
2. temporary treatment of any condition producing hypercalcemia.

Calcitonin must be given parenterally; it is probably metabolized by liver and kidney.

Insulin and Glucagon

Diabetes Mellitus

Objective 34.D.26. Describe the pathogenesis of diabetes mellitus, the role of insulin in metabolism, and the types of diabetes.

Insulin, a protein hormone from the pancreatic β cells, is used to treat diabetes mellitus. Most of the pathology associated with diabetes can be attributed to the following metabolic defects:

1. decreased utilization of glucose (i.e., inhibition of glucose entry into cells)
2. increased mobilization of fats from fat storage sites (this may be a result of decreased utilization of glucose)
3. decreased deposition of protein in tissue (this also may be secondary to decreased glucose utilization)

The earliest symptoms of diabetes are:

1. polyuria
2. polydipsia
3. polyphagia
4. loss of weight
5. lack of energy

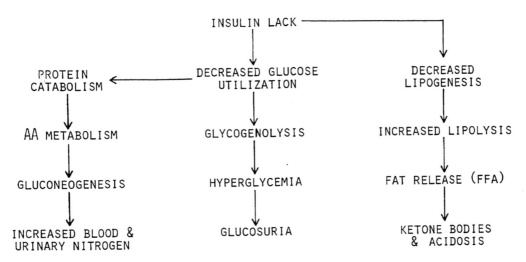

Figure 34-1. Metabolic defects caused by insulin deficiency. AA, amino acid; FFA, free fatty acid.

Metabolically the defects in diabetes are schematically outlined in Figure 34-1. Notice how the chemical changes in blood and urine can be traced to specific changes in substrate utilization.

Types of Diabetes

Objective 34.D.27. Describe two types of diabetes mellitus. Types of diabetes mellitus are:

1. juvenile-onset diabetes (insulin dependent, ketosis-prone, no beta cells present)
2. maturity onset diabetes (nonketotic, and beta cells are present).

Dental Implications of Diabetes

Objective 34.D.28. Describe the important considerations for dental treatment of the diabetic patient.

Although the dentist will not be directly involved in the medical therapy of diabetes, there are certain drugs used by dentists that can interact with sulfonylureas (see the following). In addition, there are other dental implications concerning the treatment of diabetics. The following dental implications may be cited:

1. Sugar cubes or candy should be in your emergency kit. If the diabetic patient begins to feel weak, some carbohydrate should be administered, even if the weakness is due to lack of insulin. This extra sugar will not hurt, and it may help.
2. If the problem is more serious (delirium or coma) DO NOT INJECT INSULIN; call a physician. This emphasizes the need to work closely with the physician regarding dental care. Since it is difficult to decide whether the patient is hypoglycemic (too much insulin) or hyperglycemic (not enough insulin), the best procedure is to take a blood sample which can be saved for diagnostic purposes. Then either give sugar by mouth or by IV injection (infusion of glucose in water). The sugar can do no harm, while insulin injection could be harmful, aggravating insulin shock.
3. Uncontrolled diabetics are very susceptible to infections.
4. Excessive stress may lead to release of glucocorticoids and epinephrine from the adrenals. These hormones counteract the effect of insulin by inducing hyperglycemia. Preoperative and operative "tender loving care" may be even more important for diabetic patients than for normal patients.

Insulin as a Hormone

Objective 34.D.29. Describe important features of insulin as a hormone, including mechanism of action and stimuli for release.

Insulin is a protein hormone with the following important features:

1. mechanism of action—increases transport of glucose into cells
2. stored in vesicles in pancreatic beta cells
3. stimuli for release:
   a. increased glucose in plasma
   b. signals from the GI tract, including food and GI hormones
   c. neural signals, originating from autonomic and central nervous systems
   d. amino acids, fatty acids, and ketone bodies
   e. adrenergic beta agonists (alpha agonists block)
   f. parasympathomimetics

Insulin as a Drug

Objective 34.D.30. Describe insulin as a drug.

The following points are important considerations for insulin therapy:

1. must be given parenterally because of digestion of GI tract
2. liver and kidney are responsible for degradation and excretion
3. the physician usually has to tailor the medication to the patient's needs, considering diet, insulin, oral hypoglycemics, and other factors.

Types of Insulin

Objective 34.D.31. Recognize types of insulin as short-acting, intermediate-acting, or long-acting.

Preparations of available insulin are described below:

1. short-acting (6 to 14 hours' duration)
   a. insulin injection
   b. insulin zinc, prompt suspension
2. Intermediate acting (18 to 24 hours' duration)
   a. isophane insulin suspension
   b. insulin zinc
   c. globin zinc insulin injection
3. Long-acting (36 hours' duration)
   a. protamine zinc insulin suspension
   b. extended insulin zinc suspension

Oral Hypoglycemics

Objective 34.D.32. Define oral hypoglycemic agents and recognize the class of agents used.

Oral hypoglycemic agents are drugs that lower blood sugar after oral ingestion. The major group of oral hypoglycemic agents is classified as **sulfonylureas**. The major difference between different drugs in this class is their duration of action.

Mechanism of Action and Pharmacokinetics of Sulfonylureas

Objective 34.D.33. Recognize mechanism of action and pharmacokinetics of sulfonylureas.

The mechanism of action is stimulation of beta cells to secrete insulin. All agents of this class are well absorbed from the GI tract. The liver metabolizes all sulfonylureas except chlorpropamide, which is excreted unchanged. Metabolically active products are produced by the liver when acetohexamide and tolazamide are metabolized.

The kidneys are the major organs of excretion.

Toxicity and Contraindications of Sulfonylureas

Objective 34.D.34. Recognize toxicity and contraindications of sulfonylureas.

Toxicities include:

1. leukopenia, thrombocytopenia, pancytopenia, agranulocytosis
2. paresthesias, tinnitus, and headache
3. cholestatic jaundice
4. hyponatremia
5. coma (from hypoglycemia)

Contraindications include:

1. renal or hepatic insufficiency
2. pregnancy

Names and Dental Drug Interactions of Sulfonylureas

Objective 34.D.35. Be able to name at least two sulfonylureas (set in bold type) and state their interactions with dental drugs.

Important oral hypoglycemic agents include:

1. **chlorpropamide**
2. **tolbutamide**
3. acetohexamide
4. tolazamide

Drugs that may antagonize sulfonylureas to induce hyperglycemia:

1. **glucocorticoids**°
2. **epinephrine**
3. **norepinephrine**
4. glucagon
5. thiazide diuretics

Drugs that may enhance sulfonylureas to induce hypoglycemia:

1. **sulfonamides**°
2. propranolol
3. **salicylates**
4. phenylbutazone
5. dicumarol
6. **chloramphenicol**
7. MAO inhibitors
8. alcohol
9. anabolic steroids
10. guanethidine
11. **oxytetracycline**

Glucagon Features

Objective 34.D.36. Recognize glucagon, its role in glucose control, its source, mechanism of action, stimuli for release, preparation, and use.

Glucagon is a protein hormone also secreted by pancreatic islets (but from α cells instead of β cells). The important features of glucagon are listed below:

1. mechanism of action—causes glycogenolysis.
2. stored in vesicles of pancreatic alpha cells.
3. stimuli for release are:
    a. low levels of glucose.
    b. low levels of food products in GI tract.
    c. sympathomimetics.
4. preparation—glucagon for injection

° Drugs set in bold type in these groups are those which may be used or prescribed by dentists and should be remembered.

5. use—for insulin-induced coma when glucose solutions have not relieved the coma.

E. POLYPEPTIDE HORMONES

Oxytocin

This is an octapeptide hormone that is synthesized in the hypothalamus and stored in the neurohypophysis.

Effects and Pharmacokinetics of Oxytocin

Objective 34.E.1. Recognize effects of oxytocin and its pharmacokinetics.

Effects of oxytocin on various organs are listed below.

1. Uterus: oxytocin stimulates the pregnant uterus to contract, especially during the last trimester and in the presence of estrogen.
2. Mammary glands: oxytocin causes milk ejection or milk letdown.
3. Cardiovascular system effects:
    a. with large doses, transient fall of BP with reflex tachycardia.
    b. with continuous infusion of large doses, there is a slight rise of BP after the initial decrease.
4. Kidney: oxytocin causes a slight antidiuretic effect.

Pharmacokinetics of oxytocin include the following:

1. absorption—must be given parenterally, intranasally or via buccal mucosa
2. metabolism in liver, kidney, and in lactating mammary tissue
3. excretion by the kidney

Uses of Oxytocin

Objective 34.E.2. List uses of oxytocin.

Uses of oxytocin are:

1. to induce labor at term
2. to control postpartum hemorrhage
3. to correct postpartum uterine atony

4. to cause uterine contraction after cesarean section

Vasopressin or Antidiuretic Hormone (ADH)

This is an octapeptide hormone synthesized in the hypothalamus and stored in the neurohypophysis.

ADH Deficiency and Excess Syndromes

Objective 34.E.3. Recognize the effects of deficiency and excess of vasopressin.

1. Absence of vasopressin causes diabetes insipidus.
2. Excess of vasopressin causes increased extracellular fluid volume and edema.

ADH Effects and Pharmacokinetics

Objective 34.E.4. Recognize effects and pharmacokinetics of vasopressin.

Effects of vasopressin are:

1. causes renal tubular reabsorption of water, mostly in collecting ducts of kidneys
2. large doses cause vasoconstriction with reflex bradycardia
3. large doses cause contraction of smooth muscle of GI tract and uterus

Absorption, fate, and excretion include:

1. must be given parenterally or by nasal insufflation
2. metabolism by liver and kidneys
3. excretion by kidneys

Uses of Vasopressin and Comparison to Oxytocin

Objective 34.E.5. Recognize uses of vasopressin and compare its relative potency in causing biologic effects to oxytocin.

The only use for vasopressin is in diabetes insipidus. Relative potencies are shown in Table 34-3, which relates the potencies on an arbi-

TABLE 34–3. BIOLOGIC ACTIVITY OF ADH AND OXYTOCIN

	Anti-diuretic	Pressor	Milk Ejection	Oxytocic
ADH	100	100	15	5
oxytocin	1	1	100	100

From Brazeau P: In Gilman AG, Goodman LS, Gilman A (eds): Goodman and Gilman's The Pharmacological Basis of Therapeutics, 4th ed, 1970. Courtesy of Macmillan Publishing Co.

trary scale. On the first line, the primary effects of ADH are expressed as 100, while on the second line, the primary effects of oxytocin are set at 100.

Derivatives of Vasopressin and Their Chemistries

Objective 34.E.6. Recognize the chemical difference between POR-8 and felypressin as compared to vasopressin.

Figure 34–2 shows the chemical formula (peptide sequence) of vasopressin and its numbering system.

POR-8 is an octapeptide containing the amino acid ornithine at position number 8. Felypressin (marketed in Europe under the trade name of *Octapressin*) is an octapeptide containing the amino acids phenylalanine at position number 2 and lysine at position number 8.

Dental Significance of Vasopressin Analogs

Objective 34.E.7. Describe the dental significance of POR-8 and felypressin.

These two derivatives have been used as vasoconstrictors in local anesthetic solutions. The vasopressin molecules are modified such that they are fairly potent vasoconstrictors with little or no antidiuretic activity. The reported advantages of these agents are (1) they do not interact with autonomic or antihypertensive drugs, and (2) there is very little or no risk of potentially dangerous side effects in patients with cardiovascular disease. One disadvantage is that they

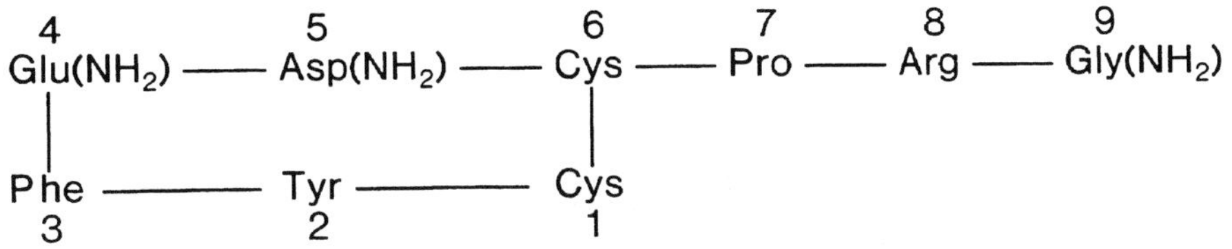

Figure 34-2. Chemical formula of vasopressin (peptide sequence). (*From Brazeau P: In Gilman AG, Goodman LS, Gilman A (eds): Goodman and Gilman's The Pharmacological Basis of Therapeutics, 4th ed, 1970. Courtesy of Macmillan Publishing Co.*)

cannot be used to help control gingival hemorrhage during certain dental surgical procedures. Therefore, the adrenergic drugs are still required.

Hypothalamic Releasing Factors

These are described under adenohypophyseal hormones (p. 356). The releasing (and inhibitory) factors isolated are polypeptides, and each polypeptide controls a specific adenohypophyseal hormone (more details are given above under each adenohypophyseal hormone).

F. AMINO ACID DERIVATIVES: THYROID HORMONES

Thyroid Deficiency and Excess Syndrome

Objective 34.F.1. Recognize symptoms of deficiency and excess of thyroid hormones.

Hypothyroidism. In adults this is often termed myxedema or Gull's disease, cretinism in infants, and juvenile myxedema in later childhood.

Myxedema is characterized by the following:

1. goiter may or may not be present
2. expressionless face that is puffy and pallid
3. skin is cold and dry, scalp is scaly
4. fingernails are thick and brittle
5. voice is husky and low pitched
6. mentality is impaired
7. heart is dilated, and cardiac output is diminished
8. prone to drowsiness and sleep
9. complaint of cold in winter but not of heat in summer

Cretinism is characterized by the following:

1. goiter may or may not be present
2. child is dwarfed, and extremities are short
3. mentally retarded and inactive
4. face is puffy and expressionless
5. enlarged tongue which may protrude
6. skin has yellowish hue and doughy appearance
7. heart rate is slow and temperature low

Hyperthyroidism. This is called thyrotoxicosis or Graves's disease in young adults and toxic nodular goiter or Plummer's disease in older adults. Most signs and symptoms arise from increased heat production, increased neuromuscular excitability, and increased sympathetic nervous system activity.

Symptoms of thyrotoxicosis are listed below:

1. skin flushed, warm, and moist
2. muscles weak and tremulous
3. increased heart rate and force of contraction
4. prominent and pounding pulse
5. increased appetite, but loss of weight
6. insomnia, anxiety, and apprehension
7. intolerance to heat
8. exophthalmos

Dental Implications

Objective 34.F.2. Describe the dental implications of hypothyroidism and hyperthyroidism.

The hypothyroid or hyperthyroid patient who is under control with drugs prescribed by a physician may be considered euthyroid and does not require special care. However, the uncontrolled patient requires special care.

The hyperthyroid patient:

1. will be hyperreactive to epinephrine (absolute contraindication)
2. should be treated with care to avoid a thyroid crisis
3. may require increased dosages of CNS depressant drugs

The hypothyroid patient:

1. will probably be hyperreactive to usual dosages of narcotic analgesics
2. may require decreased dosages of other CNS depressant drugs

Chemistry and Status

Objective 34.F.3. Recognize the chemistry and status of thyroid hormones.

There are two types of thyroid hormones. They are derivatives of the amino acid, tyrosine, which is converted by iodination and other metabolic reactions in the thryoid gland. Thyroxine (T_4) has four iodines attached to the aromatic rings, and triiodothyronine (T_3) has three iodines attached.

The status of iodine in the plasma is as follows:

1. 95% is organic, 5% ionic
2. 90 to 95% of organic iodine is T_4, and 5% is T_3
3. 99 to 99.9% of T_4 and T_3 are bound to plasma protein

Secretion and Pharmacokinetics

Objective 34.F.4. Recognize the mechanism of secretion, the pharmacokinetics, preparations, and uses of thyroid hormones.

Secretion is regulated by TSH from the adenohypophysis (see discussion above). TSH controls iodine uptake and the secretion of T_3 and T_4, which is thought to be the result of proteolysis of thyroglobulin. Excesses of T_3 and T_4 in the plasma have a negative feedback control over TSH.

Pharmacokinetics include the following:

1. T_3 better absorbed orally than T_4
2. activity of all preparations (thyroid extracts, powders, and so on) depends upon content of T_3 and T_4
3. T_3 and T_4 are highly protein bound and inactive until released
4. both T_3 and T_4 are metabolized in the liver
5. metabolites are excreted by the kidney

Preparations of thyroid hormone include:

1. thyroid extract
2. thyroglobulin
3. L-thyroxine
4. liothyronine
5. mixtures of T_3 and T_4
   (*Note:* TSH can also be used to stimulate T_3 and T_4 secretion.)

Uses of these preparations are for correction of hypothyroidism, and they must be carefully controlled by the physician to produce the euthyroid state.

Methods of Controlling Thyroid Function

Objective 34.F.5. Recognize methods of controlling excessive thyroid activity. (Remember drugs set in bold type.)

Excessive thyroid activity can be controlled by destruction of the thyroid tissue, as well as by antithyroid drugs. Removal of the tissue occurs during surgery and after ionizing radiation. Since iodine will concentrate almost entirely in the thyroid, a dose of ^{131}I can be used to destroy the gland. Smaller doses of ^{131}I (or of ^{125}I) have been used to determine thyroid gland function. After administration, the radioactive iodine will label the protein-bound iodine (PBI) pool.

Antithyroid Drugs. Each step in the formation and secretion of T_3 and T_4 theoretically is susceptible to inhibition.

Step 1. Uptake of iodide. This is inhibited by a number of anions which are chemically related to iodide, including perchlorates, thiocyanates, and nitrates. These agents are experimental and not used in human therapy. However, these compounds may occur in cabbages, rutabagas, and turnips, which may be goitrogenic if taken in sufficient quantities. **TSH** stimulates the uptake of iodide by thyroid cells.

Step 2. Formation of active iodine from iodide. This is required before tyrosine can be iodinated. This step is inhibited by **thiouracils** or thiocarbamides. Useful drugs in this class include: **propylthiouracil**, methylthiouracil, and **methimazole**. These drugs are well absorbed orally, concentrate in the thyroid gland, cross the placenta, and get into milk. They are metabolized in the liver and excreted by the kidney. The use of these drugs is for suppression of thyroid activity in hyperthyroidism, especially as a temporary treatment before thyroidectomy. Side effects of these drugs include agranulocytosis, rash, pain and stiffness of joints, headache, nausea, and hypothyroidism.

Step 3. Active iodine reacts with tyrosine in several chemical reactions, forming MIT (monoiodotyrosine) and DIT (diiodotyrosine). This step can be blocked by iodides (Step 6) but not dependably.

Step 4. MIT and DIT react to form T_3 and T_4. No inhibitors of this step are known.

Step 5. T_3 and T_4 are stored with protein-forming thyroglobulin. No inhibitors of this step are known.

Step 6. Proteolysis of thyroglobulin leads to secretion of T_3 and T_4 into blood. **Iodide** (high dose) inhibits this step, while **TSH** stimulates it. Excess iodide secondarily blocks binding of iodide into organic iodine. Iodide use is limited to preparation and temporary control of the thyroid state before surgery. Long-term use of excess iodides may result in loss of inhibition and massive release of hormone, which is known as "thyroid storm." KI or NaI are used for iodide therapy.

REFERENCES

Brazeau P: Agents affecting the renal conservation of water. In Gilman AG, Goodman LS, Gilman A (eds): Goodman and Gilman's The Pharmacological Basis of Therapeutics, 4th ed. New York, Macmillan, 1970, Ch 40, p 876

Darzenta NC, Giunta JL: Radiographic changes of the mandible related to oral contraceptives. Oral Surg 43:478, 1977

Kaufman AY: An oral contraceptive has an etiologic factor in producing hyperplastic gingivitis and a neoplasm of the pregnancy tumor type. Oral Surg 28:666, 1969

Knight GM, Wade AB: The effects of hormonal contraceptives on the human periodontium. J Periodontal Res 9:18, 1974

Lindhe J, Bjorn AL: Influence of hormonal contraceptives on the gingiva of women. J Periodont Res 2:1, 1967

Lynn BD: "The pill" as an etiologic agent in hypertrophic gingivitis. Oral Surg 24:333, 1967

Magnusson I, Ericson T, Hugoson A: The effect of oral contraceptives on the concentration of some salivary substances in women. Arch Oral Biol 20:119, 1975

Sweet JB, Butler DP: Increased incidence of postoperative localized osteitis in mandibular third molar surgery associated with patients using oral contraceptives. Am J Obstet Gynecol 127:518, 1977

BIBLIOGRAPHY

Csáky TZ: Cutting's Handbook of Pharmacology, 6th ed. New York, Appleton-Century-Crofts, 1979, Ch 32, 33, 34, 35, 36, 37, 38

Gilman AG, Goodman LS, Gilman A (eds): Goodman and Gilman's the Pharmacological Basis of Therapeutics, 6th ed. New York, Macmillan, 1980, Ch 59, 60, 61, 62, 63, 64, 65

Melmon KL, Morrelli HF (eds): Clinical Pharmacology: Basic Principles in Therapeutics, 2nd ed. New York, Macmillan, 1978, Ch 11

Meyers FH, Jawetz E, Goldfien A: Review of Medical Pharmacology, 6th ed. Los Altos, CA, Lange, 1978, Ch 33, 34, 35, 36, 37, 38, 39

QUESTIONS

1. Endocrine drugs may be used:

    A. to achieve a physiologic balance
    B. for a therapeutic effect
    C. to block a hormonal effect
    D. all of the above are correct

2. Endocrine agents are useful for:

    A. diagnosis of endocrine dysfunction
    B. attaining a new physiologic state
    C. both A and B are correct
    D. neither A nor B is correct

3. Hormones may be broadly classified as:

    A. steroids
    B. proteins
    C. polypeptides
    D. amino acid derivatives
    E. all of the above are correct

4. All of the following are protein hormones *except:*

    A. ACTH
    B. LH
    C. parathyroid hormone
    D. insulin
    E. thyroid hormone

5. Steroid hormones include all of the following *except:*

    A. glucocorticoids
    B. adrenocorticotropin
    C. estrogens
    D. androgens

6. **T F** All adrenocorticosteroids contain the 18-C steroid nucleus.

7. **T F** The 18-C steroid nucleus must be taken in with food because the body does not have the enzymes to form it.

8. **T F** While glucocorticoids are formed in the adrenal cortex, mineralocorticoids come from bone.

9. **T F** Aldosterone is controlled *mainly* by ACTH activity.

10. A deficiency of adrenal corticosteroids is called:

    A. Addison's disease
    B. Cushing's syndrome
    C. both A and B are correct
    D. neither A nor B is correct

11. The anti-inflammatory effect of glucocorticosteroids is most closely related to:

    A. gluconeogenesis
    B. lysosomal membrane stabilization
    C. inhibition of PG synthetase
    D. antagonism of insulin

12. **T F** Glucocorticoids do *not* cause salt retention.

13. Excessive administration of glucocorticoids could lead to:

    A. depletion of glycogen and hypoglycemia
    B. lipolysis which cause a generalized thin appearance
    C. salt and water elimination
    D. none of the above are correct

14. **T F** Glucocorticoids are excreted by the kidney as 17-hydroxysteroids.

15. Glucocorticoids may worsen which of the following conditions?

    A. peptic ulcer
    B. diabetes mellitus
    C. high blood pressure
    D. all of the above are correct

16. **T F** Glucocorticosteroids are indicated only in Addison's disease.

17. If a patient needs glucocorticosteroid and is edematous, the best choice of the following would be:

    A. cortisol
    B. cortisone
    C. prednisolone
    D. methylprednisolone

18. Which of the following drugs (drugs used by dentists) may interact with systemic glucocorticoid therapy?

    A. penicillins
    B. salicylates
    C. guanethidine
    D. narcotic-analgesics

19. Dental uses of glucocorticosteroids include:

    A. drug of choice for anaphylaxis
    B. topical treatment of oral ulcerations
    C. both A and B are correct
    D. neither A nor B is correct

20. Contraindications for glucocorticosteroids include:

    A. hypotension
    B. insulin excess
    C. peptic ulcer
    D. all of the above are correct

21. **T F** Mineralocorticoids may be life-saving in an addisonian crisis.

22. In glucocorticoid use, the following principles should apply:

    A. high doses of steroids for five days will probably *not* suppress the adrenal cortex
    B. the full dose should be taken each morning at 8 AM

C. both A and B are correct
D. neither A nor B is correct

23. **T F** Spironolactone is used to counteract hyperaldosteronism.

24. Natural estrogens include:

    A. estradiol
    B. diethylstilbestrol
    C. progesterone
    D. all of the above are correct

25. **T F** The action of progestins on cells is thought to occur by direct combination with ribosomal receptors to stimulate protein synthesis.

26. **T F** Increasing estrogen levels result in menstruation.

27. **T F** Estrogen levels are important in triggering LH secretion during the menstrual cycle.

28. **T F** Increasing progesterone levels block release of LH and FSH.

29. **T F** Estrogens and progestins are secreted in the kidney in the nonmetabolized form.

30. Estrogens are used in:

    A. menopause
    B. acne
    C. dysmenorrhea
    D. all of the above are correct

31. **T F** Progestins in combination with estrogens are used at term to suppress lactation.

32. Which of the following can be used as an anticancer drug?

    A. tamoxifen
    B. progesterone

C. estrogen

D. all of the above are correct

33. Oral contraceptives contain a:

A. combination of an estrogen and a progestin

B. progestin only

C. both A and B are correct

D. neither A nor B is correct

34. T F One mechanism of estrogen as an oral contraceptive is thought to be inhibition of FSH secretion.

35. A patient taking oral contraceptives may have the following systemic side effects:

A. thromboembolism

B. hypertension

C. alteration of mood

D. all of the above are correct

36. A patient taking oral contraceptives may have the following dental side effects:

A. decreased radiopacity of the mandible

B. no change in the incidence of alveolar osteitis after third molar extraction

C. gingival hyperplasia and increased gingival exudate

D. all of the above are correct

37. T F Oral contraceptive use can increase fibrinolysis, resulting in increased postoperative bleeding.

38. T F The gingival side effects of oral contraceptives are *not* worsened by poor oral hygiene.

39. T F The testes is the only source of androgens in humans.

40. T F The cellular mechanism of action of testosterone is similar to other steroidal mechanisms.

41. T F Testosterone is known to be metabolized to a compound which retains the androgenic actions.

42. Testosterone promotes:

A. aggressive sexual behavior

B. anabolic effect

C. both A and B are correct

D. neither A nor B is correct

43. T F All of the effects of testosterone therapy are pleasant.

44. Testosterone may be useful in:

A. osteosclerosis

B. hyperpituitarism

C. both A and B are correct

D. neither A nor B is correct

45. T F GH stimulates protein synthesis in all tissues.

46. GH secretion is caused by:

A. hyperglycemia

B. overeating

C. both A and B are correct

D. neither A nor B is correct

47. T F GH excess results in gigantism in the child but acromegaly in the adult.

48. T F LH is only active in females.

49. LH secretion is controlled by:

A. feedback inhibition due to rising progesterone

B. a hypothalamic releasing-factor

C. a hypothalamic inhibitory-factor

D. all of the above are correct

50. T F LH is used to treat cryptorchism in males, but only in combination with FSH.

51. **T F** FSH stimulates spermatogenesis.

52. **T F** While LH peaks in midcycle, FSH is at a low level.

53. **T F** While FSH is used to treat infertile women, LH is not.

54. **T F** TSH causes regulation of synthesis and release of thyroid hormones.

55. Protirelin is a drug recognized as:

    A. a polypeptide
    B. a hypothalamic releasing factor for TSH
    C. both A and B are correct
    D. neither A nor B is correct

56. **T F** TSH is frequently used in thyroid deficiency states to stimulate secretion of thyroid hormone.

57. **T F** ACTH controls production of cortisol but has no effect on aldosterone.

58. ACTH release is controlled by:

    A. feedback inhibition related to plasma cortisol level
    B. a hypothalamic releasing factor
    C. both A and B are correct
    D. neither A nor B is correct

59. **T F** ACTH is administered orally as a test for adrenal cortex function.

60. **T F** Prolactin secretion controls FSH levels in midcycle.

61. Prolactin secretion increases during:

    A. pregnancy
    B. nursing
    C. both A and B are correct
    D. neither A nor B is correct

62. **T F** Melanocyte-stimulating hormone is chemically related to ACTH.

63. Hypocalcemia causes:

    A. depression of nervous tissue
    B. depression of muscle spasms
    C. no threat to life
    D. none of the above is correct

64. Parathyroid hormone causes:

    A. mobilization of calcium from bone
    B. kidney secretion of calcium
    C. both A and B are correct
    D. neither A nor B is correct

65. **T F** PTH levels increase as calcium levels increase.

66. **T F** Oral PTH therapy is useful in controlling serum calcium.

67. **T F** Calcitonin has the opposite effects on serum calcium as PTH.

68. **T F** The stimulus for calcitonin secretion is the level of calcium perfusing the parathyroid gland.

69. Calcitonin's therapeutic uses include:

    A. hyperparathyroidism
    B. hypocalcemia
    C. both A and B are correct
    D. neither A nor B is correct

70. Diabetes mellitus is characterized by:

    A. decreased utilization of glucose
    B. decreased mobilization of fat
    C. increased deposition of protein in tissue
    D. all of the above are correct

71. **T F** Diabetes mellitus occurs only in adults.

72. A diabetic patient expresses a feeling of discomfort while in your office, which is followed by weakness and light-headedness.

Suspecting that this patient is experiencing a diabetic emergency, you should treat the situation in which one of the following ways?

A. administer insulin intravenously and immediately
B. administer some form of sugar
C. wait for the symptoms to subside, then continue working
D. administer a sulfonylurea drug PO

73. T F Insulin is stored in vesicles of the pancreatic α cells.

74. Release of insulin is triggered by:

A. increased blood glucose
B. beta adrenergic agonists
C. parasympathomimetics
D. all of the above are correct

75. T F Insulin preparations are now called "oral hypoglycemics."

76. The following insulin preparations are considered long acting:

A. protamine zinc insulin
B. isophane insulin suspension
C. both A and B are correct
D. neither A nor B is correct

77. T F Drugs which are orally effective in diabetes are called sulfonylureas.

78. Sulfonylureas act by:

A. stimulating pancreatic β cells to secrete insulin
B. cholinergic blockade of insulin secretion
C. adrenergic blockade of insulin secretion
D. none of the above

79. T F Sulfonylureas are free of toxic effects.

80. Tolbutamide may be used in a patient with:

A. thyrotoxicosis
B. diabetes mellitus
C. Addison's disease
D. Cushing's syndrome

81. Which one of the following drugs or drug groups is thought to antagonize tolbutamide, producing a hyperglycemia?

A. epinephrine
B. salicylates
C. sulfonamides
D. oxytetracycline

82. T F Glucagon is secreted from the pancreatic α cells.

83. T F Oxytocin is a more powerful uterine stimulant than vasopressin.

84. Oxytocin is used:

A. to induce labor at term
B. to control postpartum hemorrhage
C. both A and B are correct
D. neither A nor B is correct

85. T F A deficiency of vasopressin causes diabetes mellitus.

86. Vasopressin and oxytocin have the following in common:

A. both are secreted by the neurohypophysis
B. both are octapeptides
C. both have antidiuretic and pressor activity, but to different degrees
D. all of the above are correct

87. T F POR-8 and felypressin are chemical analogs of vasopressin and are used as vasoconstrictors.

88. **T F** Since felypressin is a noncatecholamine, nonadrenergic vasoconstrictor, epinephrine is no longer needed in dental local anesthetic solutions.

89. Hypothyroidism is characterized by:

    A. increased heart rate and force of contraction
    B. insomnia, anxiety, and apprehension
    C. both A and B are correct
    D. neither A nor B is correct

90. A patient with thyrotoxicosis may:

    A. be hyperreactive to the effects of epinephrine
    B. require higher than usual doses of sedative drugs
    C. both A and B are correct
    D. neither A nor B is correct

91. A patient with myxedema would be expected to:

    A. require decreased dosage of CNS depressant drugs
    B. be hyperreactive to usual dosages of narcotic analgesics
    C. both A and B are correct
    D. neither A nor B is correct

92. **T F** Thyroid hormone consists of two substances called T_3 and T_4, depending upon the number of iodines in the molecule.

93. Preparations of thyroid hormone include:

    A. thyroid extract
    B. thyroglobulin
    C. L-thyroxine
    D. mixtures of T_3 and T_4
    E. all of the above are correct

94. The thyroid gland can be inhibited by:

    A. excess of iodide
    B. iodide-related drugs in food (e.g., thiocyanates)
    C. both A and B are correct
    D. neither A nor B is correct

95. **T F** TSH is thought to stimulate thyroid secretion by stimulating proteolysis of thyroglobulin.

96. Excess secretion of thyroid hormone could be counteracted by administration of:

    A. high doses of iodide
    B. radioactive iodide
    C. propylthiouracil
    D. A, B, and C are correct
    E. neither A, B, nor C is correct

35
General Anesthesia

General anesthesics are not, in the normal sense, considered drugs for dental office use. Yet many of the drugs in this chapter are vitally important to the practice of dentistry, and there are many misconceptions about their use in a dental practice. First, N_2O/O_2 may be used routinely in the dental office for its sedative-amnesic and analgesic properties. The dentist using this must always use adequate oxygenation (at least 50% O_2 in the mixture), maintain contact with the patient, and properly monitor the conscious-analgesic state. Thus, the authors do not consider use of N_2O/O_2 as general anesthesia in the dental office.

Second, IV sedative drugs may also be routinely used, assuming adequate practice and again maintaining conscious contact with the sedated patient. However, this is only recommended for routine use with a single IV drug, such as diazepam, and with adequate patient monitoring.

Third, the use of more potent anesthetics, such as ultrashort-acting barbiturates or true general anesthetics (other drugs discussed in this chapter), or any mixing of drugs, such as narcotics, neuroleptic agents, and so on, should be reserved for practitioners who have had adequate

anesthesiology training, and who are working in an environment where sophisticated facilities for monitoring the patient's condition are available.

Other dentists or practitioners may have a different viewpoint, and it should be emphasized that each dentist is responsible for his own decisions in the matter of IV drug use or outpatient general anesthesia.

Dentists who continue in specialities requiring anesthesiology training will obviously require much more knowledge about general anesthetic drugs. In that case, the initial background provided in this chapter will only be the first in a long series of steps necessary to achieve the adequate knowledge required in anesthesiology training.

A. DEFINITION OF GENERAL ANESTHESIA

Objective 35.A.1. Recognize the definition of general anesthesia and distinguish it from local anesthesia and analgesia.

General anesthesia is the total loss of sensation so as to allow general surgery. General anesthetics are general CNS depressants that cause reversible unconsciousness. General anesthetics should ideally produce not only unconsciousness but also analgesia, muscular relaxation, and amnesia. At the same time, general anesthetics should have only minimal effects on vital functions. On the other hand, analgesics diminish pain while having a minimal effect on consciousness. Local anesthesia refers to loss of pain in a localized area of the body.

B. HISTORY

Objective 35.B.1. Recognize six drugs or other measures which were used before general anesthetics were introduced for surgery.

1. **Opium and narcotics.** These agents are too dangerous because they tend to cause too much respiratory depression as the patient approaches unconsciousness.
2. **Ethanol** is also dangerous for anesthesia because of respiratory depression, and the patient approaches coma and death as unconsciousness is achieved.
3. **Belladonna alkaloids.** Although these have been used in the past, the reason for their use as general anesthetics is not apparent.
4. **Asphyxia.** This state, by its very nature, is extremely dangerous and must be avoided.
5. **Cerebral concussion.** This state is not acceptable; the cure is worse than the disease.
6. **"Great Haste."** Many doctors prided themselves on their speed, but the pain had to be endured by the patient, and this caused a great amount of fear.

Objective 35.B.2. Describe the importance of two dentists in the introduction of general anesthetics.

Horace Wells. In 1845, Wells successfully used nitrous oxide to extract teeth. However, his demonstration for surgeons was unsuccessful.

W. T. G. Morton. In 1846, Morton used ether for extracting teeth and successfully demonstrated ether anesthesia to surgeons at the Massachusetts General Hospital. Actually, Crawford W. Long of Jefferson, Georgia, is credited with first

doing operations under ether starting in 1842, but his results were not publicized until after Morton's demonstration.

C. MECHANISM OF ACTION

Objective 35.C.1. Recognize six theories of the mechanism of general anesthetic action and the present status of these theories.

1. **Meyer-Overton Lipid Theory.** Meyer and Overton measured oil/water partition coefficients of anesthetics and found that the more lipid soluble an anesthetic is, the more powerful it is. This led them to believe that anesthetic action is based upon lipid solubility.

    Present status. The brain cells have a great amount of lipid, and the more lipid soluble a substance is, the more it will dissolve in the brain cells. Since a higher concentration is achieved, the anesthetics with greater lipid solubility may be more potent because of greater penetration (see 3. Ferguson Theory, under this objective).
2. **Surface Tension or Surface Adsorption Theory.** Measuring surface tension or adsorption effects of anesthetics in vitro, it was found that there is a direct correlation between anesthetic potency and either of the following: (1) the ability to lower surface tension or (2) adsorption of the anesthetic at a lipid-aqueous interface. The investigators who reported these facts believed that similar physical properties were altered in neural cells, causing altered metabolism, electron transport, permeability, or other changes that cause depressed transmission.

    Present status. See Ferguson theory, which follows.
3. **Ferguson Theory of Thermodynamic Activity.** Ferguson noted that anesthetics affect many physicochemical systems, including surface tension, adsorption, oil/water partition, and so on. He believed that anesthetics acted by altering some physical property of the cells (not by chemical reaction), so that the mere presence of anesthetic at a certain

activity level (concentration) causes the anesthetic effect.

Present status. This agrees well with the numerous diverse chemical structures that can cause general anesthesia and the increased potency of anesthetics related to increased physiochemical action. However, the theory does not help to explain anesthesia in terms of cell function.

4. **Cell Permeability Theory.** Anesthetics change permeability of neural cells, which interferes with ion movements causing stabilization and which prevents depolarization.

   Present status. This theory does not explain the selectivity of general anesthetics for certain types of brain function.

   (*Note:* local anesthetics act by membrane stabilization, see Chapter 15.)

5. **Neurophysiologic Theory.** Synaptic transmission is selectively depressed, first affecting the ascending reticular activating system (ARAS). Depression of ARAS causes sedation and sleep. Then, at progressively higher concentrations, depression spreads to cortex (causing excitement and unconsciousness), in midbrain, and, finally, the spinal cord.

   Present status. This explains selectivity and agrees well with stages of anesthesia (see Section 35-D), but does not elucidate specific cellular mechanisms.

6. **Pauling Theory of Microcrystals.** Linus Pauling proposed the theory that clathrate crystals can be formed in the intercellular spaces (synapses) by anesthetics dissolved in the intercellular water. The microcrystals could bind proteins and decrease freedom of movement, changing the electrical properties of the synapse and causing more resistance to the flow of impulses.

   Present status. There is no doubt that anesthetics induce clathrate microcrystal formation at extremely low temperatures, but further proof is needed for acceptance of formation at physiologic temperature.

Summary

This quote from Smith et al. (1980) summarizes our present lack of knowledge. "Despite a considerable effort to formulate a unitary hypothesis of mechanism of action of general anesthetics, there is yet no single theory that is generally accepted."

D. SIGNS AND STAGES

Objective 35.D.1. Recognize the signs and stages of ether anesthesia as described by Guedel.

During World War I, there was a need to train paramedics to give ether anesthesia to a large number of soldiers. Therefore, Dr. Guedel devised a simple system that allowed anesthetists to distinguish between various phases of anesthesia. This is especially important in general anesthesia because the difference between a safe dose (surgical anesthesia) and an unsafe dose is not great (low therapeutic index or margin of safety).

Dr. Guedel divided ether anesthesia into four stages (I, II, III, IV), and stage III was divided into four planes (1, 2, 3, 4). This scheme is shown in Figure 35-1 and outlined below.

Stage I. Analgesia
There is partial loss of sensation, sedation, complete or partial amnesia, and then inebriation. The patient is cooperative and responds to commands. (This is the only stage that dentists should use for N_2O/O_2 sedation).

Stage II. Delirium (or Excitement)
There is a loss of consciousness and increased voluntary movements. Reflexes are hyperreactive, and the patient must often be restrained because of violent, irregular movements. The pupils dilate; breathing is irregular and is usually compromised, resulting in hypoxia. The blood pressure is usually elevated. Vomiting is common, and secretions are profuse. There is a danger that the patient may suffocate because of excessive fluids in the respiratory passages. (Induction implies that the patient has passed through stages I and II.)

Stage III. Surgical Anesthesia

Plane 1. Respiration becomes regular and slow but is usually adequate. Involuntary movements

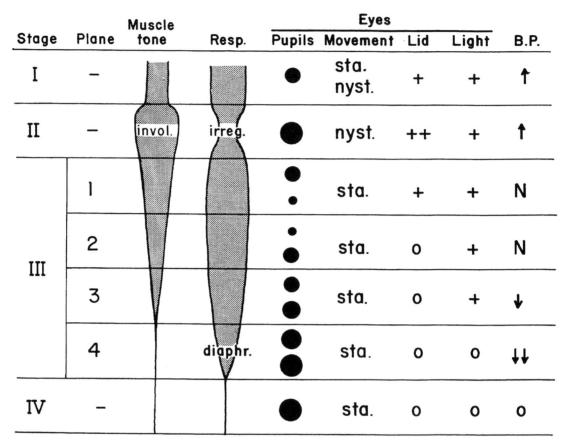

| Stage | Plane | Muscle tone | Resp. | Eyes | | | | B.P. |
				Pupils	Movement	Lid	Light	
I	–			●	sta. nyst.	+	+	↑
II	–	invol.	irreg.	●	nyst.	++	+	↑
III	1			● •	sta.	+	+	N
	2			• ●	sta.	o	+	N
	3			● ●	sta.	o	+	↓
	4		diaphr.	● ●	sta.	o	o	↓↓
IV	–			●	sta.	o	o	o

Figure 35–1. Schematic of signs of anesthesia. B.P., blood pressure; diaphr., diaphragmatic; invol., involuntary; irreg., irregular; Lid, Light, reflexes; N, normal; nyst., nystagmus; sta., stationary. (*Adapted from DiPalma JR (ed): Basic Pharmacology in Medicine, 2nd ed, 1982. Courtesy of McGraw-Hill Book Company.*)

are lost, and there is a decrease of muscle tone. The eyeballs may rove (nystagmus) and the pupils constrict.

Plane 2. Muscles relax, breathing is shallow but regular and may continue to provide adequate oxygen in the unassisted state, and the eyeballs become fixed with pupillary dilation.

Plane 3. There is abdominal breathing with only thoracic movement; respiratory assistance may be required. The blood pressure begins to fall. Pupils are fairly well dilated, but the light reflex is present (most surgical procedures are done in either plane 2 or 3).

Plane 4. Complete pupillary dilation with loss of light reflex. There is intercostal paralysis with irregular and inadequate, shallow breathing. The respiratory system is severely compromised, and artificial respiration must be employed in plane 4. This is difficult to distinguish from stage IV.

Stage IV. Respiratory and Medullary Paralysis

Respiration ceases and circulation collapses. Artificial respiration and/or circulatory support are necessary to prevent death.

It should be noted that Guedel's signs are for ether without any other drugs. These signs may vary for other anesthetics, and whenever pre-medications are used. Therefore, the anesthetist must gain experience with the anesthetics that are being employed, as well as with combinations of drugs that may be required.

E. CLASSIFICATION OF GENERAL ANESTHETICS

Objective 35.E.1. Classify, by selecting from a list, the important general anesthetics into three groups and recognize appropriate methods of administration for each group and individual agent.

Fixed Agents. These are given intravenously. This group includes water-soluble drugs that must be metabolized or excreted for termination of action. Fixed agents include:

> thiopental (*Pentothal*)
> thiamylal
> methohexital (*Brevital*)
> ketamine

The first three are ultrashort-acting barbiturates (see also, Chapter 21). Methohexital is popular in dental sedation (Bennett, 1978), but its advantage over other ultrashort-acting barbiturates has not been clearly established. Thiopental and thiamylal are metabolized to intermediate-acting barbiturates, pentobarbital and amobarbital, respectively. However, redistribution is probably more important in determining duration of ultrashort acting barbiturates, while metabolism and excretion play a lesser role (see also Chapter 21).

Ketamine is unusual because it is a stimulant rather than a depressant. By stimulating the patient, a state of "dissociation" is eventually reached, resulting in an anesthetic state. (The production of anesthesia by either depression or excitement was described in Chapter 20.) Ketamine appears useful in patients with a compromised cardiovascular system or respiratory system and sometimes in children. Ketamine's disadvantages include lack of muscular relaxation, unpleasantness of stimulatory induction, and possible hallucinations.

Volatile Liquids. These are first vaporized and then given by inhalation. Oxygen is used not only as the vaporizer but also as a carrier gas. Volatile liquids include:

> **diethyl ether**
> **chloroform**
> **halothane.**

(NOTE: Enflurane and isoflurane are very similar to halothane, and the differences are described under Section 35–H.)

See Table 35–1, A and B, for summary of properties of these agents.

Gases. Gases are given by inhalation using oxygen as a carrier. These include **nitrous oxide** and **cyclopropane.** Tables 35–1 and 35–2 give a summary of properties of these agents.

F. THE IDEAL GENERAL ANESTHETIC

Objective 35.F.1. Recognize the properties of an ideal general anesthetic.

Properties of an ideal general anesthetic include:

1. ease of administration—pleasant and nonirritating
2. smooth induction (passing through stages I and II rapidly and smoothly)
3. rapid recovery
4. stability—nonexplosive, nonflammable
5. bleeding not accentuated
6. analgesic
7. amnesic
8. muscular relaxant
9. wide margin of safety
10. no adverse effects
11. economic, inexpensive

G. COMPARISON OF USEFUL GENERAL ANESTHETICS TO THE IDEAL AGENT

Objective 35.G.1. Recognize how the representative general anesthetic agents compare to the ideal and the advantages of each agent.

TABLE 35–1. SUMMARY OF GENERAL ANESTHETICS (Part I)

	Ease of Administration	Induction	Recovery	Stability	Capillary Bleeding	Analgesia	Amnesia	Muscular Relaxation
ideal	pleasant and nonirritating	smooth and rapid	rapid	nonexplosive, nonflammable	no effect	yes	yes	yes
N_2O	pleasant and nonirritating	smooth and rapid	rapid	nonexplosive but supports combustion	no effect	good at 20–35%	good at 35–50%	none
cyclopropane	usually pleasant, slightly irritating	rapid	rapid, N, V, clouded consciousness	very explosive	accentuated	good at low concentration	delirium common	yes
diethyl ether	unpleasant and irritating, N, V, stimulates secretion	slow	slow, long duration of intensive care, N, V	highly flammable	no effect	poor	no, delirium very common	yes
chloroform	pleasant and nonirritating	rapid	rapid	nonexplosive	no effect	poor	delirium possible	yes
halothane	easy to administer no N, V, nonirritating	slow	rapid	nonexplosive	no effect	poor	supplement with adjuvant agents	adequate (but enflurane better)
thiopental	IV	smooth and rapid	usually slow, due to redistribution, metabolism and excretion	chemically unstable (mix at time of use)	no effect	none	good	requires high dose (causes respiratory depression)
ketamine	IV, also effective IM	dissociative	prolonged and unpleasant	stable solution available	minimal bleeding (slightly increased)	good	delirium	tremors and hyperreactivity

N, nausea; V, vomiting.

TABLE 35-2. SUMMARY OF GENERAL ANESTHETICS (Part II)

	Margin of Safety	Oxygenation	Adverse Effects	Economics	Uses and Evaluation
ideal	wide	allows adequate O_2	no adverse effects	inexpensive, ease of storage	if only we had one!
N_2O	wide for analgesia, sedation, or amnesia, none for anesthesia	anesthesia not possible without hypoxia	hypoxia (overdose), birth defects (chronic), brain damage (abuse)	requires tanks and necessary apparatus	amnesia, sedation, some analgesia, good adjuvant aids induction
cyclopropane	low	adequate (very potent)	CVS: hypotension and arrhythmias (due to catecholamine sensitization)	requires tanks and elaborate recovery system	good anesthetic but explosiveness makes it obsolete
diethyl ether	low	adequate	increased SNS activity, stabilized circulation in planes 2–3	difficult storage, administration by open drop method but mask may cause hypoxia	safe, irritation and flammability limit usefulness
chloroform	low	adequate	liver necrosis and cardiac arrhythmias (therefore not useful)	easy to store, administration by open drop method, mask may cause hypoxia	now considered obsolete
halothane	low	adequate	CVS: hypotension and catecholamine-induced arrhythmias, liver toxicity (allergy, repeated use)	expensive and requires elaborate machinery	popular anesthetic, (enflurane and isoflurane becoming more popular)
thiopental	low	respiratory depression	respiratory, circulatory failure at high dose	inexpensive, easy to mix and administer	rapid inducer, need to supplement with other anesthetics
ketamine	wide	excellent	hallucinations	easy to administer, expensive	useful when circulatory depression must be avoided, useful for children

CVS, cardiovascular system; SNS, sympathetic nervous system.

Tables 35–1 and 35–2 compare the useful general anesthetic agents to the ideal. As an aid to study, you should make a chart which classifies agents according to which:

1. are nonirritating
2. have smooth and rapid induction
3. have a rapid recovery
4. are nonexplosive and nonflammable
5. are analgesic
6. are amnesic
7. cause muscular relaxation
8. have a wide margin of safety
9. allow adequate oxygenation

Also list the following:

10. the most important adverse effects of each agent
11. agents that are inexpensive and/or easy to administer
12. the present medical status of each agent

H. FEATURES OF OTHER GENERAL ANESTHETICS

Objective 35.H.1. Recognize the distinguishing features of some anesthetic agents related to the representative agents.

Divinyl Ether. Like diethyl ether but more potent and having a rapid induction; liver damage is possible. May be useful in children for open drop method of administration.

Trichloroethylene. Has excellent analgesic properties, like chloroform, but is difficult to vaporize. It is nonflammable but decomposes in the presence of soda lime into the toxic compound, trichloroacetylene. TCE is now obsolete but was used for analgesia in obstetrics and in chronic pain in the past.

Other Fluorinated Compounds

1. **Enflurane.** This is a new drug, similar to halothane, but having fewer adverse effects. It is now the most popular anesthetic agent (Med Lett Drugs Ther, 1981) because of its similarity to halothane, but with less toxicity and more neuromuscular relaxation. The only major disadvantage is that it is metabolized to fluoride ion like methoxyflurane with the potential for the same type of renal toxicity. However, less fluoride ion is formed after enflurane anesthesia than after methoxyflurane. **Isoflurane** is an isomer of enflurane and is said to have less toxicity than enflurane (Med Lett Drugs Ther, 1981).

2. **Fluroxene.** Also similar to halothane, but less potent. Oxygenation is considered excellent. To date, few adverse effects have been reported. Its main use is for anesthesia when circulatory embarrassment is present.

3. **Methoxyflurane.** This drug has many properties similar to halothane. The differences are slower recovery, better analgesia, better muscle relaxation, and the formation of fluoride ion (which may cause nephrotoxicity). Methoxyflurane may induce hypotension and liver problems. Because of the nephrotoxicity, methoxyflurane is now rarely used in modern anesthesiology.

Other Barbiturates

1. **Methohexital.** This may be favored by some anesthetists, but thiopental is still more popular. All properties are similar to thiopental. More rapid recovery is claimed. Some dentists have advocated IV use of methohexital, but usually other drugs are also required (as with any ultrashort-acting barbiturate), and the practitioner must be well versed in handling anesthesia before attempting this use.

Innovar. A neuroleptic-narcotic combination consisting of **fentanyl** (narcotic analgesic) and **droperidol** (a neuroleptic drug which causes psychic indifference). The combination produces "neurolept-analgesia," but sleep does not occur unless a hypnotic or N_2O is also used. This combination has been touted by some dentists, but its use is complex because:

1. respiratory depression occurs
2. fentanyl is short acting while droperidol is long acting
3. drug interactions may occur
4. muscular rigidity may occur

This fixed-ratio combination is considered irrational, and, therefore, *Innovar* should probably be avoided completely (Med Lett Drugs Ther, 1974, 1977, 1981).

I. METABOLISM OF GENERAL ANESTHETICS

Objective 35.I.1. Describe metabolism of general anesthetics.

1. Thiobarbiturates are metabolized slowly by sulfoxidation.
2. Ketamine is rapidly metabolized and excreted by the kidney.
3. Gaseous agents (N_2O, cyclopropane) are usually inert and excreted through the lungs.
4. Liquid anesthetics are also mainly excreted by the lungs, but a small amount, especially of the fluorinated compounds, may be metabolized in the liver. Trichloroethylene is metabolized to trichloroacetic acid. Halothane is dechlorinated in the liver. Methoxyflurane (and, to a lesser extent, enflurane) is exceptional because it is highly metabolized, forming fluoride ion and organic fluorometabolites (Taves et al., 1970). The fluoride ion, fluorometabolites, and the precipitation of renal oxalic acid contribute to the nephrotoxic, adverse effect of methoxyflurane.

J. ABSORPTION, DISTRIBUTION, AND EXCRETION

Objective 35.J.1. Describe the absorption, distribution, and excretion of inhalation general anesthetics.

The anesthetic vapors are equilibrated with air in the lungs according to the physical gas laws (Boyle's law, Henry's law, law of partial pressures). The gas passes across the lung alveolar membrane, which is so thin that it is **not** a limiting factor in absorption. The blood picks up the gas according to the rate of blood flow and blood/air partition coefficient. The dissolved gas is then carried by the blood to other organs and is then distributed according to organ blood flow and tissue/blood partition coefficient. All of these processes are reversed,

and excretion occurs because of the removal of the anesthetic gas from the input side. General anesthetic gases and liquids are sometimes metabolized in the liver (mainly fluorinated compounds), and any products formed are excreted through the kidney, but the lung is the main organ of excretion for all inhalation anesthetics.

Objective 35.J.2. Recognize the definition of diffusion hypoxia and its importance in dentistry.

Gases which dissolve to a great extent (rapid inducers like N_2O) give off a great deal of gas from blood to lungs when the input is suddenly removed. According to the law of partial pressures, a great amount of anesthetic gas rushing into the alveoli from the blood would allow only a small volume for oxygen. Thus, the air that is in equilibrium with the blood has an inadequate partial pressure of O_2, resulting in hypoxia. This can be avoided by flushing the patient with 100% oxygen when N_2O is removed. Since room air has only 20% oxygen, allowing the patient to equilibrate with room air could be hazardous.

K. PREANESTHETIC MEDICATIONS

Objective 35.K.1. Recognize preanesthetic medications and their usefulness.

1. **Anticholinergics,** such as atropine, are used to reduce secretions. This is necessary for ether anesthesia because the patient could drown in his own secretions. **Scopolamine** has the same anticholinergic effect.
2. **Sedative-hypnotics,** such as barbiturates and diazepam, are used to relax the patient or cause sleep so that the patient enters the operating room without anxiety. A smaller amount of general anethetic agent is considered necessary when the subject is premedicated with sedative-hypnotics.
3. **Analgesics,** such as morphine and meperidine, are used to prevent preoperative and postoperative pain. The narcotic analgesics are also used to cause sedation-hypnosis and diminish the amount of general anesthetic

needed (see also neurolept-analgesia, *Innovar*, Objective 35.H.1.).

4. **Induction agents,** such as nitrous oxide, are often used to aid in rapid and pleasant induction in combination with a more potent anesthetic. Sometimes the combination (N_2O/O_2 and the major anesthetic) is continued in order to diminish the amount of major anesthetic needed. Thiopental is also used for anesthetic induction.

REFERENCES

Bennett CR: Conscious Sedation in Dental Practice, 2nd ed. St. Louis, Mosby, 1978, p 152

DiPalma JR (ed): Basic Pharmacology in Medicine, 2nd ed. New York, McGraw-Hill, 1982, p 63

Med Lett Drugs Ther 16:42, 1974

Med Lett Drugs Ther 19:27, 1977

Med Lett Drugs Ther 23:74, 1981

Smith TC, Cooperman LH, Wollman H: History and principles of anesthesiology. In Gilman AG, Goodman LS, Gilman A (eds): Goodman and Gilman's The Pharmacological Basis of Therapeutics, 6th ed. New York, Macmillan, 1980, p 271

Taves DR, Fry BW, Freeman RB, Gillies AJ: Toxicity following methoxyflurane anesthesia. II. Fluoride concentrations in nephrotoxicity. JAMA 214:91, 1970

BIBLIOGRAPHY

DiPalma JR (ed): Drill's Pharmacology in Medicine, 4th ed. New York, McGraw-Hill, 1971, Ch 7, 8, 9, 10

Gilman AG, Goodman LS, Gilman A (eds): Goodman and Gilman's The Pharmacological Basis of Therapeutics, 6th ed. New York, Macmillan, 1980, Ch 14

Wylie WD, Churchill-Davidson HC: A Practice of Anesthesia, 2nd ed. Chicago, Year Book, 1966, Ch 7, 8, 9

QUESTIONS

1. The essential element of general anesthesia is:

   A. unconsciousness
   B. amnesia
   C. muscular relaxation
   D. analgesia

2. **T F** Whereas local anesthesia requires loss of only the pain sensation, general anesthesia requires loss of all sensation.

3. **T F** General anesthesia is the loss of muscular activity and reflexes, allowing the performance of general surgery.

4. Which of the following would produce acceptable general anesthesia for surgery?

   A. IV administration of narcotic-analgesics
   B. inebriation with alcohol
   C. administration of belladonna alkaloids
   D. all of the above are correct
   E. none of the above is correct

5. **T F** Crawford W. Long was the first dentist to successfully demonstrate general anesthesia.

6. Physical properties which appear related to general anesthetic activity include:

   A. oil/water partition coefficient
   B. surface adsorption
   C. surface tension lowering
   D. all of the above are correct
   E. none of the above is correct

7. Which of the following theories best explains the selectivity of general anesthetics?

   A. stabilization of membranes (reducing cell permeability)
   B. progressive depression of synaptic function
   C. increasing surface adsorption
   D. decreasing surface tension.

8. **T F** Since most general anesthetics have a similar chemical structure, their action is best explained by receptor theory.

9. Surgery is usually performed in:

   A. Stage II or Stage III, plane 1
   B. Stage III, plane 1 or plane 2
   C. Stage III, plane 2 or plane 3
   D. Stage III, plane 4 or Stage IV

10. Dental office use of nitrous oxide should result in:

    A. Stage II
    B. Stage III, Plane 1
    C. Stage III, Plane 2
    D. none of the above

11. T F General anesthetics are useful because they cause no CNS excitement.

12. Dilated pupils would be usually noted in:

    A. Stage II
    B. Plane 4
    C. both A and B are correct
    D. neither A nor B is correct

13. Eyelid reflex would be missing in:

    A. Stage II
    B. Plane 2
    C. both A and B are correct
    D. neither A nor B is correct

14. Breathing would be compromised in:

    A. Plane 4
    B. Stage II
    C. both A and B are correct
    D. neither A nor B is correct

15. Respiratory and medullary paralysis is evident in:

    A. Stage III, plane 3
    B. Stage IV
    C. both A and B are correct
    D. neither A nor B is correct

16. Blood pressure would appear normal in:

    A. Stage I
    B. Stage II, plane 1
    C. both A and B are correct
    D. neither A nor B is correct

17. T F The eyes respond to light in all stages except Stage IV.

18. The general anesthetic ketamine is:

    A. a general CNS depressant
    B. not a respiratory depressant at usual doses
    C. both A and B are correct
    D. neither A nor B is correct

19. T F All general anesthetics are general CNS depressants.

20. Which of the following is not an inhalation general anesthetic?

    A. diethyl ether
    B. ketamine
    C. halothane
    D. methoxyfluorane

21. Which of the following is given by inhalation using oxygen as a vaporizing gas?

    A. N_2O
    B. cyclopropane
    C. both A and B are correct
    D. neither A nor B is correct

22. Which of the following is not expected of an ideal general anesthetic?

    A. analgesia
    B. muscular relaxation
    C. respiratory stimulation
    D. amnesia

23. All of the following are characteristic of an ideal general anesthetic *except:*

A. smooth and rapid induction

B. adequate analgesia

C. long duration after a single loading dose

D. adequate amnesia

E. inexpensive

24. Which of the following general anesthetics does *not* support combustion?

A. diethyl ether

B. cyclopropane

C. nitrous oxide

D. halothane

25. Which of the following general anesthetics does *not* provide adequate muscular relaxation in plane 2–3?

A. cyclopropane

B. diethyl ether

C. halothane

D. nitrous oxide

26. Which of the following general anesthetics does *not* allow adequate oxygenation in plane 2–3 when used as a single agent?

A. nitrous oxide

B. cyclopropane

C. diethyl ether

D. halothane

27. Which of the following are used as an adjuvant to general anesthesia for rapid induction?

A. thiopental or nitrous oxide

B. scopolamine or morphine

C. trichlorethylene or nitrous oxide

D. halothane or droperidol

28. N_2O may be effectively used for all of the following *except:*

A. producing surgical anesthesia without any other added agent

B. producing rapid induction

C. as a carrier gas to reduce the amount of the more effective anesthetic gas used

D. for production of sedation and amnesia

29–32. General anesthetics that have adequate skeletal muscular relaxation in plane 2–3 of Stage III include:

29. T F Enflurane

30. T F Diethyl ether

31. T F Halothane

32. T F Nitrous oxide

33. Which of the following provides adequate amnesia?

A. N_2O

B. cyclopropane

C. both A and B are correct

D. neither A nor B is correct

34. T F Fluroxene is an agent which allows excellent oxygenation and may be preferred over halothane for open heart surgery.

35. T F The advantage of *Innovar* is that it produces analgesia, psychic indifference, and sleep.

36. T F Ketamine is rapidly metabolized in the liver and excreted by the lung.

37. T F Halothane is dechlorinated in the liver.

38. T F Volatile anesthetics are mainly excreted by the lungs.

39. The amount of N_2O in the brain is related to all of the following *except:*

    A. blood flow to the brain
    B. brain/blood partition coefficient for N_2O
    C. oil/water partition coefficient for N_2O
    D. rate of drug metabolism in the liver

40. **T F** Nephrotoxicity of methoxyflurane is related to kidney concentration of the unaltered anesthetic.

41. **T F** Volatile general anesthetics are sometimes metabolized in the liver.

42. **T F** Gases which are poorly soluble in blood tend to cause diffusion hypoxia.

43. **T F** After N_2O sedation in the dental office, the patient should be flushed with 100% O_2 for several minutes.

44. When prescribing a preanesthetic medication, one would probably select any of the following *except:*

    A. atropine
    B. morphine
    C. N_2O
    D. thiopental
    E. amitripytiline

36

Antipsychotics

A. INTRODUCTION

The pharmacologic control of psychosis began in 1950 with the successful synthesis of chlorpromazine, a phenothiazine. Reserpine had been successfully used also, but this drug had numerous side effects, including increased suicidal tendencies in some patients. Reserpine is no longer used for this purpose, and the drug is not discussed further in this chapter. Reserpine is used as an antihypertensive drug (Chapter 31).

Phenothiazines were derived from chemical modification of antihistamines. Phenothiazines exerted a major impact on the treatment of psychosis. For example, prior to drug therapy, most or all hysterical or maniacal patients had to be restrained physically or placed in locked padded rooms so that they could not harm themselves. In addition, the psychiatrist never could establish rapport with these patients, with the result that they remained restrained for long periods of time. Conversely, phenothiazines are able to calm patients to a degree that the psychiatrist is able to establish rapport and, therefore, help patients further. Moreover, nonmaniacal patients were helped significantly as well, because jumbled thoughts are a prominent symptom of schizophrenia. Drug therapy tends to unjumble thought processes, and psychotherapy can then proceed more successfully. However, the drugs by themselves truly do have an antipsychotic effect besides their calming effect. The importance of drug therapy is further emphasized by the fact that there were about 559,000 patients (a peak level) in public mental institutions in the US in 1955. Beginning in 1956, the figure declined steadily so that by 1978, the mental patient population was estimated to be 200,000, despite the increase in the total US population.

B. CLASSIFICATION AND CHEMISTRY

Objective 36.B.1. Recognize the classification and chemistry of antipsychotic drugs and name the drugs (or classes) set in bold type.

There are five chemical classes of antipsychotic drugs: (1) **phenothiazines**, (2) thioxanthenes, (3) **butyrophenones**, (4) dibenzoxapines, and (5) dihydroindolones. The pharmacologic

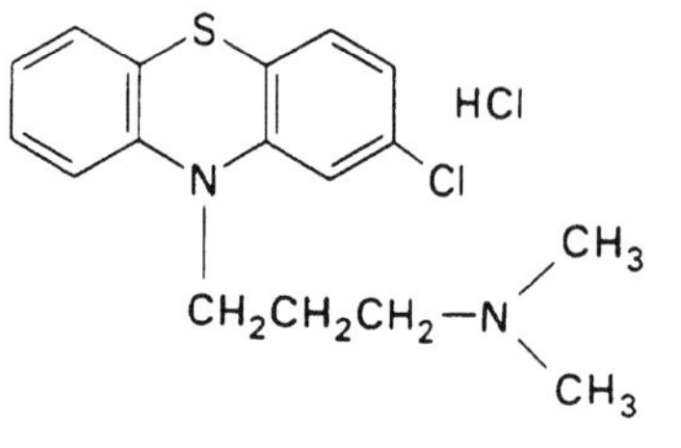

Figure 36–1. Chemical structure of chlorpromazine hydrochloride. (*From Csáky TZ: Cutting's Handbook of Pharmacology, 6th ed, 1979. Courtesy of Appleton-Century-Crofts.*)

profiles of the drugs in all five groups are so similar that we will not describe each drug or group of drugs. Only **chlorpromazine,** the prototype, will be described, and the practitioner may be assured that the pharmacology of the other drugs is essentially the same. The only major clinical differences between drugs is that there are differences in intensity of side effects and in absorption, distribution, metabolism, and excretion.

One other agent, **promethazine,** is by chemical classification a phenothiazine, but it has no antipsychotic activity. Promethazine is an antihistamine with prominent sedative and antiemetic effects, and it is most often used for these purposes (Chapters 4, 19, and 21). With regard to chemistry, only the largest group of drugs, the phenothiazines, is described.

The phenothiazines contain a fused three-ring

system, the rings being six-sided. A carbon chain, or chain and ring system, is attached to the central ring. The configuration resembles the tricyclic antidepressants (Chapter 37). The structure of chlorpromazine is given in Figure 36–1. In Table 36–1, a brief summary of names of drugs, according to chemical classification, is presented.

One other antipsychotic drug, **lithium carbonate,** is briefly described at the end of the chapter. Lithium carbonate is used exclusively for manic-depressive psychosis.

C. MECHANISM OF ACTION

Objective 36.C.1. Recognize the mechanism of action of chlorpromazine, which is thought to result in an antipsychotic effect.

The mechanism by which chlorpromazine produces an antipsychotic effect is actually unknown. However, chlorpromazine blocks brain dopamine receptors, which results in a compensatory increase in dopamine turnover rates (rate of synthesis and metabolism). Based on that evidence and other indirect evidence, it is believed that the neurotransmitter, dopamine, may be involved in the induction of psychosis.

Chlorpromazine interacts with many other specific receptors, but those receptor interactions are not known to be related to the antipsy-

TABLE 36–1. CLASSIFICATION OF ANTIPSYCHOTIC DRUGS

phenothiazines	thioxanthenes
1. aliphatic derivatives	chlorprothixene (*Taractan*)
chlorpromazine (*Thorazine*)	thiothixene (*Navane*)
triflupromazine (*Vesprin*)	
2. piperidine derivatives	butyrophenones
mesoridazine (*Serentil*)	**droperidol** (*Inapsine*)
thioridazine (*Mellaril*)	**haloperidol** (*Haldol*)
3. piperazine derivatives	
acetophenazine (*Tindal*)	dibenzoxapines
fluphenazine (*Prolixin, Permitil*)	loxapine (*Loxitane*)
perphenazine (*Trilafon*)	
piperacetazine (*Quide*)	dihydroindolones
prochlorperazine (*Compazine*)	molindone (*Moban*)
trifluoperazine (*Stelazine*)	

chotic effect. For instance, chlorpromazine blocks the following receptors: peripheral α adrenergic (and probably central), peripheral and central muscarinic, histaminergic (H_1), central dopaminergic in mesolimbic and basal ganglia regions, central serotonergic, and emetic in the chemoreceptor trigger zone (CTZ) of the area postrema. The emetic receptors are also thought to be dopaminergic. Chlorpromazine enhances peripheral β receptor activity, which could help to explain epinephrine reversal (Chapter 18, p. 168).

D. ABSORPTION, DISTRIBUTION, METABOLISM, AND EXCRETION

Objective 36.D.1. Recognize the absorption, distribution, metabolism, and excretion of chlorpromazine.

All the phenothiazines are well absorbed by all routes, and the drugs are widely distributed.

The liver microsomal enzymes are involved with the major metabolic transformations, and the kidney is the primary organ of excretion of unchanged drug and metabolites.

The loss of drug and metabolites is exceedingly slow, and drug and metabolites can be detected in the urine up to six months after cessation of chlorpromazine therapy. This slow excretion may account for the lack of production of psychologic dependence. Recently, some degree of physical dependence has been noted with the use of antipsychotic drugs.

E. PHARMACOLOGIC EFFECTS

Objective 36.E.1. Recognize the pharmacologic effects of chlorpromazine.

An outline of the pharmacologic effects is presented below.

1. CNS
   a. Psychomotor slowing, emotional quieting, and affective indifference (neuroleptic syndrome)
   b. Sedation and hypnosis with easy arousal
   c. Motor dysfunctions (central dopamine blockade)
   d. Lowered seizure threshold
   e. Blocks release of growth hormone, and of ACTH but causes release of prolactin (probably central dopamine and serotonin blockade)
   f. Disruption of temperature regulation
   g. Depression of vasomotor center and reflexes, resulting in decreased blood pressure and postural hypotension
   h. Antiemesis (CTZ blockade, central dopamine blockade)
   i. Local anesthetic activity
2. Autonomic Nervous System
   a. α Receptor blockade
   b. Enhanced β receptor activity } decreased blood pressure, postural hypotension
   c. Miosis (α blockade) or mydriasis (anticholinergic)
   d. Blurred vision (anticholinergic)
   e. Xerostomia, constipation, decreased gastric secretion, decreased GI motility (anticholinergic)
3. Kidney—diuresis due to blockade of ADH secretion
4. Cardiovascular—decreased blood pressure and postural hypotension due to CNS and autonomic effects
5. Liver—obstructive jaundice (may be allergic)
6. Antihistaminic and antiserotonergic activity

F. ADVERSE EFFECTS

Objective 36.F.1. Describe four important, dentally related, adverse effects of chlorpromazine.

There are many adverse effects noted for these drugs, most of which occur from the high doses often used and from prolonged treatment. Four important adverse effects are listed here

TABLE 36–2. ADVERSE EFFECTS OF PHENOTHIAZINES

faintness	skin rashes
palpitations	contact dermatitis
nasal stuffiness	photosensitivity
dry mouth	gray-blue pigmentation of skin
constipation	
drowsiness	opacities of the cornea and lens
hypothermia or hyperthermia	pigmentary retinoppathy
leukocytosis	increased plasma cholesterol
leukopenia	in males, erection without ejaculation
eosinophilia	
urticaria	

because of their dental significance: **xerostomia, postural hypotension, leukopenia,** and **parkinsonian syndrome.** These important adverse effects produced by antipsychotic drugs are further discussed under Implications for Dentistry, Section 36.I.1. All other adverse effects are presented in Table 36–2 (for completeness and for reference) except for the motor dysfunctions. These are of dental significance, and require a separate presentation (Table 36-3) because of their uniqueness and severity. Such motor effects are probably due to blockade of central dopamine receptors.

Interestingly, it has been known for some time that certain antipsychotic drugs (e.g., **thioridazine**) produce little or no muscle dysfunction, but the reason was unknown until recently. It was found that thioridazine not only lacks motor dysfunctional activity but also is a more potent anticholinergic drug. In fact, one method of treating parkinsonlike syndromes produced by antipsychotic agents is to administer a centrally acting anticholinergic agent (see Chapter 40 for a more comprehensive review of treatment of Parkinson's disease). However, there is good evidence to suggest that the best treatment is to reduce the dosage of the antipsychotic drug until the syndrome disappears because using anticholinergic drugs may mask the effect of an increased dose of antipsychotic drug and may produce some permanent damage in the basal ganglia, which is the site of action of this effect.

G. DRUG INTERACTIONS

Objective 36.G.1. Recognize drug interactions of antipsychotic drugs.

1. **Epinephrine.** A marked fall of blood pressure may occur (reversal).
2. **Guanethidine.** Blockade of antihypertensive effect may occur.
3. **CNS depressants.** Additive or supra-additive CNS depression occurs.
4. **Narcotic-analgesics.** An increased miotic effect and increased analgesic effect with certain phenothiazines may occur, as well as an additive or supra-additive CNS depressant effect (including respiratory depression).

H. THERAPEUTIC USES

Objective 36.H.1. Recognize the two major medical therapeutic uses.

The two major medical therapeutic uses of the antipsychotic drugs are to treat psychosis and for their antiemetic effect.

TABLE 36–3. MOTOR DYSFUNCTION CAUSED BY CHLORPROMAZINE

Parkinsonian Syndrome
Slowing of volitional movements (akinesia) with mask facies
Rigidity and tremor of upper extremities at rest
Pill-rolling movements of the thumb and fingers

Akathisia
Compelling need of the patient to be in constant movement

Acute Dystonic Reactions
Facial grimacing and twisting of the neck (torticollis)
Oculogyric crisis

Tardive Dyskinesia
(Late appearing, usually does not reverse after withdrawal of drug, difficult to treat)
Sucking and smacking of the lips
Lateral jaw movements
Fly-catching tongue movements
Purposeless, quick movements of extremities

The antiemetic effect of these agents (and promethazine) is most useful to block or reverse emesis by drugs and substances produced by microorganisms (which stimulate the CTZ). However, nausea and vomiting induced by motion sickness are an exception and should be treated by drugs with more prominent anticholinergic activity, such as scopolamine or the antihistaminic motion sickness drugs (Chapter 19). The phenothiazines are useful only if they possess potent anticholinergic activity.

I. IMPLICATIONS FOR DENTISTRY

Objective 36.I.1. List and describe dental implications of antipsychotic drugs.

1. In the presence of a hypotensive crisis of a dental patient, the practitioner must *never* use epinephrine or other adrenergic drugs that activate both α and β receptors because the blood pressure will decrease further (see above). If a pressor agent is needed, phenylephrine or norepinephrine is indicated. However, in case of an acute allergic reaction, epinephrine is probably the drug of choice, but the practitioner must be prepared for a possible marked hypotensive effect.

2. Chlorpromazine has been shown to cause a supra-additive analgesic effect when combined with narcotic analgesics (Moore and Dundee, 1961; Dundee JW et al., 1965). However, the dose of narcotic-analgesic may have to be reduced to one quarter to one half because of a probable supra-additive CNS depressant effect, especially respiratory depression.

3. Because most of these agents are potent antiemetics and since narcotic-analgesics often produce nausea and vomiting, combined use may be rational for this problem. However, as described above, the dose of narcotic analgesic should be reduced to one quarter to one half.

4. Xerostomia usually causes an increased incidence of caries (especially cervical) and promotes increased ingestion of liquids and soft foods which may be cariogenic and enhance the cariogenic situation. Further, secondary to xerostomia, patients may have increased difficulty retaining full dentures and an increased discomfort of the tissue-bearing surfaces.

5. Facial motor dysfunctions may result in difficulty in retaining full dentures (see Section 36.F).

6. The practitioner and staff must exercise caution when dismissing patients taking phenothiazines; rapid movement of the dental chair and standing erect may lead to postural hypotension.

7. The presence of leukopenia may predispose these patients to infection, especially candidiasis.

8. Some pedodontists have used chlorpromazine, in combination with other drugs (e.g., narcotic-analgesics), by IM injection for certain unmanageable children (Ripa and Barenie, 1979). This is considered controversial and should probably be used only by practitioners with experience and in a hospital situation or where the office is equipped to manage adverse reactions.

9. Phenothiazines have been shown to lower seizure thresholds. Local anesthetics are potential convulsant drugs. Therefore, extra caution is advised when treating patients taking these agents. Perhaps lower local anesthetic dosages and extra care during injection are advisable to ensure that the local anesthetics are not injected IV.

10. Phenothiazines have been used by some dentists as an oral preoperative sedative. However, we believe generally that the drugs are not the best choice for this purpose. Two reasons against their use are that patients often complain about unpleasant drowsiness and these agents have a great number of side effects, making it difficult to control the patient. Currently, the benzodiazepines are the best choice for preoperative sedation.

11. Droperidol is a butyrophenone that is used along with the narcotic-analgesic, fentanyl.

This IV combination, *Innovar*, is available for use in general anesthesia but is considered irrational (Chapter 35).

J. MANIC-DEPRESSIVE PSYCHOSIS

Lithium Carbonate (*Lithane*)

Objective 36.J.1. Recognize the specific use of lithium in medicine.

Objective 36.J.2. Describe dental implications.

Lithium ion exerts an antimanic effect, but the exact mechanism by which the effect occurs is at present unknown.

Lithium is used to treat a specific type of psychosis, namely, manic-depressive illness. Treatment actually is aimed at the manic phase, and lithium is effective in reversing or preventing the manic form of the illness. It is thought that the depressive portion of the illness is also controlled by the drug, but there is no scientific evidence to support this contention.

With the patient properly titrated, there are essentially no pharmacologic effects except an antipsychotic effect or reversal of the manic phase. Also, the drug will restore normal sleep patterns that are disrupted during mania. Certainly, one does not see all the frequent side effects noted with chlorpromazine that were outlined above.

Of course, if doses higher than therapeutic are provided, toxic effects are predictable, consisting of fatigue and muscle weakness, slurred speech, ataxia and fine tremors of the hands, nausea, vomiting, diarrhea, polyuria, polydipsia, exophthalmos, leukocytosis, and nontoxic goiters. With very high doses, there can be coma, muscle rigidity, hyperactive reflexes, marked tremors, muscle fasciculations, and seizures.

There are no important drug interactions of lithium with dental drugs.

With regard to dental implications, the feeling of dry mouth with increased thirst and the possible production of muscle dysfunctions about the face are the only two potential dental problems. These two effects are similar to those

described for antipsychotics in general. (See Sections 36.I.4. and 36.I.5.)

REFERENCES

Accepted Dental Therapeutics, 38th ed. Chicago, American Dental Association, 1979, pp 16–17

Csáky TZ: Cutting's Handbook of Pharmacology, 6th ed. New York, Appleton-Century-Crofts, 1979, p 596

Dundee JW, Moore J, Love WJ, Nicholl RM, Clarke RSJ: Studies of drugs given before anaesthesia. VI: The phenothiazine derivatives. Br J Anaesth 37:332, 1965

Moore J, Dundee JW: Alterations in response to somatic pain associated with anaesthesia. VII. The effect of nine phenothiazine derivatives. Br J Anaesth 33:422, 1961

Ripa LR, Barenie JA: Management of Dental Behavior in Children. Postgraduate Dental Handbook Series. Littleton, MA, PSG, 1979, Vol 1, pp 144–145

BIBLIOGRAPHY

Csáky TZ: Cutting's Handbook of Pharmacology, 6th ed. New York, Appleton-Century-Crofts, 1979, Ch 54

Gilman AG, Goodman LS, Gilman A (eds): Goodman and Gilman's The Pharmacological Basis of Therapeutics, 6th ed. New York, Macmillan, 1980, Ch 19

Meyers GH, Jawetz E. Goldfien A: Review of Medical Pharmacology, 7th ed. Los Altos, CA, Lange, 1980, Ch 25

QUESTIONS

1. Antipsychotic drugs may be classified chemically into:

   A. butyrophenones
   B. phenothiazines
   C. thioxanthenes
   D. all of the above are correct
   E. none of the above is correct

2. **T F** Chlorpromazine's antipsychotic effect is thought to occur by blocking central serotonin receptors.

3. **T F** Phenothiazines are well absorbed by all routes, and the liver and kidney participate in metabolism and excretion, respectively.

4. Pharmacologic effects of chlorpromazine include:

   A. cholinergic activation
   B. increased seizure threshold
   C. sedation and hypnosis with easy arousal
   D. stimulation of vasomotor centers
   E. all of the above are correct
   F. none of the above is correct

5. Adverse effects of chlorpromazine include:

   A. leukopenia
   B. postural hypotension
   C. xerostomia
   D. all of the above are correct
   E. none of the above is correct

6. **T F** An additive or supra-additive respiratory depressant effect may occur if chlorpromazine is used along with narcotic analgesics.

7. **T F** Two major medical therapeutic uses of chlorpromazine include both the treatment of psychosis and prevention of emesis.

8. **T F** Patients receiving chronic chlorpromazine therapy who have a hypotensive crisis in a dental chair should be given epinephrine to raise blood pressure.

9. **T F** Lithium carbonate is used to treat manic-depressive illness.

10. **T F** Patients taking lithium carbonate may experience xerostomia.

37
CNS Stimulants and Antidepressants

A. INTRODUCTION

This chapter describes several types of CNS stimulants and antidepressants, including xanthines (an example of mild CNS stimulants), amphetamines (an example of moderate CNS stimulants), monoamine oxidase inhibitors, which are very similar to amphetamines in effect, and tricyclics, the more specific CNS antidepressants that are the most useful group for therapeutic purposes. Potent CNS stimulants are briefly noted in Chapter 20 and are not reconsidered here.

Although mental depression is a disease of unknown cause, there are specific drugs for this problem. On the other hand, if depression is a symptom of anxiety or of neurosis, an antianxiety drug is useful. If anxiety is not the cause of the depression, antianxiety drugs by themselves will be ineffective.

B. XANTHINES—CHEMISTRY

Objective 37.B.1. Recognize the names of three xanthine drugs.

Objective 37.B.2. Recognize the chemical relationship of xanthines to uric acid and purines.

The **xanthines** consist of **caffeine, theobromine,** and **theophylline.** The agents are also sometimes referred to as the methylxanthines.

The xanthines contain a fused double-ring system and structurally resemble uric acid or the purines.

C. MECHANISM OF ACTION

Objective 37.C.1. Recognize three possible proposed mechanisms of action of xanthines.

The xanthines have been shown to inhibit the enzyme phosphodiesterase, which is the enzyme that metabolizes cyclic AMP. By inhibiting phosphodiesterase, cyclic AMP is allowed to accumulate, thus increasing its concentration. As a result, such effects occur as are seen with stimulation of β adrenergic receptors or receptors of certain hormones. Therefore, some effects produced by xanthines will mimic β adrenergic receptor activation, while cyclic AMP accumula-

397

TABLE 37–1. PHARMACOLOGIC EFFECTS OF THE XANTHINES

Effect	Caffeine	Theobromine	Theophylline
CNS stimulation	potent	mild	potent
cardiac stimulation	mild	moderate	potent
coronary dilation	mild	moderate	potent
smooth muscle re-			
laxation	mild	moderate	potent
skeletal muscle			
stimulation	potent	mild	moderate
diuretic effect	mild	moderate	potent

tion in other cells may either mimic hormonal stimulation or affect certain intracellular events (i.e., in CNS cells).

A second proposed mechanism involves a xanthine interaction with calcium that has been characterized mostly in skeletal muscle but also in cardiac muscle. Xanthines apparently increase the availability of calcium, which is involved in excitation-contraction coupling of muscle tissue.

A third, and possibly the most important, proposed mechanism of action is that the xanthines have been shown to block adenosine receptors (adenosine is a purine, too). The functional significance of activation of adenosine receptors has not been completely established, although adenosine has been shown to dilate blood vessels and to potentiate certain actions of norepinephrine.

D. ABSORPTION, DISTRIBUTION, METABOLISM, AND EXCRETION

Objective 37.D.1. Recognize the absorption, distribution, metabolism, and excretion of xanthines.

All the xanthines are poorly absorbed when administered PO, although PO preparations are available. The agents are also administered IV and, once absorbed into the bloodstream, gain access to most tissues, including the CNS.

Approximately 90% of each drug is metabolized and 10% is excreted unchanged. Little is known about the enzymatic conversion of the agents.

E. PHARMACOLOGIC EFFECTS

Objective 37.E.1. Recognize the pharmacologic effects of xanthines.

As is true of many other drug groups, caffeine, theobromine, and theophylline exert various pharmacologic effects that are qualitatively similar, but the degree of effect for each drug may differ quantitatively, depending on the organ system. Table 37–1 compares the actions of the three xanthines. The organ effects in Table 37–1 may be further described as follows:

1. **CNS.** All levels of the CNS are stimulated by xanthines. Generally, cerebral cortex stimulation is noted at a lower dose, while convulsions may be produced at extremely high doses.
2. **Cardiovascular.** The myocardium is stimulated by these agents, resulting in a positive chronotropic and positive inotropic effect. With moderate to high doses, the stimulatory effect may change the increased rate to frank arrhythmias. Systemic blood vessels and pulmonary and coronary blood vessels are dilated by the drugs, but cerebral vessels are constricted.
3. **Other Smooth Muscle.** Bronchiolar and biliary smooth muscle become relaxed under the influence of xanthines, but the GI tract smooth muscle may increase or decrease motility depending on the dose. Aminophylline, a combination of theophylline and ethylenediamine, is a recommended emergency drug for bronchiolar smooth muscle relaxation (see

also 37.H.1. and Appendix I, Emergency Drugs).

4. **Skeletal Muscle.** Xanthines cause an increase in strength of contraction, and they increase the capacity for work.

5. **Kidney.** The agents cause diuresis (increased amount of urine), possibly as a result of increased renal blood flow. There is some evidence that the xanthines inhibit the reabsorption of sodium in the renal tubule, which may contribute to the diuresis (see also Chapter 32).

6. **GI Tract.** There can be a marked increase of gastric secretion by the xanthines, and for that reason the drugs are contraindicated in patients with a history of peptic ulcer.

7. **Metabolism.** Xanthines have been shown to increase metabolic rate. They can also cause increased lipolysis, glycogenolysis, and gluconeogenesis, much like the catecholamines.

8. **Tolerance and Dependence.** Some tolerance to the agents may develop, and induction of psychologic dependence also occurs. However, there is no evidence that physical dependence is induced.

F. ADVERSE EFFECTS

Objective 37.F.1. Recognize the adverse effects of xanthines.

All the toxic effects are extensions of the pharmacologic effects and are mostly CNS, cardiovascular, and GI. Effects consist of dizziness, excitement, tremor, and convulsions (CNS); palpitations, extrasystoles, arrhythmias, and hypotension (cardiovascular); nausea, vomiting, and stomach cramps (GI); and diuresis (kidney).

G. XANTHINE CONTENT OF BEVERAGES

The following is a list of beverages that contain xanthines and their relative concentrations.

1. cocoa: average cup, 250 mg theobromine
2. coffee: average cup, 85 mg caffeine

3. cola: 12 oz bottle, 50 mg caffeine
4. tea: average cup, 50 mg caffeine

H. IMPLICATIONS FOR DENTISTRY

Objective 37.H.1. Recognize the dental implications for use of aminophylline or caffeine.

These agents have little use in dentistry, but suggested uses and indications are listed below.

1. **Aminophylline.** This highly soluble ethylenediamine salt of theophylline may be useful as an emergency drug. When administered IV, it can reverse an acute asthmatic attack or anaphylactoid reaction. Aminophylline should be used for any patient who is refractory to epinephrine's bronchorelaxant effect, especially those patients taking β blocking drugs.

2. Aminophylline may also be useful IV for an acute episode of congestive heart failure or in a patient with excessive β blockade.

3. **Caffeine** is one ingredient of many analgesic products including APC alone (aspirin, phenacetin, and caffeine), and as APC with a narcotic-analgesic. There is no rational basis for inclusion of caffeine to control dental pain or routine headache. In addition, the caffeine content is often low, 30 to 32 mg, while one cup of coffee contains 85 mg, which is closer to the therapeutic dose range.

   Caffeine is apparently useful in therapy of headache caused by hypertension, and relief is due to caffeine's cerebral vasoconstrictor effect.

I. AMPHETAMINES

Objective 37.I.1. Recognize the effects and side effects of amphetamines and their current use in therapy.

Amphetamine was discussed previously as an autonomic drug (Chapter 18) and is presented as a drug of abuse in Appendix III. Amphetamine and its relatives are basically autonomic drugs, activating α and β receptors, with a prominent

TABLE 37–2. MAOI AND TRICYCLIC ANTIDEPRESSANTS

MAOI	Tricyclic Antidepressants
— **iproniazid** (*Marsilid*)	**amitriptyline** (*Elavil, Endep*)
— **isocarboxazid** (*Marplan*)	amoxapine (*Asendin*)
pargyline (*Eutonyl*)	— **desipramine** (*Norpramin, Pertofrane*)
— **phenelzine** (*Nardil*)	doxepin (*Sinequan, Adapin*)
tranylcypromine (*Parnate*)	— **imipramine** (*Tofranil*)
	nortriptyline (*Aventyl*)
	protriptyline (*Vivactil*)
	trimipramine (*Surmontil*)

CNS stimulatory effect. Due to the latter effect, these agents were previously used for the treatment of depression and for control of obesity (anorexic effect), but they are no longer considered useful because (1) with chronic therapy, the drugs produce paranoid behavior and frank psychosis, (2) they produce tolerance and psychologic dependence, and there is some evidence that they produce physical dependence as well, and (3) superior drugs have been developed (tricyclic antidepressants). Furthermore, there is a move underway by some investigators urging the FDA to remove these agents from the market, for it is believed that amphetamines have no rational medical use.

Methylphenidate, another similar but milder CNS stimulant of this class, has also been used, but it is not recommended for depression. However, it may be useful for treating hyperkinetic children.

J. MONOAMINE OXIDASE INHIBITORS (MAOI)

Objective 37.J.1. Recognize the effects, contraindications, and dental significance of treating patients taking MAOI.

Objective 37.J.2. Recognize names of important (in bold type) MAOI presented in Table 37–2.

MAOIs are occasionally used to treat depression, but they are more frequently administered in hospitals than to ambulatory patients. However, the dentist may have an occasion to treat a patient taking an MAOI.

MAOI will inhibit MAO, but how this mechanism correlates with their CNS stimulatory effect is not known, nor can the mechanism be correlated with their hypotensive effect.

CNS effects are similar to those of amphetamine. Wakefulness, euphoria, respiratory stimulation, and excitement are frequently reported, and with high doses, convulsions and toxic psychoses have occurred.

MAOI interact with many drugs and could cause an adverse or fatal reaction. One reason for the proposed interaction is that MAOI inhibits many liver microsomal enzymes in addition to its inhibitory effect on MAO. The practitioner must take extra precautions when using or prescribing dental drugs in patients taking MAOI. In addition, the effects of MAOI continue for 10 to 14 days after cessation of therapy, and care must be exercised during that period as well. Some drugs are absolutely contraindicated, e.g., indirect-acting sympathomimetics, including tyramine contained in some beverages and food. Other drugs are relatively contraindicated, e.g. direct-acting, sympathomimetics, including epinephrine, norepinephrine, and levonordefrin. In patients taking MAOI, perhaps local anesthetics without vasoconstrictors should be used when possible. However, if vasoconstrictors must be used in patients taking MAOI, the dentist must use lower total dosages, inject very slowly (more slowly than usual), and aspirate several times during the injection to ensure that no drug is administered IV. Meperidine can cause excitation, sweating, rigidity, and hypertension or hypotension and coma in patients taking MAOI. Other narcotic-analgesics may be cautiously given, but at a reduced initial dosage. In summary, the practitioner must ensure no drug interactions by consulting various refer-

imipramine hydrochloride   chlorpromazine hydrochloride

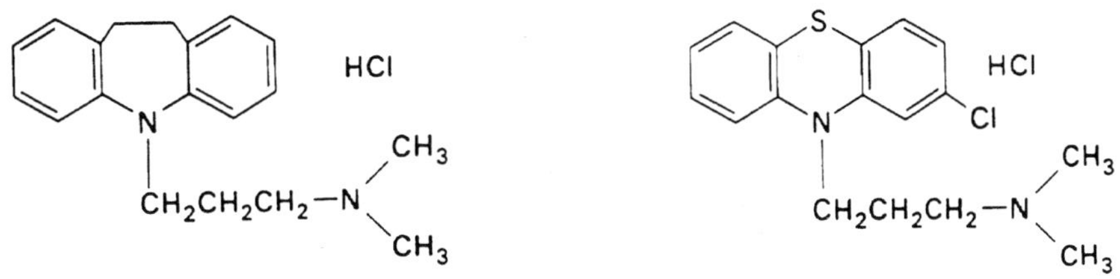

Figure 37–1. Comparison of chemical structure of tricyclic antidepressants and phen-othiazines. (*From Czáky TZ: Cutting's Handbook of Pharmacology, 6th ed., 1979. Courtesy of Appleton-Century-Crofts.*)

ence sources before prescribing dental drugs. If there is a known drug interaction with MAOI, other therapy must be used. Table 37–2 lists drugs that are either MAOI or tricyclic antide-pressants. As usual, the drugs set in bold type should be memorized.

K. TRICYCLIC ANTIDEPRESSANTS—CHEMISTRY

Objective 37.K.1. Recognize the chemical struc-ture of imipramine and compare differences of structure with chlorpromazine, an antipsychotic drug.

Objective 37.K.2. Recognize the names of im-portant tricyclics (set in bold type) presented in Table 37–2.

The tricyclic antidepressants (TCs) contain a fused three-ring system; the center ring is seven-membered and the two end rings are six-membered. A three-carbon chain is attached to the central ring and terminates with a secondary or tertiary amine (Fig. 37–1). The TCs and the antipsychotic phenothiazines are quite similar chemically (Fig. 37–1), and predictably they have many effects in common (although not their principal effect).

L. MECHANISM OF ACTION

Objective 37.L.1. Recognize the mechanism of action of tricyclic antidepressants.

The TCs block the reuptake of norepineph-rine (NE) in the autonomic nervous system and

also block the reuptake of NE and serotonin in the CNS. The latter effect is a proposed mecha-nism of antidepressant action but may not be the actual mechanism, since the mechanisms of depression are almost totally unknown at present.

M. ABSORPTION, DISTRIBUTION, METABOLISM, AND EXCRETION

Objective 37.M.1. Recognize the absorption, distribution, metabolism, and excretion of tricyclic antidepressants.

The pharmacokinetics of the TCs are not unique. They are well absorbed PO and IM, and they are distributed throughout the body, in-cluding the brain, where the agents exert their antidepressant effect.

The liver is the major site of metabolism, and the microsomal enzyme system is quite impor-tant. Active metabolites are generated in some cases, e.g., imipramine is partially metabolized to desipramine. Moreover, there is some evi-dence that the accumulation of active metabo-lites is necessary for the onset of antidepressant activity.

The kidney is the major organ of excretion of unchanged drug and metabolites.

N. PHARMACOLOGIC EFFECTS

Objective 37.N.1. Recognize the pharmacologic effects of the tricyclic antidepressants.

There is no antidepressant (mood-elevating) effect when the drugs are first administered. In fact, initially, the patient may report unhappiness and increased anxiety. Later, depressed patients do report an elevation of mood but not by CNS stimulation. Two to three weeks must elapse before the full therapeutic effects of the drugs are observed. For this reason, these agents should not be prescribed prn for depressive episodes, and drug dosage and patient compliance must be carefully monitored. Other effects include:

1. sedation
2. suppression of REM sleep
3. prominent xerostomia
4. blurred vision
5. constipation
6. urinary retention
7. tachycardia with increased incidence of arrhythmias (due to blockade of NE reuptake)
8. decreased blood pressure (due to depression of brain cardiovascular centers)
9. postural hypotension

The following facts are known about tolerance and dependence:

1. Tolerance usually develops to xerostomia, constipation, blurred vision, tachycardia, and postural hypotension.
2. With high doses for long periods, an occasional patient develops mild but definite psychologic and physical dependence.

O. ADVERSE EFFECTS

Objective 37.O.1. Recognize the adverse effects of tricyclic antidepressants.

A large number of toxic and side effects have been reported (see above). The more important ones, of dental significance, are xerostomia, postural hypotension, arrhythmias, and a mild parkinsonlike syndrome (see below).

P. DRUG INTERACTIONS

Objective 37.P.1. Recognize drug interactions of the tricyclic antidepressants, especially dental drugs.

1. TCs and MAOI combinations should be avoided.
2. Additive or supra-additive CNS depression is noted when these are combined with any CNS depressant drug.
3. Blockade of guanethidine's peripheral hypotensive effect and clonidine's central hypotensive effect occur.
4. Sympathomimetics may have an enhanced effect (this is a relative contraindication for vasoconstrictors in local anesthetic solutions).
5. Enhanced antidepressant effect occurs with thyroid preparations, amphetamines, methylphenidate, and phenothiazines.
6. Enhanced atropinelike effects occur when combined with any drug which has significant anticholinergic activity.

Q. THERAPEUTIC USES

Objective 37.Q.1. Recognize two types of depressive states and therapeutic use(s) of antidepressants in these states.

In broad terms, there are two types of depressive illness.

1. **Reactive depression.** This is a response to a readily identifiable event, e.g., death of a loved one or a major illness. The depression may become prolonged, exaggerated, and incapacitating. Psychotherapy seems to be more effective than drug therapy.
2. **Endogenous depression.** There is definite onset of symptoms, apparently unrelated to external events. Drug therapy and electroconvulsant therapy are effective.

Tricyclic antidepressants are the drugs of choice to treat mental depression; MAOI are secondary drugs and they are not commonly used; amphetamines are rarely used for this purpose.

R. IMPLICATIONS FOR DENTISTRY

Objective 37.R.1. Describe the dental implications of patients taking tricyclic antidepressants.

1. Marked xerostomia occurs, resulting in increased caries (especially cervical), difficulty retaining full dentures, and increased "sore spots" associated with dentures. There may

be an increased intake of cariogenic liquids and foods due to xerostomia, with further worsening of the cariogenic effect.

2. Care must be exercised when dismissing patients from a supine position in the dental chair because of postural hypotensive effects.

3. In the presence of a parkinsonlike syndrome, there may be an increased incidence of involuntary facial muscle movement, resulting in difficulty in retention of full dentures.

4. There is a relative contraindication to the use of vasoconstrictors in the presence of tricyclics. Perhaps plain solutions of local anesthetics should be used initially. However, if vasoconstrictors are necessary, the dentist must use a lower total dosage of vasoconstrictor, take more time to inject, and aspirate frequently to avoid intravascular injection.

   Vasoconstrictors (with a possible exception of phenylephrine) contained in local anesthetics are contraindicated in the presence of arrhythmias induced by TCs.

REFERENCE

Csáky TZ: Cutting's Handbook of Pharmacology, 6th ed. New York, Appleton-Century-Crofts, 1979, pp 596, 631

BIBLIOGRAPHY

Accepted Dental Therapeutics, 38th ed. Chicago, American Dental Association, 1979

Gilman AG, Goodman LS, Gilman A (eds): Goodman and Gilman's The Pharmacological Basis of Therapeutics, 6th ed. New York, Macmillan, 1980, Ch 19, 24, 25

Meyers FH, Jawetz E, Goldfien A: Review of Medical Pharmacology, 7th ed. Los Altos, CA, Lange, 1980, Ch 28

QUESTIONS

1. Drugs that are considered to be xanthines include:

   A. caffeine
   B. theobromine
   C. theophylline
   D. all of the above are correct
   E. none of the above is correct

2. T F Xanthines structurally resemble the purines.

3. T F Xanthines are thought to inhibit adenylate cyclase, thereby causing accumulation of cyclic AMP.

4. T F The xanthines are rapidly absorbed from the GI tract, but little drug gains access to the CNS.

5. Theophylline's effect on bronchiolar smooth muscle is thought to be:

   A. mild
   B. moderate
   C. potent
   D. none of the above

6. With regard to ability to stimulate cardiac tissue, arrange the xanthines (Column I) in correct order according to the choices below:

	Column I
A. 1, 2, then 3	
B. 2, 3, then 1	1. caffeine
C. 3, 1, then 2	2. theobromine
D. 3, 2, then 1	3. theophylline

7. T F Xanthines are capable of producing both diuresis and increased gastric acid secretion.

8. T F Toxic effect of xanthines are extensions of their pharmacologic effects and include actions on the CNS, GI tract, and cardiovascular system.

9. Theophylline (or aminophylline) is useful for:

   A. reversing an acute asthmatic attack
   B. treating peptic ulcers

...ment of postoperative dental pain, especially at 30 to 32 mg

  D. stimulating the CNS to increase respiration

10. Amphetamines are capable of:

  A. activating α and β receptors
  B. producting tolerance and dependence
  C. stimulating the CNS
  D. all of the above are correct
  E. none of the above is correct

11. **T F** Use of epinephrine as a vasoconstrictor is absolutely contraindicated in patients taking MAO inhibitors.

12. **T F** The effects of MAO inhibitors are similar to amphetamine, e.g., CNS stimulation.

13. Which one of the following drugs is classified as a tricyclic antidepressant?

  A. pargyline
  B. imipramine
  C. iproniazid
  D. tranylcypromine

14. **T F** Imipramine is chemically related to the phenothiazines.

15. **T F** The proposed mechanism for relief of depression by the tricycle antidepressants is the blockade of dopamine receptors.

16. **T F** Imipramine is well absorbed by all routes of administration, and it is distributed throughout the body.

17. **T F** Accumulation of active metabolites of imipramine may be necessary for onset of antidepressant activity.

18. Pharmacologic effects of imipramine include:

  A. antidepressant effects
  B. blurred vision
  C. sedation
  D. xerostomia
  E. all of the above are correct
  F. none of the above is correct

19. Adverse effects of imipramine include:

  A. arrhythmias
  B. postural hypotension
  C. xerostomia
  D. all of the above are correct
  E. none of the above is correct

20. **T F** Imipramine may have an additive or supra-additive effect when combined with any CNS depressant drug.

21. **T F** Tricyclic antidepressants are the drugs of choice to treat depression.

22. **T F** If dental patients taking tricyclics exhibit cardiac arrhythmias, a vasoconstrictor should not be used.

38
Antiepileptic Drugs

A. BACKGROUND OF EPILEPSY

This chapter describes the general types of epilepsy, their symptomatologies, the pharmacology of the drugs used in their treatment, and the precautions required in treating epileptic dental patients.

Current estimates place the incidence of epilepsy in the general population at 0.5 to 4% (Hammill, 1973). Of these afflicted individuals, the majority are controlled, that is, they have not experienced a seizure for two or more years. In spite of such an impressive rate of control, epileptics continue to experience difficulty in obtaining dental care, either because of financial considerations or because of the reluctance of many dentists to treat epileptics. An understanding of the disease and its manifestations, as well as the medications used to treat it, will greatly aid the clinician in providing dental care to epileptics.

Objective 38.A.1. List five reasons why the dentist should understand epilepsy and antiepileptic drugs.

The dentist should be familiar with the symptomatology of epilepsy as well as the pharma-

cotherapeutics of the disease for several reasons:

1. The dentist may be the first health care professional to recognize the disorder in a previously untreated patient.
2. The dentist must know how the disease and the drugs used to treat it can modify his delivery of dental care (e.g., drug interactions).
3. The dentist may be alerted to the presence of epilepsy from the current medications of the patient.
4. The dentist should be able to offer dental care to epileptics.
5. The dentist should be able to handle epileptic emergencies should they arise in his office.

Objective 38.A.2. Be able to list conditions which may predispose to epilepsy; describe the manner in which a seizure begins in the brain and spreads and the clinical manifestations of the various types of seizures.

Epilepsy may be associated with pathologic lesions of the brain, including brain tumors, abscesses, and vascular disorders. Similarly, metabolic disturbances, such as alterations of blood CO_2 content or pH, may cause an epileptogenic focus to discharge, but in the majority of cases, the underlying cause of the disease remains idiopathic. An epileptic seizure can be described as a sudden discharge of neurons in a localized area of the brain. This area, which is termed a **focus,** can result in the patient sensing the onset of a seizure. The initial sensation, termed an **aura,** is part of the seizure and may consist of olfactory, gustatory, or other unusual sensory alterations. Once initiated at the focus, the intense neural discharge results in excitation of adjacent brain areas. The areas to which this "storm" of discharge spreads determine the clinical symptoms of the seizure. A generalized, grand mal type seizure (with involvement of nearly all muscle groups of the body) indicates a general spread of seizure activity over the entire motor cortex.

Objective 38.A.3. Recognize a broad classification of epilepsy into (1) generalized seizures and (2) partial seizures. Recognize symptomatology of two types of generalized and two types of partial seizures.

A brief description of some of the more common types of epileptic seizures follows. It should be noted that this is not a complete classification and that only the most common types of epilepsy were selected for further discussion. The reader is referred to Gilman et al. (1980) for the full classification.

1. Generalized Seizures

Grand Mal (Tonic-Clonic Seizures). The grand mal seizure is one that is usually associated with the term "epilepsy" and involves a sequence of maximal tonic spasms of all muscles followed by clonic muscle jerking. The muscle activity is often accompanied by spontaneous micturition or defecation and is followed by post-seizure central nervous system depression in which the patient may exhibit confusion, ataxia, or sleep. In cases in which drugs have been used to bring the seizure under control, the post-seizure depression may be more severe due to the additional central depression caused by the drugs, and respiratory assistance may be indicated.

Petit Mal (Absence Seizures). Petit mal epilepsy usually occurs in children, and such seizures may go unnoticed, since they are very brief and are manifested as short staring spells in which the child may fix his eyes briefly and loses touch with his surroundings (but not his consciousness). Tonic and clonic muscle contractions are not characteristic of this type of epilepsy.

2. Partial Seizures (Focal Seizures)

Cortical Focal. In this type of seizure, muscle contractions are usually confined to single limbs or muscle groups. As in other types of epilepsy, this seizure activity may spread over the entire motor cortex, resulting in a grand mal episode. Muscles involved in this type of seizure depend on the particular area of the cerebrum in which the discharge is occurring.

Psychomotor (Temporal Lobe). These attacks consist of confused, inappropriate episodes of behavioral changes, and the patient can easily be misdiagnosed as being psychotic. For example, the patient may fumble with his/her clothing while ignoring activity in the surroundings. Amnesia occurs following the seizure, and this type of seizure activity may also proceed to a grand mal episode.

B. ANTIEPILEPTIC DRUGS

Objective 38.B.1. Identify four major groups of primary antiepileptic drugs and the representative drugs of each group and describe their indications and side effects.

Some of these drug categories are limited to the treatment of one type of seizure, e.g., those used to treat petit mal epilepsy. Other classes of drugs can be used in a variety of seizure types, and it is not unusual to see two or even three different types of drugs used in a single patient. This is because of the highly individualized nature of drug therapy of epilepsy, based on the many different types of seizures, the frequency of seizures, and the severity of the side effects caused by the primary drug.

Major Classes of Antiepileptic Drugs (Primary Drugs)

1. Hydantoins. **Phenytoin** (*Dilantin*) is now the most widely used anticonvulsant for the treatment of grand mal epilepsy and is useful in other types of epilepsy as well. Its major advantage over phenobarbital (see barbiturates below) is that it produces very little sedation and has a wide margin of safety. Occasionally, the dose of phenobarbital being used in a patient is reduced, and therapy is supplemented with phenytoin. The adverse effects of phenytoin include various central nervous system disturbances (nystagmus, ataxia), gastric irritation, hirsutism in young females, occasional allergic reactions, and gingival hyperplasia. The gingival hyperplasia produced by phenytoin is a severe problem in some patients and occurs in approximately 20% of patients who take the drug. Poor oral hygiene aggravates this problem, and gingivectomy is frequently required on a periodic basis. Vitamin therapy does not appear to provide relief from this condition. Other antiepileptic hydantoins are listed in Section 38.B.2.

2. Barbiturates. **Phenobarbital** is by far the oldest and most widely used barbiturate in the treatment of epilepsy. Phenobarbital is effective at relatively low doses compared to other barbiturates because phenobarbital has a specific anticonvulsant effect. In comparison with phenytoin, phenobarbital yields a more consistent biologic half-life. Phenobarbital is used in the treatment of grand mal and cortical focal seizures but may actually worsen petit mal and psychomotor seizures. The major side effect of the barbiturates when used to treat epilepsy is sedation, which is occasionally counteracted by the concomitant administration of an amphetamine. Other side effects include various allergic reactions (rashes, pruritus, urticaria) and aggravation of the condition known as acute intermittent porphyria. Barbiturates can cause gastrointestinal irritation and an increase in the rate of metabolism of certain drugs handled by the liver, thereby altering drug effectiveness and dosage requirements. Sudden withdrawal of an epileptic from the barbiturate regimen can precipitate seizures. In terms of dental therapy, the use of a barbiturate by an epileptic may result in potentiation of central nervous system depressants, such as narcotic-analgesics and sedatives. Extreme care must be exercised in administering such drugs to *any* patient taking *any* barbiturate.

3. Primidone (*Mysoline*). **Primidone** is a deoxybarbiturate which is often considered a primary drug for therapy of epilepsy and has a spectrum of activity similar to phenobarbital.

4. Succinimides. **Ethosuximide** (*Zarontin*) is the most widely used succinimide and is used almost exclusively in the treatment of petit mal epilepsy. Its adverse effects include anorexia, nausea and vomiting, drowsiness, motor disturbances, headaches, and, in some severe cases, blood dyscrasias.

Secondary Drugs

Objective 38.B.2. Identify secondary antiepileptic drugs.

The drugs in the following list are secondary agents, in that they are largely used to supplement the drugs described above or are used in cases that are refractory to the drugs described above.

Oxazolidinediones. **Trimethadione** (*Tridione*) and paramethadione (*Paradione*) are two such compounds that are used in petit mal epilepsy. Because these drugs can cause bone marrow depression and renal damage, they have been supplanted by the succinimides in most cases, especially if such side effects occur. (Trimethadione was formerly the drug of choice for petit mal epilepsy.) These drugs may also cause drowsiness, motor disturbances, and various visual disturbances, including hemeralopia, in which viewed objects appear to have a cloudy, white halo.

Hydantoins. Mephenytoin (*Mesantoin*) is an alternate to phenytoin.

Barbiturates. Mephobarbital (*Mebaral*), a long-acting barbiturate, is metabolized to phenobarbital.

Succinimides. These are alternate agents for ethosuximide, but have no particular advantage:

    methsuximide (*celontin*)
    phensuximide (*milontin*)

Phenacemide (Phenurone). This is used in psychomotor seizures but is very toxic. It may be useful when other combinations fail.

Acetazolamide (Diamox). This is a carbonic anhydrase inhibitor (see Chapter 32, Diuretics), used in several types of epilepsy.

Carbamazepine (Tegretol): **Carbamazepine** is discussed below under Objective 38.B.3.

Valproic Acid (Depakene). This is used in Europe and was recently introduced into the U.S.

Benzodiazepines. These are used primarily as sedative and antianxiety agents (see Chapter 22) and include:

    clonazepam (*Clonopin*)
    diazepam (*Valium*)

Objective 38.B.3. Describe the role of **carbamazepine** (*Tegretol*) in antiepileptic therapy and in trigeminal neuralgia, including side effects.

Carbamazepine is an antiepileptic drug which is used in cases of epilepsy refractory to other drugs. Recently, its use in relieving trigeminal and glossopharyngeal neuralgias has become popular. It is important to note that this drug is neither an antipyretic-analgesic, like aspirin or acetaminophen, nor an anti-inflammatory compound. Carbamazepine should be used in treating neuralgias only when indicated and only with an understanding of the potential risks involved. The mechanism of action of carbamazepine in relieving trigeminal neuralgia is not completely known, although it appears to involve an action that reduces the occurrence of antidromic nerve impulses (reflected waves) in the trigeminal nerve. Carbamazepine, when used to treat trigeminal neuralgia, is given in doses of 100 to 200 mg twice daily. It produces symptomatic relief in approximately 70% of patients, although its adverse effects can necessitate its discontinuation in 5 to 20% of patients. Carbamazepine should not be used in patients taking monoamine oxidase inhibitors and must be used with great caution in patients taking tricyclic antidepressants. Its many side effects include adverse reactions of the hematopoietic system (e.g., aplastic anemia, leukopenia), hepatocellular and cholestatic jaundice, acute oliguria, hypertension, acute left ventricular failure, a variety of central nervous system effects (diplopia, blurred vision, drowsiness, ataxia, nystagmus, tinnitus), and gastrointestinal irritation. Patients taking this drug must be carefully monitored for the development of serious side effects by routine blood analysis and also by liver and kidney function tests.

C. DRUG INTERACTIONS

Objective 38.C.1. List possible interactions between antiepileptic drugs and other agents.

CNS Depressants. The following agents, which are used in dentistry, will show enhanced degrees of central nervous system depression in patients taking anticonvulsants and should be used with caution: sedatives, hypnotics, antianxiety drugs, antipsychotic drugs, narcotic-analgesics, muscle relaxants, and antihistamines.

Alterations of Drug Metabolism. Barbiturate-type anticonvulsants tend to enhance the rate of metabolism of drugs that undergo biotransformation by the liver. The hydantoin compounds are also capable of causing this effect, which can reduce the effectiveness of other drugs, both related and unrelated (e.g., corticosteroids can be accelerated in their clearance rate from the body).

Blood Clotting. Anticonvulsants may alter the ability of the patient to form blood clots in several ways: (1) barbiturates can impair the formation of vitamin K-dependent clotting factors in the liver, (2) some anticonvulsants, e.g., valproic acid, can also inhibit platelet aggregation, and (3) such drugs as the succinimides and oxazolidinediones can alter blood clotting by producing blood dyscrasias, such as thrombocytopenia. Any indication of abnormal blood clotting, such as epistaxis or petechial hemorrhages, should be immediately reported to the physician who is treating the epileptic patient.

D. SIDE EFFECTS

Objective 38.D.1. Describe "benign" and "serious" side effects of antiepileptic drugs.

The drugs used in the treatment of epilepsy can exert two general categories of side effects: benign (e.g., mild central nervous system disturbances and gastrointestinal irritation) and serious (e.g., blood dyscrasias, allergy, nephrotoxicity). Benign side effects are usually dealt with by reduction in dosage of antiepileptic drug and supplementation with another drug, or other simple measures. Serious side effects necessitate withdrawal of the offending drug and replacement with an alternative agent.

E. DENTAL TREATMENT OF THE EPILEPTIC PATIENT

Objective 38.E.1. Describe principles of dental office treatment of epileptic patients.

There are several principles of antiepileptic drug therapy to keep in mind when treating the epileptic patient in the dental office (Westphal, 1972).

1. The treatment of epilepsy is symptomatic, so that while drug therapy may eradicate the seizures, the pathologic process responsible for their occurrence is still present and may become overtly active during the stress of a dental appointment.
2. Drugs are the backbone of epilepsy treatment. It is, therefore, important to ensure that the patient is in full compliance with his/her drug regimen before undertaking dental treatment.

3. Drug therapy is long-term, daily, and self-administered. In view of this fact, the dentist should be careful not to interfere with the antiepileptic drug regimen through his dental treatment and should monitor the patient for the presence of serious side effects resulting from the use of anticonvulsant medication.

Objective 38.E.2. Describe three precautions that should be taken in treating epileptic dental patients.

Unfortunately, many epileptics do not receive adequate dental care because of a reluctance of some practitioners to treat them. The following guidelines should assist the dentist in recognizing and successfully treating the epileptic dental patient.

1. Recognition of the epileptic patient. Approximately 0.5 to 4% of the general population is afflicted with epilepsy, and it is important for the dental practitioner to be able to recognize affected individuals through a complete family and health history. In many cases, epileptics are reluctant to disclose their condition for fear of discrimination. In cases in which the patient does not voluntarily disclose his condition, a family history of epilepsy or the use by the patient of any of the antiepileptic drugs described above should alert you to the possibility of epilepsy.
2. Consultation. Once epilepsy has been recognized in the dental patient, it is important to consult with the patient's physician before undertaking treatment. Several pieces of information should be obtained: (1) ascertain whether or not the patient's seizures are controlled and, if so, to what degree (an uncontrolled epileptic is a poor risk) (2) if the patient is under an acceptable degree of control (good control is one or two seizures per year, complete control is considered to be a seizure-free period for two years or more), determine the type of seizures the patient has and what factors seem to trigger them, and (3) obtain a complete drug profile of the patient, including all medications, dosage regi-

mens, side effects, and a medical opinion of those drugs which must be avoided in the patient.

3. Precautions during dental therapy. Once accepted for dental treatment, the epileptic should be treated with due caution. Above all, stress and pain must be avoided, as well as specific stimuli which have been known to trigger seizures in the past. Appointments should be scheduled at a time of day that is most comfortable for the patient. Local anesthetics are not contraindicated in the controlled epileptic, although excessive doses should be avoided, as in any patient. Vasoconstrictors can be used with local anesthetics in the controlled epileptic patient and contribute to a more reliable depth and duration of anesthesia. When prescribing postoperative medications, attention should be given to the possibility of drug interactions, and the patient should be advised **exactly** as to the dosage regimen used by specific labeling of the medication. Some anticonvulsants, especially valproic acid, can cause increased bleeding and necessitate caution prior to, during, and following surgical procedures.

Objective 38.E.3. Describe the measures to be used when an emergency situation arises due to an epileptic seizure.

When possible, the patient should be instructed to warn the dentist and/or dental assistant if an aura is occurring, so that preparations for a seizure can be made. If a seizure of the convulsive type occurs without warning, take the following steps:

1. Move trays and instruments from the immediate vicinity of the patient and place the patient in a reclined position. The most important thing is to prevent the patient from injuring himself during the seizure. Place a mouth prop between the teeth to prevent biting of the tongue, and do not move the patient from the chair nor use **forceful** restraint. Gentle restraint to keep the patient from falling or striking nearby objects is recommended.
2. When objects remain in the mouth, those that are loose and in danger of being aspirated should be removed, while those that are held firmly should be left in place until they can be removed easily. Forceful removal of an object from the patient's mouth may cause breakage of the object and aspiration or injury to the patient. In the case of impression materials, the tray and impression material should be allowed to set before removal is attempted. Failure to observe this rule may result in the aspiration of the impression material. An impression tray should never be forcefully removed during tonic jaw muscle contraction. If vomiting occurs, the vomitus should be cleared from the accessible areas of the patient's mouth with suction to minimize possibility of aspiration into the lungs.
3. If the seizure is prolonged, it may be necessary to terminate the convulsion with a drug. The drug of choice for status epilepticus is diazepam (*Valium*) IV at a dose of 2 to 20 mg in adults. Oxygen should also be administered.
4. In the postseizure period, the dentist should be prepared to administer respiratory assistance, especially if the postseizure depression is enhanced by the prior use of an anticonvulsant drug. Generally, the patient must be allowed to rest after a seizure. When a status seizure (prolonged) has occurred, the possibility of recurrence must be considered.

REFERENCES

Hammill JF: Role of the Nurse in the Understanding and Treatment of Epilepsy. Washington, DC, Epilepsy Foundation of America, 1973, p 1

Westphal P: Dental care of epileptics. Epilepsia 13:233, 1972

BIBLIOGRAPHY

Gilman AG, Goodman LS, Gilman A (eds): Goodman and Gilman's The Pharmacological Basis of Therapeutics, 6th ed. New York, Macmillan, 1980, Ch 20

QUESTIONS

1. An epileptic seizure begins as a discharge in a localized area of the brain known as a (Select one.):

   A. aura
   B. focus
   C. lesion
   D. septum

2. Epileptic seizure patterns which occur primarily in children and involve brief, frequent, staring spells are termed (Select one):

   A. grand mal seizures
   B. cortical focal seizures
   C. psychomotor seizures
   D. none of the above

3. Phenytoin (Dilantin) is the most widely prescribed agent for the treatment of which of the following types of epileptic seizures?

   A. grand mal
   B. cortical focal
   C. psychomotor
   D. none of the above

4. Ethosuximide (Zarontin) is used primarily in the treatment of which one of the following types of epileptic seizures?

   A. grand mal
   B. petit mal
   C. psychomotor
   D. none of the above

5. Which one of the following is a characteristic, serious side effect of carbamazepine (Tegretol)?

   A. eighth cranial nerve damage
   B. blood dyscrasias, e.g., aplastic anemia
   C. peptic ulcer
   D. none of the above

6. Serious side effects of antiepileptic drugs usually require which one of the following measures?

   A. reduction of dosage
   B. use of additional agents to treat the side effect
   C. discontinuation of the drug
   D. alteration in the time of drug ingestion

7. Which one of the following is a valid principle of the treatment of epileptic patients in the dental office?

   A. drug administration usually eradicates the pathologic lesion responsible for seizures, so that epileptics do not require special handling
   B. the dentist should increase the dose of the patient's medication prior to the dental appointment as a preventive measure
   C. the dentist should make sure that the patient is in full compliance with his or her antiepileptic drug regimen prior to treatment
   D. none of the above

8. Which one of the following statements correctly describes precautions to be taken during dental treatment of epileptic patients?

   A. no vasoconstrictors should be used to avoid possible CNS stimulation
   B. specific stimuli known to trigger seizures should be avoided
   C. an intravenous line must be maintained at all times
   D. prophylactic antibiotic regimens must be employed

9. Which one of the following is the drug of choice for terminating prolonged epileptic seizures in the dental office?

   A. pentothal sodium
   B. pentylenetetrazol
   C. diazepam
   D. phenobarbital

39

Alcohol

A. ALCOHOLISM

Ethyl alcohol (ethanol) is used and abused by most societies, although an exception is the Islamic society. Alcoholism is a socioeconomic problem that can threaten one's own health, family, job, credit, and credibility. The chronic alcoholic may suffer from malnutrition and avitaminosis. Thus, the alcoholic patient may have oral lesions associated with these two problems. In addition, the alcoholic is usually more susceptible to infections.

Chronic ethanol ingestion leads to tolerance and dependence, both physical and psychologic. It is the only drug of dependence that can be legally purchased without a prescription. The loss of life, limb, and property (under its influence) and the loss of work (due to hangover) is estimated to be in the hundreds of millions of dollars per year.

B. CHEMISTRY

Objective 39.B.1. Recognize the chemistry and availability of alcohols.

An alcoholic group ($R—CH_2OH$) can be synthesized or attached to most organic compounds. However, in this chapter we are most interested in ethanol, with a minor emphasis on methyl alcohol and isopropyl alcohol. Another higher alcohol (ethchlorvynol) was briefly discussed in Chapter 21 as a nonbarbiturate sedative hypnotic.

The ethanol content of various products is given in Table 39–1.

C. MECHANISM OF ACTION

Objective 39.C.1. Recognize the mechanism of action of ethanol.

The exact mechanism of action of ethanol on the CNS (its major site of action) is unknown. Several mechanisms have been proposed, including injury to cells by precipitating proteins and blockade of conduction in nerve cells. In many respects, the action of ethanol on the CNS resembles the action of barbiturates, and there is cross-tolerance and cross-dependence between ethanol and other sedative-hypnotic drugs.

TABLE 39-1. ETHANOL CONTENT OF COMMONLY CONSUMED FERMENTED PRODUCTS

Beverage	Source	% Ethanol
beer	cereals	3.5 to 6
ale	cereals	6 to 8
hard cider	apples	8 to 12
wine	grapes	10 to 22
whiskey	cereals	40 to 55
brandy	wine	40 to 55
rum	molasses	40 to 55
gin	ethanol	40 to 55
vodka	ethanol	40 to 55

From Csáky TZ: Cutting's Handbook of Pharmacology, 6th ed, 1979. Courtesy of Appleton-Century-Crofts.

D. ABSORPTION, DISTRIBUTION, METABOLISM, AND EXCRETION

Objective 39.D.1. Recognize factors involved in the absorption of ethanol.

Ethanol is readily absorbed from the stomach, small intestine, colon, and the lungs (by inhalation of ethanol vapors). Absorption may be delayed by the presence of food, especially milk, and if ethanol is rapidly absorbed initially, a decreased rate of absorption eventually develops. Beer is generally absorbed more slowly, compared to other forms of ethanol.

Absorption from the small intestine is always rapid; food, motility and intestinal emptying time do not seem to influence absorption rate.

Objective 39.D.2. Recognize the distribution of ethanol.

Ethanol is distributed freely throughout the body to all tissues and fluids. It readily crosses the placenta, resulting in significant levels in the fetus as well.

Objective 39.D.3. Recognize the metabolism of ethanol.

At least 90% of ethanol is metabolized (oxidized) and sometimes as much as 98%. The metabolism of ethanol is somewhat unique in that it does not follow first-order kinetics. Ethanol is metabolized always at the same rate (zero-order kinetics); metabolism is not dependent on concentration (as in first-order kinetics). Ethanol is metabolized at a rate of about 10 ml/hr or 8 gm/hour, which is approximately equal to the ethanol in ⅔ oz of 100 proof whiskey or 8 oz of beer.

The liver initially, then other tissues are the sites of ethanol metabolism. The initial step is the transformation to acetaldehyde (by alcohol dehydrogenase), then to acetate or acetyl CoA by acetaldehyde dehydrogenase (see Scheme 1 under Drug Interactions). Eventually, the acetyl CoA is oxidized to carbon dioxide and water.

Objective 39.D.4. Recognize the excretion of ethanol.

From 2 to 10% of ingested ethanol is excreted unchanged; the remainder is metabolized and excreted as metabolites. The kidney and lungs are the major organs of excretion of ethanol, and excretion from the lungs is the basis of the respiratory test for drunkenness. The test is based on the fact that the concentration of ethanol in the expired air is 0.05% of blood concentration.

E. PHARMACOLOGIC EFFECTS

Objective 39.E.1. Recognize the pharmacologic effects of alcohol.

Behavioral Effects
Blood concentrations of ethanol are thought to produce the following behavioral effects:

50 mg/100 ml: initial motor disturbances and euphoria
60 mg/100 ml: additional motor disturbances
80 mg/100 ml: altered driving ability
100–150 mg/100 ml: grossly altered motor function
200–300 mg/100 ml: very drunk
300–350 mg/100 ml: coma
350–600 mg/100 ml: death

Central Nervous System
The overall effects on the CNS are quite similar to those of the classic sedative-hypnotic drugs, and, in fact, most pharmacologists classify eth-

anol as a sedative-hypnotic agent. The behavioral stimulatory effect also is similar to the sedative-hypnotics, and it occurs by the agent depressing inhibitory outflow (disinhibition), thus allowing enhancement of excitatory outflow.

The initial susceptible sites of ethanol in the CNS are the RAS and some cortical sites. With release of cortical integrated control, there is jumbled thought and disturbances of motor function.

The personality often changes, sometimes for the better, but often it becomes worse. The individual perceives increased capabilities under the influence of alcohol, but all tests reveal that motor and mental functions worsen.

With increased dose, there is increased CNS depression, with the result that general anesthesia can be attained, and with further increases, coma and death. Ethanol is not useful as a general anesthetic because the anesthetic dose is too close to the lethal dose.

Analgesia does occur with ethanol, as significant increases in pain threshold have been reported. However, ethanol is not recommended for analgesia, nor is it recommended as a hypnotic, even though many persons use ethanol for the latter purpose.

Central control of respiration may be stimulated or depressed by ethanol, but excessive doses invariably depress respiration. The agent shows some anticonvulsant activity at certain dosages, but this is not useful clinically.

Cardiovascular System

Low to moderate doses of ethanol do not produce any adverse effects on myocardial function, but with increased dose, there is myocardial depression, which is at first central in origin, and later direct CVS depression occurs.

In moderate doses, cutaneous vasodilation occurs, giving the person a "warm feeling." Because of this effect, many people drink ethanol in the cold outdoors in an effort to warm up. This is a mistake, because cutaneous vasodilation leads to increased loss of body heat, and the subject will lose even more heat. The vasodilating effect is thought to originate centrally.

Ethanol has been reported to produce a relief of pain from angina pectoris, but this effect is due to central depression, not to coronary vasodilation. Ethanol does produce cerebral vasodilation, especially at higher doses, but this action is not useful clinically.

GI Tract

Ethanol's effects on the GI tract can be variable, depending on the presence of food, type of food, status of motility at the time of ethanol exposure, and other factors.

Salivary and gastric secretions are increased by ethanol, via psychic and reflex mechanisms, the latter by stimulation of sensory nerve endings of the oral and gastric mucosa. Ethanol apparently causes a direct stimulation of gastric acid via local histamine release. For these reasons, alcoholic beverages are absolutely contraindicated for patients with peptic ulcers.

In higher concentrations, ethanol is a direct irritant to the gastric mucosa and, in addition to the increased gastric acid release, can cause erosive gastritis.

Liver

The habitual use of ethanol leads to fatty liver. This is thought to occur by increased release of fat from fat depots, increased esterification of triglycerides, and inhibition of triglyceride release from liver stores.

Hepatitis and cirrhosis of the liver are prominent effects in alcoholics, but the exact cause of these dysfunctions is not known.

Acute ethanol intoxication tends to inhibit liver microsomal enzymes, while chronic intoxication seems to stimulate liver microsomal enzymes.

Kidney

Ethanol has a diuretic effect. It will produce increased urine flow due to increased ingestion of fluid, but it also inhibits release of antidiuretic hormone (ADH). However, with repeated doses, there is evidence of an antidiuretic effect.

Sexual Function

Ethanol generally produces an increased desire but a decreased function or performance, especially in males.

Endocrine Effects

Ethanol produces a decreased uptake of catecholamines and, hence, an increased excretion. The blockade occurs mostly in the CNS and adrenal medulla.

Blood

Anemias can occur and may be due to malnutrition, but there is evidence that ethanol is also a weak folic acid antagonist. Thrombocytopenia and vacuolization of red and white blood cells occurs, probably due to depression of bone marrow. There is depression of leukocyte migration into inflamed areas.

F. TOLERANCE AND DEPENDENCE

Objective 39.F.1. Recognize the induction of tolerance or dependence by ethanol.

The chronic ingestion of ethanol leads to tolerance and physical and psychologic dependence. Sudden withdrawal leads to symptoms that resemble withdrawal from sedative-hypnotic drugs. Because of cross-tolerance, sedative-hypnotic drugs can be substituted in the alcohol-dependent patient and vice versa. During withdrawal, the alcoholic goes through a phase commonly known as the DTs (delirium tremens), which is characterized by confusion, disorientation, and tremulousness. Often during withdrawal, the alcoholic will hallucinate, and a common hallucination is seeing crawling insects. In contrast to narcotic withdrawal, alcohol withdrawal is more frequently fatal because of postconvulsive respiratory depression (Appendix III).

G. CONTRAINDICATIONS

Objective 39.G.1. Recognize contraindications to the use of ethanol.

Contraindications to the use of ethanol are hepatic or severe renal disease, peptic ulcer or evidence of increased gastric activity, epilepsy, infections of the urinary tract, and, especially, providing it to patients with a prior history of dependence.

H. DRUG INTERACTIONS

Objective 39.H.1. Recognize drug interactions for ethanol, especially dental drug interactions.

Interactions include:

1. oral anticoagulants: increased or decreased anticoagulant effect
2. antidiabetic agents: increased hypoglycemia and/or disulfiramlike reaction
3. all CNS depressants: additive or supra-additive CNS depression
4. disulfiram: metabolic interference which may be fatal
5. guanethidine: increased postural hypotension
6. methotrexate: hepatotoxicity
7. nitroglycerin: increased hypotension
8. salicylates: enhanced GI erosion and bleeding
9. acetaminophen: increased hepatotoxicity

I. DISULFIRAM

Objective 39.I.1. Recognize the mechanism by which disulfiram interacts with ethanol.

Disulfiram (Fig. 39–1) is a drug that is often prescribed by the physician for the alcoholic. The drug blocks the enzyme aldehyde dehydrogenase and results in the accumulation of a toxic product, acetaldehyde. The reason for the block by disulfiram is its metal-binding ability, due to the concentration of sulfur groups (note reac-

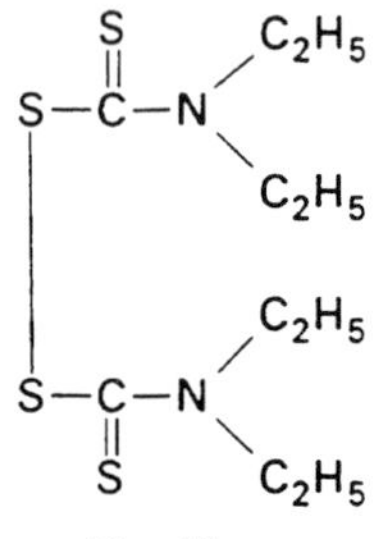

Disulfiram

Figure 39–1. Chemical Structure of Disulfiram. (*From Csáky TZ: Cutting's Handbook of Pharmacology, 6th ed, 1979. Courtesy of Appleton-Century-Crofts.*)

$$CH_3CH_2OH \xrightarrow[\text{dehydrogenase}]{\text{alcohol}} CH_3CHO \xrightarrow[\text{dehydrogenase}]{\text{aldehyde}} CH_3COO^-$$

Scheme 39-1. See text.

tion, Scheme 39–1). Normally, acetaldehyde is rapidly converted to acetate, which is not a rate-limiting reaction. However, disulfiram effectively blocks this step (aldehyde dehydrogenase). Disulfiram has practically no other effect than the one just described.

The disulfiram reaction (also known as the acetaldehyde syndrome) consists of vasodilation, initially over the face and then spreading over the entire body, an intense throbbing of the head, nausea, vomiting, sweating, thirst, chest pain, respiratory difficulties, hypotension, syncope, weakness, vertigo, and blurred vision. The intensity of the reaction is dependent on how much ethanol the patient ingests, and the duration of the reaction is also related to the amount ingested. Very severe reactions can be fatal. Needless to say, as long as the alcoholic takes disulfiram, he will hesitate to have another drink.

J. IMPLICATIONS FOR DENTISTRY OF ETHANOL

Objective 39.J.1. Describe dental implications of ethanol, including alcoholism, drug interactions, and uses.

1. Chronic alcoholism is a socioeconomic problem which may make the patient difficult to manage. The practitioner may have an increased number of broken appointments, or there may be difficulty collecting fees because supporting the habit may be relatively expensive. On the other hand, if the dentist becomes an alcoholic, he and his family may become the socioeconomic issue.
2. An increased incidence of oral lesions due to malnutrition and/or avitaminosis may be noted in these patients. In addition, these patients may have increased difficulty retaining full or partial dentures on the tissue-bearing

surfaces because of the increased incidence of sore spots.
3. There may be an increased incidence of infections.
4. There is generally an increased incidence of fractured jaws and teeth from falling or fighting.
5. There may be an additive or supra-additive CNS depressant effect when ethanol is taken concurrently with any other CNS depressant drug. However, in the chronic alcoholic, the patient may need increased dosages of CNS depressants due to liver enzyme induction.
6. Salicylates should be avoided because of the increased ulcerogenic effect when combining salicylates and ethanol. In addition, the alcoholic will probably be more susceptible to acetaminophen hepatotoxicity due to prior liver damage from alcohol ingestion.
7. Acute effects of alcohol ingestion result in disorientation and inebriation, and excessive use can cause coma and death. For these reasons, it would be unwise to use ethanol as a dental office peroral medication (or for any other reason).
8. Uses: ethanol has two uses in dental practice: (1) as a diluent for certain drugs (tinctures) and (2) in 70% concentration as a disinfectant (Appendix IV).

K. METHYL ALCOHOL

Objective 39.K.1. Recognize the adverse effects and lethal dose of methanol.

Methyl alcohol (methanol, wood alcohol) is of toxicologic interest only, for it has no therapeutic use in the practice of medicine or dentistry.

Methanol does induce some CNS depression; the generation of the metabolites formaldehyde and formic acid is entirely responsible for its toxic effect. Apparently, the same enzymes that metabolize ethanol also metabolize methanol, and methanol is changed to the same chemical classes of products, i.e., an aldehyde and an acid.

Formic acid produces a marked and potentially lethal systemic acidosis, while formaldehyde is thought to be responsible for blindness. However, the acidotic state produced by formic acid potentiates formaldehyde's effects on the eye. Inhalation of methanol can produce eye changes.

Treatment of acute intoxication (accidental or intentional ingestion) often includes administering ethanol, which is the preferred substrate for the enzyme, thereby preventing the generation of toxic methanol products.

Ingestion of 80 to 150 ml is often fatal, and a lesser amount can produce blindness. Denatured alcohol is ethanol with additives, making it unfit for human consumption. The additive is usually mostly methanol, and denaturation makes the substance not only tax exempt but also very toxic.

L. ISOPROPYL ALCOHOL

Objective 39.L.1. Recognize the use, toxic effect, and lethal dose of isopropyl alcohol.

Isopropyl alcohol can be used in a 70% concentration as an antiseptic or disinfectant because it precipitates bacterial proteins.

The major toxic effect when ingested is renal damage, and the lethal dose is between 120 and 240 ml in humans.

REFERENCE

Csáky TZ: Cutting's Handbook of Pharmacology, 6th ed. New York, Appleton-Century-Crofts, 1979, pp 641, 643

BIBLIOGRAPHY

Accepted Dental Therapeutics, 38th ed. Chicago, American Dental Association, 1979, pp 20–21

DiPalma JR (ed): Drill's Pharmacology in Medicine, 4th ed. New York, McGraw-Hill, 1971, Ch 15

Gilman AG, Goodman LS, Gilman A (eds): Goodman and Gilman's The Pharmacological Basis of Therapeutics, 6th ed. New York, Macmillan, 1980, Ch 18

Goth A: Medical Pharmacology, 10th ed. St. Louis, Mosby, 1981, Ch 26

Meyers FH, Jawetz E, Goldfien A: Review of Medical Pharmacology, 7th ed. Los Altos, CA, Lange, 1980, Ch 24

QUESTIONS

1. **T F** Ethanol is a 2 carbon alcohol.

2. **T F** The exact mechanism of action of ethanol on the CNS is unknown.

3. **T F** Ethanol is readily absorbed from most parts of the GI tract and from the lungs.

4. **T F** Ethanol is distributed freely throughout the body.

5. **T F** Ethanol's metabolism follows first order kinetics, i.e., ethanol's rate of metabolism is dependent on concentration.

6. **T F** The kidneys and lungs are the major organs of excretion of ethanol.

7. Pharmacologic effects of ethanol include:

   A. analgesia
   B. general anesthesia
   C. increased salivary and gastric secretion
   D. diuresis
   E. all of the above are correct
   F. none of the above is correct

8. **T F** Chronic ingestion of ethanol results in psychologic and physical dependence.

9. Contraindications to use of ethanol include:

   A. epilepsy
   B. hepatic disease
   C. infections of the urinary tract

D. all of the above are correct

E. none of the above is correct

10. **T F** An additive or supra-additive CNS depressant effect can occur when ethanol is ingested with any other CNS depressant.

11. **T F** The combination of ethanol and aspirin can lead to enhanced GI erosion and bleeding.

12. **T F** Disulfiram blocks the enzyme aldehyde dehydrogenase, and the blockade results in the accumulation of acetaldehyde.

13. Dental implications of chronic ethanol use include:

A. difficulty collecting fees

B. increased incidence of infections

C. increased incidence of oral lesions

D. all of the above are correct

E. none of the above is correct

14. **T F** Ingestion of 80 ml of methanol in man could lead to blindness or death.

15. **T F** Isopropyl alcohol (70%) may be used as an antiseptic.

40

Antiparkinson Drugs

A. INTRODUCTION: SYMPTOMS AND CAUSE OF PARKINSON'S DISEASE

Objective 40.A.1. Recognize the symptoms of Parkinson's disease.

Objective 40.A.2. Recognize the cause of Parkinson's disease.

Parkinson's disease (or paralysis agitans) is a chronic and progressive motor dysfunction. Weakness or loss of motor function, rigidity (including rigidity to the jaws), and tremor are present, and a pill-rolling muscle activity of the thumb and fingers is noted. Moreover, patients with Parkinson's disease have difficulty initiating movements.

The cause of the disease is the result of damage to dopaminergic neurons that project from the substantia nigra to the putamen and globus pallidus, and there is an indirect dopaminergic connection from the substantia nigra to the caudate nucleus as well. The former dopaminergic pathway is an inhibitory neuronal pathway. It makes connections with and is antagonistic to an excitatory pathway that is known to contain acetylcholine (ACh). In the normal state, the excitatory and inhibitory output are balanced, and coordinated muscle movement results. In the presence of Parkinson's disease, where there is damage to dopaminergic neurons, the excitatory, ACh-containing neurons become dominant, and the motor dysfunctions previously described become evident. In addition, some other cholinergic symptoms are common and include sialorrhea, seborrhea, and hyperhidrosis.

B. GOAL OF PHARMACOTHERAPY IN PARKINSON'S DISEASE

Objective 40.B.1. Recognize two methods of pharmacologic treatment of Parkinson's disease.

In general terms, pharmacologic intervention is aimed at either restoring dopaminergic function (with dopaminergic drugs) or at inhibiting the dominant cholinergic outflow (with anticholinergic agents). Obviously, the patient must be titrated to restore a balance of tone, with the ultimate goal of controlling muscular coordination and movement.

421

C. ANTICHOLINERGIC DRUGS (ATROPINELIKE DRUGS)

Objective 40.C.1. Recognize antiparkinson drugs with an anticholinergic effect and list one drug from each category.

Anticholinergic drugs were the first to be used to treat Parkinson's disease. They are still used today, but to a much lesser degree since the advent of levodopa. However, in certain instances, these agents are used in combination with levodopa.

The useful anticholinergic drugs must be capable of crossing the **blood-brain barrier** so that they can have an effect in the brain. Therefore, charged drugs (drugs that are in an ionic form at body pH) are not useful.

The following outline lists some useful antiparkinson drugs with anticholinergic effects.

1. **Parasympatholytics**
   a. **benztropine** (*Cogentin*)
   b. **biperiden** (*Akineton*)
   c. **cycrimine** (*Pagitane*)
   d. **procyclidine** (*Kemadrin*)
   e. **trihexphenidyl** (*Artane* and so on)
2. **Antihistamines**
   a. chlorphenoxamine (*Phenoxene*)
   b. **diphenhydramine** (*Benadryl*)
   c. orphenadrine (*Disipal, Norflex*)
3. **Phenothiazines** (chemically, but having no antipsychotic effect)
   a. ethopropazine (*Parsidol*)
   b. **promethazine** (*Phenergan*)

The pharmacology of these agents is not given in this chapter, since they were described in Chapters 17, 19, and 36. Also refer to Chapters 16 and 21.

D. MECHANISM OF ACTION OF LEVODOPA

Objective 40.D.1. Recognize the mechanism of action of levodopa.

Levodopa is currently the most important antiparkinson drug. Interestingly, it is essentially inert pharmacologically until it is metabolized. Most if not all of its effects and side effects occur after conversion to dopamine (DA), norepinephrine (NE), or epinephrine (E). It has been found that more than 95% of levodopa is decarboxylated in the periphery after only one circulation through the body, and probably less than 1% reaches the CNS.

The mechanism of antiparkinson effect is that the drug crosses the **blood-brain barrier,** apparently penetrates the remaining viable DA neurons, is converted to DA, stored, and released like the natural transmitter. Of course, the agent can gain access to NE and epi neurons, both centrally and peripherally, and can be converted to the appropriate transmitter, stored, and released as well.

The use of DA itself is of no value clinically, since it is a highly charged molecule which does not cross the **blood-brain barrier.** However, the precursor, levodopa (the official name for L-dopa), readily crosses the **blood-brain barrier.**

The biochemical machinery that generates DA is quite similar, if not exactly the same, as the synthetic pathway for the generation of NE or E. The major difference between synthesis of NE or E and the DA synthetic pathway in the brain is that these neurons lack dopamine β-hydroxylase (to convert DA to NE) and also lack the enzyme, phenylethanolamine N-methyltransferase, that converts NE to epi (Chapter 18). Thus, only DA is generated, and it is stored for future release. Scheme 40–1 for generation of dopamine was presented in Chapter 18 but is repeated here for sake of completeness.

E. PHARMACOLOGIC EFFECTS OF LEVODOPA

Objective 40.E.1. Recognize the major pharmacologic effects of levodopa, and the proposed mediator of each effect.

1. Amelioration of parkinsonian symptoms (due to conversion of levodopa to DA in brain)
2. CNS stimulation and elevation of mood (probably by generation of increased brain levels of DA and NE)

$$\text{Tyrosine} \xrightarrow{\frac{\text{tyrosine}}{\text{hydroxylase}}} \text{L-dopa} \xrightarrow{\frac{\text{L-aromatic}}{\text{amino acid decarboxylase}}} \text{dopamine}$$

Scheme 40-1. Generation of dopamine (see text).

3. Weak peripheral α and β agonist activity (due to conversion to DA, NE, or epi in the periphery)
4. Centrally mediated hypotension and postural hypotension (unknown cause, but possibly due to increased accumulation of NE centrally)
5. Nausea and vomiting (conversion to DA centrally; DA is thought to mediate emesis in the chromoreceptor trigger zone of the area postrema)
6. Minimal increased secretion of growth hormone (conversion to DA; DA is thought to mediate growth hormone release)
7. Decreased release of prolactin (conversion to DA; DA is thought to mediate the release of prolactin inhibitory releasing factor or hormone)

F. ADVERSE EFFECTS (USUALLY FROM HIGH DOSES)

Objective 40.F.1. Recognize adverse effects of levodopa and the proposed mediator for the effect (if known).

1. Arrhythmias (due to increased peripheral levels of NE and E)
2. Abnormal involuntary movements (unknown cause)
3. Psychiatric disturbances (unknown cause, but may be due to increased accumulation of DA in the mesolimbic projection)

G. DRUG INTERACTIONS

Objective 40.G.1. Describe drug interactions of levodopa with dental drugs.

1. Pyridoxine (vitamin B_6) antagonizes levodopa by causing an increased rate of metabolism to DA in the periphery. Pyridoxine is a neces-

sary cofactor for the decarboxylation reaction.
2. Sympathomimetics are contraindicated.
3. Antipsychotic and tricyclic antidepressants may be antagonized.
4. Diazepam antagonizes antiparkinson action.

H. CARBIDOPA

Objective 40.H.1. Recognize the mechanism of action of carbidopa.

Objective 40.H.2. Recognize the advantages of using carbidopa in conjunction with levodopa therapy.

Carbidopa is a drug that blocks the enzyme, L-aromatic amino acid decarboxylase, in the periphery, allowing more levodopa to reach the CNS (carbidopa is a charged drug, and it does not cross the **blood-brain barrier**). Therefore, the accumulation of NE and E peripherally is essentially eliminated, including many effects or side effects (see section 40.E.1. and 40.E.2). By using a combination of levodopa and carbidopa, the dose of levodopa may be reduced by as much as 75%. In addition, the following advantages have also been noted:

1. nausea and vomiting are almost entirely eliminated
2. cardiac side effects are essentially eliminated
3. pyridoxine therapy does not antagonize levodopa's effect
4. the number of divided doses may be reduced, and there is much better control of symptoms of Parkinson's disease
5. improved success rate of treatment is achieved

A 1:10 mixture of carbidopa:levodopa is available and is marketed under the trade name *Sinemet*. Carbidopa (*Lodosyn*) has recently been approved and is marketed as a single agent.

I. IMPLICATIONS FOR DENTISTRY

Objective 40.I.1. Describe dental implications concerning patients taking levodopa.

1. The practitioner or his office personnel must be careful when dismissing patients seated in a dental chair, due to the postural hypotensive effect.
2. It may be difficult to take impressions of patients' dental arches because of the marked incidence of nausea and vomiting that occurs with levodopa therapy. However, in combination with carbidopa, there should not be a problem.
3. If arrhythmias are present, vasoconstrictors contained in local anesthetic solutions should probably be avoided, with the possible exception of phenylephrine. Those patients taking the combination of levodopa and carbidopa should be free of cardiac effects.
4. Involuntary movements may be present, and full denture patients may report difficulty of retention of their dentures.
5. All the benzodiazepines, including diazepam, should be avoided. If sedation is required, perhaps a sedative-hypnotic (see Chapters 3 and 21) should be used.

J. OTHER DOPAMINERGIC DRUGS

Objective 40.J.1. Recognize amantadine and its mechanism of action as an antiparkinson drug.

Amantadine (*Symmetrel*) is an antiviral drug that is useful for the prophylactic treatment of influenza A viruses (see Chapter 30). Amantadine causes an antiparkinson effect apparently by increasing release of DA from the remaining viable dopaminergic neurons. The drug is best given with levodopa.

K. DRUGS THAT WORSEN PARKINSON'S DISEASE OR PRODUCE A PARKINSONLIKE SYNDROME

These are **dentally important** because the dentist may be consulted regarding **mandibular immobility** as part of the syndrome.

Objective 40.K.1. Describe the drugs that worsen Parkinson's disease.

Objective 40.K.2. Recognize the reason for the aggravation.

1. Reserpine depletes many brain amines, including dopamine.
2. Antipsychotic drugs (including phenothiazines and others, see Chapter 36): this occurs by dopamine receptor blockade.
3. Methyldopa: its structural similarity to levodopa causes mutual competition for (1) intestinal absorption sites, (2) **blood-brain barrier** transport sites, and (3) uptake into dopaminergic neurons.

Objective 40.K.3. Recognize a drug that can be used in an emergency situation to alleviate parkinsonian akinesia.

Diphenhydramine's antiparkinsonian effect has been used for emergency treatment of drug-induced akinesia (see also Chapter 36). The probable mechanism is the prominent anticholinergic effect of diphenydramine, which relieves the extrapyramidal stimulation caused by such drugs as chlorpromazine.

BIBLIOGRAPHY

Gilman AG, Goodman LS, Gilman A (eds): Goodman and Gilman's The Pharmacological Basis of Therapeutics, 6th ed. New York, Macmillan, 1980, Ch 21
Goth A: Medical Pharmacology, 10th ed. St. Louis, Mosby, 1981, Ch 12
Meyers FH, Jawetz E, Goldfien A: Review of Medical Pharmacology, 7th ed. Los Altos, CA, Lange, 1980, Ch 30

QUESTIONS

1. T F Parkinson's disease typically shows weakness or loss of motor function, rigidity, and tremor.

2. T F The cause of Parkinson's disease is thought to be damage to cholinergic neurons, thereby allowing enhancement of dopaminergic outflow.

3. Pharmacologic methods of treating Parkinson's disease include the use of:

    A. adrenergic drugs
    B. cholinergic drugs
    C. dopaminergic drugs
    D. noradrenergic drugs

4. All of the following drugs are classified as parasympatholytics *except:*

    A. benztropine
    B. biperiden
    C. cycrimine
    D. diphenhydramine
    E. procyclidine

5. The mechanism by which levodopa has an antiparkinson effect is by:

    A. blockade of L-aromatic amino acid decarboxylase
    B. blockade of tyrosine hydroxylase
    C. conversion to dopamine in the brain
    D. conversion of epinephrine in the brain
    E. conversion to norepinephrine in the brain

6. Major pharmacologic effects of levodopa include:

    A. amelioration of Parkinson's symptoms
    B. centrally mediated postural hypotension
    C. CNS stimulation
    D. nausea and vomiting
    E. all of the above are correct
    F. none of the above is correct

7. Toxic effects of levodopa include:

    A. abnormal involuntary movements
    B. arrhythmias
    C. psychotic disturbances
    D. all of the above are correct
    E. none of the above is correct

8. T F Levodopa may produce additive effects with other sympathomimetics that patients may be taking.

9. T F Pyridoxine antagonizes levodopa by causing an increased rate of metabolism of levodopa to dopamine in the periphery.

10. Carbidopa blocks:

    A. L-aromatic amino acid decarboxylase
    B. dopamine β-hydroxylase
    C. tyrosine hydroxylase
    D. phenylethanolamine N-methyltransferase

11. T F The dose of levodopa may be reduced by as much as 75% when levodopa and carbidopa are taken concurrently.

12. Dental implications concerning patients taking levodopa include:

    A. diazepam should be avoided
    B. if arrhythmias are present, all vasoconstrictors should be avoided except phenylephrine
    C. full denture patients may have difficulty retaining their dentures
    D. all of the above are correct
    E. none of the above is correct

13. Drugs that may aggravate Parkinson's disease include:

    A. antipsychotic drugs
    B. methyldopa
    C. reserpine
    D. all of the above are correct
    E. none of the above is correct

14. T F Drugs that aggravate Parkinson's disease do so by interfering with the uptake, storage, and receptors for dopamine.

41
Antineoplastic Drugs

A. PRINCIPLES OF ANTICANCER THERAPY

Objective 41.A.1. Recognize two reasons for the difficulty in finding a magic bullet in cancer chemotherapy.

Objective 41.A.2. Recognize two hypotheses that may be useful in explaining the mechanisms of action of anticancer drugs, including their present status.

Objective 41.A.3. Relate side effects of anticancer drugs to their therapeutic effects.

Objective 41.A.4. State the three most susceptible human systems which display side effects when anticancer drugs are used.

Developing anticancer drugs has been one of the biggest challenges for pharmacologists. There appears to be no **magic bullet** to specifically kill cancer cells because (1) the host accepts cancer cells as **self**, so that immunologically there is only minimal defense against the cancer, and (2) the cancer cells use the same metabolic pathways as the normal cells.

Although specificity did not seem possible, one point of attack of cytotoxic drugs on cancer cells appears to be the rapid rate of metabolism and new cell formation (mitosis) in some cancerous tissue. It is known, for example, that ionizing radiation and certain classes of chemotherapeutic agents have a greater effect on rapidly dividing cells than on slowly dividing ones. Unfortunately, in most common tumors, the cell turnover is actually less rapid than for some normal tissues, especially tissues of the: (1) bone marrow, (2) epithelia (especially gastrointestinal mucosa), and (3) reproductive cells. We can expect, therefore, that any drug which depends on differences in rates of turnover for its cytotoxic action will have side effects related to suppression of these tissues. A more recent explanation for specificity is that repair of damage to nuclear material may be less efficient in cancer cells than in normal cells. Therefore, the attack of the cytotoxic drugs on nuclear material would be valid if the cancerous cells have a slower rate of repair than normal cells. Irrespective of mechanism, the cytotoxic drugs have many side effects related to cytotoxicity in proliferating tissues.

B. CLASSIFICATION OF ANTICANCER DRUGS

Objective 41.B.1. Be able to match the drugs set in bold type to the major drug group to which they belong.

1. **Alkylating agents**
   (nitrogen mustards, ethyleneimines, sulfonate esters)
   a. chlorambucil (*Leukeran*)
   b. cyclophosphamide (*Cytoxan*)
   c. mechlorethamine (*Mustargen*)
   d. melphalan (*Alkeran*)
   e. triethylene thiophosphoramide (*Thiotepa*)
   f. **busulfan** (*Myleran*)
2. **Antimetabolites**
   a. aminopterin
   b. **methotrexate**
   c. **mercaptopurine** (*Purinethol*)
   d. **cytarabine Ara-C** (*Cytosar*)
   e. **fluorouracil, 5-FU**
3. **Antibiotics**
   a. puromycin
   b. **actinomycin D, dactinomycin** (*Cosmegen*)
   c. **mitomycin C**
   d. **doxorubicin** (*Adriamycin*)
   e. **daunorubicin** (*Cerubidine, Daunoblastina*)
   f. **bleomycin** (*Blenoxane*)
4. **Plant alkaloids**
   a. vinblastine (*Velban*)
   b. **vincristine** (*Oncovin*)
   c. epipodophyllotoxin (also called etoposide or VP 16–213)
   d. VM-26 (a derivative of podophyllotoxin, also called teniposide)
   e. vindesine
5. **Nitrosoureas**
   a. **carmustine,** BCNU (*BiCNU*)
   b. **lomustine,** CCNU (*CeeNU*)
   c. **semustine,** ME-CCNU (*Methyl-CCNU*)
   d. streptozotocin
6. **Miscellaneous**
   a. Cis-diamine-dichloroplatinum, **cisplatin** (*Platinol*)
   b. **dacarbazine** (*Dtic-Dome*)
   c. hydroxyurea
   d. L-Asparaginase
   e. **procarbazine** (*Matulane*)

7. **Hormones**
   a. **cortisone, prednisone,** and other corticosteroids
   b. **sex hormones**
   c. **tamoxifen** (*Nolvadex*)

C. MECHANISMS OF ACTION AND USES

Objective 41.C.1. Be able to match the drugs or drug types (set in bold type) to their mechanisms of action and uses.

Alkylating Agents. These act by forming alkyl bonds with reactive groups on DNA, RNA, and proteins. The chemical bonds formed are irreversible. Bonding inhibits cellular function and sometimes causes cellular death (cytotoxic effect). The alkylating agents are radiomimetic, mutagenic, cytotoxic, and carcinogenic. The alkylating agents are used in Hodgkin's disease, leukemia, and lymphoma, and are sometimes tried in lung or other cancers of epithelial origin.

Antimetabolites. These act by interfering with specific steps in production of necessary precursors of key chemicals, such as DNA or RNA. The folic acid mechanism for forming thymidine is a susceptible step which can be blocked by folic acid antagonists, such as methotrexate (e.g., by block of dihydrofolate reductase) or 5-FU (e.g., by block of thymidine synthetase). Purine antimetabolites (e.g., mercaptopurine) act on adenine-adenosine enzymes, whereas cytarabine probably acts in the pyrimidine pathway. Antimetabolites are used for leukemia and choriocarcinoma and in difficult cases of psoriasis (a nonmalignant skin condition). 5-FU is still widely used in the treatment of adenocarcinomas. Methotrexate is useful in head and neck cancer, sarcomas, and in combination with other drugs in breast cancer and leukemia.

Antibiotics.

1. Puromycin inhibits protein synthesis during ribosomal assembly and chain growth. Puromycin is so toxic that it is used only experimentally.

2. **Actinomycin D** combines with and inactivates DNA, which is needed for RNA synthesis. Actinomycin D is used in Wilms' tumor, sarcomas, and experimentally in other cancers.

3. **Mitomycin C** is inhibitory by its action on DNA and is used mainly in adenocarcinomas of the gastrointestinal tract and other solid tumors.

4. **Doxorubicin** (*Adriamycin*) binds with DNA, inhibiting its template activity. Doxorubicin is effective in leukemias, lymphomas, and in solid tumors and has perhaps the broadest spectrum of activity of any cancer chemotherapeutic agent in clinical use today.

5. **Daunorubicin** is very similar in chemical structure and mechanism of action to doxorubicin, although there may be a small difference in metabolic disposition. Clinically, daunorubicin is used in acute leukemias.

6. **Bleomycin** is used in squamous cell carcinomas of the head and neck, lymphomas, and testicular cancer.

Plant Alkaloids. Plant alkaloids (vinca alkaloids) are active by arresting mitosis in metaphase. Plant alkaloids are investigational for use in Hodgkin's disease, lymphocytic leukemia, and choriocarcinoma resistant to other agents. They may be tried in other carcinomas. VP 16–213 is active against small (or oat) cell carcinomas of the lung and potentially against other tumors. VP 16–213 probably acts by a different mechanism (which is not entirely clear) than do the vinca alkaloids.

Nitrosoureas. While the exact mechanism of action of the nitrosoureas (**BiCNU, CCNU,** and **Me-CCNU**) is unknown, they probably exert their effects in a manner similar to that of alkylating agents. They have been used to treat hematologic malignancies, brain tumors, and adenocarcinomas. Streptozotocin is often effective against islet cell tumors and malignant carcinoid.

Miscellaneous Agents.

1. **Cisplatin** is active against tumors of the genitourinary tract (testes, bladder, ovary, prostate), head and neck tumors, and other tumors of epithelial origin.

2. **Carbazines** are used for Hodgkin's disease and other lymphomas. **Procarbazine** and **dacarbazine** act by inhibiting DNA, RNA, and protein synthesis, but the exact mechanism is unknown.

3. **Hydroxyurea** is used for chronic granulocytic leukemia and other myeloproliferative disorders.

4. **L-Asparaginase** is used for acute lymphocytic anemia. Its mechanism of action is interesting; it is the only enzyme used that has anticancer action. Depletion of asparagine adversely affects some cancer cells because they cannot synthesize asparagine since they lack asparagine synthetase.

Hormones. Corticosteroids in high doses cause protein catabolic effects and may inhibit cancer cells by inhibiting cell division. Corticosteroids are sometimes used in acute lymphocytic leukemia and lymphomas, in combination with other agents. Sex hormones are used to suppress tumors of secondary sex organs. Androgens are used for suppression of breast cancer, and estrogens are useful for prostatic carcinoma and breast cancer. Tamoxifen is an antiestrogenic agent of low toxicity that is active in hormonally responsive breast cancer.

D. TOXICITY

Objective 41.D.1. Recognize the side effects of cytotoxic anticancer drugs.

Objective 41.D.2. Recognize the side effects of hormonal anticancer agents.

Many, though not all, cytotoxic anticancer agents produce nausea (N), vomiting (V), and diarrhea (D), due to GI irritation and action upon the CNS. Another side effect is local irritation at the site of injection. Myelosuppression and immunosuppression occur; in addition to these being serious problems by themselves, they often result in bacterial, viral, and fungal infections which can cause death. Thrombocytopenia can result in bleeding or bruising.

In addition, some agents have unique dose-limiting toxicity affecting certain organ systems, e.g., doxorubicin (cardiac toxicity), **cisplatin** (nephrotoxicity), and vincristine (neurotoxicity).

The side effects of hormonal anticancer agents are related to the type of hormone used. Corticosteroid use causes pituitary-adrenal suppression, increased susceptibility to infections, electrolyte and metabolic disturbances, cushingoid syndrome, and hirsutism. The sex steroids generally emphasize the corresponding sexual characteristics; estrogens feminize the male, and androgens masculinize the female. Estrogens may cause hypercalcemia in breast cancer patients—a serious side effect which may lead to confusion, coma, or kidney damage if not detected early. All steroids may cause fluid retention and precipitate a worsening congestive heart failure or hypertension in susceptible individuals.

E. CITROVORUM FACTOR (CF, LEUCOVORIN) RESCUE

Objective 41.E.1. Describe the leucovorin rescue technique.

A very high dose of methotrexate is first given in an attempt to kill cancer cells that might otherwise be resistant to methotrexate at conventional doses. Then calcium leucovorin (or folinic acid), which is a nutritional supplement, is given, usually every 6 hours, up to 24 to 48 hours after the methotrexate infusion. This regimen must be combined with forced hydration in order to prevent renal toxicity and to facilitate the renal clearance of the massive doses of methotrexate. Patients must be closely monitored during this period. If the rescue is properly carried out, the patient will not suffer the toxic effects of methotrexate on folate metabolism and hence on DNA, RNA, and protein synthesis. However, the use of high-dose methotrexate with CF rescue has been limited in recent years by the finding that it is no more ef-

fective for many cancers than conventional dose methotrexate without rescue (since CF will, to an extent, rescue the malignant cells as well as the normal cells). Furthermore, it is extremely expensive and requires hospitalization and close monitoring of the patient.

F. COMBINATION CANCER CHEMOTHERAPY

Objective 41.F.1. Recognize the goals and principles of combination cancer chemotherapy.

Combinations of drugs with anticancer action are often used. Usually, three or four different drugs are chosen with different mechanisms of action and nonoverlapping toxicities. The goals are to attack different points of cell proliferation to achieve greater cancer cell kill without excessive toxicity. Most importantly, it is hoped that the use of several agents will prevent or slow down the development of drug resistance (one of the major causes of treatment failure).

An important criterion for inclusion of a drug in any combination is that it should have shown activity against the cancer in question as a single agent.

G. DENTAL IMPLICATIONS

Objective 41.G.1. Describe the dental implications of cancer chemotherapy.

1. The patient may have oral cancer, which will require antineoplastic therapy. The patient's overall condition and needs should be considered by a health team, while an oncologist should prescribe and administer the necessary chemotherapeutic agents. The dentist not only participates on the team but also may have the responsibility to make an initial oral diagnosis. The oropharynx should be examined carefully at each visit whether the patient is cancer-suspect or not. After chemotherapy and/or radiation therapy is started, a complete blood count (including platelets) is recommended prior to all dental procedures. It is advisable to consult with the

oncologist(s) in charge of the patient's overall cancer management.

2. Patients taking anticancer drugs may have bacterial, viral, or fungal infections in the oral cavity, which become especially serious because of immune suppression. In addition, drug-induced stomatitis (especially with methotrexate, bleomycin, or 5-FU) may result in a breakdown of the normal mucosal barrier, as well as a compromise in the nutritional status of the patient. Early diagnosis and treatment of oral infections may prevent disastrous systemic complications. Low platelet counts secondary to chemotherapy may cause spontaneous gingival bleeding or bleeding after minor trauma (e.g., toothbrushing). A platelet count should be obtained prior to any dental manipulation in a patient on chemotherapy, since the platelet count may be inadequate for hemostasis (because of the cancer chemotherapy).

3. Drug interactions with anticancer drugs are uncommon clinically, despite the large number of potential interactions that exist. Methotrexate may be potentiated by phenytoin, salicylates, sulfonamides, and PABA. The mechanism is thought to be competition for protein-binding sites. Alcohol and anticoagulants are mutually synergistic with methotrexate, but the mechanism is not understood. Aminoglycoside antibiotics (e.g., streptomycin) should not be used in patients who have received cisplatin because of the increased nephrotoxicity that may result. Another interaction is allopurinol potentiation of mercaptopurine and azathioprine by interference with their metabolic degradation. Succinylcholine's action and CNS depressants may be enhanced by various specific anticancer drugs (especially cyclophosphamide and other alkylating agents).

All drug interactions should be noted by checking authoritative sources. Generally, the information is found in other chapters under the specific dental drugs that one plans to use. Refer to Appendix II of this book and the package insert, and consult the patient's physician whenever the patient is undergoing cancer chemotherapy.

4. Patients undergoing radiation therapy may develop salivary gland degeneration with chronic dry mouth (xerostomia), rapid progression of periodontal recession, and massive root caries. The situation may be relieved by frequent use of a lubricating solution and fluoride treatments of any exposed root dentin (see also Appendix V). The mouth should be restored to the healthiest state possible and plaque control initiated.

5. During cancer therapy, healing may be difficult and susceptibility to infection increased because the therapy inhibits the rapidly proliferating healing tissue. If possible, any major extractions should be done before therapy (especially in areas to be included within radiation fields) or during periods of remission when drugs and radiation are not being used. Ideally, whenever possible, patients who are to undergo chemotherapy should have a complete examination, with prophylaxis and correction of any existing problems prior to beginning chemotherapy. Periodontal disease or dental abscesses may become sources of septicemia or other infections in patients with neutropenia secondary to chemotherapy.

6. Prophylactic antibiotics may be recommended for dental procedures in immunosuppressed patients, especially those with hematologic malignancies (i.e., multiple myeloma, chronic lymphocytic leukemia, and acute myelogenous leukemia or preleukemia), which predispose them to bacterial infection.

H. TABLE OF THERAPEUTIC USES OF CANCER CHEMOTHERAPEUTIC AGENTS

Table 41–1 is presented to reemphasize the major uses of the drugs and the frequent and varied use of combinations. For dentists and dental students, the table is presented only as a reference; there is no need to commit it to memory. However, Objective 41.C.1. should be reinforced by reference to Table 41–1.

TABLE 41-1. MAJOR USES OF DRUGS AND DRUG COMBINATIONS[a]

Drug	Primary Drug for:	Secondary Drug for:	Combination Therapy with:
vincristine (Oncovin)	acute lymphocytic leukemia Hodgkin's disease non-Hodgkin's lymphoma Burkitt's lymphoma Wilms' tumor embryonic rhabdomyosarcoma	Ewing's sarcoma breast cancer	prednisone, asparaginase, doxorubicin, mechlorethamine, procarbazine, cyclophosphamide, methotrexate, dactinomycin
epipodophyllotoxin (etoposide, VP 16-213)	small cell carcinoma of lung	—	—
VM-26 (teniposide)	—	acute lymphocytic leukemia	—
vindesine	nonsmall cell carcinoma of lung	—	—
BiCNU, carmustine	brain tumors	Hodgkin's disease non-Hodgkin's lymphoma multiple myeloma	—
CCNU, lomustine	brain tumors	Hodgkin's disease non-Hodgkin's lymphoma	cytoxan
Me-CCNU, **semustine**	colorectal adenocarcinoma	—	5-FU
streptozotocin	Islet cell carcinoma	carcinoid tumors pancreatic adenocarcinoma	mitomycin C 5-FU
cis-diamine-dichloroplatinum (cisplatin)	testicular cancer other cancers of the genitourinary tract nonsmall cell lung cancer	osteogenic sarcoma squamous carcinoma of the head and neck	vinblastine, bleomycin, doxorubicin, dactinomycin, cyclophosphamide
dacarbazine	Ewing's sarcoma malignant melanoma	Hodgkin's disease	cyclophosphamide, doxorubicin, bleomycin, vinblastine
hydroxyurea	chronic granulocytic leukemia	myeloproliferative disorders	—
L-asparaginase	acute lymphocytic leukemia	non-Hodgkin's lymphomas	vincristine, prednisone
procarbazine (Matulane)	Hodgkin's disease non-Hodgkin's lymphoma	nonsmall cell lung cancer	mechlorethamine, vincristine, prednisone, cyclophosphamide
prednisone	acute lymphocytic leukemia Hodgkin's disease non-Hodgkin's lymphoma	breast cancer	vincristine, asparaginase, doxorubicin, mechlorethamine, procarbazine, cyclophosphamide, methotrexate
sex hormones	breast cancer prostate cancer	renal cell carcinoma endometrial carcinoma	—
tamoxifen (Nolvadex)	breast cancer	prostate cancer	—
chlorambucil (Leukeran)	chronic lymphocytic leukemia	non-Hodgkin's lymphoma	corticosteroids
cyclophosphamide (Cytoxan)	non-Hodgkin's lymphoma small-cell carcinoma of lung ovarian and breast cancer	acute lymphocytic leukemia (ALL) multiple myeloma	doxorubicin, vincristine, prednisone, procarbazine, methotrexate, dacarbazine, dactinomycin, fluorouracil, vinblastine, bleomycin cisplatin
mechlorethamine (Mustargen)	Hodgkin's disease	control of malignant effusions	vincristine, procarbazine, prednisone
melphalan (alkeran)	multiple myeloma	osteogenic sarcoma testicular cancer ovarian cancer	—
triethylene thiophosphoramide (Thiotepa)	bladder carcinoma (by intravesicular instillation)	—	—
busulfan (Myleran)	chronic granulocytic leukemia	—	—
methotrexate	acute lymphocytic leukemia non-Hodgkin's lymphoma Burkitt's lymphoma osteogenic sarcoma breast cancer choriocarcinoma	Burkitt's lymphoma embryonal rhabdomyosarcoma testicular cancer	mercaptopurine, cyclophosphamide, vincristine, prednisone, doxorubicin, leucoverin rescue, fluorouracil
mercaptopurine (Purinethol)	acute lymphocytic leukemia	—	methotrexate

(Continued)

TABLE 41–1. (*Continued*)

Drug	Primary Drug for:	Secondary Drug for:	Combination Therapy with:
cytarabine (*Cytosar*)	acute myelogenous leukemia	—	daunorubicin, thioguanine
fluorouracil (*5-FU*)	breast cancer Gastrointestinal adenocarcinomas	other adenocarcinomas	cyclophosphamide, methotrexate, doxorubicin, mitomycin C
actinomycin D	childhood sarcomas Wilm's tumor	testicular carcinoma	cylcophosphamide, vincristine, adriamycin
mitomycin C	gastric and pancreatic adenocarcinomas	osteogenic sarcoma breast cancer	adriamycin, 5-fluorouracil ("FAM")
doxorubicin (*Adriamycin*)	acute lymphocytic leukemia non-Hodgkin's lymphoma Ewing's sarcoma embryonal rhabdomyosarcoma osteogenic sarcoma breast cancer testicular cancer	Hodgkin's disease Wilms' tumor other adenocarcinomas	vincristine, prednisone, cyclophosphamide, dacarbazine, dactinomycin, methotrexate, leucovorin rescue, fluorouracil, bleomycin, cisplatin, vinblastine
daunorubicin	acute leukemia	—	—
bleomycin (*Blenoxane*)	testicular cancer	Hodgkin's disease non-Hodgkin's lymphoma choriocarcinoma squamous cell carcinomas of head and neck	vinblastine, cisplatin, doxorubicin, dactinomycin, cyclophosphamide, dacarbazine (DTIC)
vinblastine (*Velban*)	testicular cancer	Hodgkin's disease breast cancer choriocarcinoma	bleomycin, cisplatin, doxorubicin, dactinomycin, cyclophosphamide, dacarbazine (DTIC)

[a] Drugs having moderate or minor activity can be found in the reference, Med Lett, 1980.

BIBLIOGRAPHY

Dorr RT, Fritz WL: Cancer Chemotherapy Handbook. New York, Elsevier, 1980, Ch 4

Med Lett Drugs Ther 22:101, 1980

Devita VP, Hellman S, Rosenberg SA: Cancer: Principle and Practice of Oncology. Philadelphia, Lippincott, 1982

QUESTIONS

1–4. Regarding the antineoplastic effects of drugs, answer True or False to the following statements:

1. T F Host accepts cancer cells as self.

2. T F Cancer cells may not be able to repair DNA as well as normal cells.

3. T F Cancer cells have a faster cell turnover than all host cells.

4. T F Most current cancer chemotherapy is based upon build-up of the body's normal defense mechanisms.

5. T F The most productive point in attacking cancer cells by chemotherapy is to depend on the faster rate of turnover and metabolism of cancer cells compared to normal cells.

6. T F Side effects of anticancer drugs are high in number and severity because bone marrow, GI tract and epithelia are suppressed.

7. Anticancer drugs cause the greatest acute adverse effects in which of the following:

   A. gingiva
   B. developing blood cells
   C. salivary glands
   D. skin

8. Which of the following drugs act on cancer cells by alkylation?
   A. busulfan
   B. methotrexate
   C. both A and B are correct
   D. neither A nor B is correct

9. Which of the following drugs act on cancer cells as an antimetabolite?

   A. fluorouracil
   B. actinomycin D
   C. cyclophosphamide
   D. L-asparginase

10. A male patient has a malignant tumor of the prostate, and it is decided to use a steroid to suppress it. The best choice would be:

    A. vincristine
    B. cortisone
    C. testosterone
    D. estrogen

11-15. Which of the following antibiotics are considered active antineoplastic drugs?

11. T F chlortetracycline

12. T F puromycin

13. T F streptomycin C

14. T F actinomycin D

15. T F amphotericin B

16. The chemical bonds formed by alkylating agents are:

    A. reversible
    B. irreversible
    C. competitive
    D. ionic

17. Methotrexate acts by blocking:

    A. purine enzymes
    B. pyrimidine enzymes
    C. DNA polymerase
    D. dihydrofolate reductase

18. Vinca alkaloids are thought to act by arresting mitosis in:

    A. prophase   C. anaphase
    B. metaphase   D. GI synthesis

19-22. Match the best drug in Column 2 to the condition in Column 1.

Column 1

19.____brain tumor
20.____head and neck cancer
21.____Islet tumor
22.____lymphoma

Column 2

A. DTIC dacarbazine
B. streptozotocin
C. BCNU
D. methotrexate

23. T F A specific side effect of cisplatin is nephrotoxicity.

24. Nephrotoxicity is characteristic of:

    A. doxorubicin
    B. vincristine
    C. both A and B are correct
    D. neither A nor B is correct

25. Myelosuppression and immunosuppression are characteristic of:

    A. cytotoxic anticancer drugs
    B. hormonal anticancer drugs
    C. both A and B are correct
    D. neither A nor B is correct

26. T F Hormonal anticancer drugs produce cytotoxic side effects.

27. All of the following are characteristic of leucovorin rescue except:

    A. it has not been more effective for many cancers than conventional dose methotrexate..
    B. the malignant cells may be rescued as well as the normal cells.
    C. forced hydration is necessary to prevent renal toxicity
    D. easy to perform, inexpensive, and can be done on an outpatient basis.

28. T F In combination cancer therapy a drug is often chosen that has no effect against the specific cancer cells when used alone.

29. The dentist has the responsibility to:

    A. initiate cancer chemotherapy in a patient with oral malignancy
    B. diagnose cancer of the oral mucosa if he sees the patient first
    C. radiate the oral cancer
    D. refer xerostomia problems after radiation therapy to a physician

SECTION IV
APPENDICES: SPECIAL PROBLEMS OF DRUG USE IN DENTAL PRACTICE

—— APPENDIX I. ——

Emergency Drugs

A. INTRODUCTION

1. The best way of dealing with dental office emergencies is by **prevention.** Prevention of office emergencies is based upon:
   a. knowing the patient (through health history, and so on)
   b. knowing the medications you are using
   c. knowing the warning signs of an impending emergency
2. Principles of emergency use of drugs:
   a. Drug therapy is **symptomatic.**
   b. Drug therapy is a **temporary** measure.
   c. Never substitute drug therapy for **simpler** methods.
   d. Drugs must be regularly **updated** according to expiration dates.
   e. Side effects must not outweigh the benefit of the drug (**risk:benefit ratio**).
   f. Drugs should be one part of an **emergency plan.**
3. Suggested office emergency plan:
   a. Every dentist and auxiliary should take a course in **cardiopulmonary resuscitation.**

   b. The dentist should instruct each of his auxiliaries in his or her exact role during an emergency (The Office Plan). The dentist is leader of the emergency team and should supervise the performance of all suggested steps until a physician (or other qualified expert) arrives.
   c. Cardiopulmonary procedures should be reviewed periodically by study and refresher courses, including actual practice.
   d. The Office Plan should be reviewed at least once a month with all personnel.
   e. The Office Plan should include ready access to phone numbers of physicians or cardiopulmonary emergency teams who can be enlisted for help.

B. DEALING WITH THE DENTAL EMERGENCY SITUATION

1. General procedures for all emergencies
   a. reposition patient
      (usually supine)

TABLE AI-1. DENTAL EMERGENCY DRUGS

Drug[a]	Indication(s)	Adult Dose[b] and Route	Mechanism of Action
epinephrine (Adrenalin HCl)	anaphylaxis acute asthma laryngeal edema	0.3–0.5 mg IV, IM, sc[c] 0.3–0.5 mg IM, sc 0.3–0.5 mg IM, sc	beta-mediated broncho-dilation
aminophylline	asthma	250 mg to 500 mg (over 20 min) IV	direct bronchial relaxation
mephentermine (Wyamine)	acute hypotensive crisis	10–30 mg IM or sc	direct and indirect stimulation of cardiac beta and vascular alpha receptor
nitroglycerin	angina pectoris	0.3 mg tablet sublingual	vasodilation, reduced cardiac work
amyl nitrite	angina pectoris	crush Vaporole and allow patient to inhale vapor	vasodilation, reduced cardiac work
diazoxide (Hyperstat)	acute hypertension	100–150 mg IV (rapid)	direct vasodilation
diphenhydramine (Benadryl)	mild or delayed allergy secondary drug in anaphylaxis	50 mg IM	H_1 receptor blockade
methylprednisolone (Solu-Medrol)	acute allergy (adjunct) adjunct in shock	125 mg IV over 1 minute	suppression of inflammatory response and reduction of capillary permeability
spirits of ammonia	syncope	crush Vaporole, allow patient to inhale vapor	Chemical irritation of respiratory tract, reflex stimulation of CNS
diazepam[d] (Valium)	status epilepticus local anesthetic-induced convulsions	2–20 mg, titrated slowly IV	neural depression
naloxone	narcotic overdose	0.4 mg IV, IM or sc	opiate receptor blocker
50% dextrose solution	acute hypoglycemia accompanied by partial or total loss of consciousness	50 ml slowly by IV	direct elevation of blood glucose
sugar cubes	acute hypoglycemia with unimpaired consciousness	oral ingestion prn	direct elevation of blood glucose
morphine sulfate[d]	adjunct to relieve pain of myocardial infarction	5 to 15 mg sc	central analgesia and sedation
nitrous oxide	adjunct to relieve pain of myocardial infarction	inhalation of 50% N_2O/50% O_2 via nasal hood	central analgesia and sedation
oxygen	variety of emergencies in which respiratory difficulty present (100% O_2 not to be used in emphysemic patients)	inhalation of 100% O_2 by mask or with positive pressure ventilation by trained personnel	saturation of alveolar spaces with oxygen

TABLE AI-1. (*Continued*)

Drug[a]	Indication(s)	Adult Dose[b] and Route	Mechanism of Action
glucagon	acute hypoglycemia accompanied by partial or total loss of consciousness	0.5–1.0 unit sc or IM	increased blood glucose level by promotion of liver glycogen mobilization

[a] This list includes representative drugs and commonly recognized proprietary names and is not intended to exclude the use of other equivalent products and generic preparations when they are indicated.
[b] Child doses must be calculated according to manufacturer's recommendations.
[c] sc, subcutaneously.
[d] Morphine and diazepam are controlled substances and require special inventory and disposal and double-locking.

b. Airway patent?
  neck extended
  mandible and tongue anterior
c. Breathing OK?
  if breathing OK, administer oxygen with mask and bag
  if not, administer mouth-to-mouth resuscitation
d. Circulation OK?
  check pulse (radial, carotid)
  check heart and blood pressure
  external cardiac massage, if necessary (patient on hard surface)
e. Call for help!
  (as soon as possible)

C. TABLE OF DENTAL EMERGENCY DRUGS

Table AI–1 contains a list of emergency drugs that may be useful to the dentist. It contains only the drugs that are considered life-saving or preventive of further complications in certain specific emergency situations. It is deemed ad-visable for the dentist to have these drugs available in his emergency kit, and the dentist should become familiar with the use of these agents by studying them in the appropriate chapters of this book and in other reference sources.

The dentist may wish to have other emergency drugs in his emergency kit for use after a medical team arrives. Antiarrhythmic drugs are an example; when used with proper medical care and patient monitoring, such drugs may be extremely useful, but the dentist is usually unprepared (in a private office situation) to handle such emergencies. In such cases, it is best to content oneself with the basics of CPR until a medical team is available.

BIBLIOGRAPHY

Gilman AG, Goodman LS, Gilman A (eds): Goodman and Gilman's The Pharmacological Basis of Therapeutics, 6th ed. New York, Macmillan, 1980, Ch 8, 20, 32, 63

Malamed SF: Handbook of Medical Emergencies in the Dental Office. St. Louis, Mosby, 1978

APPENDIX II.
Drug Interactions

A. INTRODUCTION

Drug interactions can occur at any site in the body, and, in fact, drug incompatibilities are a type of interaction which can occur before drugs enter the body. An example of drug incompatibility involves mixing drugs in solution; due to chemical or physical interaction, a precipitate may form. The resulting mixture may not only be harmful but also lack pharmacologic activity.

B. MECHANISMS OF DRUG INTERACTION

An exhaustive list of mechanisms of drug interaction is not presented, since we are only concerned with dental drug interactions. Additional details, if needed, can be found in the publications listed in the Bibliography or drug package inserts.

The following is a list of known mechanisms of dental drug interactions.

1. Receptor interactions include:
   a. pharmacologic antagonism
   b. physiologic antagonism
   c. antibiotics binding at the same site on a ribosome
2. Additive or complementary interactions (effects) include:
   a. two drugs with the same effect, producing an additive or supra-additive effect
   b. combination of two complementary adverse effects
3. GI interactions include:
   a. presence of food markedly decreasing absorption
   b. alteration of GI motility
   c. drug interference of GI absorption
   d. inhibition of enteric, vitamin K-producing bacteria
4. Enzyme interactions include:
   a. induction of liver microsomal enzymes
   b. inhibition of liver or other enzyme systems
5. Renal interactions include:
   a. inhibition of active renal secretion
   b. alteration of urine pH to cause increased or decreased renal excretion or to increase the incidence of crystalluria

TABLE AII–1. DRUG INTERACTIONS

Dental Drug[a]	Second Agent	Possible Response[b]
aminoglycosides (e.g., streptomycin)	ethacrynic acid	↑ ototoxicity; ↑ nephrotoxicity
	furosemide	↑ ototoxicity; ↑ nephrotoxicity
	cephalosporins	↑ nephrotoxicity
aminophylline	propranolol	reversal of propranol effect
anticholinergic	amantadine	confusion, hallucinations
	tricyclic antidepressants	↑ xerostomia
	levodopa	↓ levodopa effect
	methotrimeprazine	↑ extrapyramidal effect
	phenothiazines	↑ xerostomia
propantheline only	food	↓ propantheline absorption
	digoxin (slow dissolving)	↑ absorption of digoxin
	digitalis	antagonizes vagomimetic response of digitalis
barbiturates	oral anticoagulants	↓ anticoagulant effect
	tricyclic antidepressants	↓ antidepressant effect
	β blockers	↓ β blocking effect
	promethazine	↑ CNS depression
	ethanol	↑ CNS depression
	oral contraceptives	↓ contraception
	corticosteroids	↓ corticosteroid effect
	digitalis	↓ digitalization
	griseofulvin	↓ absorption of griseofulvin
	narcotic analgesics	↑ CNS depression
	monoamine oxidase inhibitors	↑ barbiturate effect
	phenothiazines	↑ CNS depression or ↓ antipsychotic effect
	phenytoin	↓ phenytoin effect
	primidone	↑ barbiturate effect
	quinidine	↓ quinidine effect
	rifampin	↓ barbiturate effect
	doxycycline	↓ doxycycline effect
	theophylline	↓ theophylline effect
carbamazepine	oral anticoagulants	↓ anticoagulant effect
	monoamine oxidase inhibitors	excitation, hyperpyrexia, convulsions
	doxycycline	↓ doxycycline effect
cephalosporins	probenecid	↑ cephalosporin effect
	aminoglycosides, colistin, furosemide, ethacrynic acid	↑ nephrotoxicity
	erythromycin, lincomycins, tetracycline, chloramphenicol	probably antagonize cephalosporins
choral hydrate	sedatives[c]	↑ CNS depression
	oral anticoagulants	↑ anticoagulant effect
chloramphenicol	oral anticoagulants	↑ or ↓ anticoagulant effect
	tolbutamide	↑ hypoglycemia
	iron	interferes with erythropoiesis
	penicillins and cephalosporins	antagonizes penicillins and probably cephalosporins
	vitamin B_{12}	interferes with erythropoiesis
	phenytoin	↑ phenytoin effect

TABLE AII–1. (*Continued*)

Dental Drug[a]	Second Agent	Possible Response[b]
clindamycin	erythromycin	mutually antagonistic
	penicillins and cephalosporins	probably antagonize penicillins and cephalosporins
corticosteroids	oral anticoagulants	ulcerogenic with ↑ bleeding
	antidiabetic	loss of antidiabetic control
	chlorthalidone	↑ potassium loss
	ephedrine	↓ corticosteroid response
	ethacrynic acid	↑ potassium loss
	furosemide	↑ potassium loss
	indomethacin	↑ ulcerogenic effect
	phenytoin	↓ corticosteroid effect
	rifampin	↓ corticosteroid effect
	salicylates	↑ ulcerogenic effect
	tetracycline	↑ incidence of superinfection
	thiazide diuretics	↑potassium loss
benzodiazepines	sedatives[c]	↑ CNS depression
diazepam only	levodopa	↓ levodopa effect
diphenhydramine	aminosalicylic acid	↓ aminosalicylic acid effect
	sedatives[c]	↑ CNS depression
ephedrine	guanethidine	loss of antihypertensive control
	monoamine oxidase inhibitors	hypertensive crisis
epinephrine	tricyclic antidepressants	may result in increased blood pressure; exercise caution
	antidiabetic	may cause hyperglycemia
	propranolol	↑ blood pressure; exercise caution
	monoamine oxidase inhibitors	may result in ↑ blood pressure; exercise caution
erythromycin	lincomycin	mutually antagonistic
	clindamycin	mutually antagonistic
	penicillins and cephalosporins	antagonizes penicillins and cephalosporins
	theophylline	↑ theophylline effect
ethchlorvynol	oral anticoagulants	↓ anticoagulant effect
	sedatives[c]	↑ CNS depression
glutethimide	oral anticoagulants	↓ anticoagulant effect
	sedatives[c]	↑ CNS depression
hydroxyzine	sedatives[c]	↑ CNS depression
norepinephrine	tricyclic antidepressants	may result in increased blood pressure; exercise caution
	guanethidine	may result in increased blood pressure; exercise caution
	methyldopa	may result in increased blood pressure; exercise caution
	monoamine oxidase inhibitors	may result in increased blood pressure; exercise caution
levonordefrin	There are few or no reports in the literature describing drug interactions with levonordefrin. However, since this drug is so similar to epinephrine and norepinephrine, both chemically and pharmacologically, the practitioner should refer to the statements for epinephrine and norepinephrine.	

TABLE AII–1. DRUG INTERACTIONS (*Continued*)

Dental Drug[a]	Second Agent	Possible Response[b]
lincomycin	food	↓ absorption lincomycin
	cyclamates	↓ absorption lincomycin
	erythromycin	mutually antagonistic
	koalin–pectin	↓ absorption lincomycin
	penicillins and cephalosporins	probably antagonizes penicillins and cephalosporins
meprobamate	sedatives[c]	↑ CNS depression
methaqualone	sedatives[c]	↑ CNS depression
narcotic-analgesics	monoamine oxidase inhibitors	excitation, sweating, rigidity, hypertension; or hypotension and coma
	sedatives[c]	↑ CNS depression
methadone only	rifampin	↓ methadone effect
penicillins	chloramphenicol	penicillin antagonism
	erythromycin	penicillin antagonism
	lincomycins	penicillin antagonism
	food	↓ absorption of penicillins (except amoxicillin)
	probenecid	↑ penicillin effect
	oral neomycin	↓ absorption of penicillin V
	tetracycline	penicillin antagonism
oxacillin only	sulfonamides	↓ absorption of oxacillin
phenylephrine	tricyclic antidepressants	possible pressor effect; exercise caution
	guanethidine	possible pressor effect; exercise caution
	monoamine oxidase inhibitors	possible pressor effect; exercise caution
procaine	echothiophate iodide	↓ metabolism of procaine
	sulfonamides	antagonize sulfas
promethazine	sedatives[c]	↑ CNS depression
propoxyphene	oral anticoagulants	↑ anticoagulant effect
	carbamazepine	↑ carbamazepine effect
	food	↓ absorption propoxyphene
salicylates	ethanol	↑ gastrointestinal bleeding
	p-aminosalicylic acid (PAS)	↑ PAS toxicity
	ammonium chloride	↑ renal reabsorption of salicylates
	oral anticoagulants	↑ anticoagulant effect
	antidiabetic	↑ hypoglycemia
	corticosteroids	↑ ulcerogenic effect
	food	delayed analgesia
	heparin	↑ anticoagulant effect
	methotrexate	↑ methotrexate effect
	phenytoin	↑ phenytoin effect
	probenecid	↓ uricosuric effect
	sulfinpyrazone	↓ uricosuric effect
sulfonamides	PABA local anesthetics	antagonize sulfa effect
	oral anticoagulants	may ↑ anticoagulant effect
	antidiabetic	↑ hypoglycemia
	methenamine	↑ crystalluria
	methotrexate	↑ methotrexate effect

TABLE AII–1. (*Continued*)

Dental Drug[a]	Second Agent	Possible Response[b]
sulfonamides (*Cont.*)	oxacillin	↓ absorption oxacillin
	paraldehyde	↑ crystalluria
tetracyclines	antacids	↓ absorption tetracycline
	oral anticoagulants	possible ↑ anticoagulant effect
	corticosteroids	possible severe suprainfection
	diuretics	elevated BUN
	milk and dairy products	↓ absorption tetracycline
	iron	↓ absorption tetracycline
	zinc	↓ absorption tetracycline
	penicillins and cephalosporins	antagonize penicillins and cephalosporins
oxytetracycline only	antidiabetic drugs	↑ hypoglycemia
doxycycline only	alcohol	↑ metabolism of doxycycline
	barbiturates	↑ metabolism of doxycycline
	carbamazepine	↑ metabolism of doxycycline
	phenytoin	↑ metabolism of doxycycline
trimethoprim	oral anticoagulant	may disturb anticoagulant effect
	sulfamethoxasole or antidiabetic	↑ hypoglycemia

[a] Drug group names instead of individual drug names are used for aminoglycosides, anticholinergics, barbiturates, cephalosporins, corticosteroids, benzodiazepines, narcotic-analgesics, penicillins, salicylates, sulfonamides, and tetracyclines.

[b] Possible response: response may or may not occur, or if it does occur, the severity may be variable.

[c] Sedatives include all drugs having a sedative effect, especially antianxiety drugs, antihistamines, barbiturate and non-barbiturate sedative-hypnotics, ethanol, narcotic-analgesics, antipsychotics, and tricyclic antidepressants.

6. Miscellaneous interactions include:
   a. displacement from plasma protein-binding sites
   b. antibiotic protein synthesis inhibitors antagonize antibiotic cell wall synthesis inhibitors

C. DENTAL DRUG INTERACTIONS

Drug interactions for each dental drug are summarized in Table AII–1. This is not intended to cover every drug interaction; rather, the list involves only drug interactions for drugs which dentists use. Because we list two agents as causing a drug interaction, it is not implied that their use together is an absolute contraindication. In some cases, the interaction may be a relative contraindication, requiring only a precaution or reduction of dosage. The practitioner is urged to refer to package inserts concerning absolute ("warnings") and relative ("cautions" or "precautions") contraindications. Moreover, the list does not include most beneficial interactions, such as the administration of penicillin G and streptomycin which produces a synergistic, bactericidal effect. Finally, the list does not include the following: (1) drug interactions that require no special precaution, (2) interactions that have been reported only one time or are not well documented, (3) interactions that occur only when the agent is given by a route not usually used by a dentist (e.g., IV lidocaine), and (4) interactions for agents that are used solely by anesthesiologists in a hospital operating room (e.g., succinylcholine).

BIBLIOGRAPHY

Gilman AG, Goodman LS, Gilman A (eds): Goodman and Gilman's The Pharmacological Basis of Therapeutics, 6th ed. New York, Macmillan, 1980

Hansten PD: Drug Interactions, 4th ed. Philadelphia, Lea & Febiger, 1979

APPENDIX III:
Drug Abuse

A. INTRODUCTION

The importance of the dentist's understanding of the abuse of drugs is underscored by its increasingly wide occurrence in the general patient population and also within the profession. Recognition of the characteristics, both physical and affective, of various types of drug abuse in dental patients will enable the dentist to better handle this situation when it presents in his office, not only in terms of avoiding dangerous drug interactions and serious medical emergencies but also in curtailing the illicit procurement of drugs through the abuse of dental prescriptions.

B. GLOSSARY OF TERMS

Drug Abuse. Self-administration of a drug in a nonprescribed manner, leading to abnormal behavior and mental states and, in many cases, to tolerance and dependence.

Psychologic Dependence. A condition in which the effects produced by a drug or the conditions

associated with its uses are necessary to maintain an optimal state of well being (equivalent to "habituation").

Tolerance. A condition in which repeated administration of a drug results in a given dose producing progressively reduced effects or results in increasingly larger doses required to produce the same effect.

Physical Dependence. An altered physiologic state produced by repeated administration of a drug which necessitates continued use of the drug to prevent the occurrence of a withdrawal syndrome. (Tolerance and physical dependence usually develop concurrently but are not necessarily associated.)

Cross-Dependence. The ability of one drug to suppress the withdrawal syndrome of another drug while maintaining a state of tolerance and dependence (may be **partial** or **complete**). For example, all narcotic-analgesics (opiates or opioids) display cross-dependence with each other but not with sedative-hypnotics (alcohol, barbiturates, and nonbarbiturate sedative-hypnotics), and vice versa.

445

Addiction. A behavioral pattern of compulsive drug use which involves overwhelming involvement with the procurement and use of a drug and a high tendency to relapse if the drug is withdrawn. Addiction is not equivalent to physical dependence, and the terms "addiction" and "addict" are so poorly defined that other, better defined terms should be used, e.g., dependence, habituation.

Withdrawal. The removal of an abused drug from a dependent patient. During the withdrawal period, there may be mild to severe physical and psychologic signs and symptoms, depending on the drug that was taken, its dose, the duration of its abuse, and the psychologic state of the abuser.

Abstinence Syndrome. The group of signs and symptoms that is characteristic of withdrawal from a specific type of abused drug.

C. CAUSES OF DRUG ABUSE

Positive Euphoria. A state induced in the individual that causes a feeling of well-being or elation (getting high); euphoria is characteristic of cocaine and amphetamine abuse.

Negative Euphoria. A state of coming down from a drug-induced high or, simply, a disposition to calm down after an excited state, especially with sedative abuse.

Escape from Reality. The state of an individual who can no longer cope with his present situation; the action of the drug is thought to psychologically dissociate the subject from his environment.

Social Peer Pressure. A characteristic of drug abuse, often seen among younger people, where the drug is abused simply because it is the thing to do and other members of the peer group use it. The drug may be any one of the drugs of abuse, depending on group preference.

D. CLASSES OF DRUGS OF ABUSE AND THEIR CHARACTERISTICS

Opiates and Opioids (synthetic narcotic-analgesics)

1. Strong psychologic and physical dependence
2. Rapid development of tolerance
3. Produce euphoria
4. Lethal dose increases with tolerance
5. Produce toxic abstinence syndrome
   a. Early symptoms (10 to 12 hours) are exaggerated autonomic responses, including dilated pupils, diaphoresis, rhinitis, yawning, gooseflesh, tremor, and elevation of temperature; also, crying, loss of appetite, insomnia, weakness, and restlessness.
   b. Late symptoms (24 hours) are vomiting, diarrhea, agitated movements, mania, abdominal cramps, weight loss, high fever, and possibly death.
   c. Recovery occurs in 3 to 4 days.
6. Commonly abused opiates
   a. morphine—important narcotic-analgesic, produces drowsiness and euphoria
   b. heroin—preferred by narcotic abusers for slightly greater euphorogenic properties than morphine; initial euphoria when mainlined; later, the drug becomes necessary for maintenance of a feeling of normalcy
   c. meperidine (*Demerol*)—widely used synthetic narcotic-analgesic; primary narcotic of abuse by medical professionals
   d. codeine—important analgesic and cough suppressant; tolerance develops more slowly than with morphine
7. Street names
   a. Heroin—dope, skag, horse, big H
   b. Heroin + cocaine—speedball
   c. Heroin + amphetamine + tuinal—bombita
8. Dental complications
   a. Tolerance to ordinary analgesic doses of narcotics

b. Potentiation of sedative drugs and other depressants
c. Additive respiratory depression following local anesthetic toxicity
d. Precipitation of withdrawal syndrome if pentazocine, butorphanol, or nalbuphine are used
e. High percentage of abusers are hepatitis carriers (5% of heroin abusers)
f. Prone to other systemic infections
g. Frequent attempts to obtain narcotic prescriptions from dental practitioners

Sedative-Hypnotic Drugs Including Barbiturates, Alcohol, and Nonbarbiturate Sedative-Hypnotics

1. Strong psychologic and physical dependence
2. Requires prolonged and intense abuse for dependence development
3. Tolerance develops before dependence
4. Lethal dose does not increase with tolerance
5. Produce sedation, depression, "high" with lower dose and inebriation with higher dose
6. Withdrawal syndrome more toxic than opiate withdrawal (15% death rate)

    The withdrawal syndrome after alcohol abuse is often referred to as **delirium tremens** (DTs) and is characterized by hallucinations, tremors, nervousness, increases of blood pressure, heart rate, and respiratory rate, nausea, vomiting, and potential development of severe grand mal-type convulsive seizures, with dangerous postseizure respiratory depression. Barbiturate withdrawal may result in a similar type of syndrome.
7. Street names of abused barbiturates
    a. amobarbital—goof balls, blue heavens
    b. tuinal (amobarbital + secobarbital)—tuies, Christmas trees, rainbows
    c. glutethimide—cibas
    d. methaqualone—ludes, sopars, 714s
    e. pentobarbital—yellow jackets
    f. phenobarbital—purple hearts

g. secobarbital—reds, red birds, red devils
8. Dental complications of alcohol and barbiturate abuse
    a. Potentiation of CNS depressants, including narcotic analgesics
    b. Possible reduction of sedative effect of preoperative medications due to tolerance or induction of drug-metabolizing enzymes
    c. Attempts to obtain illicit prescriptions from dental practitioner
    d. Alcohol-induced liver dysfunction, with potentiation of toxic effects of narcotic-analgesics, amide-type local anesthetics, and other drugs

CNS Stimulants, Including Amphetamines and Cocaine

1. Euphoric excitement, feeling of increased endurance
2. Sexual arousal and enhancement of sexual pleasures
3. Produce psychologic dependence
4. Cocaine produces tolerance very slowly, amphetamines more rapidly
5. Amphetamines may or may not produce physical dependence, cocaine probably does not
6. CNS stimulation is followed by depression and fatigue, or the so-called crash, which necessitates further abuse
7. Commonly abused CNS stimulants
    a. amphetamines—sympathomimetic with potent CNS excitement
    b. cocaine—only local anesthetic with abuse potential
        (1) Frequently causes necrosis of nasal septum due to intense vasoconstriction (SNS mimetic effect)
        (2) Death can result from respiratory depression during depressive state
        (3) Frequent development of psychosis
    c. decongestants (*Dristan* inhaler, ephedrine, *Wyamine*)
    d. methylphenidate (*Ritalin*)

8. Street names of CNS stimulants
   a. amphetamine—uppers, bennies, splash, peaches
   b. dextroamphetamine—dexies, copilots, oranges
   c. amphetamine + dextroamphetamines —footballs
   d. methamphetamine—meth, crystal, speed
   e. cocaine—coke, cake, snow, big C, candy, girl, charlie
9. Dental complications of stimulant abuse
   a. Patient restlessness, irritability
   b. Hypertension, possible hypertensive crisis, cerebral hemorrhage, worsening of vasoconstrictor toxicity
   c. Increased tendency toward convulsions, worsening of local anesthetic-induced convulsions
   d. Attempts to obtain illicit prescriptions
   e. Systemic infections associated with intravenous abuse

Psychotogens (Hallucinogens, Includes LSD and Mescaline)

1. Produce tolerance
2. Physical dependence does not occur
3. Signs of abuse include hypertension, accelerated heart rate, tremor, fever
4. Subject-dependent euphoria or dysphoria (variable effects depend on psychologic state of user)
5. Schizophrenic-like perceptual effects, primarily visual hallucinations, disorientation, sedation can be produced
6. Frequently diluted (cut) with other agents
7. Mind-body detachment (bad trip)
8. Creativity not enhanced; mental processes are impaired and confused
9. Street names of psychotogens
   a. LSD (lysergic acid diethylamide)—acid
   b. mescaline—white light, blue caps, pink wedge, peyote
   c. phencyclidine—angel dust, peace pill, DOA

   d. diethyltryptamine—DET
   e. dimethyltryptamine—DMT
   f. dipropyltryptamine—DPT
   g. 2,5-dimethyl-4-methyl amphetamine —STP, DOM
   h. 3-methoxy-4,5-methylenedioxy amphetamine—love pill, MDA
10. Dental complications of psychotogen abuse
    a. Patient disorientation, panic reaction, psychotic behavior
    b. Flashbacks to psychosis can be triggered by administration of CNS drugs, including narcotic analgesics, sedatives
    c. Possible hypertensive crisis, worsening of vasoconstrictor toxicity

Nitrous Oxide

Recent epidemiologic surveys have indicated that the abuse of nitrous oxide in dental offices is on the increase. Abuse occurs by the self-administration of nitrous oxide by dentists and auxiliary personnel and by after-hours abuse by maintenance personnel. The dangers of nitrous oxide abuse are outlined below.

1. Severe hypoxia with possible coma and death: this is especially likely when the drug is abused by a lone individual (without monitoring by an accomplice) who can become drowsy and then become unconscious
2. Peripheral neuropathies associated with prolonged exposure (Layzer, 1978): this diffuse polyneuropathy occurs following the self-administration of N_2O, as well as in dentists who are inadvertently exposed to high ambient gas concentrations, e.g., through leaky gas tubing. The syndrome is predominantly sensory, rather than motor, and while removal from N_2O abuse or the N_2O environment may result in a gradual reversal of symptoms, some of the damage may be permanent.

Marijuana

1. Physical dependence does not occur.
2. Varying degrees of psychologic depen-

dence and tolerance may occur, depending on the extent of the habit and the psychologic state of the abuser.

3. Affective responses vary greatly, usually reported as a euphoria.
4. Central effects
   a. sedation
   b. psychogenic (mind-altering, possible hallucinations)
   c. euphoriant
   d. psychotic-like symptoms, including time-space distortion, loss of memory, flashbacks, depersonalization
   e. vertigo, postural instability
5. Cardiovascular effects:
   a. increased heart rate
   b. conjunctival injection
6. Other side effects
   a. bronchitis
   b. asthma

E. AGENTS USED IN TREATMENT OF DRUG DEPENDENCE

1. Naloxone (narcotic-antagonist) is the drug of choice for reversing acute narcotic toxicity. Its short duration of action may require repeated injection. This agent must be used cautiously in patients with opioid dependence because it causes a severe withdrawal syndrome.
2. Nalophorine was the first narcotic antagonist but has been largely replaced by naloxone.
3. Methadone
   a. Orally effective synthetic narcotic
   b. Satisfies craving for drugs; produces less euphoria. Methadone, when taken during therapy, blocks euphoric effect of heroin.
   c. Allows gradual withdrawal and normal performance of tasks during therapy.
4. Disulfiram (Antabuse)
   a. Preventive therapy in alcoholism
   b. Blocks metabolism of alcohol (acetaldehyde cannot be converted to acetate)
   c. Ingestion of alcohol during therapy causes nausea, vomiting, and chest pain due to acetaldehyde build-up
5. Chlordiazepoxide (Librium), diazepam (Valium), or flurazepam (Dalmane) is frequently used as an alcohol replacement and then gradually withdrawn.
6. Pentobarbital (Nembutal) or phenobarbital (Luminal) is frequently used as a replacement drug for patients who are dependent on barbiturate or nonbarbiturate sedative-hypnotics. After replacement therapy is complete, the replacement drug is gradually withdrawn.
7. Benzodiazepine withdrawal is usually gradually performed, using the benzodiazepine of dependence.

F. RECOGNITIONS OF DRUG ABUSE IN THE DENTAL PRACTICE

The recognition of the abuse of drugs in the dental practice is important to prevent life-threatening drug interactions, patient management problems, and attempts to use the dentist to illicitly obtain drugs. The following guidelines will assist the recognition of the drug-abusing patient:

1. Health and family history
   a. note patient condition
   b. ask patient about drug abuse if suspected
   c. history of past pain syndromes which were treated with narcotic analgesics
   d. history of past psychiatric therapy treated with CNS depressants or stimulants
   e. history of insomnia treated with CNS depressants
2. Note important physical signs
   a. Heart rate, blood pressure, and pupil size
   b. sedation or central stimulation (restlessness, and so on)
   c. odor
   d. signs of self-administered injections
   e. systemic infections (especially hepatitis)

3. Note suspicious requests for medications
   a. patient reports severe pain but never seems to make appointments
   b. out-of-town patient requests narcotic analgesics over the phone, cannot appear at office
   c. patient reports pain that is greatly out of line with severity of procedure
   d. patient requests "special preference" drugs, stronger than required

REFERENCE

Layzer RB: Myeloneuropathy after prolonged exposure to nitrous oxide. Lancet 313:1227, 1978

BIBLIOGRAPHY

Gilman AG, Goodman LS, Gilman A (eds): Goodman and Gilman's The Pharmacological Basis of Therapeutics, 6th ed. New York, Macmillan, 1980, Ch 23.

APPENDIX IV.

Antiseptics and Disinfectants

One of the most important requirements of a dental practice is protection of the patient and operators from spread of infection. This requires proper use of sterilizing procedures (which kill all forms of life) as well as disinfection, asepsis, antisepsis, cleanliness, and hygienic care of skin. Whenever possible, autoclaving is the preferred method, since steam heat under pressure at high temperatures is the best method of killing microbes. Sterilization is an absolute requirement for any instrument that will enter human tissues. The subject of sterilization is not covered in detail in this text. These details can be found in textbooks of microbiology and in handbooks of operating procedures.

Although autoclaving is preferred, it is not always possible, so there is still a need for other methods of controlling microbial growth. Chemical antiseptics and disinfectants are, therefore, important, as are the proper use of asepsis, cleanliness, and hand cleaning. In this appendix, we review chemical antiseptics and disinfectants and attempt to define their usefulness in dental practice.

A. DEFINITIONS

Antiseptic. A substance which, when used on living tissue, kills or prevents growth of microbes.

Disinfectant. A substance which, when used on inanimate objects, destroys pathogenic microbes.

Sterilization. Complete destruction of all forms of life by physical or chemical means. (*Note:* it is possible to achieve sterilization with a disinfectant, although any use of disinfectants is discouraged when physical sterilization is possible).

Germicidal. Indicates an action that kills microbes (including bactericidal, fungicidal, virucidal actions). Chemical disinfectants often cause stasis at low concentrations but sometimes are cidal at higher concentrations.

Asepsis. The technique of preventing introduction of microbes into a sterile field.

451

TABLE AIV-1. FEATURES OF ANTISEPTICS AND DISINFECTANTS

Group Name Agent Name	Activity and Spectrum	Degree of Activity	Agents that Deactivate	Stability
Phenols phenol	0.2% static 1.0% bactericidal 1.3% fungicidal	intermediate to low	soap glycerin lipids	good
cresol (methyl substituted phenol)	about 4 × more active than phenol	intermediate	same as phenol	good
hexachlorophene (halogen substituted phenol)	3% kills gram-positive in 15–30 seconds, primarily gram-positive, long time required for full spectrum	low	compatible with soap	good
parabens (benzoic acid derivatives: methyl, ethyl, propyl, butyl)	active at 1/200–1/500	low	pus	good
Alcohols ethanol	70% optimal, kills 90% of skin bacteria in 2 minutes	intermediate	none	good (flammable)
isopropyl	70–90% slightly better than ethanol	intermediate	none	good (flammable)
Aldehydes formaldehyde	3–8% needed; slow (20–30 minutes needed)	high to intermediate	organic matter	volatile, pungent
glutaraldehyde	better than formaldehyde; 2% kills in 10 minutes except spores (10 hours)	high	acid stabilizes but lowers activity	14-day shelf-life (polymerizes)
Halogens iodine	cidal, rapid and potent, wide spectrum	intermediate	none	good
povidone-iodine (neutral polymer which releases I)	less active than tincture; 10% → 1% I	intermediate to low	none	good

452

Agent	Comments		Inactivators	
Oxidizing agents				
hydrogen peroxide	$H_2O_2 \rightarrow H_2O + O$, 3% on skin or 1.5% on mucosa, kills anaerobes	low	catalase; organic matter	low
urea peroxide (carbamide peroxide)	10% in glycerol is equal to 3% H_2O_2	low	catalase; organic matter	moderate
sodium hypochlorite	dissolves pulpal tissue and organic matter, released chlorine is germicidal	high	none	low
Bisguanides				
chlorhexidine	wide spectrum but not vs spores; 4% better than povidone-iodine, equal to 3% hexachlorophene for cumulative effect	high	none	high
alexidine	same as chlorhexidine	high	none	high
Mercury compounds				
inorganics	wide but no effect on spores or TB bacilli	low	tissue, organic matter	good
thimerosal (merthiolate)	wide but no effect on spores or TB bacilli	low	tissue, organic matter	sunlight
Quaternary ammonium compounds (benzalkonium, cetylpyridinium or benzethonium chlorides)	surface active cationic detergents, gram-positive and gram-negative, resistant organisms grow well in the cold sterilizing solution, slow action (7 minutes) for 50% kill on skin, 7 hours for 98% kill of E. coli	low	organic matter, anionic detergents and soaps	good

TABLE AIV–2. FEATURES OF ANTISEPTICS AND DISINFECTANTS

Group Name Agent Name	Corrosive or Destructive	Expense	Therapeutic Index	Comments
Phenols phenol	tissue (penetrates well)	low	low	used in mouthwash, local anesthesia, cavity sanitation, instrument disinfection, root canal sterilization
cresol (methyl substituted phenol)	same as phenol	low	better than phenol, still irritating	used in formocresol for root canal sterilization
hexachlorophene (halogen substituted phenol)	none	low	high tissue acceptability	in *Septisoft* (hand antiseptic); activity builds up and retained with repeat washings; withdrawn from OTC market because of brain damage in infants; may be teratogenic (pregnant staff)
parabens (benzoic acid derivatives: methyl, ethyl, propyl, butyl)	none	high	high	allergenic and cross-allergenic; used in pharmaceutical preparations as preservatives
Alcohols ethanol	coagulates tissue	low	not for use on open wounds	potentiates hexachlorphene or chlorhexidine; keep moist for maximum activity as a skin scrub
isopropyl	coagulates tissue	low	not for use on open wounds	same as ethanol; used as wipe for skin; also on immovable and non-autoclavable equipment between patients
Aldehydes formaldehyde	precipitates protein in higher concentration	low	causes tissue necrosis and dermatitis	used in instrument sterilization, can be combined (3–4%) in isopropyl alcohol; should not be used for tooth desensitization (irritant)
glutaraldehyde	carbon steel (after 24 hours), dissimilar metals (electrolysis)	moderate	irritates eyes and skin; wash instruments before use	may sensitize; best all purpose cold sterilizer; (USCDC[a]) excellent for rubber, tubing, plastics, and bonded materials

Agent	Effect on materials/tissue	Toxicity	Germicidal activity	Comments
Halogens				
iodine	clothing may stain, stains acrylic, silicate, or porcelain	low	high; good on skin and open wounds; allergenic	2% tincture with 2.4% NaI is best agent for skin or mucosa; use as a surgical preparation or on open wounds. Also used as disclosing agent
povidone-iodine (neutral polymer which releases I)	does not stain skin, stains clothing	moderate	high; cross-allergenic with I	used for surgical preparation; does not sting or irritate; used as preinjection scrub and on wounds
Oxidizing Agents				
hydrogen peroxide	breaks down newly granulating tissue; may decalcify tooth on prolonged use	low	high	foaming action (due to catalase) causes wound cleansing; used to cleanse and treat infected root canals; also as mouthwash in ANUG; causes hairy tongue (rarely)
urea peroxide (carbamide peroxide)	same as H_2O_2	moderate	high	source of H_2O_2; widely advertised to dentists for control of gingivitis; causes hairy tongue (rarely)
sodium hypochlorite	metals	low	low; do not apply to skin or mucosa	used in root canal therapy
Bisguanides				
chlorhexidine	none	low	high, can be used on open wounds	antiseptic handwash; surgical scrub and skin wound cleaner; effective vs plaque but stains teeth and may be allergenic; not approved for plaque control
alexidine	none	high	high	claimed to cause less stain; not approved for plaque control
Mercury compounds				
inorganics	none	low	cause skin allergy, systemic toxicity	no longer used, too toxic
thimerosal	none	low	well tolerated by tissue	scrub or use on wounds
Quaternary ammonium compounds (benzalkonium, cetylpyridinium or benzethonium chlorides)	none	low	high (but may cause allergy and sloughing)	used in mouthwash, gargles, lozenges; reacts with aluminum (of anesthetic cartridges); hard water may inactivate, disadvantages outweigh advantages

[a] Center for Disease Control.

Cleansing. Proper use of cleaners, such as soaps, detergents, surfactants, sonicators, and scrubs, is important because it is almost impossible to sterilize, disinfect, or use antiseptics effectively in the presence of foreign matter.

B. PROPERTIES OF AN IDEAL AGENT

Properties of an Ideal Disinfectant
1. germicidal activity
2. wide spectrum: sporicidal, fungicidal, virucidal
3. rapid activity
4. penetration of organic matter
5. cidal in presence of organic matter
6. compatible with soaps, detergents, and so on
7. chemically stable
8. noncorrosive to surgical instruments and nondestructive of other materials involved
9. pleasant odor and color and nonstaining
10. inexpensive, especially when used in large quantities

Properties of an Ideal Antiseptic
1. high degree of germicidal activity
2. wide spectrum of activity (narrower spectrum may be useful for specific indications)
3. cidal rather than static
4. low surface tension
5. active in presence of body fluids
6. rapid and sustained activity
7. high therapeutic index
8. low allergenicity

C. CLASSIFICATION BY CHEMICAL STRUCTURE AND COMPARISON TO IDEAL PROPERTIES

1. Tables AIV-1 and AIV-2 describe the important features of most antiseptic and disinfectant agents. The considerations for each agent include activity and spectrum, degree of activity, agents which deactivate, stability, corrosive or destructive, expense, therapeutic index, and comments.

2. Other important agents (not included in the tables) and their features are presented here.
   a. Miscellaneous phenols
      (1) Thymol, chlorothymol, and eugenol are essential oils with low antimicrobial activity. They are used in dentistry (especially eugenol) as anodynes and, combined with zinc oxide, for temporary fillings, as pulp coverings (on the nonexposed pulp), and in periodontal packs. These oils are irritants and caustic at moderate to high concentrations.
      (2) Parachlorophenol (PCP) is more potent than phenol. Combined with camphor, it has been recommended for root canal therapy. It is ineffective in the presence of pus and less effective than sodium hypochlorite.
      (3) Triclosan is a new antiseptic used in soaps and antiseptic solutions for skin disinfection and is also used in dermatologic conditions.
      (4) LPH is a mixture of phenols used to spray bench tops and fixed equipment.
   b. Iodoform is triiodomethane and has mild antiseptic and analgesic activity. It has been used as a dusting powder for open wounds, and it may be impregnated into gauze for insertion as a dressing into dry sockets (infected extraction sites). Other dressings for dry socket include preparations containing benzocaine, eugenol, iodine, chlorobutanol, guaiacol (a phenol derivative), and balsam of Peru.

D. CHOICE OF ANTISEPTICS AND DISINFECTANTS FOR DENTISTRY

The following methods of antisepsis and disinfection are preferred by the authors for the situations listed, although this does not preclude choices by other authorities.

1. Preferred germicidal methods
   a. Autoclave or dry heat methods

  b. Ethylene oxide—used industrially
  c. Ultraviolet light
2. Hand scrub or hand rinse
  a. Hexachlorophene soap or lotion
  b. Chlorhexidine rinse (*Hibistat*)
  c. Chlorhexidine scrub (*Hibiclens*)
  d. Povidone-iodine
3. Cold sterilization of nonautoclavable items
  a. Glutaraldehyde (*Cidex*)
4. Skin preparation and instrument wipe
  a. 70% Isopropyl alcohol
  b. povidone-iodine
5. Surgical preparation
  a. Chlorhexidine (*Hibitane*)
  b. Tincture of iodine
  c. povidone-iodine
6. Root canal antiseptic
  a. sodium hypochlorite (5.25%)
7. Operatory wipe and spray
  a. LPH spray
8. Anesthetic cartridges
  a. Sterile set-up—can be autoclaved (Parker, 1977)

  b. Aseptic technique—wipe diaphragm with tincture of iodine or soak in alcohol (10 minutes maximum)

REFERENCES AND BIBLIOGRAPHY

Accepted Dental Therapeutics, 38th ed. Chicago, American Dental Association, 1979, pp 63–79, 223–239

AMA Drug Evaluations, 3rd ed. Littleton, MA, Publishing Sciences Group, 1977, pp 883–884

Harvey SC: Antiseptics and disinfectants. In Gilman AG, Goodman LS, Gilman A (eds): Goodman and Gilman's The Pharmacological Basis of Therapeutics, 6th ed. New York, Macmillan, 1980, pp 964–981

Parker RL: The Effect of Autoclaving on the Stability of Epinephrine Contained in Lidocaine Solutions. M.S. Thesis, Medical College of Georgia, 1977, 31 pp

Willet HP: Sterilization and disinfection. In Joklick WK, Willet HP, Amos DB (eds): Zinsser's Microbiology, 17th ed. New York, Appleton-Century-Crofts, 1980, pp. 278–301

APPENDIX V.

Xerostomia-Producing Drugs

Many drugs produce xerostomia (dry mouth) as a primary or side effect. Table AV–1 contains a list of drugs reported to produce xerostomia as an effect.

The use of drugs for short-term xerostomia, such as during a dental procedure, has no known adverse effects on teeth or supporting structures. However, xerostomia induced by chronic drug therapy can be a destructive situation because the well-known protective qualities of saliva are lost. The same conditions and treatments could apply for radiation-induced xerostomia as for chronic drug-induced xerostomia.

Preventive dentistry is especially important in those patients with chronic xerostomia. The following list outlines some of the factors that should be considered in the management of these patients.

1. Insure that the patient is instructed in proper and thorough brushing and flossing of teeth.
2. Recommend that the patient brush and floss thoroughly after each meal, after snacks, and at bedtime.
3. Advise that affected patients be seen at three or four month recalls (rather than six months).
4. Advise a thorough scaling, prophylaxis, and fluoride treatment at every recall period.
5. Recommend the use of an ADA-recommended fluoride toothpaste and fluoride mouth rinse or gel (see also Chapter 11).
6. Recommend the use of an imitation saliva (e.g., *Xero-Lube*).
7. Counsel the patient concerning the use of cariogenic foods and beverages. This type of patient will often overuse such items as chewing gum, hard candies, lozenges, soft drinks, and so on, in an effort to keep the mouth moist. Since saliva may be reflexly stimulated in that manner, the method may be useful; however, sugarless items should be identified and used for this purpose.
8. Identify denture patients with xerostomia. They usually complain of more sore spots and problems with retention of dentures than do regular patients. Several of the items already mentioned above may help, but denture adhesives may also have to be used.

459

TABLE AV–1. DRUGS WITH THE POTENTIAL OF PRODUCING XEROSTOMIA

Antianxiety Drugs
 diazepam (*Valium*)
 flurazepam (*Dalmane*)
 prazepam (*Verstran*)

Anti-arrhythmics
 disopyramide (*Norpace*)
 procainamide (*Pronestyl*)
 quinidine

Anticholinergics
 anisotropine (*Valpin*)
 atropine
 belladonna alkaloids
 clidinium (*Quarzan*)
 cyclopentolate (*Cyclogyl*)
 dicyclomine (*Bentyl*)
 diphemanil (*Prantal*)
 glycopyrrolate (*Robinul*)
 hexocyclium (*Tral*)
 isopropamide (*Darbid*)
 mepenzolate (*Cantil*)
 methantheline (*Banthine*)
 methixene (*Trest*)
 oxyphencyclimine (*Daricon*)
 oxphenonium (*Antrenyl*)
 piperidolate (*Dactil*)
 propantheline (*Pro-Banthine*)
 scopolamine
 thiphenamil (*Trocinate*)
 tridihexethyl (*Pathilon*)
 tropicamide (*Mydriacyl*)

Antiemetics
 prochlorperazine (*Compazine*)
 promethazine (*Phenergan*)
 thiethylperazine (*Torecan*)
 triflupromazine (*Vesprin*)

Antihistamines
 antazoline (*Vasocon-A*)
 brompheniramine (*Dimetane*)
 carbinoxamine (*Clistin*)
 chlorpheniramine (*Chlor-Trimeton*)
 cyclizine (*Marezine*)
 cyproheptadine (*Periactin*)
 dimenhydrinate (*Dramamine*)
 diphenhydramine (*Benadryl*)
 hydroxyzine (*Atarax, Vistaril*)
 meclizine (*Antivert, Bonine*)
 promethazine (*Phenergan*)
 pyrilamine (*Neo-Antergan*)
 tripelennamine (*PBZ*)

Antihypertensives
 clonidine (*Catapres*)
 methyldopa (*Aldomet*)
 pargyline (*Eutonyl*)
 reserpine (*Serpasil*)

Antineoplastics
 procarbazine (*Matulane*)
 vinblastine (*Velban*)

Antiparkinson Drugs
 amantadine (*Symmetrel*)
 benztropine (*Cogentin*)
 biperiden (*Akineton*)
 chlorphenoxamine (*Phenoxene*)
 cycrimine (*Pagitane*)
 ethopropazine (*Parsidol*)
 levodopa (*Larodopa*)
 orphenadrine (*Disipal*)
 procyclidine (*Kemadrin*)
 trihexyphenidyl (*Artane*)

Antipsychotics
 acetophenazine (*Tindal*)
 chlorpromazine (*Thorazine*)
 chlorprothixene (*Taractan*)
 fluphenazine (*Permitil, Prolixin*)
 haloperidol (*Haldol*)
 lithium (*Lithane*)
 loxapine (*Daxolin, Loxitane*)
 mesoridazine (*Serentil*)
 molindone (*Lidone, Moban*)
 perphenazine (*Trilafon*)
 piperacetazine (*Quide*)
 thioridazine (*Mellaril*)
 thiothixene (*Navane*)
 trifluoperazine (*Stelazine*)
 triflupromazine (*Vesprin*)

Antitubercular
 isoniazid

CNS Stimulants and Antidepressants
 amitriptyline (*Elavil*)
 amoxapine (*Asendin*)
 amphetamine
 carbamazepine (*Tegretol*)
 desipramine (*Norpramin, Pertofrane*)
 doxepin (*Adapin, Sinequan*)
 imipramine (*Tofranil*)
 isocarboxazid (*Marplan*)
 maprotiline (*Ludiomil*)

TABLE AV-1. DRUGS WITH THE POTENTIAL OF PRODUCING XEROSTOMIA (*Continued*)

CNS (*Cont.*)
  nortriptyline (*Aventyl, Pamelor*)
  phenelzine (*Nardil*)
  protriptyline (*Vivactil*)
  tranylcypromine (*Parnate*)
  trimipramine (*Surmontil*)

Diuretics
  bendroflumethiazide (*Naturetin*)
  benzthiazide (*Exna*)
  chlorothiazide (*Diuril*)
  chlorthalidone (*Hygroton*)
  cyclothiazide (*Anhydron*)
  ethacrynic acid (*Edecrin*)
  furosemide (*Lasix*)
  hydrochlorothiazide (*Hydrodiuril*)
  hydroflumethiazide (*Saluron*)
  methyclothiazide (*Enduron*)
  metolazone (*Zaroxolyn*)
  polythiazide (*Renese*)
  quinethazone (*Hydromox*)
  spironolactone (*Aldactone*,

  triamterene (*Dyrenium*)
  trichlormethiazide (*Naqua*)

Ganglionic Blockers
  hexamethonium
  mecamylamine (*Inversine*)
  trimethaphan (*Arfonad*)

Muscle Relaxant
  baclofen (*Lioresal*)

Narcotic-Analgesics
  meperidine (*Demerol*)
  methadone (*Dolophine*)
  morphine
  nalbuphine (*Nubain*)
  pentazocine (*Talwin*)

Nonbarbiturate Sedative-Hypnotics
  glutethimide (*Doriden*)
  hydroxyzine (*Atarax, Vistaril*)
  methaqualone (*Quaalude, Sopor*)
  promethazine (*Phenergan*)

BIBLIOGRAPHY

Gilman AG, Goodman LS, Gilman A (eds): Goodman and Gilman's The Pharmacological Basis of Therapeutics, 6th ed. New York, Macmillan, 1980

Kastrup EK (ed): Facts and Comparisons, 1980 ed. St. Louis, Facts and Comparisons, 1980

Physicians' Desk Reference, 35th ed. Oradell, NJ, Medical Economics, 1981

OTC Dental Drugs and Devices

The following is based upon a 5-year review (1973–1978) of dentifrices and dental care agents by an FDA-appointed panel of experts, the Dentifrices and Dental Care Agents (DDCA) Panel. DDCA was charged with review of all products contained in dental OTC drugs except for antiseptics and mouthwashes, which were assigned to a second panel, the OTC Oral Cavity Panel. This report considers only the work of the DDCA Panel; the Oral Cavity Panel report was not available at the time of this report.

Before this review, industrial firms or other interested parties were asked, through an announcement in the Federal Register (January 5, 1972, 37FR85) to submit any data on OTC products contained in dentifrices and dental care products except mouthwashes and oral antiseptics. After preliminary review of submitted products, the DDCA classified dentifrices and dental care ingredients into the following types of products:

1. Denture aids
2. Dental plaque-disclosing agents
3. Agents for oral mucosal injury

4. Agents for the relief of oral discomfort
5. Anticaries agents

Although the Panel was charged with categorizing each ingredient as to its safety, effectiveness, and other conditions (such as labeling), the official categorization is not presented here because it is not final at the time of this publication.

A brief report on each class of ingredients is presented because this may aid the dentist in the evaluation and use of OTC dental care products by dental patients.

A. DENTURE AIDS

After DDCA convened, all denture aids were classified as devices, and the DDCA recommendations were referred to the Bureau of Medical Devices and Drug Products (BMDD). The BMDD will decide on the ultimate classification of all such products based on review by another panel. Table AVI–1 indicates the current status of various OTC denture aids.

TABLE AVI-1. STATUS OF DENTURE AIDS AND PLAQUE-DISCLOSING AGENTS

Composition	Problems and Disadvantages	Advantages	Status
Denture Adhesives			
acacia, karaya sodium carboxymethylcellulose ethylene oxide homopolymer, polyvinyl methyl ether maleate	must be thoroughly cleaned may prolong use of ill-fitting dentures (excessive bone loss) adhesive is poor substitute for correct seal	aids during adjustment temporary aid until new denture can be made seal may require adhesive	deferred (Devices Panel)
Denture Cleansers			
oxygen releasors (usually peroxides, perborates or hypochlorites)	irritate if left on denture	patient preference	deferred (Devices Panel)
Denture Cushions			
paraffin wax, butylmethacrylate	prolongs use of ill-fitting dentures (irreversible bone loss)	patient preference	deferred (Devices Panel)
Denture Reliner and Repair Kit			
acrylics or glues	irreversibly alters denture base impossible to fit properly documented irreversible bone loss should be removed from marketplace	none could be found	deferred (Devices Panel)
Plaque-disclosing Agents			
FD and C ingestable dyes	require adequate tests of effectiveness FDC status used as safety standard	visualization of plaque OTC availability may promote plaque control	deferred (Devices Panel)

TABLE AVI-2. STATUS OF AGENTS FOR ORAL MUCOSAL INJURY

Composition	Problems and Disadvantages	Advantages	Status
Oral Wound Cleansers			
hydrogen peroxide (3% in aqueous solution), carbamide peroxide (10% in glycerin solution), sodium perborate	no OTC claim for periodontitis or gingivitis professional advice for use on wounds or lesions other extravagant claims have been made	temporary use (7 days or less) cleansing of minor oral irritation, minor injury following dental procedures, irritation of dental appliances, gum irritation around erupting teeth	hydrogen peroxide and carbamide peroxide acceptable for OTC use; sodium perborate considered high risk for benefit obtained
Oral Wound Healing Agents			
allantoin (0.4–2%), carbamide peroxide (10%), chlorophyllins (0.2%), and hydrogen peroxide (3%)	mechanism of action unknown uncertainty that O_2 tension increases in the wound, needs evaluation	temporary use (7 days or less)	recommended for further study

B. DENTAL PLAQUE-DISCLOSING AGENTS

DDCA also referred these products as dental devices to BMDD. The status of these agents at the time of deferral is outlined in Table AVI-1.

C. AGENTS FOR ORAL MUCOSAL INJURY

This classification of OTC drugs includes oral wound cleansers and oral wound healing agents. The agents within this classification and their evaluations are outlined in Table AVI-2. Although such agents have been on the market for years, they were never classified as such. This new classification is presented to aid discussion and for proper labeling. Antimicrobial agents, which might also influence oral mucosal injury by a different mechanism, were deferred to the Oral Cavity Panel. Agents for relief of oral discomfort (protectives, anesthetics, counterirritants) are related drugs and are presented separately below (D).

Definitions of Subclassifications
Oral Wound Cleansers. Agents that do not delay wound healing and physically or chemically assist in removal of foreign material from small superficial oral wounds. *Labeling:* "Discontinue use and see your dentist or physician promptly if irritation persists, inflammation develops, or if fever and infection develop." Sodium perborate is not acceptable because of possible borate toxicity.

Oral Wound Healing Agents. These are nonirritating agents that aid in the healing of small superficial oral wounds by means other than cleaning and irrigating or serving as a protectant. It was felt by the Panel that wound healing acceleration could be realistically accomplished during the stage of reorganization or remodeling but not during inflammatory and proliferative stages. *Labeling:* "For temporary use to aid healing of minor soft tissue wounds due to injury."

D. AGENTS FOR RELIEF OF ORAL DISCOMFORT

Agents in this classification include oral mucosal protectants, toothache relief agents, tooth desensitizers, oral mucosal analgesics, and counterirritants.

TABLE AVI-3. STATUS OF AGENTS FOR RELIEF OF ORAL DISCOMFORT

Composition	Problems and Disadvantages	Advantages	Status
Oral Mucosal Protectant			
benzoin compound or tincture; myrrh (fluid extract)	could seriously delay treatment of a dangerous condition (see warnings) use in aphthous ulceration on advice of practitioner	temporary relief of discomfort of minor burns, minor injuries, or irritations	benzoin and its compound tincture acceptable; myrrh safe but requires more studies for effectiveness
Toothache Relief Agent			
eugenol or clove oil; thymol; benzocaine or butacaine; capsicum; methyl salicylate; iodine; phenol or creosote; beeswax, myrrh, and sandarac	caustic preparations burn the oral mucosa and cause pulpal irritation large placebo effect; few reports on effectiveness cavity fillers (block the flow of fluids and gases) dehydrating agents may increase dentin permeability use may delay dental appointment	sufficient target population needing temporary relief of toothache needed when dentist not available	eugenol acceptable; all other agents need more study
Tooth Desensitizers			
Dentifrices containing fluoride: 1.4% formalin (*Thermodent*), 5% potassium nitrate (*Denquel* or *Promise*), 10% strontium chloride (*Sensodyne*), citric acid/sodium citrate/pluronic F127 gel (*Protect*), sodium ededate (EDTA)	difficulty of diagnosis large placebo effect difficulty of evaluation different times for effectiveness	OTC medication sufficient target population	all of the dentifrices were recommended for further OTC testing except *Protect* (a new drug) and sodium EDTA (unsafe)

Oral Mucosal Analgesics

5–20% Benzocaine; 4% butacaine sulfate; 0.25–1.5% phenol; up to 3% benzyl alcohol; 0.25 to 1% cresol; camphor; methyl salicylate; menthol	for temporary relief of minor irritation	butacaine must be limited to 30 mg dosage phenol (and probably cresol) implicated as cocarcinogens; temporary use at low concentrations considered safe local irritation limits safe upper limit possibility of allergy	benzocaine and phenol acceptable; butacaine acceptable with dosage limit, benzyl alcohol and cresol require further testing; camphor, methyl salicylate, and menthol are irritants and not acceptable

Counterirritants

capsicum only ingredient submitted (as a poultice)	placebo effect and sensation of heat poultice dosage form allows counterirritant to be placed on healthy tissue	mechanism unknown large placebo effect studies not available avoid in presence of inflammation remove poultice at bedtime to prevent aspiration	recommended for further testing

467

Definitions of Subclassifications

Oral Mucosal Protectants (Table AVI–3). These are agents that are insoluble, pharmacologically inert substances that form adherent, continuous, flexible, or semirigid coats when applied to the oral mucous membranes. These coatings help to protect the irritated areas of the mouth from further irritation from chewing, swallowing, and other mouth activity. When applied locally to the oral mucous membranes, they can provide temporary relief of discomfort of minor thermal or chemical burns, irritation, or ulcerations resulting from mechanical trauma and aphthous ulceration (canker sores).

Since the use of the protectant might delay dental care (e.g., in early cancer), the following warnings were recommended: "Not to be used for a period exceeding 7 days," and "Discontinue use and see your dentist or physician if irritation persists, inflammation develops, or if fever and infection develop."

Toothache Relief Agents (Table AVI–3). These are applied into an open tooth cavity to provide temporary relief of pain arising from the tooth pulp. Such medications have been on the market for a long period of time; they probably had their origin in empiric medicine. *Labeling* includes: "Do not use these medications in a tooth with intermittent pain." "Such use may cause irreversible damage to the tooth." "See your dentist immediately."

Tooth Desensitizers (Table AVI–3). Such preparations are used to treat hypersensitive (ultrasensitive) dentin. The diagnosis is difficult to make especially for the consumer, and treatment usually requires professional care. However, the Panel still considered it useful to have tooth desensitizer dentifrices on the OTC dental market for temporary use until a dentist can be seen or following recommendation of the dentist. *Labeling* includes: "See your dentist as soon as possible whether relief is obtained or not." "Sensitive teeth may indicate a serious problem." "Continue use beyond 2 weeks **only** under supervision of a dentist."

Oral Mucosal Analgesics (Table AVI–3). These are surface or topical anesthetics and are used as dental care agents by surface application to provide temporary relief of oral discomfort. *Labeling* includes: "Not to be used for a period exceeding 7 days." "Discontinue use and see your dentist or physician promptly if irritation persists, inflammation develops, or if fever and infection develop."

Counterirritants (Table AVI–3). These are irritating drugs that are applied locally to the skin or oral mucosa for relief of pain originating from a structure other than the site of application. For example, an irritant drug might be applied in a dental poultice to the mucosa surrounding a tooth with a painful pulpitis. These are often supplied as dental poultices, which are topical dosage forms confined to porous bags and are applied to the healthy oral mucous membrane in order to supply medication in the presence of heat and moisture.

E. ANTICARIES AGENTS

Ingredients Considered and Disposition

1. Anticaries food additives—food claim
   Includes DCPD (dicalcium phosphate dihydrate) and CASP (calcium sucrose phosphate).
2. Fluorides—active
   The Panel was aware of the great contributions of fluoride dentifrices as a partial aid in caries control and of recent evidence that fluoride mouthwashes could also aid to prevent caries. The Panel made recommendations which would allow laboratory testing of fluoride dentifrices instead of clinical studies which were no longer deemed necessary. The Panel also recommended that certain fluoride rinses be available for daily OTC use.
3. Abrasives—inactive ingredients
   The Panel recommended that any dentifrice with an RDA abrasivity level (Hefferen, 1976) of 250 or less would be satisfactory for daily use and that a higher abrasivity level would incur additional risk without a substantial increase in ben-

efit. All known, currently available dentifrices met the safety standard when the DDCA report (1978) was completed.

4. Control of fluoride/abrasive incompatibilities

Because the abrasive is considered a possible inactivating agent for fluoride dentifrices, the Panel recommended laboratory profiles or tests for each fluoride source/abrasive combination. The profiles include:

a. for all dentifrices: total fluoride (ppm), soluble fluoride (ppm), pH, and specific gravity
b. special tests: Sn^{++} for stannous fluoride dentifrice; soluble MFP as F and ionic F for MFP dentifrices
c. biological tests: ESR (enamel solubility reduction), animal caries tests, and fluoride uptake

Values of the chemical tests must fall within limits of known caries active fluoride/abrasive combinations. Two out of three biologic tests must be available to support the product's effectiveness.

5. New fluoride sources—considered new drug entities

6. Ingredients ineffective as anticaries agents

These may be present as pharmaceutical necessities (e.g., abrasives). Generally, there were no data to indicate effectiveness. These include:

a. inorganic phosphates
b. sodium bicarbonate

Specific Recommendations on Fluorides as OTC Anticaries Agents

1. Mouthrinses: any fluoride mouth rinse which provides an effective fluoride ion concentration of 0.02% is a safe and effective dental rinse for OTC use as an anticaries agent. These included:

a. acidulated phosphate fluoride
b. sodium fluoride
c. stannous fluoride powder (for making a rinse)

2. Dentifrices (must meet laboratory testing profiles above):

a. sodium fluoride (dentifrice): 0.22% sodium fluoride (0.1% fluoride ion)
b. sodium monofluorophosphate (NaMFP dentifrice), containing 0.76% sodium monofluorophosphate
c. stannous fluoride dentifrice (containing 0.4% stannous fluoride)

Recommendation on Labeling for Fluoride Anticaries Agents

1. Indications. "Aids in the prevention of dental caries (decay or cavities)."
2. Warnings. "Dental rinses. Limited to topical use in the mouth. Do not swallow. Developing teeth in children 5 years of age and under may become permanently discolored if excessive amounts of fluoride are swallowed."
3. Directions.
   a. Dentifrices. "Brush teeth thoroughly at least once daily as directed by dentist. Children under 5 years should be supervised in the use of this product. Use approximately 1 gm per brush." (Manufacturer will specify how 1 gm is measured).
   b. Dental rinses. "Adults and children from 6 years of age use 10 ml once daily as a rinse by swishing between the teeth for at least 1 minute. Then, do not eat or drink for 30 minutes. Children under 12 years should be supervised in the use of this product. For children under 5 years of age there is no recommended dosage except under the advice and supervision of a dentist or physician."
4. Package limit. "Package should not contain more than 120 mg total fluoride."

Special Instructions for Individual Products

1. Stannous fluoride dentifrice labeling. "Improper brushing will result in a light brown stain on the teeth."

2. Stannous fluoride rinse.
   a. The solutions must be mixed from a dry powder or tablet just before rinsing (manufacturer will supply instructions).
   b. This product may produce staining on the teeth. Adequate toothbrushing may prevent these stains which are not harmful or permanent and may be removed by your dentist.

REFERENCES

Hefferren JJ: A laboratory method for assessment of dentifrice abrasivity. J Dent Res 55:563, 1976

Proposed Review of OTC Drugs. Fed Reg, Jan 5, 1972, 37FR85

Report of Council and Bureaus: Council classified fluoride mouth rinses. J Am Dent Assoc 91:1250, 1975

BIBLIOGRAPHY

Gangarosa LP, Aleo JJ, Hurst V, Plein JB, Raymond PE, Scholle RH, Van Kirk LE: Denture aids and plaque disclosants in OTC Dentifrices and Dental Care Agents Report filed with the Commissioner, Food and Drug Administration, pp. 1–47. Noted in Fed Reg 43(85): Tues, May 2, 1978

Gangarosa LP, Aleo JJ, Hurst V, Plein JB, Raymond PE, Scholle RH, Van Kirk LE: OTC drugs for oral mucosal injury. OTC Dentifrices and Dental Care Agents Report filed with the Commissioner of FDA, pp. 1–160. Modified for inclusion in the Federal Register under the title, Oral mucosal injury drug products for over-the-counter human use; establishment of a monograph; proposed rulemaking. Fed Reg 44(214):63270–63290, 1979

Gangarosa LP, Aleo JJ, Hurst V, Plein JB, Raymond PE, Scholle RH, Van Kirk LE: Anticaries OTC drugs. OTC Dentifrices and Dental Care Agents Report filed with the Commissioner of FDA, pp. 1–145B, 1978. Modified for inclusion in the Federal Register, under the title, Establishment of a monograph on anticaries drug products for over-the-counter human use; proposed rulemaking. Fed Reg 45(62):20666–20691, 1980

Gangarosa LP, Aleo JJ, Hurst V, Plein JB, Raymond PE, Scholle RH, Van Kirk LE: Over-the-counter drugs for the relief of oral discomfort. OTC Dentifrices and Dental Care Agents Panel Report Filed with the Commissioner, Food and Drug Administration, pp. 1–204. Modified for inclusion in the Federal Register, under the title Drug Products for the Relief of Oral Discomfort for Over-the-Counter Human Use, Fed Reg 47(101):22712–22759, 1982

Further References will be supplied on request.

Iontophoresis in Dental Practice

Iontophoresis is a well-recognized method of drug application for surface tissues. Since many dental treatments are at a surface of the body (teeth and oral mucosa), a number of iontophoresis treatments have been developed for dentistry as listed in Table A.VII–1. Note in the table that each drug has an ionic charge and thus can be introduced onto the surface by an electrode of the same charge. An electrode pad of the opposite charge to the drug is soaked with sodium nitrate and placed at any other indifferent site on the body.

Although iontophoresis is an old method and has been used with extremely poor technology for a number of years by dentists, some recent studies from the Medical College of Georgia and some modern technology from the University of Utah have provided a new technique for iontophoresis that is safe and effective and is based upon sound scientific principles, making the application of iontophoresis practical for routine dentistry.

In order to properly perform iontophoresis three considerations are important: (1) a safe and effective source of direct current supplying between 0 and 45 volts is needed, (2) a flexible system of electrodes is needed so that the dentist can reach all of the different surfaces of the teeth and mouth, and (3) consideration must be given to insulation, since electrical current follows the path of least resistance. It is especially important to insulate metal restorations, since electrode contact to the metal will serve as a current sink and will prevent entry of current into the desired tissues.

The exact techniques for performing iontophoresis in dental practice are outlined by one of the authors (LPG) in his monograph and instruction manual (see Bibliography). It would now be helpful to outline each of the four major uses of iontophoresis in dental practice.

A. TREATMENT OF HYPERSENSITIVE TEETH

All dentists are aware of the problem of hypersensitive teeth in dental practice. Because all previous methods of treatment have been so undependable and often irrational, the dentist now

TABLE AVII-1. DENTAL IONTOPHORESIS

Condition	Drug	Charge on Drug
sensitive teeth	fluoride	negative
aphthous ulcers	methylprednisolone sodium succinate[a]	negative
local anesthesia	lidocaine HCl	positive
	epinephrine HCl	positive
herpes simplex	idoxuridine[b]	negative

[a] Solu-Medrol, Upjohn Co., Kalamazoo, MI.
[b] Stoxil, SKF Labs, Philadelphia, PA.

shrugs his shoulders when the problem arises. We would rather that the problem disappear, but as much as "we hope and pray" for this, it continues to reappear in patient after patient. Sometimes the patient may blame the problem on the dentist. After all, when he came to you, the problem either was not evident or it didn't exist! After restoration or surgery, suddenly the mouth is uncomfortable even though the "operation was a success."

If we had good methods of diagnosis and treatment, the dentist would start to look for the problem and program any care needed into the patient's treatment plan. It should be an axiom in this modern day of therapy never to work on a tooth that is already sensitive until the condition is under control. To violate this axiom is to court problems!

The author has developed not only a useful system of treating all types of dentin exposure but also new methods of diagnosis. Since accurate diagnosis must precede treatment, it is recommended that the dentist perform a very simple test of blowing cold air on each suspected hypersensitive surface, along with his other diagnostic procedures, at **every** oral examination. An air spray tip is placed in a standardized manner near the labial surface while covering adjacent teeth with the fingers. The surface is then tested with a 1 second air blast (several blasts or a constant stream causes more discomfort). The patient rates the discomfort according to the scale in Table AVII-2.

These data along with other tests, such as explorer probing, ice water tests, or acrid juices,

are charted on a record. The complete air test with charting consumes only 2 to 3 minutes and is used as the basis of treatment planning to correct any hypersensitivity which the patient had before arriving in your office. Once corrected, the treatment is permanent, and the dentist can proceed with other therapy with confidence.

Questions should be asked regarding history of sensitivity especially after previous restorative or operative procedures. Patients who respond positively should be tested as described above but with extra care. In addition, special precautions should be taken to prevent sensitivity by treating the dentin when it is exposed. Otherwise, your patient will be complaining about thermal sensitivity under an amalgam or gold restoration, and you will be fumbling for words trying to explain it!

Now that the importance of diagnosis and prevention has been placed in proper perspective, the treatment will be considered. First one needs the proper methodology for fluoride iontophoresis. Most dentists have the impression that the equipment can be put together in the garage on a Saturday afternoon. Some companies continue to market underpowered, clumsy, and ill-conceived systems (hand-held

TABLE AVII-2. DISCOMFORT SCALE

0 = normal
1 = mild discomfort
2 = moderate
3 = severe, but transient
4 = intolerable, severe and lasting

models) and even provide improper directions for use. Once the dentist learns that such equipment is unsuitable, the proper adaptation of safe and effective instrumentation can be carried out.

The new methodology recommended by the author is useful for treating any type of dentin exposure. Furthermore, this technology makes it so simple that any dentist, hygienist, and even a well-trained assistant (the latter two under dentist supervision) can quickly and easily perform these procedures. Since these have been adequately described in the author's monograph and can be learned by all dentists with a minimum of effort and study, only a brief overview is presented here.

Our studies and the experience of many other researchers and dentists indicate that an immediate and profound desensitization occurs after fluoride iontophoresis. This treatment is permanent when the dentist properly applies fluoride ions to the exposed dentin. Single teeth are desensitized in 2 minutes, while three or four teeth can be desensitized in a 20 to 30 minute appointment. The methodology includes provisions for single tooth treatment by means of a plastic-tip technique or a brush technique, as well as multiple tooth desensitization by a tray technique. Upper and lower arch can be desensitized in about 40 minutes, with an assistant spending the entire time and the dentist about 20 minutes. Another adaptation of the tray technique is used to treat multiple crown preparations.

Not only is the fluoride iontophoresis the ideal method of desensitization, but also, as a bonus, the method adds fluoride to the tooth, causing the fluoride to penetrate deeper and at a higher concentration than with any other method. Thus, fluoride iontophoresis adds to the health of the tooth by reinforcing the tooth mineral using fluoride catalysis of remineralization. This reasoning has led us to propose iontophoresis as a method of fluoride application to protect cavity preparations, crown preparations, exposed root surfaces, and even natural tooth structure, especially to protect fissures, pits, and demineralized areas.

B. APHTHOUS ULCERS AND OTHER NONSPECIFIC INFLAMMATORY LESIONS

Before the new ideas in iontophoresis were introduced, there was no acceptable therapy for this type of lesion. Corticosteroids appeared to be the best drugs for the condition, but use by ointment or gel application is only modestly effective and may be ineffective if the vehicle does not adhere to the lesion. Systemic corticosteroids are sometimes used for massive involvement, but a method of local application with assurance of penetration is highly desirable.

Aphthae (either major or minor) are best treated by direct iontophoretic application of the charged steroid, methylprednisolone sodium succinate (*Solu-Medrol*). The powdered drug must be diluted just prior to use because it is unstable after mixing. The drug is soaked onto cotton contained in a large plastic tip which is placed over the lesion, and a negative current forced through the cotton carries a high concentration of ionic drug into the diseased tissue.

Results are an immediate relief of discomfort, with rapid elimination of inflammation and promotion of rapid healing. The healing time is reduced at least 50%, and healing occurs without further pain. Although this provides a great benefit for the patients, it unfortunately does not prevent recurrences. Presently, our program at the Medical College of Georgia involves treating large, painful lesions by iontophoresis and follow-up considerations of the patient's systemic health status for prevention of recurrences.

C. ANTIVIRAL THERAPY

Currently there is no topical therapy that is useful in herpes simplex (HSV) orolabialis. Many practitioners are recommending idoxuridine, vidarabine or acyclovir ointments but these should not be used topically on the lip because they have been proven ineffective by topical application. There is a further disadvantage that a small amount of drug might promote induction of viral resistance. Thus, no therapy is better than application of these topical preparations.

However, we have found that electrical assistance greatly increases the penetration of certain antiviral drugs into skin, including idoxuridine. This drug has now been used safely in human eye disease for over 20 years and is accepted all over the world as a treatment for HSV infection. Since the drug has this safe record when used topically and since its penetration can be greatly increased by iontophoresis, we recommend iontophoretic application of idoxuridine ophthalmic solution (*Stoxil*) under certain conditions. These conditions involve risk:benefit considerations. First, we would like the patient to obtain a positive benefit from the treatment. This means we do not encourage patients to receive the therapy if they have only a simple lesion less than once a year and which heals uneventfully. Second, we exclude pregnant women because the package insert advises that idoxuridine is teratogenic in certain animal studies. Third, allergy to idoxuridine or history of resistance would be considered contraindications. One other precaution should be to inform the patient that idoxuridine is mutagenic and might be cancer-inducing. However, the virus itself is believed to be a greater threat for induction of cancer than is the drug. In the author's experience, almost all patients will accept the treatment after these considerations are explained except pregnant women. Since they are excluded anyway, there is usually no problem except with patients who are excluded because of infrequent lesions who often still request therapy.

The idoxuridine iontophoresis is indicated in primary herpes, immune-compromised patients having recurrences, massive attacks involving one quarter or more of the lip, spreading, increasing frequency of recurrence, interference with one's profession, and in subjects who are in contact with infants or immune-compromised patients. This is also helpful in patients who need dental therapy, since it is inadvisable to perform any dental treatment on a patient with herpes orolabialis unless the virus is first controlled.

The technique is very similar to treatment of aphthae except that the antiviral drug instead of the steroid is placed on the cotton. Idoxuridine is forced into the lesion with negative current. The results are extremely dramatic: immediate relief of discomfort, rapid changes in the lesion which indicate promotion of healing, and a much reduced severity and healing time. There is lack of spreading and discomfort during healing, and, best of all, our studies indicate a reduced rate and severity of recurrences. Further research is planned to document all of these results.

D. LOCAL ANESTHESIA

Topical mucosal anesthesia is less than satisfactory with all available topical ointments, solutions, sprays, and so on. However, lidocaine and epinephrine can be administered with electrical assistance into the oral mucosa, causing a deep topical anesthesia through the thickness of the mucosa. This has been used for extraction of loose deciduous teeth, as a preinjection topical, for biopsies, and for skin anesthesia prior to IV needle insertion.

Preinjection topicals by iontophoresis will greatly aid in patient cooperation. Many patients refuse the dental encounter because of subconscious or conscious fear of the needle. The preinjection topical requires 3 to 5 minutes and a trained auxiliary can perform this before the dentist injects the anesthetic. We recommend this for any palatal injection or other infiltration into fixed tissue, such as mucobuccal or lingual infiltration. Use of this technique will greatly increase the esteem of your patients and should result in practice building by referrals.

BIBLIOGRAPHY

Gangarosa, LP Sr: Monograph: Iontophoresis in Dental Practice. Chicago, Quintessence Publishing, 1982
Gangarosa LP Sr: Instruction Manual ElectroAppli-

cator System Model C-2 for Iontophoresis in Dental Practice. Augusta, GA, Dentelect Corp., 1981

Gangarosa LP, Park NH: Practical considerations in iontophoresis of fluoride for desensitizing dentin. J Prosthet Dent 39:173, 1978

Gangarosa LP Sr: Iontophoretic Application of Fluoride by a tray technique for desensitization of multiple teeth. J Am Dent Assoc 102:50, 1981

Carlo GT, Ciancio SG, Seyrek SK: An evaluation of iontophoretic application of fluoride for tooth desensitization. J Am Dent Assoc, 105:452, 1982

Gangarosa LP, Merchant HW, Park NH, Hill JM: Iontophoretic application of idoxuridine for recurrent herpes labialis. Report of preliminary clinical trials. Methods Findings Exp Clin Pharmacol 1:105, 1979

Other references available on request.

Answers to Text Questions

CHAPTER 12

Answer	Objective	Answer	Objective
1. D	12.A.1.	12. A	12.F.2.
2. B	12.B.1.	13. C	12.F.3.
3. D	12.C.1.	14. T	12.G.1.
4. F	12.D.1.	15. T	12.G.2.
5. T	12.D.2.	16. F	12.G.3.
6. F	12.E.1.	17. B	12.H.1.
7. D	12.E.2.	18. B	12.H.2.
8. F	12.E.3.	19. B	12.I.1.
9. A	12.E.4.	20. F	12.I.2.
10. F	12.E.5.	21. F	12.I.3.
11. T	12.F.1.	22. F	12.I.4.
		23. T	12.I.5.
		24. T	12.I.6.
		25. B	12.J.1.

CHAPTER 13

Answer	Objective	Answer	Objective
1. F	13.A.1.	6. B	13.B.1.
2. D	13.B.1.	7. F	13.B.1.
3. C	13.B.1.	8. T	13.C.1.
4. A	13.B.1.	9. F	13.C.1.
5. E	13.B.1.	10. F	13.C.1.

CHAPTER 13 (*Cont.*)

Answer	Objective	Answer	Objective
11. B	13.C.3.	34. F	13.I.1.
12. D	13.C.3.	35. A	13.I.1.
13. C	13.C.3.	36. B	13.I.1.
14. C	13.C.6.	37. B	13.I.1.
15. D	13.C.4.	38. T	13.I.1.
16. A	13.C.4.	39. D	13.J.1.
17. B	13.C.4.	40. E	13.J.1.
18. F	13.C.5.	41. E	13.J.1.
19. B	13.C.5.	42. B	13.J.1.
20. D	13.C.6.	43. C	13.J.1.
21. B	13.D.1.	44. A	13.J.1.
22. T	13.D.1.	45. E	13.J.1.
23. D	13.D.2.	46. E	13.J.1.
24. D	13.D.3.	47. E	13.J.1.
25. T	13.D.4.	48. E	13.J.1.
26. F	13.F.1.	49. C	13.J.2.
27. F	13.F.2.	50. E	13.J.2.
28. T	13.F.2.	51. T	13.K.1.
29. B	13.F.3.	52. F	13.K.1.
30. F	13.F.3.	53. F	13.K.1.
31. F	13.G.1.	54. T	13.K.1.
32. T	13.H.1.	55. F	13.L.1.
33. F	13.H.1.	56. C	13.L.2.

CHAPTER 13 (*Cont.*)

Answer		Objective	Answer		Objective
57.	B	13.L.2.	60.	C	13.M.2.
58.	F	13.M.1.	61.	T	13.M.2.
		13.L.1.	62.	T	13.M.2.
59.	T	13.M.2.	63.	A	13.M.2.

CHAPTER 14

Answer		Objective	Answer		Objective
1.	C	14.A.1.	9.	F	14.B.5.
2.	B	14.A.2.	10.	F	14.B.6.
3.	T	14.A.3.	11.	T	14.C.1.
4.	F	14.A.3.	12.	F	14.C.2.
5.	A	14.B.1.	13.	F	14.C.3.
6.	T	14.B.2.	14.	C	14.C.4.
7.	C	14.B.3.	15.	F	14.C.5.
8.	D	14.B.4.	16.	T	14.D.1.

CHAPTER 15

Answer		Objective	Answer		Objective
1.	B	15.A.1.	10.	D	15.E.1.
2.	C	15.A.2.	11.	C	15.E.2.
3.	C	15.A.3.	12.	B	15.E.3.
4.	A	15.B.1.	13.	A	15.E.4.
5.	A	15.B.2.	14.	D	15.F.1.
6.	B	15.C.1.	15.	B	15.G.1.
7.	C	15.D.1.	16.	A	15.H.1.
8.	B	15.D.2.	17.	C	15.I.1.
9.	C	15.D.3.	18.	D	15.J.1.

CHAPTER 16

Answer		Objective	Answer		Objective
1.	F	16.A.1.	15.	F	16.J.1.
2.	F	16.A.1.	16.	F	16.K.2.
3.	T	16.A.1.	17.	T	16.N.1.
4.	F	16.A.1.	18.	T	16.B.2.
5.	F	16.A.2.	19.	F	16.B.2.
6.	T	16.A.2.	20.	F	16.B.2.
7.	F	16.C.1.	21.	T	16.B.2.
8.	T	16.I.2.	22.	D	16.B.1.
9.	F	16.I.2.	23.	C	16.C.1.
10.	T	16.I.2.	24.	D	16.E.1.
11.	T	16.I.2.			16.E.2.
12.	F	16.I.2.			16.E.3.
13.	T	16.I.2.	25.	D	16.F.1.
14.	F	16.I.3.	26.	D	16.G.1.

CHAPTER 16 (*Cont.*)

Answer		Objective	Answer		Objective
27.	A	16.G.1.	45.	A	16.L.2.
28.	D	16.I.1.	46.	B	16.L.1.
29.	D	16.K.1.	47.	C	16.M.1.
30.	A	16.L.1.	48.	A	16.M.1.
31.	A	16.H.1.	49.	A	16.J.2.
32.	A	16.H.1.	50.	B	16.J.2.
33.	A	16.H.1.	51.	D	16.J.2.
34.	B	16.H.1.	52.	D	16.N.2.
35.	B	16.H.1.	53.	D	16.O.2.
36.	A	16.B.1.	54.	B	16.O.1.
37.	D	16.C.1.	55.	D	16.O.3.
38.	C	16.D.1.	56.	D	16.M.1.
39.	C	16.D.2.	57.	B	16.M.1.
40.	B	16.D.3.	58.	C	16.M.2.
41.	C	16.G.1.	59.	A	16.M.1.
42.	B	16.G.2.	60.	B	16.M.1.
43.	C	16.J.1.	61.	B	16.M.1.
44.	C	16.J.1.	62.	D	16.M.1.

CHAPTER 17

Answer		Objective	Answer		Objective
1.	T	17.A.1.	24.	T	17.B.2.
2.	T	17.A.1.	25.	A	17.B.3.
3.	F	17.A.1.	26.	F	17.B.3.
4.	F	17.A.1.	27.	T	17.B.3.
5.	C	17.A.1.	28.	B	17.C.1.
6.	F	17.A.1.	29.	T	17.C.1.
7.	C	17.A.1.	30.	T	17.C.1.
8.	B	17.A.2.	31.	F	17.C.1.
9.	A	17.A.2.	32.	A	17.C.2.
10.	B	17.A.2.	33.	C	17.C.2.
11.	B	17.A.2.	34.	A	17.C.2.
12.	B	17.A.2.	35.	D	17.C.2.
13.	F	17.A.2.	36.	D	17.C.2.
14.	F	17.A.3.	37.	T	17.C.3.
15.	F	17.A.3.	38.	T	17.C.4.
16.	B	17.A.3.	39.	B	17.C.4.
17.	C	17.A.3.	40.	C	17.C.4.
18.	C	17.A.4.	41.	D	17.C.4.
		17.C.9.	42.	T	17.C.5.
19.	D	17.A.4.	43.	T	17.C.5.
20.	B	17.A.4.	44.	F	17.C.6.
21.	A	17.B.1.	45.	T	17.C.6.
22.	C	17.B.2.	46.	T	17.C.4.
23.	B	17.B.2.			17.C.6.

CHAPTER 17 (*Cont.*)

Answer	Objective	Answer	Objective
47. B	17.C.7.	54. D	17.C.10.
48. T	17.C.7.	55. A	17.C.10.
49. F	17.C.7.	56. F	17.C.10.
50. T	17.C.7.	57. T	17.C.10.
51. B	17.C.8.	58. D	17.C.10.
52. F	17.C.8.	59. B	17.C.10.
53. D	17.C.9.		

CHAPTER 18

Answer	Objective	Answer	Objective
1. F	18.A.1.	18. C	18.C.1.
2. D	18.A.2.	19. A	18.C.1.
3. D	18.A.2.		18.C.2.
4. D	18.A.3.	20. A	18.C.2.
5. F	18.A.4.	21. B	18.C.3.
6. A	18.A.5.	22. B	18.C.3.
7. B	18.A.5.	23. B	18.C.3.
8. C	18.B.1.	24. A	18.C.4.
	18.B.2.	25. T	18.C.4.
9. A	18.B.1.	26. F	18.C.4.
10. T	18.B.1.	27. C	18.C.6.
11. F	18.B.1.	28. B	18.D.1.
12. B	18.B.1.	29. C	18.D.2.
	18.B.2.	30. A	18.D.2.
13. B	18.B.1.		18.D.3.
14. D	18.B.1.	31. T	18.D.2.
15. D	18.B.1.		18.D.3.
16. D	18.B.1.	32. D	18.D.2.
17. C	18.B.2.		18.D.3.
	18.D.3.		

CHAPTER 19

Answer	Objective	Answer	Objective
1. T	19.A.1.	10. A	19.B.1.
2. B	19.A.1.	11. D	19.B.1.
	19.A.4.		19.G.2.
3. C	19.A.1.		19.I.4.
4. B	19.A.2.	12. C	19.B.2.
5. C	19.A.2.	13. B	19.B.3.
	19.A.3.	14. B	19.B.3.
6. D	19.A.3.	15. T	19.B.3.
7. T	19.A.4.		19.G.1.
8. A	19.A.4.	16. D	19.C.1.
9. E	19.B.1.	17. A	19.C.1.

CHAPTER 19 (*Cont.*)

Answer	Objective	Answer	Objective
18. A	19.C.1.	32. T	19.G.1.
19. F	19.C.2.	33. T	19.G.1.
20. F	19.C.2.	34. D	19.G.2.
	19.C.3.	35. D	19.H.1.
21. D	19.C.3.	36. T	19.H.2.
22. C	19.C.3.	37. F	19.H.2.
23. D	19.C.3.	38. A	19.H.2.
24. D	19.C.4.		19.H.4.
25. T	19.C.4.	39. C	19.H.3.
26. C	19.D.1.	40. A	19.H.4.
27. D	19.E.1.	41. D	19.B.1.
28. B	19.F.1.		19.H.4.
29. D	19.F.2.	42. F	19.I.1.
30. C	19.F.3.	43. F	19.I.2.
31. D	19.A.4.	44. D	19.I.2.
	19.B.1.	45. F	19.I.3.
	19.F.2.	46. T	19.I.4.
	19.G.1.	47. C	19.I.4.
	19.H.4.		

CHAPTER 20

Answer	Objective	Answer	Objective
1. D	20.B.1.	9. A	20.E.1.
2. T	20.B.1.	10. D	20.F.1.
3. T	20.C.1.	11. B	20.G.1.
4. C	20.C.2.	12. B	20.H.1.
5. T	20.D.1.	13. T	20.I.1.
6. C	20.D.2.	14. F	20.I.1.
7. F	20.D.3.	15. F	20.I.1.
8. F	20.D.3.	16. T	20.I.1.

CHAPTER 21

Answer	Objective	Answer	Objective
1. F	21.A.1.	11. T	21.F.4.
2. F	21.B.1.	12. T	21.G.1.
3. T	21.B.1.	13. F	21.H.1.
4. B	21.C.1.	14. T	21.H.1.
5. T	21.D.1.	15. E	21.I.1.
6. T	21.D.1.	16. T	21.J.1.
7. F	21.E.1.	17. T	21.K.1.
8. C	21.F.1.	18. C	21.L.1.
9. T	21.F.2.	19. E	21.M.1.
10. E	21.F.3.		

CHAPTER 22

Answer	Objective	Answer	Objective
1. F	22.B.1.	7. D	22.F.1.
2. T	22.C.1.	8. T	22.G.1.
3. T	22.D.1.	9. T	22.H.1.
	22.D.2.	10. D	22.I.1.
	22.D.3.	11. D	22.J.1.
	22.D.4.	12. T	22.J.1.
4. A	22.D.3.	13. F	22.K.2.
5. D	22.E.1.	14. B	22.K.1.
6. T	22.E.1.		

CHAPTER 23

Answer	Objective	Answer	Objective
1. T	23.A.1.	12. A	23.E.1.
2. B	23.B.1.	13. T	23.F.1.
3. A	23.C.1.	14. F	23.F.2.
4. F	23.C.2.	15. F	23.F.3.
5. F	23.C.3.	16. F	23.G.1.
6. D	23.C.4.	17. A	23.H.1.
7. F	23.C.5.	18. D	23.I.1.
8. F	23.C.6.	19. T	23.J.1.
9. D	23.D.1.	20. F	23.J.2.
10. C	23.D.2.	21. C	23.K.1.
11. F	23.D.3.		

CHAPTER 24

Answer	Objective	Answer	Objective
1. B	24.A.1.	17. F	24.B.2.
2. E	24.A.1.	18. C	24.B.3.
3. C	24.A.1.	19. T	24.B.4.
4. B	24.A.1.	20. T	24.B.4.
5. F	24.A.1.	21. T	24.B.4.
6. F	24.B.1.	22. D	24.B.5.
	24.B.4.	23. T	24.B.5.
7. T	24.B.1.	24. T	24.B.6.
8. T	24.B.1.	25. F	24.B.6.
9. F	24.B.1.	26. F	24.C.1.
10. F	24.B.1.	27. F	24.C.1.
11. T	24.B.1.	28. F	24.D.1.
12. T	24.B.1.	29. F	24.C.1.
13. F	24.B.1.	30. C	24.C.1.
14. A	24.B.2.	31. C	24.D.1.
15. C	24.B.2.	32. T	24.D.1.
16. T	24.B.2.	33. F	24.D.1.

CHAPTER 24 (*Cont.*)

Answer	Objective	Answer	Objective
34. F	24.D.1.	40. T	24.D.1.
35. T	24.D.1.	41. T	24.D.1.
36. T	24.D.1.	42. F	24.D.1.
37. T	24.D.1.	43. C	24.D.1.
38. T	24.D.1.	44. B	24.D.1.
39. F	24.D.1.	45. B	24.D.1.

CHAPTER 25

Answer	Objective	Answer	Objective
1. T	25.B.1.	8. T	25.E.1.
2. F	25.B.1.	9. T	25.E.2.
3. T	25.B.1.	10. A	25.F.1.
4. E	25.B.2.	11. A	25.G.1.
	25.B.3.	12. B	25.H.1.
5. C	25.C.1.	13. D	25.I.1.
6. B	25.D.1.	14. D	25.J.1.
	25.D.2.	15. T	25.K.1.
7. D	25.D.3.	16. E	25.L.1.

CHAPTER 26

Answer	Objective	Answer	Objective
1. C	26.B.1.	17. F	26.I.2.
	26.B.2.	18. T	26.I.1.
2. D	26.B.3.	19. D	26.J.1.
3. C	26.C.1.	20. T	26.J.1.
4. F	26.C.2.	21. T	26.K.1.
5. T	26.C.3.	22. T	26.K.1.
6. F	26.D.2.	23. F	26.L.1.
	26.D.3.	24. F	26.I.2.
7. T	26.D.2.	25. D	26.I.1.
	26.D.4.	26. F	26.I.1.
8. T	26.D.2.	27. F	26.M.2.
	26.D.3.	28. T	26.M.1.
9. B	26.D.5.	29. F	26.M.1.
10. T	26.E.1.	30. E	26.M.2.
11. F	26.F.1.	31. E	26.M.2.
12. F	26.G.1.	32. F	26.M.3.
13. T	26.D.1.	33. F	26.M.3.
14. D	26.I.1.	34. F	26.M.3.
15. T	26.I.1.	35. D	26.N.1.
16. D	26.I.1.	36. C	26.N.1.

CHAPTER 27

Answer	Objective	Answer	Objective
1. E	27.A.1.	24. T	27.P.1.
2. T	27.B.1.	25. T	27.P.2.
3. F	27.C.1.	26. T	27.Q.1.
4. F	27.C.2.	27. T	27.R.1.
5. T	27.C.3.		27.R.2.
6. T	27.D.1.	28. F	27.S.1.
7. F	27.D.1.	29. T	27.S.1.
8. D	27.E.1.	30. D	27.T.1.
9. T	27.F.1.	31. T	27.U.1.
10. T	27.G.1.	32. T	27.U.1.
11. F	27.G.1.	33. T	27.V.1.
12. F	27.H.1.	34. T	27.V.2.
13. T	27.H.2.	35. D	27.V.3.
14. T	27.H.3.	36. F	27.V.2.
15. F	27.I.1.	37. F	27.W.1.
16. D	27.J.1.	38. T	27.W.2.
17. T	27.K.1.	39. B	27.W.3.
18. T	27.K.1.	40. T	27.W.3.
19. T	27.L.1.	41. T	27.X.1.
20. T	27.M.1.	42. F	27.X.1.
	27.M.2.	43. E	27.X.1.
21. T	27.N.1.	44. T	27.X.1.
22. T	27.O.1.	45. T	27.X.1.
23. T	27.O.1.		

CHAPTER 28

Answer	Objective	Answer	Objective
1. T	28.B.1.	8. T	28.E.1.
	28.B.2.	9. T	28.E.1.
2. B	28.C.1.	10. B	28.E.1.
3. F	28.C.2.	11. T	28.E.1.
4. F	28.C.3.	12. T	28.F.1.
5. F	28.D.1.	13. F	28.G.1.
6. D	28.D.1.	14. E	28.G.1.
7. T	28.D.1.	15. T	28.H.1.

CHAPTER 29

Answer	Objective	Answer	Objective
1. T	29.B.1.	6. T	29.F.1.
2. T	29.C.1.	7. T	29.G.1.
3. T	29.D.1.	8. T	29.G.1.
4. B	29.D.1.	9. T	29.H.1.
5. D	29.E.1.	10. T	29.I.1.

CHAPTER 30

Answer	Objective	Answer	Objective
1. D	30.A.1.	12. T	30.I.2.
2. C	30.A.2.	13. F	30.J.1.
	30.A.3.	14. T	30.K.1.
3. F	30.B.1.	15. F	30.L.1.
	30.B.2.	16. D	30.L.2.
4. C	30.C.1.	17. F	30.L.3.
5. T	30.C.2.	18. D	30.N.1.
6. F	30.D.1.	19. A	30.N.1.
7. T	30.E.1.	20. B	30.N.2.
8. T	30.F.1.	21. T	30.N.2.
9. E	30.G.1.	22. E	30.N.2.
10. T	30.H.1.	23. D	30.N.2.
	30.H.2.	24. F	30.N.2.
11. F	30.I.1.		

CHAPTER 31

Answer	Objective	Answer	Objective
1. A	31.A.1.	26. C	31.C.4.
2. T	31.A.2.	27. B	31.C.5.
3. B	31.A.3.	28. F	31.C.6.
4. A	31.A.4.	29. F	31.C.7.
5. D	31.A.5.	30. F	31.C.8.
6. B	31.A.6.	31. T	31.D.1.
7. B	31.A.6.	32. T	31.D.2.
8. T	31.A.7.	33. F	31.D.3.
9. T	31.A.8.	34. D	31.D.4.
10. F	31.A.9.	35. T	31.D.5.
11. T	31.A.10.	36. C	31.D.6.
12. F	31.B.1.	37. B	31.D.7.
13. F	31.B.2.	38. D	31.E.1.
14. F	31.B.3.	39. A	31.E.2.
15. F	31.B.4.	40. C	31.E.3.
16. T	31.B.5.	41. T	31.E.4.
17. T	31.B.6.	42. C	31.E.5.
18. A	31.B.7.	43. A	31.E.6.
19. C	31.B.8.	44. B	31.E.7.
20. D	31.B.9.	45. F	31.E.8.
21. D	31.B.10.	46. T	31.E.9.
22. C	31.B.11.	47. T	31.E.10.
23. B	31.C.1.	48. T	31.E.11.
24. D	31.C.2.	49. A	31.E.12.
25. C	31.C.3.		

CHAPTER 32

Answer	Objective	Answer	Objective
1. A	32.B.1.	8. C	32.G.1.
2. B	32.C.1.	9. C	32.H.1.
3. B	32.D.1.	10. B	32.H.1.
4. C	32.E.1.	11. T	32.H.2.
5. D	32.F.1.	12. D	32.I.1.
6. C	32.G.1.	13. A	32.J.1.
7. F	32.F.2.		

CHAPTER 33

Answer	Objective	Answer	Objective
1. F	33.B.1.	12. T	33.E.1.
2. D	33.B.2.	13. F	33.E.1.
3. T	33.B.3.	14. C	33.G.1.
4. F	33.B.4.	15. C	33.G.2.
5. T	33.C.1.	16. B	33.G.4.
6. C	33.C.1.	17. D	33.G.5.
7. T	33.C.2.	18. B	33.H.1.
8. D	33.D.1.	19. A	33.1.2.
9. T	33.D.1.	20. D	33.J.1.
10. T	33.D.1.	21. A	33.J.2.
11. T	33.E.1.	22. C	33.K.1.

CHAPTER 34

Answer	Objective	Answer	Objective
1. D	34.B.1.	23. T	34.C.16.
2. C	34.B.2.	24. A	34.C.17.
3. E	34.B.3.	25. F	34.C.18.
4. E	34.B.3.	26. F	34.C.19.
5. B	34.B.3.	27. T	34.C.19.
6. T	34.C.1.	28. T	34.C.20.
7. F	34.C.1.	29. F	34.C.21.
8. F	34.C.2.	30. D	34.C.22.
9. F	34.C.3.	31. T	34.C.23.
10. A	34.C.4.	32. D	34.C.24.
11. B	34.C.5.	33. C	34.C.25.
12. F	34.C.6.	34. T	34.C.25.
13. D	34.C.6.	35. D	34.C.26.
14. T	34.C.7.	36. C	34.C.27.
15. D	34.C.8.	37. T	34.C.28.
16. F	34.C.9.	38. F	34.C.28.
17. D	34.C.10.	39. F	34.C.29.
18. B	34.C.11.	40. T	34.C.30.
19. B	34.C.12.	41. T	34.C.31.
20. C	34.C.13.	42. C	34.C.32.
21. T	34.C.14.	43. F	34.C.33.
22. C	34.C.15.	44. D	34.C.34.

CHAPTER 34 (Cont.)

Answer	Objective	Answer	Objective
45. T	34.D.1.	72. B	34.D.28.
46. D	34.D.2.	73. F	34.D.29.
47. T	34.D.3.	74. D	34.D.29.
48. F	34.D.4.	75. F	34.D.30.
49. D	34.D.5.	76. A	34.D.31.
50. T	34.D.6.	77. T	34.D.32.
51. T	34.D.7.	78. A	34.D.33.
52. F	34.D.8.	79. F	34.D.34.
53. F	34.D.9.	80. B	34.D.35.
54. T	34.D.10	81. A	34.D.35.
55. C	34.D.11.	82. T	34.D.36.
56. F	34.D.12.	83. T	34.E.1.
57. F	34.D.13.	84. C	34.E.2.
58. C	34.D.14.	85. F	34.E.3.
59. F	34.D.15.	86. D	34.E.4.
60. F	34.D.16.		34.E.5.
61. C	34.D.17.	87. T	34.E.6.
62. T	34.D.18.	88. F	34.E.7.
63. D	34.D.19.	89. D	34.F.1.
64. A	34.D.20.	90. C	34.F.2.
65. F	34.D.21.	91. C	34.F.2.
66. F	34.D.22.	92. T	34.F.3.
67. T	34.D.23.	93. E	34.F.4.
68. F	34.D.24.	94. C	34.F.5.
69. A	34.D.25.	95. T	34.F.5.
70. A	34.D.26.	96. D	34.F.5.
71. F	34.D.27.		

CHAPTER 35

Answer	Objective	Answer	Objective
1. A	35.A.1.	17. F	35.D.1.
2. T	35.A.1.	18. B	35.E.1.
3. F	35.A.1.	19. F	35.E.1.
4. E	35.B.2.	20. B	35.E.1.
5. F	35.B.2.	21. D	35.E.1.
6. E	35.C.1.	22. C	35.F.1.
7. B	35.C.1.	23. C	35.F.1.
8. F	35.C.1.	24. D	35.G.1.
9. C	35.D.1.	25. D	35.G.1.
10. D	35.D.1.	26. A	35.G.1.
11. F	35.D.1.	27. A	35.G.1.
12. C	35.D.1.	28. A	35.G.1.
13. B	35.D.1.	29. T	35.G.1.
14. C	35.D.1.	30. T	35.G.1.
15. B	35.D.1.	31. T	35.G.1.
16. D	35.D.1.	32. F	35.G.1.

CHAPTER 35 (*Cont.*)

Answer		Objective	Answer		Objective
33.	A	35.G.1.	39.	D	35.J.1.
34.	T	35.H.1.	40.	F	35.J.1.
35.	F	35.H.1.	41.	T	35.J.1.
36.	F	35.I.1.	42.	F	35.J.2.
37.	T	35.I.1.	43.	T	35.J.2.
38.	T	35.I.1.	44.	E	35.K.1.

CHAPTER 36

Answer		Objective	Answer		Objective
1.	D	36.B.1.	6.	T	36.G.1.
2.	F	36.C.1.	7.	T	36.H.1.
3.	T	36.D.1.	8.	F	36.I.1.
4.	C	36.E.1.	9.	T	36.J.1.
5.	D	36.F.1.	10.	T	36.J.2.

CHAPTER 37

Answer		Objective	Answer		Objective
1.	D	37.B.1.	13.	B	37.J.2.
2.	T	37.B.2.			37.K.2.
3.	F	37.C.1.	14.	T	37.K.1.
4.	F	37.D.1.	15.	F	37.L.1.
5.	C	37.E.1.	16.	T	37.M.1.
6.	D	37.E.1.	17.	T	37.M.1.
7.	T	37.E.1.	18.	E	37.N.1.
8.	T	37.F.1.	19.	D	37.O.1.
9.	A	37.H.1.	20.	T	37.P.1.
10.	D	37.I.1.	21.	T	37.Q.1.
11.	F	37.J.1.	22.	T	37.R.1.
12.	T	37.J.1.			

CHAPTER 38

Answer		Objective	Answer		Objective
1.	B	38.A.2.	6.	C	38.D.1.
2.	D	38.A.3.	7.	C	38.E.1.
3.	A	38.B.1.	8.	B	38.E.2.
4.	B	38.B.1.	9.	C	38.E.3.
5.	B	38.B.3.			

CHAPTER 39

Answer		Objective	Answer		Objective
1.	T	39.B.1.	9.	D	39.G.1.
2.	T	39.C.1.	10.	T	39.H.1.
3.	T	39.D.1.	11.	T	39.H.1.
4.	T	39.D.2.	12.	T	39.I.1.
5.	F	39.D.3.	13.	D	39.J.1.
6.	T	39.D.4.	14.	T	39.K.1.
7.	E	39.E.1.	15.	T	39.L.1.
8.	T	39.F.1.			

CHAPTER 40

Answer		Objective	Answer		Objective
1.	T	40.A.1.	8.	T	40.G.1.
2.	F	40.A.2.	9.	T	40.G.1.
3.	C	40.B.1.	10.	A	40.H.1.
4.	D	40.C.1.	11.	T	40.H.2.
5.	C	40.D.1.	12.	D	40.I.1.
6.	E	40.E.1.	13.	D	40.K.1.
7.	D	40.F.1.	14.	T	40.K.2.

CHAPTER 41

Answer		Objective	Answer		Objective
1.	T	41.A.1.	15.	F	41.B.1.
2.	T	41.A.1.	16.	B	41.C.1.
3.	F	41.A.1.	17.	D	41.C.1.
4.	F	41.A.1.	18.	B	41.C.1.
		41.A.2.	19.	C	41.C.1.
5.	T	41.A.2.	20.	D	41.C.1.
6.	T	41.A.3.	21.	B	41.C.1.
7.	B	41.A.4.	22.	A	41.C.1.
8.	A	41.B.1.	23.	T	41.D.1.
9.	A	41.B.1.	24.	D	41.D.1.
10.	D	41.B.1.	25.	A	41.D.1.
11.	F	41.B.1.	26.	F	41.D.2.
12.	T	41.B.1.	27.	D	41.E.1.
13.	F	41.B.1.	28.	F	41.F.1.
14.	T	41.B.1.	29.	B	41.G.1.

Index

Food, interaction of, with nonnarcotic analgesics, 225
Food and drug administration, 91
Formaldehyde, 452, 454
Frank-Starling ventricular function curves, 304
FSH (Follicle-stimulating hormone), 358
5-FU, 428
Furosemide, 332, 334

GABA (ɤ-aminobutyric acid), 193
Gallamine, 157
Gantanol (sulfamethoxazole), 289
Ganglionic blocking drug(s), 154, 156–157. *See also* specific drugs
  action of, 140
  side effects of, 156–157
  xerostomia- producing, 461
Ganglionic stimulants, 157
  action of, 140
Gantrisin (sulfisoxazole), 289
Gastric antacid(s). *See also* specific drugs
  indications for, 341
  side effects of, 341
Gastrointestinal drug. *See* GI drugs
General anesthesia, 375–384
  definition of, 375
  history of, 376
  mechanism of action in theories of, 376–377
  preanesthetic medications and, 383–384
  signs of, 377–379
  stages in, 377–379
General anesthetic(s). *See also* specific agents
  absorption of, 383
  classification of, 379
  distribution of, 383
  excretion of, 383
  features of, 379–383
  fixed agents in, 379
  gases in, 379
  metabolism of, 383
  summary of, 380–381
  volatile liquids in, 379
Generic drug names, for prescriptions, 66
Genetic variations, and drug metabolism, 75
Geocillin (carbenicillin), 49
Germicidal, definition of, 451
GH (growth hormone), 356–357
GI drug(s)
  antacid, 340–341
  anticholinergic, 341–342
  antidiarrheal, 342–343
  antiemetic, 343

  antihistamine, 342
  cathartic, 342
  emetic, 343
  laxatives, 342
Gingiva
  hemorrhage of, drugs for, 12
  oral contraceptive effects on, 354–355
  pregnancy effects on, 354
  retraction of, drugs in, 12
  tissues of, vasoconstriction of, 12
Gingivitis, 244
Glaucoma, and parasympatholytic drugs, 155
Glucagon, 360, 437
  features of, 363
Glucocorticosteroid(s), 348, 363
  action mechanism of, 349
commonly used, activities of, 351
  contraindications for, 351
  dental uses of, 351
  drug interactions with, 350
  effects of, 349–350
  medical uses of, 350
  pharmacokinetics of, 350
  principles of usage of, 352
  toxicity of, 350
Glutamic acid, 193
Glutaraldehyde, 452, 454
Glutethimide, 206
  drug interactions involving, 441
  interaction of, with oral anticoagulants, 315
Glycine, 193
Glycopyrrolate, 342
Gram-negative spectrum, definition of, 240
Gram-positive spectrum, definition of, 240
Grand mal seizure, 406
Growth hormone
  effects of, 356–357
  secretion of, 357
  syndromes involving, 357
Guaifenesin, 339
Guanethidine, 170–171
  action mechanism of, 322–323
  as adrenergic blocking agent, 170–171
  interaction of, with antipsychotics, 392
  side effects of, 324
Guedel, Dr., 377–379

Haldol (haloperidol), 390
Half-life, biologic, 86
Halogens, 452, 454
Haloperidol, 390
Halothane, 379, 380, 381